# Science and Soccer

Now in a fully revised and updated fourth edition, *Science and Soccer* is still the most comprehensive and accessible introduction to the science behind the world's most popular sport. Offering important guidance on how science translates into practice, the book examines every key facet of the sport, with a particular focus on the development of expert players. The topics covered include:

- anatomy, physiology, psychology; sociology and biomechanics;
- principles of training;
- nutrition;
- physical and mental preparation;
- injury;
- decision-making and skill acquisition;
- coaching and coach education;
- performance analysis;
- talent identification and youth development.

*Science and Soccer: Developing Elite Performers* is a unique resource for students and academics working in sports science. It is essential reading for all professional support staff working in the game, including coaches at all levels, physiotherapists, conditioning specialists, performance analysts, club doctors and sports psychologists.

**A. Mark Williams, PhD** is a Professor and Senior Research Scientist at The Institute for Human & Machine Cognition (IHMC) in Florida, USA.

**Paul R. Ford, PhD** is a Senior Lecturer in the School of Sport, Exercise and Applied Sciences at St Mary's University, UK.

**Barry Drust, PhD** is an Applied Exercise Physiologist and an Industrial Professorial Fellow in the School of Sport, Exercise and Rehabilitation Sciences at the University of Birmingham, UK.

# Science and Soccer

Developing Elite Performers

**Fourth Edition**

# Edited by A. Mark Williams, Paul R. Ford, and Barry Drust

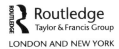

LONDON AND NEW YORK

Cover image: Stanislaw Pytel

Fourth edition published 2023
by Routledge
605 Third Avenue, New York, NY 10158

and by Routledge
4 Park Square, Milton Park, Abingdon, Oxon, OX14 4RN

*Routledge is an imprint of the Taylor & Francis Group, an informa business*

© 2023 selection and editorial matter, A. Mark Williams, Paul R. Ford, and Barry Drust; individual chapters, the contributors

The right of A. Mark Williams, Paul R. Ford, and Barry Drust to be identified as the authors of the editorial material, and of the authors for their individual chapters, has been asserted in accordance with sections 77 and 78 of the Copyright, Designs and Patents Act 1988.

All rights reserved. No part of this book may be reprinted or reproduced or utilised in any form or by any electronic, mechanical, or other means, now known or hereafter invented, including photocopying and recording, or in any information storage or retrieval system, without permission in writing from the publishers.

*Trademark notice*: Product or corporate names may be trademarks or registered trademarks, and are used only for identification and explanation without intent to infringe.

First edition published by Willan 2008
Third edition published by Routledge 2013

ISBN: 978-0-367-70895-5 (hbk)
ISBN: 978-1-032-46030-7 (pbk)
ISBN: 978-1-003-14841-8 (ebk)

DOI: 10.4324/9781003148418

Typeset in Times
by codeMantra

# Contents

| | |
|---|---|
| *Preface* | viii |
| *List of figures* | xiii |
| *List of tables* | xvii |
| *List of contributors* | xx |

**SECTION A**
**Biological Sciences** — 1

**1 Physical preparation** — 3
T. STRUDWICK

**2 Resistance training** — 15
CONALL MURTAGH, DAVID RYDINGS AND BARRY DRUST

**3 Aerobic and anaerobic training** — 34
LIAM ANDERSON AND BARRY DRUST

**4 Soccer in the heat: Performance and mitigation** — 52
CAROLINE SUNDERLAND, STACEY COWE, AND RACHEL MALCOLM

**5 Nutrition for match play and training** — 67
JAMES P. MORTON, LIAM ANDERSON, HANNAH SHERIDAN
AND GRAEME L. CLOSE

**6 Recovery strategies** — 90
WARREN GREGSON, GREGORY DUPONT, ABD-ELBASSET ABAIDIA AND
ROBIN THORPE

**SECTION B**
**Social and Behavioural Sciences** — 109

**7 Psychological characteristics of players** — 111
GEIR JORDET AND TYNKE TOERING

vi *Contents*

**8 Anticipation and decision-making** 124
A. MARK WILLIAMS, JOSEPH L. THOMAS, GEIR JORDET, AND PAUL R. FORD

**9 Skill acquisition: Player pathways and effective practice** 141
PAUL R. FORD AND A. MARK WILLIAMS

**10 Sociological influences on the identification and development of players** 155
MATTHEW J. REEVES AND SIMON J. ROBERTS

**11 Player wellbeing and career transitions** 168
CAROLINA LUNDQVIST AND DAVID P. SCHARY

**12 Developing (adaptive) coaching expertise** 183
CHRISTOPHER J. CUSHION AND ANNA STODTER

**SECTION C**
**Sports Medicine and Biomechanics** 197

**13 Injury epidemiology, monitoring, and prevention** 199
IAN BEASLEY

**14 Infectious diseases** 223
MONICA DUARTE MUÑOZ AND TIM MEYER

**15 Biomechanical assessments** 238
MARK A. ROBINSON, KATHERINE A.J. DANIELS, AND JOS VANRENTERGHEM

**SECTION D**
**Analysing and Monitoring Performances** 251

**16 Analysis of physical performance in match-play** 253
CHRISTOPHER CARLING AND NAOMI DATSON

**17 Technical and tactical match analysis** 273
ALLISTAIR P. McROBERT, JAVIER FERNÁNDEZ-NAVARRO, AND LAURA SETH

**18 Monitoring training** 292
BARRY DRUST AND LAURA BOWEN

**19 Utilising training and match load data** 309
PATRICK WARD AND BARRY DRUST

*Contents* vii

**SECTION E**
**Talent Identification, Growth, and Development** 327

**20 Growth and maturation** 329
SEAN P. CUMMING, MEGAN HILL, DAVID JOHNSON, JAMES PARR,
JAN WILLEM TEUNNISEN, AND ROBERT M. MALINA

**21 Talented or developmentally advanced? How player evaluation can be improved** 346
STEPHEN COBLEY, CHRIS TOWLSON, SHAUN ABBOTT,
MICHAEL ROMANN AND RIC LOVELL

**22 Talent identification and talent promotion** 363
ARNE GÜLLICH AND PAUL LARKIN

**23 Modern approaches to scouting and recruitment** 382
DAVID PIGGOTT AND BOB MUIR

**SECTION F**
**Some Key Organizational Roles at Clubs** 395

**24 Working as a director of sports science or high-performance director** 397
TONY STRUDWICK

**25 Working as a sporting director** 414
DANIEL PARNELL, REBECCA CAPLEHORN, KEVIN THELWELL,
TONY ASGHAR AND MARK BATEY

*Index* 429

# Preface

## Science and Soccer (4<sup>th</sup> Edition)

### *Developing Elite Performers*

This fully revised fourth edition of *Science and Soccer* includes 25 chapters grouped into two parts and six different sections. The chapters are written by some of the leading authorities globally in their respective fields, particularly regarding the focus on soccer. In recruiting authors, we made concerted efforts to try and include both academics and practitioners in efforts to better translate research into practice. While acknowledging that there remains far less research on women and special population groups in soccer, we tasked authors with integrating this information into each chapter where possible. The book testifies to the increasing role played by scientists in supporting the work undertaken by practitioners and coaches in soccer, particularly in the professional environment.

The book is not intended as an encyclopaedia of science and soccer, and we acknowledge that some important topics are not covered in the book, such as, for example, child development and safeguarding, and the role of soccer in promoting health and physical activity in non-elite populations. These are all important topics, but space is limited, and the focus in this book is strongly geared towards the more elite end of the soccer pyramid. Moreover, the book is not intended as an exhaustive course text per se, but rather may be seen as a reference source that provides background reading for students on sports science related degree programs and research academics, as well as for practitioners and coaches, particularly those working at the elite level.

The first part of the book is somewhat mono-disciplinary in scope. Three sections are presented which focus respectively on the role played by the biological sciences, the social and behavioural sciences, and sports medicine and biomechanics in enhancing scientific understanding of soccer. The second part of the book is more multi-disciplinary in nature focusing on three separate themed areas. The three themed areas are analysing and monitoring performance, talent identification, growth, and development, and finally, an overview of some of the key organisational roles performed by sports science and medicine practitioners in professional clubs. The overall aim of the book is to highlight the varied and significant role played by science in enhancing player performance in soccer.

In the opening section, we consider the role played by the biological sciences in the training and preparation of players for competition. First, Strudwick highlights the importance of how players should warm-up prior to match play and training. The chapter presents a scientific approach to designing effective warm-up routines for training and competition. He provides insights into training methods and regimens relevant to real working practices in elite professional soccer. In the second chapter, Murtagh, Rydings, and Drust consider the importance of resistance training in soccer. They answer questions related to the why, when, and what of resistance training at the elite level. A model is presented to guide resistance training in elite soccer and some of the practicalities in implementing such an approach are discussed. In similar vein, Anderson and Drust consider the importance of aerobic and anaerobic training to high-level performance in soccer. The authors highlight the relative importance of both energy systems and present some practical examples as to how components of fitness may be developed in training. Next, Sunderland, Cowe, and Marshal highlight how performance in soccer is influenced in warm climates. They discuss some of the mechanisms involved when adapting to playing and training in the heat and present several mitigation strategies that can be used to minimise any adverse effects on performance. Morton and colleagues outline the nutritional requirements associated with performing at the highest level. They present guidelines for the consumption of carbohydrates, protein, fluids, micronutrients, and nutritional supplements and how these should fluctuate relative to training and match-play demands. They consider practical considerations in implementing good nutritional practices in the professional game and discuss the importance of recovery after match-play. Finally, Gregson and colleagues highlight the physiological and psychological mechanisms involved in recovery and review the evidence supporting various methods proposed to facilitate the process. These methods include, amongst others, the use of stretching, massage, cryotherapy, compression garments, and hot-water immersion.

In Section 2, we explore how the social and behavioural sciences have advanced understanding of the factors underpinning successful performance in soccer. First, Jordet and Toering highlight how certain psychological characteristics are associated with superior performance and enhanced player development and present examples of how these factors may be evaluated in youth and adult players. The authors provide a compelling argument for greater interaction between coaches and scientists in exploring the psychological characteristic that underpin elite player development and how psychological skills may be developed through targeted interventions. Williams, Thomas, Jordet and Ford then discuss the importance of anticipation and decision-making in soccer. They review published work that has identified the skills that underpinning superior game intelligence. They highlight how these skills may be measured and suggest interventions that can be used to enhance the acquisition of 'game intelligence'. Notably, they highlight the importance of coaching and instruction and the potential of using virtual reality and other forms of technology to increase opportunities for practice. Next, Ford and Williams explore some key concepts underlying skill acquisition in soccer. They identify the typical developmental history profiles of elite players, highlighting the pre-eminence of an early-engagement pathway, and review video-based, time-use analysis of coaching sessions to identify the types of practice activities that may be most beneficial. The authors close by briefly highlighting recent conceptual developments in the field of skill acquisition and how these could be integrated into the coaching curriculum. Reeves and Roberts focus more so on the sociological factors that impact on talent development. They highlight the important roles played by families, including siblings, and the importance of coach-athlete relationships in player development. Moreover, they review research that has explored x *Preface*

the importance of culture and socio-economic background, highlighting significant changes in the landscape of professional soccer over recent decades. Lundqvist and Schary explore what has hitherto been an under-researched topic in soccer, that is, mental health and wellbeing. The authors highlight different interventions that may be used to reduce the risks associated with mental health and increase wellbeing. Notably, they touch on the challenges involved when players transition from a professional career into retirement and how players can be supported through this process. Finally, to close the section, Cushion and Stodter consider the crucial role played by coaches in player development. The authors differentiate between routine and adaptive expertise and discuss the importance of formal and informal learning in coach education. They highlight shortcomings with existing methods of coach education and present several suggestions as to how the process could be improved to develop more adaptive experts.

In Section 3, chapters focus on sports medicine and the role of biomechanics in soccer. First, Beasley reviews the most common types of injuries in soccer. He outlines how these injuries occur, how they are diagnosed, and the types of treatments that are typically undertaken. Moreover, he contrasts the types of injuries that occur in the men's and women's' game, and highlights increasing awareness of the impact of concussion on player health. Next, Muñoz and Meyer consider what impact infectious diseases such as COVID-19 may have on health and performance in soccer. They discuss the frequency, diagnosis, and treatment of infectious diseases and what precautions may be taken to prevent infection. Guidelines are provided for returning to training and match-play post infection. Robinson, Daniels, and Vanrenterghem close this section by considering how biomechanical assessments may be used in a professional soccer setting. The authors argue that the role of biomechanics in soccer has shifted focus over time away from technique analysis and more towards providing measures that support medical and rehabilitation monitoring. They highlight the increased availability of portable and low-cost biomechanical assessments and discuss how such measures can help in injury prevention and performance enhancement.

In Section 4, our first themed area, we explore several topics related to analysing and monitoring player performance. First, Carling and Datson review the research carried out on motion analysis in soccer. They highlight the physical demands of match-play and how this differs across player position. Also, they consider how motion analysis data may be used to monitor player workloads across periods in a match and how such data may be used to develop player-specific training programmes as well as to identify risks of injury. Next, McRobert, Fernández-Navarro, and Seth highlight the key role played by technology in enhancing our tactical and technical understanding of the game. They illustrate how performance analysis has become a crucial weapon in the coach's armoury. The authors review how performance analysis is used to shape modern approaches to the game and helps coaches develop key performance indicators to evaluate team and individual development. Drust and Bowen then review the methods available for measuring and monitoring training load in elite players. They highlight the importance of using valid measures and some of the practical difficulties associated with monitoring, as well as the importance of building effective lines of communication with coaches and players. Next, Ward and Drust discuss how data gathered through the player monitoring process can be used to guide the implementation of relevant training interventions. The authors present a framework that may be used to facilitate better efforts at identifying and answering relevant applied questions. While the framework is presented in the context of addressing questions around

*Preface* xi

training workload, the approach is translatable as a working framework that may be used across discipline areas. The authors highlight different approaches when analysing and presenting data to coaches.

In Section 5, the theme is talent identification, growth, and development in soccer. In the opening chapter, Cumming and colleagues explore the key factors underpinning growth and maturation and how these factors can impact negatively the talent and identification process. The authors highlight how maturity status impacts on training and risk of injury and suggest several approaches that may be used to monitor and mediate the potential risks associated with overtraining and burnout in youth players. Cobley and colleagues then review the extant literature focusing on the relative age effect in soccer. That is, the tendency of scouts and coaches to select players advanced in chronological age relative to the selection year. They highlight the extent of the problem and suggest some strategies that may be employed to alleviate the systematic bias that exists in soccer, including the role of bio-banding. Next, Güllich and Larkin present a comprehensive and critical review of existing research focusing on talent identification. They highlight the generally low predictive utility of talent identification programmes and argue that more resources should be devoted to promoting the development of talent rather than on trying to identify markers of 'potential' that may have limited value. The authors highlight the negative factors associated with early talent identification programmes and suggest alternative emphases for practitioners. Finally, Pigott and Muir discuss the tole of talent scouts in professional soccer, with a particular emphasis on the international game. The authors highlight the paucity of research examining the thought processes and observational skills used in scouting and outline how they worked with a national association to develop a more systematic and structured scouting process.

In the final section, we consider some of key the organisational roles at clubs. First, Strudwick highlights the many roles and responsibilities that may be held when working as a Director of Sports Science both at club and international level. He outlines the different in structures employed by clubs as well as the varying nature and emphases of the role. Finally, Parnell and colleagues consider the role of Sporting Directors at professional clubs. The role is comparatively new, yet many clubs at the highest echelons of the sport are now embracing this management structure. The authors highlight the potential responsibilities of the Sporting Director and discuss some of the challenges faced in the role. A couple of case studies are used to provide examples of how such a role has already worked successfully in professional clubs in Europe.

Our intention in pulling this book together was to highlight the significant progress made in our scientific understanding of soccer over the last decade, notably since the last edition of this book was published in 2012. The number of scientists undertaking research on soccer and working as practitioners in professional clubs or within national associations has mushroomed. By way of example, when the Premier League launched in 1993, there were barely a handful of sports scientists working in the club setting in England, whereas these days many of the elite clubs have sports science and medicine units that are larger than the average university department in this field. The same pattern of growth in the field is exhibited globally, albeit with some variance depending on the financial resources available to clubs and national associations. Our now long-passed former colleague, Professor Thomas Reilly, who had the vision to edit the first edition of this book, and co-edited the second edition with the current book's lead editor, could never have envisaged the extent to which his dream became

xii   *Preface*

a reality for those that have followed. Yet, while celebrating scientific progress, we acknowledge that soccer at the highest level remains an art form that expresses human creativity, skill, and imagination in its greatest form. In editing this book, we have attempted to illustrate how the art of soccer can be informed and enhanced by science, and in this regard, we hope it inspires future generations of scientists to continue to explore the limits of performance in soccer. However, scientists working in isolation cannot create solutions to real-world problems, and in many instances are not always aware of the questions of interest. What remains crucial is the need for continuous interaction and dialogue between scientists, practitioners, and coaches in efforts to ensure that soccer as a sport continues to impact positively on society across the globe.

A. Mark Williams, Ph.D.
Florida Institute of Human and Machine Cognition

Paul R. Ford, Ph.D
St Mary's University, London

Barry Drust, Ph.D.
University of Birmingham

# Figures

| | | |
|---|---|---|
| 2.1 | The ability to produce, apply, and tolerate power/powerful actions is considered paramount to successful soccer performance at the elite playing level | 16 |
| 2.2 | The table displays the cost associated with resistance training exercises in each specific category | 18 |
| 2.3 | The repeated bout effect is a key concept to inform the detailed prescription process | 20 |
| 2.4 | An illustration of the processes utilised when prescribing resistance training interventions for the elite soccer players | 22 |
| 2.5 | Real-world prescription process for player 1 in different match play formats | 28 |
| 2.6 | Real-world prescription process for player 2 in different match play formats | 29 |
| 2.7 | Real-world prescription process for player 3 in different match play formats | 29 |
| 3.1 | An overview of energy system training guidelines, physiological adaptations, and performance changes for soccer players | 38 |
| 3.2 | Some typical training drills for the aerobic energy system | 40 |
| 3.3 | Some typical training drills for the anaerobic energy system | 42 |
| 4.1 | The total distance covered in a simulated soccer match in control (18°C) and hot (30°C) environmental conditions (control vs hot: $P < 0.05$). Redrawn from Aldous et al. (2015) | 53 |
| 4.2 | The sprint distance covered in a simulated soccer match in control (18°C) and hot (30°C) environmental conditions (control vs hot: $P < 0.05$). Redrawn from Aldous et al. (2015) | 54 |
| 4.3 | The high-speed running distance completed during a soccer match in control (21°C) and hot (43°C) environmental conditions (control vs hot: $P < 0.05$). Redrawn from Mohr et al. (2012) | 54 |
| 4.4 | The baseline level response times for visual search. (Data are mean ± SD. Pre: prior to the match simulation, HT: half time and FT: full time. Main effect of trial, $P < 0.01$ and trial*time interaction, $P < 0.01$.) Redrawn from Malcolm (2018) | 56 |
| 4.5 | The proportion correct on the baseline level of the visual search test. | 56 |
| 5.1 | The energy expenditure of elite soccer players, as assessed using the doubly labelled water method | 68 |

xiv *Figures*

| | | |
|---|---|---|
| 5.2 | (A) Resting metabolic rate (RMR), (B) fat-free mass, (C) fat mass, and (D) percent body fat between in adolescent male soccer players (U12–U23 age groups; $n$ = 99) from an English Premier League academy | 79 |
| 6.1a and 6.1b | Recovery of knee flexor isometric force, counter movement jump height (1a) and ratings of subjective muscle soreness and creatine kinase concentrations (1b) throughout the 72-h period following match-play. Redrawn from Silva et al. (2018) | 92 |
| 6.2 | An example of an active recovery strategy | 95 |
| 6.3 | An example of a foam rolling exercise | 97 |
| 6.4 | Cold-water immersion | 99 |
| 6.5 | Compression garments | 100 |
| 7.1 | The number of peer review articles from a search with keywords "psychology" and "soccer", registered in bibliographic database SPORT Discus between 2001 and 2020 | 112 |
| 7.2 | The 11-model. Behavioural outcomes that are important to successfully transition from youth academy to professional first team. Adapted from Jordet, 2016 | 118 |
| 8.1 | A scan (filmed from the position of the ball), where a player's face is temporarily directed away from the ball. Photo credit: Karl Marius Aksum and Lars Brotangen | 126 |
| 8.2 | Some images from eye tracking goggles worn by a central midfielder in an 11 *vs.* 11 match, with the small circle indicating the player's foveal gaze location in a scan (scan starting at 1, ending at 5). Photo credit: Karl Marius Aksum and Geir Jordet | 127 |
| 8.3 | The penalty-taker as presented in a temporal-occlusion condition where information is available up to foot-ball contact (left side) and a spatial occlusion condition where only the hips are presented (right side) (from Causer & Williams, 2015) | 128 |
| 9.1 | Hours per week in soccer practice and play across the development of (a) 14 national team and (b) 15 Bundesliga players in Germany | 143 |
| 9.2 | The continuum of representativeness for common practice activities with the ball in soccer | 146 |
| 10.1 | Parents' experiences of the youth soccer academy parenting journey. Source: Adapted from Newport et al. (2020) | 157 |
| 11.1 | An overview of mental health as an umbrella term for both well-being and illbeing | 170 |
| 11.2 | Classifications of interventions based on their overall target and risk-factors (based on Barry, 2001; Jacobsson & Timka, 2015) | 172 |
| 11.3 | Overview of essential factors for players' well-being | 177 |
| 13.1 | Hamstring injury | 201 |
| 13.2 | Meniscal tear | 205 |
| 13.3 | Meniscal cyst | 205 |
| 13.4 | Degenerative change after meniscectomy | 206 |
| 13.5 | ACL rupture coronal | 206 |
| 13.6 | ACL rupture sagittal | 207 |
| 13.7 | Ankle injury | 209 |
| 13.8 | Wobble board | 209 |
| 13.9 | Patellar tendinopathy | 211 |

*Figures* xv

| | | |
|---|---|---|
| 13.10 | Patellar tendinopathy with Doppler © 2022 Christoph Spang, Lorenzo Masci and Håkan Alfredson https://www.mdpi.com/1648-9144/58/5/601/htm | 211 |
| 13.11 | Jones fracture | 213 |
| 13.12 | Pocket Concussion recognition tool-5 | 217 |
| 14.1 | The risk of URTI is lower with moderate levels of physical activity when compared to more sedentary people. The risk of URTI increases progressively with higher levels of physical activity. Adapted from Nieman, 1994 | 227 |
| 15.1 | The processing stages of a raw EMG signal | 243 |
| 15.2 | An isokinetic dynamometer set up for right knee testing | 244 |
| 15.3 | (Left) Visualisation of the joint moment, angle, and angular velocity profiles for a concentric-concentric Quadriceps-Hamstrings protocol with the isokinetic phase highlighted. (Right) Calculation of a 10-point moving average joint moment-angle profile for the multiple trials | 246 |
| 16.1 | Physical match performance in professional male and female soccer players (adapted from Bradley et al., 2013; Datson et al., 2017) | 255 |
| 16.2 | A summary of the numerous factors influencing soccer match-play running performance | 260 |
| 16.3 | High-intensity match-running performance in elite youth soccer players according to age group (data adapted from Saward et al., 2016) | 263 |
| 17.1 | The coaching process (adapted from Maslovat & Franks, 2008) | 275 |
| 17.2 | The five moments of play (Hewitt, 2016) | 277 |
| 17.3 | Soccer teams styles of play. Attacking styles of play: (A) factors 1 and 6, (B) factors 3 and 4. Defensive styles of play: (C) factors 2 and 5 | 282 |
| 18.1 | A schematic representation of the role on monitoring training in supporting the training process | 293 |
| 18.2 | Some theoretical and practical considerations in monitoring training | 295 |
| 18.3 | A female player's physical "profile" compared to the squad average | 301 |
| 18.4 | An example well-being report illustrating colour coding and marks to help inform player readiness | 303 |
| 18.5 | A graphical representation of the progressive increase of a player's chronic high-speed running (training load metric) over the course of 8 weeks | 304 |
| 19.1 | The Problem, Plan, Data, Analysis, and Conclusion (PPDAC) cycle | 311 |
| 19.2 | The normal distribution represented as a density plot and a box plot | 318 |
| 19.3 | Some examples of common data visualization approaches | 322 |
| 19.4 | Visualizing analysis of weekly change scores (A) for an entire team, (B) for a single individual from week-to-week, or (C) for an individual player for each week relative to baseline | 323 |
| 19.5 | An example of a run chart for a professional soccer player | 324 |
| 19.6 | (A) Astronomical point above or below the three SD control limits (B) Two out of three points above or below the two SD control limits. (C) Six or more points on the same side of the centre line. (D) Six or more points all going in the same direction | 325 |
| 20.1 | The Percentages of Male Academy Players by Maturation Status Across Competitive Age Groups. Adapted from Johnson et al., 2017 | 334 |

xvi  *Figures*

20.2a and 20.2b  Heat maps showing the combined effects of growth rate and POAH on estimated (A) injury likelihood and (B) injury burden  338

20.3  Use of percentage of predicted adult stature to determine location in adolescent growth curve in young athletes  338

21.1a and b  The relationship between chronological and relative age with (a) the agility (T-test) and (b) with the multi-stage fitness test (20-m MFST) in UK soccer academy players ($N = 969$; Towlson et al., 2018)  349

21.2a and b  The relationship between maturity status (YPHV) with (a) the agility (T-test) and (b) with the multi-stage fitness test (20-m MFST) in UK soccer academy players ($N = 969$; Towlson et al., 2018)  350

22.1  Proportions of members of youth soccer academies and under-age national teams persisting in the programme through subsequent age categories (grey lines) and proportions of senior first Bundesliga/Premier League players involved in youth academies and of senior national team players involved in under-age national teams through previous age categories (black lines). Aggregated data from Anderson & Miller, 2011; Güllich, 2014, 2019; Grossmann & Lames, 2015; Hornig et al., 2016; and Schroepf & Lames, 2017  375

23.1  A three-phase approach to talent reporter CPD  387

23.2  The new talent reporter framework  388

23.3  An example of performance problems by position (central defender)  389

24.1  Example organisational model associated with the operation of a modern elite soccer team  405

24.2  A typical sports science performance management model  406

24.3  Model showing a potential periodisation strategy for player and team preparation for a international soccer team  411

25.1  A football management structure where the Sporting Director reports to a CEO  415

25.2  A football management structure where the Sporting Director, Head Coach, and CEO report to the Governance Board/Chair/Owner  416

25.3  A simplified football management structure where the Sporting Director would take responsibility for player recruitment  417

# Tables

| | | |
|---|---|---|
| 1.1 | The rational for warming-up prior to match-play | 5 |
| 1.2 | Some examples of movement-based stretching exercises | 6 |
| 1.3 | An example of an elite soccer-specific warm-up | 8 |
| 1.4 | A typical squad warm-up/activation circuit | 10 |
| 1.5 | A hamstring strengthening programme following injury performed twice a week as part of a pre-training routine | 12 |
| 1.6 | An adductor strengthening programme following groin injury performed twice a week as part of a pre-training routine | 12 |
| 1.7 | A quadriceps muscle group strengthening programme following a quadriceps injury performed twice a week as part of pre-training routine | 12 |
| 1.8 | A calf strengthening programme following calf injury performed twice a week as part of a pre-training routine | 12 |
| 2.1 | The relationship between factors affecting fixture schedule demands and the opportunity for resistance training exposures in soccer players in starts and squad players | 26 |
| 3.1 | Physical testing results of non-elite and elite soccer players | 36 |
| 5.1 | An overview of CHO recommendations for soccer match play and training | 69 |
| 5.2 | A suggested practical model of the "fuel for the work required" CHO periodisation paradigm as applied to professional soccer players during a one-game-per-week schedule with match day on Saturday. Representative loads are taken from Anderson et al. (2015) | 73 |
| 5.3 | An overview of specific vitamin and minerals that have been highlighted as a potential cause for concern for soccer players (Collins et al., 2021), including their physiological function, recommended nutrient intake (RNI), typical food sources, and potential supplement strategy if required | 82 |
| 5.4 | An overview of supplements that may be ergogenic to soccer-specific physical performance | 83 |
| 8.1 | The average hours per year in three soccer activities for soccer players aged 18 years in the six years prior to the perceptual-cognitive test (Williams et al., 2012) | 132 |
| 9.1 | The main soccer activities in which players participate. Nb. The main intentions of a small set of individual players within the activity might differ compared to the main intention | 142 |

xviii  *Tables*

9.2 Some examples of manipulations to the rules of small-sided games (e.g., 3 *vs.* 3) that may reduce the difficulty of the sport for learners — 148

9.3 Some examples of manipulations to the rules of small-sided games (e.g., 4 *vs.* 4) so that players practice specific perceptual-motor skills more frequently than normal — 150

11.1 A summary of various subdimensions of hedonic and eudaimonic perspectives on well-being (based on Diener. 2009; Keyes, 1998; Ryff, 2014) — 171

13.1 The POLICE/PRICE guidelines to initial/first-aid treatment — 202

13.2 Summary of information on CRT-5 form — 216

14.1 Prevention of vector-borne infectious diseases (*Tickborne Encephalitis,* 2022; *Yellow Fever,* 2022) — 225

14.2 Preventive measures — 226

14.3 CDC recommendations for athletes for prevention of spread of MRSA (MRSA, 2019) — 227

14.4 Infectious diseases to consider in traveling athletes — 229

15.1 A schematic overview of commonly used jump evaluation approaches — 239

16.1 Influence of playing position on match physical activity profile in elite female soccer players (data adapted from Datson et al., 2017, 2019) — 257

16.2 Total distance covered (m) by soccer players during first and second halves of competitive match-play — 258

16.3 Mean recovery duration between sprints using individualised speed thresholds and frequency of recovery periods according to the time elapsed between consecutive sprints, collectively and in relation to positional role in German Bundesliga players (data adapted from Schimpchen, et al., 2016) — 262

18.1 Potential approaches for training load monitoring including outcome measures — 298

19.1 Some examples of different forms of validity that a sport scientist might encounter in the applied environment (Thomas, Nelson, Silverman, 2015) — 313

19.2 Example of calculating typical error measurement and minimal difference for a test-retest trial — 314

19.3 An example of transforming raw scores into percentile rank, z-score, and t-scores — 349

21.1 Modelled differences in physiological performance indices according to relative age between two hypothetical youth male soccer players at the entry point to the talent development process (i.e., under 10 age-group) — 349

21.2 Modelled differences in physical qualities according to biological maturity between two elite-youth male soccer players within the same chronological age (14.3-years old; i.e., under 15 age-group) — 351

21.3 Agility test performance according to 'top-five ranked', 'relatively youngest', and 'lowest maturation status' youth academy football players (under 13 years). Relative age and maturity status *corrective adjustment procedures* determined adjusted performance scores and ranks based on the relatively oldest (*) and most mature male player (†), respectively — 355

*Tables* xix

| | | |
|---|---|---|
| 21.4 | Multi-stage fitness test performance according to 'top-five' ranked', 'relatively youngest', and 'lowest maturation status' youth academy football players (under 13 years). Relative age and maturity status *corrective adjustment procedures* determined adjusted performance scores and ranks based on the relatively oldest (*) and most mature male player (†), respectively | 356 |
| 22.1 | The effect sizes for studies investigating predictive effects of potential talent indicators of youth soccer players on their later playing performance | 367 |
| 22.2 | An overview of predictive effects of potential talent indicators of youth soccer players on their later playing performance (references reported in Table 22.1) | 368 |
| 22.3 | Some impediments to reliable talent identification in youth soccer (following Güllich & Cobley, 2017) | 369 |
| 22.4 | The effects (Cohen's *d*) of the age of selection for a talent promotion programme on later junior and adult playing performance | 373 |
| 22.5 | The annual player turnover in TPPs and the proportion of identical players in a squad after 3 and 5 years | 374 |
| 23.1 | An example short report (for a YDP player) [team names redacted] | 391 |
| 23.2 | Extracts of reports of the same player (U21 #9) under the old and new systems | 392 |
| 24.1 | Some of the key responsibilities of a High-Performance Director | 399 |
| 24.2 | High-performance status of elite players | 401 |
| 24.3 | Some key challenges at an international level of competition | 409 |
| 25.1 | Some challenges facing the Sporting Director in practice and the skills and competencies required to address them | 424 |

# Contributors

**Shaun Abbott** is at The University of Sydney, Australia.

**Abd-Elbasset Abaidia** is at University of Sfax, Tunisia.

**Liam Anderson** is at Crewe Alexandra Football Club, UK.

**Tony Asghar** is at Dundee United Football Club, UK.

**Mark Batey** is at Manchester Metropolitan University, UK.

**Ian Beasley** is at Queen Mary University of London, UK.

**Laura Bowen** is at Southampton Football Club, UK.

**Rebecca Caplehorn** is at Tottenham Hotspur Football Club, UK.

**Christopher Carling** is at French Football Federation; and French Institute of Sport, France.

**Graeme L. Close** is at Liverpool John Moores University, UK.

**Stephen Cobley** is at The University of Sydney, Australia.

**Stacey Cowe** is at Nottingham Trent University, UK.

**Sean P. Cumming** is at University of Bath, UK.

**Christopher J. Cushion** is at Loughborough University, UK.

**Katherine A. J. Daniels** is at Manchester Metropolitan University, UK.

**Naomi Datson** is at University of Chichester, UK.

**Barry Drust** is at University of Birmingham, UK.

**Monica Duarte Muñoz** is at Saarland University, Germany.

**Gregory Dupont** is at Liverpool John Moores University, UK.

**Javier Fernández-Navarro** is at Liverpool John Moores University, UK.

**Paul R. Ford** is at St Mary's University, UK.

**Warren Gregson** is at Manchester Metropolitan University, UK.

**Arne Güllich** is at Technical University of Kaiserslautern, Germany.

**Megan Hill** is at Southampton Football Club; University of Bath; and Leeds Beckett University, UK.

**David Johnson** is at AFC Bournemouth; and University of Bath, UK.

**Geir Jordet** is at Norwegian School of Sport Sciences, Norway.

**Paul Larkin** is at Victoria University, Australia.

**Ric Lovell** is at Western Sydney University, Australia.

**Carolina Lundqvist** is at Linköping University, Sweden.

**Robert M. Malina** is at University of Texas, USA.

**Allistair P. McRobert** is at Liverpool John Moores University, UK.

**Tim Meyer** is at Saarland University, Germany.

**Rachel Malcolm** is at Nottingham Trent University, UK.

**James P. Morton** is at Liverpool John Moores University, UK.

**Bob Muir** is at Leeds Beckett University, UK.

**Conall Murtagh** is at Liverpool Football Club, UK.

**Daniel Parnell** is at University of Liverpool, UK.

**James Parr** is at Manchester United Football Club, UK.

**David Piggott** is at Leeds Beckett University, UK.

**Matthew J. Reeves** is at University of Central Lancashire, UK.

**Simon J. Roberts** is at Liverpool John Moores University, UK.

**Mark A. Robinson** is at Liverpool John Moores University, UK.

**Michael Romann** is at Swiss Federal Institute of Sport Magglingen, Switzerland.

**David Rydings** is at Liverpool Football Club, UK.

**David P. Schary** is at Winthrop University, USA.

**Laura Seth** is at The Football Association, UK.

**Hannah Sheridan** – Tottenham Hotspur Football Club, UK.

**Anna Stodter** – Leeds Beckett University, UK

**Tony Strudwick** – Arsenal Football Club, UK

**Caroline Sunderland** – Nottingham Trent University, UK

**Jan Willem Teunnisen** – Bruges University, Belgium.

**Joseph L. Thomas** is at Real Salt Lake, USA.

**Chris Towlson** is at University of Hull, UK.

**Kevin Thelwell** is at Everton FC, UK.

xxii  *Contributors*

**Robin Thorpe** is at Liverpool John Moores University, UK.

**Tynke Toering** is at Hanze University of Applied Sciences, The Netherlands.

**Jos Vanrenterghem** is at KU Leuven, Belgium.

**Patrick Ward** is at Seattle Seahawks, USA.

**A. Mark Williams** is at The Institute for Human & Machine Cognition, Florida, USA.

# Section A

# Biological Sciences

# 1 Physical preparation

*T. Strudwick*

## Introduction

The key objective of this chapter is to provide a comprehensive account of the parameters that impact upon the physical preparation of elite players. This chapter will help coaches and practitioners use current scientific information in designing effective activation and warm-up routines for training and competition.

In the first section, a brief theoretical background about the importance of effective match-day routines will be given. The second section is mostly focused on applying the principles of activation and warm-up strategies, with a special insight into training methods and regimens relevant to real working practices in professional soccer.

## Preparation

The physiological demands on the modern soccer player are more variable and complex than in many individual sports and are dependent on many factors such as positional role, style of employed by the team, and the level of the opposition. It's clear that contemporary players are required to not only produce actions, but also to repeat them throughout the duration of competition while maintaining a low fatigue index. Soccer consists of high-intensity movements that include sprints, jumps, intermittent movement direction, and speed changes with many acceleration and deceleration actions. These kinds of activities require appropriate preparation to enable athletes to show their full physical potential from the very beginning of a competition (Pagaduan et al., 2012).

At the elite level of play, there has been a shift towards systematic methods of preparing players for match-play. While the formal 'warm-up' has not always been a tradition within the soccer community, current day players have been exposed to a more robust and scientific approach prior to competitive match-play and high-intensity training sessions. Moreover, it is now widely accepted that warming-up prior to exercise is vital for the attainment of optimum performance.

A warm-up refers to the execution of physical exercise prior to the main activity in training or competition (Hedrick, 1992). Coaches and conditioning practitioners routinely use warm-up routines to facilitate the increase in body temperature, the acceleration of metabolism, and elevated oxygen uptake kinetics. Independently of the increase in muscle temperature, a warm-up can potentially increase performance by 'pre-conditioning' the muscle (Racinais et al., 2017). This phenomenon called

DOI: 10.4324/9781003148418-2

## 4  *T. Strudwick*

post-activation potentiation (PAP) is generally obtained by performing a maximal or near maximal contraction and has been suggested to have additional benefits relative to a traditional warm-up to improve performance in explosive activities (Güllich & Schmidtbleicher, 1996; Tillin & Bishop, 2009).

Recently, a new concept of PAP has been proposed to be more in-line with the timeline of peak voluntary performance enhancement (Silva et al., 2020). Thus, post-activation performance enhancement (PAPE) occurs when a high-intensity voluntary conditioning contraction leads to enhancement of subsequent involuntary muscular performance without confirmatory evidence of classical PAP (Cuenca-Fernandez et al., 2017). The PAPE effect can be explained with the increase of muscle temperature, fibre water content, and activation, but inhibited by residual fatigue and motor pattern interference (Blazevich & Babault, 2019). Therefore, the PAPE effectiveness depends on the balance between potentiation and fatigue, and this should be taken into consideration when designing warm-up routines (Silva et al., 2020).

The application of evidence-based preparation strategies has a self-evident role in improving elite performance. In general, individuals and teams that adopt a strategic approach have been rewarded with success by gaining an advantage over competitors. However, it has taken some time for the accumulation of scientific-based knowledge to be translated into a form usable by practitioners. McGowan et al. (2015) provided research-based support for the physiological and neural responses to passive and active warm-up strategies.

Passive warm-up strategies are those techniques used to increase body temperature without depleting energy substrate stores. Active warm-up strategies, on the contrary, induce greater metabolic changes, leading to increased preparedness for a subsequent exercise task. According to McGowan and colleagues (2015), the following key points pertaining to the use of a warm-up are supported in the literature.

- Passive and active warm-ups markedly influence subsequent exercise performance via increase in adenosine triphosphate turnover, muscle cross-bridge cycling, and oxygen uptake kinetics, which enhance muscular function.
- An active warm-up, consisting of a brief (<15 min) aerobic portion and completion of four to five activation sprints/race-pace efforts, PAP exercises, or small-sided games, elicits improvements in performance.
- Passive heat maintenance techniques can preserve the beneficial temperature effects induced via active warm-up during lengthy transition phases.

It is important that the warm-up is well planned. The routine needs to be specific and objective, taking into consideration the player's potential and rate of development. It is apparent that there are many components that need to be incorporated into the routine. These include a full range of activities such as individual and team preparation, match rehearsal, activation modalities, and injury prevention strategies, in addition to the more obvious warming-up. The design of the routine should be based on individual training philosophy and specificity to match performance per se. The need to isolate match performance components and to control workload intensity is achieved by a series of activities conducted within the period.

All warm-up routines should incorporate elements of muscular activation and warming up to facilitate the appropriate recruitment of muscle fibres associated with the correct sequencing and timing of soccer-specific activities. Speed preparation

*Physical preparation*  5

should follow with adequate recovery time between repetitions and sets to allow continual energy resynthesis. Subsequent stimulation of the aerobic systems should then be performed via specific drills with the ball involving changes of speed, direction, and specific movement patterns typical of those performed during match play. Exercises such as small-sided games (SSG) and shooting are often employed by coaches in the warm-up routine. These exercises can potentially boost performance through priming neural pathways and increased neuromuscular activation while maintaining a link to technical and tactical principles (Silva et al., 2020).

## Match day routines

In addition to the physiological rationale for warming-up prior to match-play, some of the main reasons for warm-up activities are listed in Table 1.1. First, the term warm-up signifies that the objective is to raise body temperature so that subsequent performance potential is enhanced. As muscles utilize energy during contraction, less than a ¼ of the energy goes towards producing mechanical work, leaving the remainder to generate heat within the muscle cells. Muscular performance is improved as temperature rises, but only up to a point. An increase in body temperature of one degree [Celsius] is sufficient to maximize the ergogenic effect on the active muscles (Reilly & Waterhouse, 2005). Clearly, the most effective means of generating the necessary internal heat is via different modes of movement and running.

When designing a warm-up routine, coaches should take into consideration several factors, such as duration, volume, intensity, and the sequencing of the selected exercises (Silva et al., 2020). In contemporary elite soccer, the warm-up is frequently performed over an extended period (>20 min), which may promote fatigue and inhibit performance enhancement. While a shorter warm-up appears to have similar benefits as a longer warm-up (Mujika et al., 2012), some players report the need for longer warm-up periods to feel psychologically prepared for competition (Yanci et al., 2019). It may well be that future pre-match routines will involve an educational shift to shorter duration and hence less physiologically taxing routines, while at the same time satisfying high-intensity stimulation and psychological readiness.

Regardless of exercise sequence, the warm-up should progress in intensity, preparing for the specific tasks of the sport, and finishing with tasks of maximum intensity (Silva et al., 2018). The specific skill tasks should be related to game situations to promote transfer to match actions. Within the framework, coaches may design shooting and tactical combinations to replicate positional attacking patterns. Where appropriate,

*Table 1.1* The rational for warming-up prior to match-play

| | |
|---|---|
| Elevate body temperature | Increase range of motion |
| Increase muscle temperature | Familiarize with environment |
| Reduce muscle tightness | Potentiate neuromuscular system |
| Decrease risk of injury | |
| Activate neuromuscular system | |
| Match rehearsal | |
| Increase arousal levels | |
| Rehearse game skills | |

6   T. Strudwick

skill tasks with opposition should be included to replicate the competitive demands of match-play. To maximize preparation effectiveness, it makes sense to include warm-up exercises that combine physical demands with a technical and tactical purpose, in-line with the context of the upcoming competitive match (Silva et al., 2020).

Historically, the warm-up routine consisted of a jog around the pitch, static, and dynamic flexibility exercises, and speed, agility, and quickness activities. In this respect, the mode of activity is important. Stretching the main muscles used during the subsequent performance via eccentric contractions results in a transient increase in flexibility. This enhanced range of motion improves the capability of the muscle to yield under the anticipated strain. The stretching activity is generally promoted as a way of improving flexibility and preventing injuries. Dynamic and static stretching are the two major types of stretching interventions. Dynamic stretching involves the execution of a muscle group to a full range of motion without the help of an external force. On the contrary, static stretching uses the assistance of an external force to achieve the full range of motion of a muscle group (Pagaduan et al., 2012).

Stretching the main thigh muscles is especially important prior to evening matches and in cold winter conditions. Particular attention should be directed toward the hamstrings and hip adductor muscles. Tightness in these muscle groups is often prevalent in elite soccer players and is associated with an increased predisposition to injury. Table 1.2 provides a selection of movement-based stretching that can form the basis on which to progress to a more dynamic exercise selection.

Flexibility exercises form an essential component of the warm-up, although the method of exercises designed to increased range of motion may vary due to individual philosophy. Although contemporary scientific research supports dynamic stretching routines over traditional methods like static stretching, some practitioners are still reluctant to totally discontinue traditional methods. Dynamic flexibility refers to the ability to move part or parts of the body quickly. Intuitively, including exercises designed to move the body quickly should form an integral component of pre-match routines.

Previously, researchers have reported that static stretching leads to reduced knee extensor power and jump performance compared to dynamic stretching (Costa et al., 2010; Hough et al., 2009; Yamaguchi & Ishii, 2005; Cornwell et al., 2002). However,

*Table 1.2* Some examples of movement-based stretching exercises

| | |
|---|---|
| Forward high knee march | Maintain tall posture. Bring thigh up and flex knee maximally. |
| Forward lunge walking | Keep hand on hips. Lunge far forward to get a stretch. Stand up and bring the opposite hip up to 90° before lunging again. |
| Jack-knife walk | Push-up position. Walk the feet towards your hands (keep legs straight). Maintain flat heels and flat hands. Walk the hands forward. Repeat. |
| Lateral lunge | Step out to right and squat by sitting back and down on right leg. Keep left leg straight. |
| Backward lunge with a twist | Step back with right leg into a lunge. Arch back while twisting torso over left leg and reaching right hand to sky. |
| Drop lunge | Turn hips to left and reach back with left foot until it is about 0.75 m to the outside of right foot, left toes pointing to right heel. Rotate hips so facing forward and square. Drop into full squat. |
| Inverted hamstring | Balance on right foot and bend at waist. |

*Physical preparation* 7

when static stretching is incorporated with other dynamic activities (e.g., jogging), similar jump performance with dynamic stretching and dynamic activities is observed (Vetter, 2007; Chaouachi et al., 2010). Other authors have reported deleterious effects of static stretching on sprint performance despite being combined with dynamic stretching or an aerobic warm-up (Sim et al., 2009; Winchester et al., 2008; Fletcher & Annes, 2007).

While it is not suggested that static stretching should be eliminated from pre-match routines, the scientific community supports the concept of a more dynamic approach to warm-up regimens. These dynamic routines emphasize progressive, whole-body, continuous movement and are typically performed in running drills that include forward, lateral, and changes of direction. Some examples of dynamic warm-up exercises include lunges, squats, hops, jumps, high knees, high kicks, and leg swings. Moreover, these routines have the potential to bolster the execution of match-play activities that involve jumping or rapid body movement.

New scientific methods for exercise preparation also point to the role of the warm-up in injury prevention (FIFA 11+). Injury prevention strategies are most effective when the warm-up activities are specific to the sport. This principle implies that the warm-up routines include unorthodox modes of running, sprinting, turning, and jumping as well as intense muscular bursts such as accelerations and decelerations. All these efforts exacerbate the physiological strain imposed on players and contribute to high physical workloads during subsequent competition, so caution should be made to ensure the warm-up routine is neither too exhaustive or prolonged. There is a balance to be struck between the arousal and activation benefits on the one hand and the induction of fatigue on the other. Most elite teams have a total preparation time of around 30 min taking into consideration climatic conditions. Moreover, in cold winter conditions, more focus should be placed on elevating body temperature in the form of running-based exercises compared to warm climatic conditions.

The intensity and duration of the warm-up should be reduced when the weather is hot. In contrast to the beneficial effects of warming-up, the development of whole-body hyperthermia impairs neuromuscular function, with alterations occurring at both the central and peripheral level (Racinais et al., 2017). The goal of the warm-up in hot climates is to optimize physiological readiness through the activation of predominant energy systems and movement patterns, without producing unnecessary metabolic heat that may become more performance-limiting toward the end of the competition (González-Alonso et al., 2008).

There are specific effects of the warm-up on the neuromuscular system. Among the more obvious consequences are the likely psychological benefits of match-play rehearsal, such as passing and shooting skills. There are also the PAP effects of stimulating the nervous system by means of brief, highly intense muscular efforts prior to competition (Tillin & Bishop, 2009). However, the effect is thought to decay after only a few minutes (Wilson et al., 2013).

A final consideration is the timing of the warm-up so that its benefits are not negated prior to the start of the game. Muscle and body temperature will remain elevated for some minutes after exercise is finished. It would therefore be prudent to terminate the warm-up 10 min prior to the start of competition to facilitate a short recovery and allow for psychological preparations. This information is also relevant for the management of substitutes, as these players must be ready to enter the field of play at any given moment. It is therefore advisable to instruct substitutes to warm-up every

8　*T. Strudwick*

*Table 1.3* An example of an elite soccer-specific warm-up

| | |
|---|---|
| KO – 40 min | Leave dressing room |
| KO – 38 min | Individual preparation |
| KO – 35 min | Start of dynamic movements/stretching |
| KO – 29 min | 4 v 4 + 2 (work 60 s: rest 30 s × 2) |
| KO – 26 min | Attacking shape |
| KO – 21 min | Finishing 90 s each side |
| KO – 17 min | Individual/corners/free kicks |
| KO – 12 min | Sprints |
| KO – 10 min | Re-enter dressing room |
| KO – 2 min | Leave dressing room |

Active warm-up induces greater metabolic changes, leading to increased preparedness for a subsequent exercise task.

20 min throughout match-play for approximately 5–10 min. The half time interval also provides an excellent opportunity to raise body temperature and increase match readiness. Once again, climate plays an important role in the management of substitutes, where cold winter conditions necessitate the need to extend working periods and ensure muscle temperature is optimal. An example of a typical elite soccer-specific warm-up prior to elite participation is provided in Table 1.3.

Over the past decade, it has become common for elite teams to conduct a re-warmup to protect against physiological changes and reductions in exercise performance due to a passive recovery during the half-time period (Yanaoka et al., 2021). Previously, researchers reported that intermittent team-sport players perform a lower amount of high-intensity running during the first 15 min of the second half compared to the first half (Mohr et al., 2005). This finding is surprising given the fact that players have a passive recovery during the half-time period. Lack of preparation and/or activation for the second half may be a reason for the reduced amount of high intensity, as players warm-up before matches, but not during half-time (Silva et al., 2018). It is, therefore prudent for coaches to administer a re-warm up before the onset of the second half to maximize performance after half time. This would include match-specific movements as well as high-intensity explosive actions.

## Training routines

In recent years, match analysis data have clearly demonstrated that the game includes more explosive events than ever before (Bradley et al., 2009). These increased demands mean that players require the strength, power, and speed to perform actions repeatedly, such as kicking, accelerating, maximal velocity sprinting, decelerating, changing direction, tackling, and jumping. At all competitive levels, these high-powered actions can prove to be the difference between winning and losing. Therefore, it is prudent for practitioners to utilize player preparation time and/or the warm-up/activation routines for multi-lateral physical development and injury prevention.

Modern-day elite players should undergo valid and reliable assessment or testing protocols to ascertain their movement competency, strength, and power performance status. Player-specific programmes can then be prescribed and delivered via preparation/activation routines to improve many aspects of movement competency or athleticism, strength, and power where a player has a particular weakness or deficit.

*Physical preparation* 9

Increasing a player's movement competency in key movements such as squatting, lunging (in multiple planes), hip hinging, bracing, and rotating is a component of many contemporary training warm-up regimens and can assist in the important goals of reducing injury incurrence and increasing physical performance. Moreover, players who are sufficiently competent in specific movement patterns can then be trained to express force maximally or explosively.

In the preparation of elite soccer players, practitioners have a responsibility to implement a comprehensive and planned training programme that allows for gym-based injury prevention strategies. The player must be trained in such a way that the body will be prepared for optimum response to the physical demands of training and competition. Strength training has been increasingly employed in the holistic management of contemporary soccer players and has become more evident in the training day warm-up and activation routines. In simple terms, strength training involves increasing the ability of the athlete to apply force. The ultimate objectives of strength training are to develop the capacity to reproduce forceful bursts of energy and withstand the forces of physical impact, landing, and deceleration. Following specific screening protocols for local muscles, as well as joints and lower back/pelvis, preventative gym-based programmes in the form of core stability, balance, proprioception, muscular strength, and power should be implemented to address the increasing issues of muscle strains in contemporary elite soccer.

Training that prepares the muscle and muscle cells for the trauma and damage caused by repeated high-force generation has become an area of increased attention in the training of elite soccer players. Friden and Leiber (1992) suggest that eccentric activity, given the relatively small amount required to induce muscle damage and adaptation, may have a valuable role to play in a training regime. It follows that eccentric training in the form of gym-based activation/preventative exercises may be an effective way to promote resistance to muscular damage. Therefore, a training programme should include periodic and systematic exposure to activities involving the generation of large muscle forces to stimulate changes in the cytoskeletal system. Clearly, for this type of adaptation to be transferable to soccer, one must ensure that the high-force activities fully exploit the muscles and motor units, the range of motion, and the contraction velocity typical of movements performed.

While there are many components that need to be incorporated into gym-based activation/injury prevention programmes, the following areas may be included in the physical preparation programme of elite players.

1   Mobilization/activation
2   Core stability and rotational strength
3   Power exercises
4   Eccentric exercises
5   Reactive exercises
6   Balance/proprioception
7   Strength exercises
8   Stretching

A recommended warm-up/activation circuit conducted prior to training twice a week is provided in Table 1.4. Players may work for 5 min in each group and then move to the next group. Exercise selection, sets, reps, and resistance will depend upon the age

10   *T. Strudwick*

*Table 1.4* A typical squad warm-up/activation circuit

|  | Area | Rationale | Sample exercises |
|---|---|---|---|
| Activity 1 | Glut activation/ movement mechanics | Strengthen the gluts, groins & hamstrings with functional movements using light or no resistance. The inability to activate gluteal group is associated with injuries such as lower back pain, hamstring strain and anterior knee pain. | Glut mini-band walks, med ball squat, lunge, lateral squat, single leg RDL. |
| Activity 2 | Torso Stability/ Strengthening | To improve the players' ability to transfer force from the ground to the extremities, while preventing uncontrolled movements of spine/pelvis. | **Torso stability:** Front & side plank exercises and variations, Posterior stability exercises. **Torso Strengthening:** (a) Anti-extension exercises; movements of arm and leg with limited movement of torso, (b) Rotational and anti-rotational exercises; producing and resisting against rotary force. |
| Activity 3 | Proprioception/ landing mechanics | To improve the ability of the body to land and stabilize correctly yet provide a foundation from which to progress to more explosive plyometric movements. A recurrence of inadequate landings may lead to ankle, knee, and hip joint injury. | Bilateral landings in place, bilateral landings with movement, unilateral landings in place, unilateral landings with movement. intensity can be increased by increasing height/ resistance/ surface instability. |
| Activity 4 | Hip mobility | The ability to maintain strength through a range of motion is important for soccer players to prevent injury and to provide a platform to produce power. | Hurdle overs (Hip flexion/ extension), hurdle adduction/ abduction (bent/straight leg), resisted leg swings (front–back, side–side), hurdle unders, slideboard adduction. |

and experience of the player and stage of season. An outline of this strategy, with the rationale for exercise selection, is also provided in Table 1.4.

More recently, the FIFA 11+ has gained popularity as a strategy to develop the physical capacities of players and assist in injury prevention. The FIFA 11+ injury prevention programme was developed by an international group of experts based on their practical experience with various injury prevention programmes for amateur players aged 14 or older (Bizzini & Junge, 2016). It is a complete warm-up package that is recommended to replace the typical warm-up before training for amateur teams (Bizzini et al., 2013).

The FIFA 11+ has three parts.

- **Part 1**: Running exercises at a slow speed combined with active stretching and controlled partner contacts.
- **Part 2**: Six sets of exercises focusing on core and leg strength, balance, and plyometrics, and agility, each with three levels of increasing difficulty.
- **Part 3**: Running exercises at moderate to high speed combined with planting and cutting movements.

The key point of the programme is to use the correct technique during all the exercises. Players must pay full attention to correct posture and good body control, including straight leg alignment, knee-over-toe position, and soft landings (Bizzini & Junge, 2016).

A study of more than 1,500 youth female players reported that performing the FIFA 11+ regularly reduced training injuries by 37% compared with performing a standard warm-up (Soligard et al., 2008). More recently, a large randomized controlled study in male soccer players (NCAA Divisions I and II) found fewer training and match injuries in teams practicing the FIFA 11+ as a warm-up routine (Silvers et al., 2015). Other authors have found improvements in static and dynamic balance and thigh muscle strength in male soccer and futsal players after they performed the FIFA 11+ programme (Brito et al., 2010; Daneshjoo et al., 2012; Reis et al., 2013).

Re-injuries constitute 12% of all soccer injuries and cause longer absences than other injuries (Ekstrand et al., 2011). Although no definitive evidence suggests that strengthening previously injured areas alone prevents reinjury, it has recently been demonstrated that increasing eccentric hamstring strength is associated with reduced risk of future hamstring injury in a cohort of previously injured Australian soccer player (Opar et al., 2015). Therefore, it makes sense for strength and conditioning practitioners to develop a supportive programme for soccer players to allow for opportunities within the pre-training day routine when they return to training, and, thereafter, to work on key areas of development. This area will depend on each player's injury history and nature. For some previous serious injury history, the player may continue this area of development throughout his/her career. All routines should consist of concentric–eccentric and isometric contractions working across the force-velocity continuum. Some examples of development protocols for a player who is fully rehabilitated from hamstring, adductor, quadriceps, and calf muscle group strains are presented in Tables 1.5–1.8, respectively.

## Future directions and conclusions

Traditionally, warm-up routines were developed largely on a trial-and-error basis, utilizing coach and athlete experiences rather than scientific evidence. However, over the past decade or so, new research has emerged, providing greater insight into how and why warm-up influences subsequent performance. In future, match preparation routines will continue to develop to maximize performance from the onset of competitive match-play.

While there is a lack of research pertaining to the mental areas of pre-match routines, the next decade will explore how physical and psychological techniques will run in parallel as part of the same preparation strategy. The role of the performance

12   T. Strudwick

Table 1.5 A hamstring strengthening programme following injury performed twice a week as part of a pre-training routine

| Exercise | Sets | Sample exercises |
| --- | --- | --- |
| Nordic hamstring lowers | 2 or 3 | 4–6 |
| Single-leg RDL (resisted) | 2 or 3 | 6 On injured leg |
| Slide board hamstring curl | 2 or 3 | 8–10 |
| Single-leg hamstring bridge | 2 or 3 | 6 On injured leg |
| Single-leg speed hop | 2 or 3 | $5 \times 2$ Each leg |

Table 1.6 An adductor strengthening programme following groin injury performed twice a week as part of a pre-training routine

| Exercise | Sets | Sample exercises |
| --- | --- | --- |
| Single-leg squat | 2 or 3 | 5 Each leg |
| Hip adduction | 2 or 3 | 6 Each leg |
| Eccentric slide board adduction | 2 or 3 | 6 Each leg |
| Kossacks | 2 or 3 | 8–10 |
| Side plank with leg movements | 2 or 3 | 6–8 With injured leg |

Table 1.7 A quadriceps muscle group strengthening programme following a quadriceps injury performed twice a week as part of pre-training routine

| Exercise | Sets | Sample exercises |
| --- | --- | --- |
| Single-leg squat | 2 or 3 | 5 Each leg |
| Rear raised lunge | 2 or 3 | 6 Each leg |
| Lateral speed skater hop & hold | 2 or 3 | 8–10 Each leg |
| Single-leg speed hop | 2 or 3 | $5 \times 2$ On injured leg |
| Single-leg 90-degree ISO hold | 2 or 3 | 30 secs On injured leg |

Table 1.8 A calf strengthening programme following calf injury performed twice a week as part of a pre-training routine

| Exercise | Sets | Sample exercises |
| --- | --- | --- |
| Eccentric calf lower | 2 or 3 | 6–8 On injured leg |
| Calf raise | 2 or 3 | 8–10 |
| Low box hold and freeze | 2 or 3 | 8–10 |
| Bouncing calf raise | 2 or 3 | 6–8 Each leg |
| Single-leg speed hop | 2 or 3 | $5 \times 2$ On injured leg |

psychologist will become more influential, employing techniques such as managing emotions, performance focus, and technical/tactical imaging. Thus, the focus may shift from not only preparing the muscular system, but also the mind to facilitate winning performance.

Now more than ever, the significance of the warm-up pre-match and after half-time has been identified. The volume, intensity, and sequencing of activities will be further explored when designing warm-up routines. In addition, practitioners will search for solutions to create the appropriate balance between potentiation and fatigue, and the future of the warm-up may look at quality vs quantity in attempts to maximize performance.

## References

Bizzini, M., & Junge, A. (2016). Injury frequency and prevention. In Tony Strudwick (Ed.), *Soccer Sci*, pp. 337–364. Australia: Human Kinetics.

Bizzini, M., Junge, A., & Dvorak, J. (2013). Implementation of the FIFA 11+ football warm up program: how to approach and convince the Football associations to invest in prevention. *Br J Sports Med*, 47, 803–806.

Blazevich, A. J., & Babault, N. (2019). Post-activation potentiation versus post-activation performance enhancement in humans: Historical perspective, underlying mechanisms, and current issues. *Front Physiol*, 10, 1359.

Bradley, P. S., Sheldon, W., Wooster, B., Olsen, P., Boanas, P., & Krustrup, P. (2009). High intensity running in English FA premier league soccer matches. *J Sports Sci*, 27, 159–168.

Brito, J., Figueredo, P., Fernandes, L., & Seabra, A. (2010). Isokinetic strength effects of FIFA's "The 11+" injury prevention training programme. *Isokin Exe Sci*, 18(4), 211–215.

Chaouachi, A., Castagna, C., Chtara, M., Brughelli, M., Turki, O., Galy, O., Chamari, K., & Behm, D. G. (2010). Effect of warm-ups involving static or dynamic stretching on agility, sprinting, and jumping performance in trained individuals. *J Strength Cond Res*, 24, 2001–2011.

Cornwell, A., Nelson, A., & Sidaway, B. (2002). Acute effects of stretching on the neuromechanical properties of the triceps surae muscle complex. *Eur J Appl Physiol*, 86, 428–434.

Costa, P. B., Ryan, E. D., Herda, T. J., Walter, A. A., Hoge, K. M., & Cramer, J. T. (2010). Acute effects of passive stretching on the electromechanical delay and evoked twitch properties. *Eur J Appl Physiol*, 108, 301–310.

Cuenca-Fernandez, F., Smith, I. C., Jordan, M. J., MacIntosh, B. R., Lopez- Contreras, G., Arellano, R. (2017). Non-localized post activation performance enhancement (PAPE) effects in trained athletes: a pilot study. *Appl Physiol Nutr Metab*, 42, 1122–1125.

Daneshjoo, A., Mokhtar, A. H., Rahnama, N., & Yusof, A. (2012). The effects of comprehensive warm-up programs on proprioception, static and dynamic balance on male soccer players. *PLoS ONE*, 7(12), e51568.

Ekstrand, J., Haggluned., & Walden., (2011). Epidemiology of muscle injuries in professional football (soccer). *Am J Sports Med*, 39(6), 1226–1232.

Fletcher, I. M., & Annes, R. (2007). The acute effects of combined static and dynamic stretch protocols on fifty-meter sprint performance in track-and-field athletes. *J Strength Cond Res*, 21, 784–787.

Friden, J., & Leiber, R. L. (1992). Structural and mechanical basis of exercise-induced muscle injury. *Med Sci Sports Exe*, 24, 521–530.

González-Alonso, J., Crandall, C. G., & Johnson, J. M. (2008). The cardiovascular challenge of exercising in the heat. *J Physiol*, 586, 45–53.

Güllich, A., & Schmidtbleicher, D. (1996). MVC-induced short-term potentiation of explosive force. *New Studies Athletics*, 11, 67–81.

Hedrick, A. (1992). Physiological responses to warm -up. *J Strength Cond Res*, 14, 25–27.

Hough, P. A., Ross, E. Z., & Howatson, G. (2009). Effects of dynamic and static stretching on vertical jump performance and electromyographic activity. *J Strength Cond Res*, 23, 507–512.

McGowan, C. J., Pyne, D. B., Thompson, K. G., & Rattray, B. (2015). Warm-up strategies for sport and exercise: Mechanisms and applications. *Sports Med*, 45(11), 1523-46.

Mohr, M., Krustrup, P., & Bangsbo, J. (2005). Fatigue in soccer: A brief review. *J Sports Sci*, 23, 593–599.

Mujika, I., de Txabarri, R. G., Maldonado-Martin, S., & Pyne, D. B. (2012). Warm-up intensity and duration's effect on traditional rowing time-trial. *Int J Sports Physiol Perform*, 7, 186–188.

Opar, D. A., Williams, M. D., Timmins, R. G., Hickey, J., Duhig, S. J., & Shield, A. J. (2015). Eccentric hamstring strength and hamstring injury risk in Australian footballers. *Med Sci Sports Exe*, 47(4), 857–865.

Pagaduan, J. C., Pojskic, H., Uzicanin, E., & Babajic, F. (2012). Effect of various warm-up protocols on jump performance in college football players. *J Human Kin*, 35(1), 127–132.

Racinais, S., Cocking, S., & Periard, J. D. (2017). Sports and environmental temperature: From warming-up to heating up. *Temperature*, 4(3), 227–257.

Reilly, T., & Waterhouse, J. (2005). *Sport, Exercise and Environmental Physiology*. Edinburgh: Elsevier.

Reis, I., Rebelo, A., Krustrup, P., & Brito, J. (2013). Performance enhancement effects of federation internationale de football association's "The 11+" injury prevention training program in youth futsal players. *Clin J Sport Med*, 23, 318–20.

Silva, L. M., Neiva, H. P., Marques, M. C., Izquierdo, M., & Marinho, D. A. (2018). Effects of warm-up, post-warm-up, and re-warm-up strategies on explosive efforts in team sports: A systematic review. *Sports Med*, 48, 2285–2299.

Silva, N., Travassos, B., Goncalves, B., Brito, J., & Abade, E. (2020). Pre-match warm-up dynamics and workload in elite futsal. *Front Psych*, 11, 584602.

Silvers, H., Mandelbaum, B., Adeniji, O., & Insler, S. (2015). Efficacy of the FIFA 11+ injury prevention program in the collegiate male soccer player. *Am J Sports Med*, 43(11), 2628–2637.

Sim, A.Y., Dawson, B.T., Guelfi, K.J., & Wallman, K.E. (2009). Effects of Static Stretching in Warm-Up on Repeated Sprint Performance. *J Strength Cond Res*, 23(7), 2155–2162.

Soligard, T., Myklebust, G., & Steffen, K. (2008). Comprehensive warm-up programme to prevent injuries in young female footballers: Cluster randomised controlled trial. *BMJ*, 337, a2469.

Tillin, N. A., & Bishop, D. (2009). Factors modulating post-activation potentiation and its effect on performance of subsequent explosive activities. *Sports Med*, 39, 147–166.

Vetter, R. E. (2007). Effects of six warm-up protocols on sprint and jump performance. *J Strength Cond Res*, 21, 819–823.

Wilson, J. M., Duncan, N. M., Marin, P. J., Brown, L. E., Loenneke, J. P., & Wilson, S. M. (2013). Meta-analysis of postactivation potentiation and power: effects of conditioning activity, volume, gender, rest periods, and training status. *J. Strength Cond Res*, 27, 854–859.

Winchester, J. B., Nelson, A. G., Landin, D., Young, M. A., & Schexnayder, I. C. (2008). Static stretching impairs sprint performance in collegiate track and field athletes. *J Strength Cond Res*, 22, 13–19.

Yamaguchi, T., & Ishii, K. (2005). Effects of static stretching for 30 seconds and dynamic stretching on leg extension power. *J Strength Condit Res*, 19, 677–683.

Yanaoka, T., Iwata, R., Yoshimura, A., & Hirose, N. (2021). A 1-minute re-warm up at high-intensity improves sprint performance during the lough borough intermittent shuttle test. *Front Physiol*, 11, 616158.

Yanci, J., Iturri, J., Castillo, D., Pardeiro, M., & Nakamura, F. Y. (2019). Influence of warm-up duration on perceived exertion and subsequent physical performance of soccer players. *Biol Sport*, 36, 125–131.

# 2 Resistance training

*Conall Murtagh, David Rydings and Barry Drust*

## Introduction

Soccer players will always be judged by what they do on the pitch and not in the gym. More specifically, the perceived success of any individual player is determined by his/her accomplishments during competitive match play. When we investigate the detail of soccer match play from a physical perspective, explosive actions are performed nearly once every minute (81 ± 18 maximal actions during a 90-min game) (Murtagh et al., 2019), and 83% of goals are preceded by at least one powerful action (Faude et al., 2012). The ability to produce maximal power, apply this power during complex motor tasks and repeatedly tolerate the performance of such explosive actions throughout a match(es), may therefore be considered paramount to successful performance at the elite level. Optimising such capabilities could therefore improve the chances of the player having a successful career.

Researchers have documented that a variation of specific resistance training (defined as any training modality that requires a muscle contraction against an external load) methods can enhance the ability to produce (Loturco et al., 2016), apply (Mendiguchia et al., 2020), and tolerate (Petersen, Thorborg, Nielsen, Budtz-Jørgensen, & Hölmich, 2011) force during powerful soccer actions. When rationalised in this context (specific definitions of this training model are displayed in Figure 2.1), it seems logical that resistance training should play a role in the physical development of an elite soccer player. However, resistance training comes at a cost to the player and can initially cause acute neural fatigue, metabolic fatigue, and/or micro-damage in the muscle-tendon unit, all of which are specific to the chosen training modality (Draganidis et al., 2013). As soccer is a unique sport which often requires elite players to operate for up to 49 weeks per season, with weekly micro-cycles that can often contain two to three games per week alongside continued training, recovery becomes extremely important. Further intense training (such as resistance training) during these periods has the potential to blunt the recovery process and lead to non-functional over-reaching, sub-optimal performance, injury, or illness (Doeven, Brink, Kosse, & Lemmink, 2018). Similarly, intense training during taper periods leading into matches may cause fatigue and compromise match performance levels. While resistance training may help soccer players achieve more successful careers, the prescription should complement and not compete with the pitch/match training loads.

It is imperative when prescribing resistance training, those practitioners have an insight into the individual player's training load-recovery profile and consider several other factors, such as the upcoming game schedule. The practitioner should rationalise

DOI: 10.4324/9781003148418-3

their programming by being specific about what they are trying to achieve (i.e., our model suggests identifying which of the following areas they are trying to improve: the production, application, and/or tolerance of/to powerful soccer-specific actions), and therefore, which physiological adaptations are being targeted. The goal of the practitioner must be to optimise the balance between providing the appropriate training stimulus to enhance or maintain a physical capacity, but not impede recovery, thus reducing injury risk while maximising physical performance levels in competitive games.

In the current chapter, we present a novel systematic process for the prescription of resistance training for the soccer player. We aim to answer three questions: Why resistance training may be important in the training of soccer players? What are the most optimal prescription models, and what are the challenges to their implementation? How may we navigate the challenges to implement this process in the real world?

## Why? The production, application, and tolerance model

### Model rationale

The ability to produce (i.e., during strength and jump assessments, Murtagh, Nulty et al., 2018; Murtagh et al., 2017) and apply (i.e., during more specific actions such as sprinting, Haugen, Tønnessen, & Seiler, 2013; Murtagh, Brownlee et al., 2018) force/power may determine elite soccer playing status and provide an advantage during decisive moments of competitive games. Furthermore, the capacity to tolerate a high volume of explosive actions over 90 min, often twice per week, is an important characteristic for the elite player. Subsequently, it appears the ability to produce, apply, and tolerate power/powerful actions is imperative for the elite soccer performer; hence, we have developed a novel soccer-specific resistance training model based on this concept (Figure 2.1).

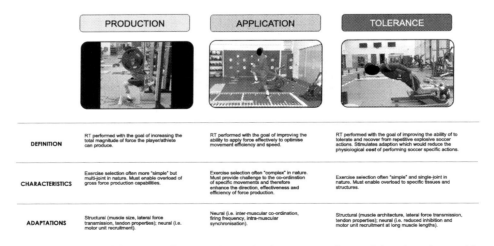

*Figure 2.1* The ability to produce, apply, and tolerate power/powerful actions is considered paramount to successful soccer performance at the elite playing level.

### Production

Given that the ability to produce force is a determinant of sporting performance (Cometti, Maffiuletti, Pousson, Chatard, & Maffulli, 2001; Murtagh et al., 2017), it is important to understand how to develop this attribute in applied practice. A key factor underpinning the capacity to produce force is the development of muscular strength. The most effective (non-pharmacological) means by which to enhance muscular strength is a resistance training exercise. Numerous researchers have shown that when the ability to produce force is increased via resistance training, there is an associated performance improvement in key actions such as accelerating, sprinting, and jumping (Channell & Barfield, 2008). This improvement supports the notion that the ability to produce large forces underpins performance and provides an indication that resistance training may provide a potent stimulus to enhance such task performance.

Resistance training results in the radial growth of skeletal muscle and the promotion of neural adaptations that result in enhanced force output. The application of different resistance training exercise, and any associated loading patterns, will impose diverse physiological stresses on an athlete's neuromuscular system. These stresses will, in turn, influence both the resultant adaptive signal and the accumulated level of fatigue (Killen, Gabbett, & Jenkins, 2010). Typically, a resistance training exercise programme aimed at maximising muscle strength (or the ability to produce force) in athletes would involve performing traditional compound resistance training exercises (e.g., back squat), training at intensities of 85% of 1 repetition maximum (1RM) or greater, performing resistance exercise at least 2 days per week, and completing a mean training volume of 8 sets per muscle group (Peterson, Rhea, & Alvar, 2004).

Although resistance exercise is an effective strategy to increase skeletal muscle strength (or the ability to produce force), it is important to recognise that resistance exercise training imparts acute skeletal muscle damage and neuromuscular fatigue. This damage and fatigue results in a transient decrement in force production and an increase in pro-inflammatory signalling molecules. While this may not be of consequence for the average exerciser, in elite soccer, managing the recovery from resistance exercise is critical. The literature would agree with anecdotal evidence that performing the resistance training necessary to enhance force production (utilising loads >85% 1 RM) can take over 48 h to recover from (Draganidis et al., 2013). If the practitioner wants to maximise training opportunities to improve production but wants to minimise the cost to the player, they often must think a little more outside of the box. We suggest where traditional methods are inappropriate alternative options could be to prescribe concentric only or an isometric exercise. We have categorised the cost of different types of production exercises in Figure 2.2 and elaborated on how such information can be applied in the considerations "cost" section.

### Application

Soccer players at the elite level are required to produce high levels of force/power during complex motor tasks such as accelerating, sprinting, changing direction, and attempting to maintain or gain possession of the ball while exerting physical force against an opponent (Bloomfield, Polman, & O'Donoghue, 2007). An athlete's movement strategy for a specific action can determine the speed of execution and, if suboptimal, can cause the biomechanical overload of specific tissues, thus elevating injury risk (King et al., 2018; Mendiguchia, Castano-Zambudio et al., 2021). To apply force

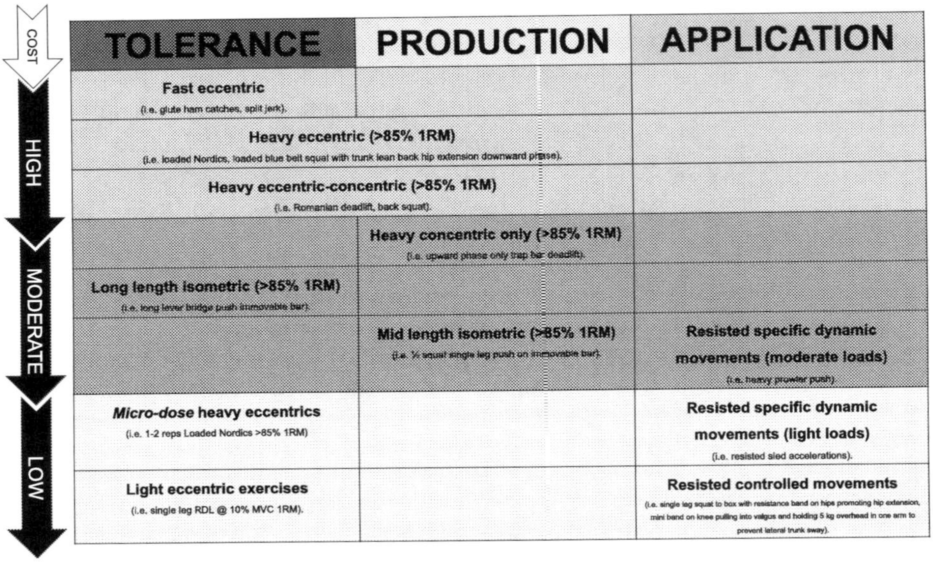

*Figure 2.2* The table displays the cost associated with resistance training exercises in each specific category.

efficiently in any complex movement, we should aim to minimise energy leakage, reduce the risk of tissue overload and subsequent injury via the improved alignment and coordination of specific movements. It, therefore, seems that resistance training should be considered in a player's training schedule.

Researchers using bony palpation methods observed that 92.5% of soccer players are suffering from multiple innominate malalignments (Elumalai, Declaro, Sanyal, Bareng, & Mohammad, 2015). Such imbalances around the pelvis can potentially lead to sub-optimal biomechanics with compensatory patterns causing asymmetrically greater workload, stress, and strain in specific muscles/tendons. Although there is limited evidence to document that optimal biomechanics exist for many dynamic soccer-specific actions, specific movement dysfunctions have previously been associated with elevated injury risk. For example, excessive pelvic and trunk motion during the swing phase of high-speed running is associated with soccer players who sustained a first hamstring injury. More specifically, hamstring injury has been associated with significantly greater anterior pelvic tilting and thoracic side-bending during acceleration (Daly, McCarthy Persson, Twycross-Lewis, Woledge, & Morrissey, 2016; Schuermans, Van Tiggelen, Palmans, Danneels, & Witvrouw, 2017). The current body of literature (although limited with small sample sizes) suggests that team sport athletes who appear to be more vulnerable to hamstring injury suffer from lacking proximal control and insufficient dissociative capacity within the lumbo-pelvic-hip complex, which may be further exacerbated by the repetitive nature of soccer actions. There is, therefore, sufficient evidence to suggest that sub-optimal force application increases injury risk in soccer players.

Recently, researchers have documented that application training modalities can be effective at improving biomechanics and improving performance in such actions. A specific intervention programme, including a focus on application training, was shown to be effective in reducing anterior pelvic tilt kinematics during gait (Mendiguchia, Gonzalez De la Flor et al., 2021). Moreover, similar interventions have resulted in faster sprint performance while continuing to alter the biomechanics towards a more efficient movement strategy which is thought to reduce the risk of hamstring injury (Mendiguchia, Castano-Zambudio et al., 2021) and athletic groin pain (King et al., 2018). Heavy sled sprint training has previously been shown to improve acceleration, and sprint performance, via the improved ability to orientate horizontal force applied to the ground during acceleration (Morin et al., 2017), thus implying that there were positive biomechanical alterations. Furthermore, when sprint "application" training (oriented around improving sprint mechanics) was performed (in addition to soccer training) in elite players, not only were there improvements in sprint mechanics (greater maximal horizontal force and ratio of force) and sprint performance but also in measures of muscle architecture of the hamstring muscles (i.e., increased fascicle length). Considering it has been shown in previous case studies that the ability to produce horizontal force during acceleration can change prior to a hamstring injury (Mendiguchia et al., 2016), and that shorter biceps femoris fascicle lengths increase hamstring injury risk (Timmins et al., 2016), the inclusion of specific "application" training oriented around acceleration and sprint actions could provide a stimulus to improve performance and reduce injury risk in elite soccer players (Mendiguchia et al., 2020). There is, therefore, sufficient evidence to show that application training can lead to improvements in explosive soccer performance and, by reducing dysfunctional movement and energy leakage during soccer-specific tasks, lowering the risk of overuse injuries.

For application training to be effective at improving movement, it is extremely important that the exercise prescribed requires the player to operate at similar joint angles and/or velocities to the specific movement(s) on the soccer pitch. We have categorised application training into three types according to the speed and resistance/external load (see Figure 2.2). As inter-muscular coordination is the primary physiological adaptation, application training in its most complex format would be considered as neurally demanding but low/moderate cost from a structural perspective. While there is not much literature investigating the cost associated with specific application training, ballistic resistance training (i.e., jump squat and lunges at 50% 1 RM), which may be classified as application training if performed in a specific context, did not show any prolonged suppression of performance (countermovement jump, 10 m and 20 m sprint) or perceptual recovery parameters (delayed onset muscle soreness, total quality recovery, Brazilian mood scale scores) 24 h post-training. Such information supports anecdotal evidence suggesting that light/moderate load, high-speed resistance training doesn't impede on any performance or perceptual recovery parameters 24 h post-training (Goulart et al., 2020). Therefore, when performed with the optimal volume (depending on pitch loads, player training status), application training can be prescribed most days within the microcycle, even close to games. Regular exposure to such stimuli increases the chances of making a positive impact on the player's movement profile.

### *Tolerance*

While applying force more efficiently is thought to reduce the risk of overuse injury, the ability of the muscle-tendon unit to tolerate a high volume of repetitive forceful actions performed at high speeds may decrease the risk of significant microtrauma

## THE REPEATED BOUT EFFECT
### A KEY CONCEPT FOR PRACTITONERS TO UNDERSTAND.

If an athlete engages in unaccustomed, strenuous physical exercise which requires the muscle to lengthen while it is active (close to the end range), they can experience stiff or sore muscles, usually apparent for 24-72 hr after exercise. Known as eccentric contractions, such activities are strongly associated with structural disruption of sarcomeres, disturbed excitation-contraction coupling and calcium signalling, leading to an inflammatory response and the activation of several muscle protein degradation pathways. This process is called exercise induced muscle damage and is normally accompanied by a swelling and temporary reduction in both maximum strength and range of motion. If recovery and regeneration is optimal, a certain amount of muscle damage is a positive stimulus for muscle-tendon unit restructuring, hypertrophy, and strength gains. The cell remodelling and adaptation that occurs after such eccentric exercise also allows the tissue to be become more resilient to damage when performing similar movements in the future. This is known as the repeated bout effect.

*Figure 2.3* The repeated bout effect is a key concept to inform the detailed prescription process.

and subsequent tissue failure. Soccer actions often require the muscle to operate eccentrically at long muscle lengths and fast contraction velocities. Such contractions are associated with the highest levels of muscle damage (Barreto, de Lima, Greco, & Denadai, 2019). Researchers have documented that there is a prolonged impairment of lower-limb strength for as long as 60 (Draganidis et al., 2015) and 72 h (Trecroci et al., 2020) post-soccer game. Further eccentric activities at long muscle lengths (such as soccer-specific explosive actions) during such periods could increase risk of tissue overload and injury. However, if recovery and regeneration are optimal, a certain amount of muscle damage is a positive stimulus for muscle-tendon unit restructuring, hypertrophy, and strength gains (Roig et al., 2009). Known as the repeated bout effect (see Figure 2.3), the cell remodelling and adaptation that occurs after such eccentric exercise allows the tissue to become more resilient to damage when performing similar movements in the future, hence, improving tissue tolerance.

It has been well documented that specific resistance training interventions with an eccentric focus can improve the tissue's ability to tolerate eccentric actions at long muscle lengths. Researchers have shown that eccentric overload resistance training in different formats leads to structural (i.e., increased fascicle length (Presland et al., 2018), lateral force transmission (Erskine et al., 2011), physiological cross-sectional area (Erskine, Fletcher, & Folland, 2014), tendon compliance at the muscle end of the tendon (Baar, 2017)) and neural ((i.e., overcoming neural regulatory mechanism that limits the recruitment and/or discharge rate of motor units exists during maximal voluntary eccentric muscle contraction (Aagaard et al., 2000; Duclay et al., 2008); muscle activation at longer muscle lengths (Hegyi et al., 2019)) adaptation that makes the tissue less likely to tear or micro-tear when put under the stress and strain associated with elite soccer training and more specifically, match-play. A number of prospective studies report that eccentric strength training performed at long muscle lengths reduces the risk of hamstring injury in soccer players (Askling. Tengvar, & Thorstensson, 2013;

Petersen et al., 2011). It is therefore thought that training to improve tissue tolerance at the neural and structural level in elite soccer players should have an eccentric component and can be maximised when ensuring the muscle operates at long muscle lengths and at a variety of contraction speeds.

From the real-world perspective, it must be considered that to gain such desirable adaptations, eccentric strength training modalities come at high physiological cost to the player (fast eccentric exercise induces greater muscle damage compared to slow eccentric exercise (Barreto et al., 2019)) and can initiate a cascade of catabolic processes within the neuro-muscular system that lead to elevated muscle soreness and reductions in power/speed outputs. Moreover, structural adaptation, such as increased fascicle length, has been shown to return to baseline after 2 weeks of detraining (Presland et al., 2018), meaning such a stimulus needs to be applied frequently in-season. It is challenging to regularly include traditional eccentric strength training in elite soccer, especially at clubs who experience congested fixture schedules. However, it has been documented that various other training protocols associated with lower cost, such as micro-dosing of two reps of maximal eccentric contractions (Nosaka et al., 2001), light, eccentric exercises ($6 \times 5$ reps at 10% MVC) (Lavender & Nosaka, 2008), and maximal isometric contractions (greater protection when performed at long muscle lengths (Lima & Denadai, 2015)), all offer a protective "tolerance" effect to subsequent exercise. More specifically, the body of literature suggests that maximal isometric contractions at long muscle lengths in small doses (i.e., 2–10 maximal isometric contractions) performed 2–4 days prior to fast or slow eccentric exercise protocols can significantly attenuate exercise-induced muscle damage symptoms (Barreto et al., 2019) and therefore acutely improve the tolerance of the muscle-tendon unit. Such training modes can also be classed as moderate/low cost tolerance training (see Figure 2.2) and could be useful for the soccer practitioner aiming to maximise training opportunities in close proximity to competitive matches.

With injury rates continuing to increase in elite soccer (Ekstrand, Waldén, & Hägglund, 2016) and fixtures regularly scheduled when the player's recovery markers (such as hamstring strength) haven't returned to baseline (Trecroci et al., 2020), it seems that many elite players would benefit from tolerance training with a view that prevention is the best form of cure. However, such training generally comes at a high cost, and the implementation needs to be strategically planned into the elite player's programme; especially if specific circumstances don't allow this stimulus to be performed regularly.

## What? The most optimal resistance training prescription

Production, application, and tolerance resistance training interventions could benefit the elite player by improving their chances of staying healthy and achieving more successful match play performance. However, the implementation of such interventions can be challenging in soccer and is often a point of contention amongst player support staff. We present a novel systematic approach for the prescription of resistance training in elite soccer players that can be applied in clubs at various playing levels, who employ different weekly training periodisation structures and engage in contrasting fixture schedules. The process involves three key stages before the detail of the resistance training session is finally prescribed and monitored accordingly (Figure 2.4).

22  *Conall Murtagh et al.*

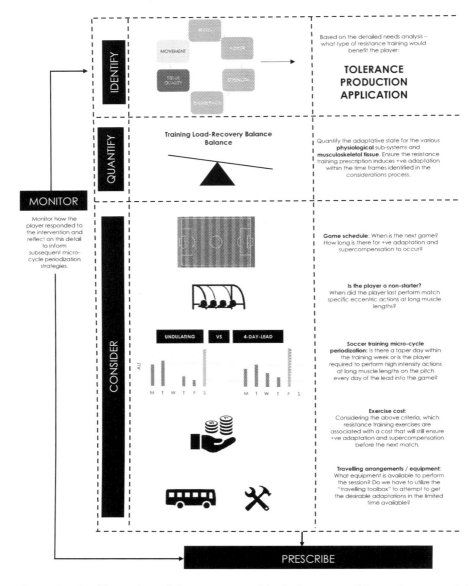

*Figure 2.4* An illustration of the processes utilised when prescribing resistance training interventions for the elite soccer players.

## *Identify – How can resistance training help this player?*

The most important element of player programming is to perform a detailed needs analysis of the player and sport. An example of a needs analysis that could be used for the elite soccer player is detailed in Figure 2.4. The need analysis is a constant process that should be performed regularly to determine effectiveness of the programme and indicate of any adjustments/changes that should be prescribed. From a resistance training perspective, the outcome of the needs analysis is to ascertain which of the resistance training goals the player should prioritise at that moment and time (production, application, and/or tolerance).

### Quantify – What is the player's current training load-recovery balance?

When planning resistance training interventions, the practitioner should always consider the individual player's training load-recovery balance. Such analyses provide an indication or estimation of the adaptative state the player is in for the various physiological sub-systems and musculoskeletal tissue. This information (although it is always an informed estimation regardless of the most recent technology available), should guide the practitioner not only to which specific training methods the player should perform to gain a positive adaptive response, but which training stimuli may further stress a sub-system or tissue that is already broken down and weakened leading to a mal-adaptive response. The practitioner should attempt to quantify every individual player's training *stimulus* and, considering specific load-adaptation pathway timeframes, the subsequent response. Such an insight is crucial when prescribing the detail of resistance training intervention.

#### Quantifying the stimulus?

When a soccer player engages in any form of physical training stimulus, internal biochemical stresses simultaneous to internal mechanical stresses to the various musculoskeletal tissues utilised during the activity. Based on the specificity of the training stimulus and the time course of any subsequent physical stimuli (further stress), the physiological sub-systems and tissues adapt. The authors believe that the most optimal way of quantifying the stimulus (or training load) of the training load-recovery balance is to use a theoretical framework in which physiological and biomechanical load-adaptation pathways are considered separately. Practitioners need to be very aware that load-adaptation pathways have different response rates, which has consequences for the planning of resistance training interventions (Vanrenterghem et al., 2017). Soccer match play, training, and resistance training all induce biochemical and biomechanical stress and initiate a cascade of specific physiological and structural/ functional adaptative processes, respectively. If specific time frames are respected before the next stimulus, positive adaptation occurs, known as supercompensation. Biomechanical adaptations have a longer response rate and adaptation time frame compared to physiological adaptations.

While quantifying the biochemical and biomechanical stress on physiological subsystems and musculoskeletal tissue from resistance training and prescribed pitch-based running sessions is relatively straight forward, quantifying the complex, unorthodox explosive actions performed during pitch based team training and match play provide more of a challenge for the practitioner. It is clear we still cannot accurately quantify the actual "stress" the players' body is exposed to during training or match play. Estimating the adaptative state is also made difficult by the fact that players will respond to the same loading stimuli in different ways, which has recently been supported by research showing that muscle damage is related to genetic profile (Baumert, 2019). Moreover, adaptation rates are highly dependent on the player's training status. When estimating biomechanical adaptation rates relative to the player's training status, the

24    *Conall Murtagh et al.*

repeated bout effect is an important concept for the practitioner to understand. While it is important to consider the physiological adaptation profile when prescribing any training intervention for the player, as the biomechanical load and subsequent adaptation profile provide an insight into the structural and functional status of each specific skeletal tissue, it is extremely important that this is considered when prescribing the specificity of resistance training.

*Quantifying the response?*

The response to training load can be measured by several commercially available wellness devices which measure player sleep profiles and heart rate variability, providing an insight into to the general recovery state of a player. Moreover, subjective questionnaires can be used to provide an insight into levels of fatigue or muscle soreness. If possible, the fitness team should be liaising closely with the medical department, who can assess a player to provide further insight into whether any tissue is still in a state of adaptation. Assessments of range of motion, single joint isometric strength at long muscle lengths or direction-specific power assessments can also provide the practitioner with valuable information regarding the adaptation profile of joints or muscle-tendon complexes. Once the practitioner has quantified the training stimulus, the subsequent response, and considered the player's training status (with reference to the repeated bout effect) and natural ability to tolerate eccentric exercise (Newton et al., 2008), they have should have a good insight into which tissues are underloaded, and if any tissue is overloaded. This information is crucial to the detailed prescription process.

*The training load-recovery balance after match play*

Competitive matches typically represents the highest physiological and biomechanical stress on the player's body. It is crucial that the practitioner respects the recovery time frames post-match when prescribing resistance training interventions. Several researchers have investigated the recovery kinetics of muscle force production after a soccer match, with some studies demonstrating lower limb strength levels remained impaired up to 12–24 h from a match (Krustrup et al., 2011), with complete recovery reached from 36 to 48 h. However, these studies only measured knee extensor (quadriceps) function when it is well known that the knee flexors (hamstrings) are the most frequently injured muscle in elite soccer. Other studies, which included assessment of knee flexor strength, showed a more prolonged impairment of lower-limb strength until 60 (Draganidis et al., 2015) and 72 h (Trecroci et al., 2020). This would suggest that whilst the tissue responsible for producing peak force in knee extension activities may be adapted and ready for another stimuli (i.e., knee extensor dominant resistance training exposure) 48 h post-game, the knee flexors (hamstrings) may not be fully recovery until 60–72 h post-game. Engaging in hamstring dominant eccentric activities at long muscle lengths, such as resistance-specific training or maximal soccer-specific explosive actions in a training or game format, during this time frame post-game, could increase the risk of injury and compromise the safety and well-being of players.

From an individual player perspective, the magnitude of the decline in knee flexor strength and countermovement jump performance may be affected by the total number of explosive actions (Nedelec et al., 2014). Such observations are supported by anecdotal evidence from practitioners, which suggests that when a player achieves statistically greater physical outputs compared to their average, physiological and perceptual recovery markers are compromised, and it takes longer to return to baseline post-game. The quantification analyses of the training load-recovery balance are extremely important if the practitioner is to effectively maximise training windows for the individual player, especially during congested fixture periods.

*The non-starter*

It is well known amongst practitioners that a recent good rhythm of games may provide protection to the skeletal muscle from strength attenuation and enhance recovery following a game. However, even the highest level of team training lacks the competitiveness and intensity of matches. When the player hasn't been exposed to a game recently (i.e., a non-starter), it is imperative that specific gym-based interventions initiate adaptations which offer a protective effect for when the player engages in their next bout of maximal eccentric activity (which in soccer players is generally a competitive game). Physiological adaptations in untrained individuals who start playing soccer (Jakobsen et al., 2012) and anecdotal evidence suggests that performing multiple maximal explosive actions in a match format improves the tolerance of specific tissue. Anecdotally, the player will always perform more extreme actions at longer muscle lengths during competitive games, possibly due to the competition component and other factors such as pressure from the crowd and the stakes/rewards of winning. Therefore, a key challenge for the fitness practitioner is to maintain and/develop match-specific fitness but, more specifically, the tissue tolerance status of the players who do not start games. Players that lack "game" rhythm are more prone to under-performance and injury when they are next selected to play a competitive match. Tolerance training that requires eccentric contractions at similar speeds and muscle lengths to extreme actions in a competitive game, is very important for "non-starters". Such training provides optimal stimulus for the tissue to maintain/develop the ability to tolerate match-specific volumes and intensities of explosive actions. The question of: "does the player have a lack of match exposure" is, therefore, a key a consideration in the resistance training prescription process.

## Consider – Which "future" circumstances could impact the prescription?

Once we have identified what area the player needs to improve and have an insight into his/her current training load-recovery balance profile, numerous other considerations will impact upon the detailed prescription process.

*Match schedule*

In every circumstance, other than a youth development player for which long-term development is prioritised over optimising match performance levels, performance during match play should be prioritised in any training regime. First and foremost, recovery from games should be respected, but the practitioner needs to consider the fixture schedule and when the next competitive game(s) will be played. Unlike some Olympic sports, where the athletes are required to peak two or three times a year, in soccer, senior players are required to peak for every competitive match (perhaps

## 26  Conall Murtagh et al.

*Table 2.1* The relationship between factors affecting fixture schedule demands and the opportunity for resistance training exposures in soccer players in starts and squad players

| TRAINING / MATCH FACTORS | PREMIER LEAGUE TEAM (TOP 4) | | PREMIER LEAGUE TEAM MID-TABLE | | ENGLISH CHAMPIONSHIP | | BUNGESLIGA TEAM | |
|---|---|---|---|---|---|---|---|---|
| Champion league qualification | YES | | NO | | N/A | | NO | |
| National Cup progression | YES | | NO | | NO | | YES | |
| Over % of team full internationals | YES | | NO | | NO | | YES | |
| Pitch training periodization Undulating at 4 day intensity lead in | 4 day intensity | | Undulating | | Undulating | | 4 day intensity | |
| Pre-season game schedule x 3 games per week | YES | | YES | | YES | | No | |
| | STARTER | ROUND PLAYER | STARTER | ROUND PLAYER | STARTER | ROUND PLAYER | STARTER | ROUND PLAYER |
| Number of matches in season | 42 | 34 | 42 | 21 | 62 | 25 | 47 | 23 |
| HIGH COST RESISTANCE TRAINING EXPOSURES | 18 | 21 (10 point game) | 42 | 12 (20 point game) | 38 | 12 (24 point game) | 21 | 44 (23 point game) |
| MODERRATE COST RESISTANCE TRAINING EXPOSURES | 15 | 32 (12 point game) | 37 | 47 (10 point game) | 48 | 52 (12 point game) | 31 | 43 (12 point game) |
| LOW COST RESISTANCE TRAINING EXPOSURES | 145 | 178 | 138 | 178 | 138 | 176 | 145 | 178 |

including pre-season friendlies where players are competing for their starting place in the 1st match of the season). Some players can be required to produce peak physical performance levels for up to 49 weeks of the year (see Table 2.1). The fixture demands can also fluctuate for the team and individual player during the season as Cup competitions finish or the team gets knocked out in earlier rounds, and players could be selected to play more or less frequently. Players and practitioners who have operated in different teams with contrasting fixture and pitch training demands would argue that from a resistance training prescription perspective, the demands and factors are so contrasting, it is like working in different sports. A systematic approach is, therefore, vital to enable practitioners to prescribe an appropriate training stimulus while allowing adequate timing for a certain level of super-compensation, thus optimising performance levels whilst reducing injury risk. Resistance training periodisation and prescription is, therefore, highly dependent on the fixture schedule.

### Pitch training micro-cycle periodisation

Although the match is the highest physical stimulus the player is ever exposed to, the pitch training loads provide significant biochemical and biomechanical stress. The periodisation of the pitch training micro-cycles is an important consideration when planning the detail of resistance training interventions. There are many micro-cycle periodisation models employed in elite soccer. Within each of these models, there is a certain amount of variation for each coaching team employing the specific model. As we won't cover this topic in detail in the current chapter, we have simplified micro-cycle periodisation strategies to two different types: An undulating week whereby there is a day off or unloading taper day during the week, usually 2 (or sometimes 3) days before the game; and a 4-day week which has no specific unloading day (other than a volume taper the day or 2 days before the game) and the players are required to train with high/maximal intensities for 4 days leading into the game (i.e., some application of the Tactical Periodisation Model; Jankowski, 2016). The strategy for prescribing resistance training can change based on different micro-cycle periodisation strategies. In theory, when the player has an unloading day during the week, it is easier to implement high-cost resistance training exercise as the unloading day, rather than a pitch training session with explosive actions, helps the player adapt (super-compensate) quicker and eradicate any residual fatigue or soreness from resistance training before the next game.

### The cost of resistance training

A consideration of the cost of the resistance training intervention is a crucial part of the prescription process. Training status and genetic profile (Baumert, 2019) can impact upon the muscle damage, adaptation rates, and cost associated with resistance training exercise. This can make it somewhat difficult to predict the exact time frame which the player requires to adapt. Nevertheless, due to the possibility of congested fixture schedules and prioritisation of pitch training in elite soccer, it is always important for the practitioner to be able to manipulate the cost associated with the resistance training stimulus. Choosing exercises methodically according to their cost can help maximise training opportunities, avoid overload of a tissue/system that is in an adaptative state whilst still allowing the player to be in peak physical condition for the up-and-coming match. Whilst respecting the individual response to resistance training, we have provided a guide of exercise types of varying cost for each specific resistance category (i.e., production, application tolerance). Such guidelines allow the practitioner to manipulate the cost of the resistance training exposure whilst still prescribing a stimulus specific to the goals identified in the needs analysis process (see Figure 2.2).

### Equipment available and travel arrangements

To optimise player physical performance levels, the practitioner needs to maximise windows of training opportunity. Often for teams with congested fixture schedules, the training opportunity comes immediately after the match (see Table 2.1). With the training-load recovery balance in mind and ensuring supercompensation occurs before the next competitive game, often immediately after the match, is the only opportunity for players to be exposed to a resistance training session that is oriented around tolerance or production goals. However, especially at away games, there is rarely the available facilities to lift the heavy loads required to perform production and tolerance exercises. In such cases, the practitioner needs to have their post-match strategies in place to optimise this training window. Exercises such as eccentric hamstring slide outs (resisted), Nordics and reverse Nordics, which expose the player to a tolerance stimulus at long muscle lengths, have been shown to be effective and time efficient. Flywheel devices can be utilised and are relatively compliant with team travelling procedures. Adjustable weighted dumbbells can also be useful, and prescribing single leg training allows higher intensities with less load. As this is also often an optimal time for energy systems conditioning and an exposure to biomechanical load on the pitch, all the chosen interventions for the specific player need to be time efficient and compatible to provide the optimal stimulus to the tissue. The practitioners "travelling toolbox" is essential to optimise training windows and player performance levels, and the extent of toolbox impacts upon the prescription process.

## How? Does this all work in practice

### The system in practice

We have presented our framework for systematically prescribing resistance training prescription in elite soccer clubs. To show how such a systematic process works in practice, Figures 2.5–2.7 depict three real-world case studies which use specific principles to overcome various challenges and provide the most optimal training stimulus for the player.

### Exposure and impact

The systematic, detailed prescription of resistance training can help the soccer player have a more successful career. We believe that the system presented in this chapter ensures that the practitioner can maximise training opportunities and have a positive impact on player match physical performance levels. Table 2.1 illustrates that the fixture schedule, starting status and training micro-cycle periodisation can largely dictate the type of resistance training exposures the player can be exposed to throughout a season in different regimes. Our analysis shows there are many opportunities for the player to be exposed to specific resistance training interventions. Analysing the resistance training exposures for specific groups of players shows which types of interventions the practitioner can prioritise in their resistance training programming. For example, a regular starter for a Champions League or English Championship team should invest his time in the most effective low-cost resistance training interventions

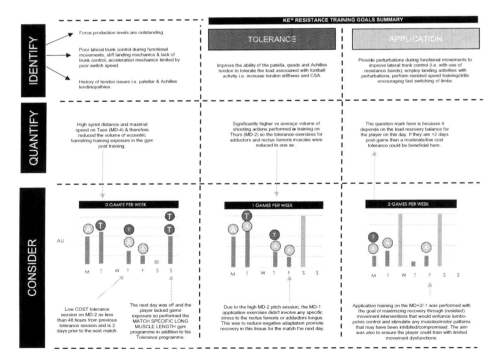

*Figure 2.5* Real-world prescription process for player 1 in different match play formats.

Resistance training 29

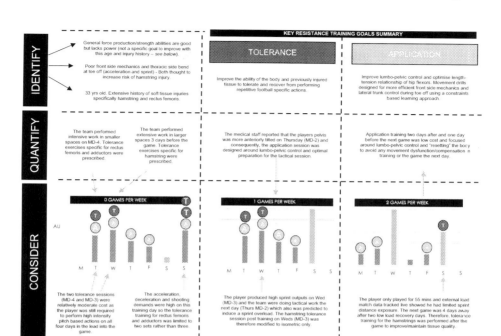

*Figure 2.6* Real-world prescription process for player 2 in different match play formats.

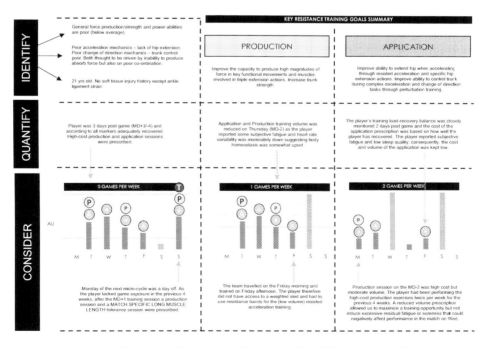

*Figure 2.7* Real-world prescription process for player 3 in different match play formats.

to improve the player's physical profile. If most of this training is to come through low and moderate intensity application training (which can be performed regularly during congested fixture periods), it would be a good idea for this player to perform regular detailed biomechanical assessments to ensure the programming is as specific as possible and is being regularly monitored. In contrast, for a squad player who needs to improve tissue tolerance as he is over 30 years old, regularly sustains soft tissue injuries, and many of his exposures must be after the game, he/she needs to be prescribed the most optimal "travel and changing room friendly" exercises. We must also highlight that as player and team circumstances can change quickly in soccer, a player's regime can also change, which is why the ability to operate a systematic approach (as we have presented in the chapter) ensures that every player gets an individual service which allows them to maximise their physical potential.

## Future directions and conclusions

Soccer is a sport where players could be required to be in peak physical condition one to two times per week for up to 49 weeks in the year. The diverse fixture and pitch training demands make resistance training periodisation and planning a challenge for practitioners. The inclusion of resistance training interventions can help players reduce injury risk and maximise physical performance levels. However, for the practitioner to maximise physical performance in competitive games, the prescription process should be systematic and detailed. We have presented a prescription model whereby the soccer practitioner can identify how resistance training could help the player, continually quantify the player's training load-recovery balance, and then go through a checklist of considerations before providing the most specific and detailed prescription of resistance training, which attacks the player's deficiencies and builds on their strengths. Future developments may enhance methods which enable a greater understanding of the specific, individual, responses to both training and match play. This would, in turn, better empower practitioners to make both faster and more informed decisions around a player's current training load-recovery balance in order to optimally prescribe resistance training programmes. Further to this, the ongoing development of strategies to provide a resistance training stimulus whilst "on the road" and/or during periods of fixture congestion, may enhance the practitioner's ability to optimise resistance training prescription under these challenging, "real-world" scenarios. Such a specific process should allow super-compensation to occur before the next match(es), which will increase the player's chances of successful performance and, in the long term, a healthy career whereby the player can maximise their physical potential.

## References

Aagaard, P., Simonsen, E. B., Andersen, J. L., Magnussen, S. P., Halkjaer-Kristensen, J., & Dyhre-Poulsen, P. (2000). Neural inhibition during maximal eccentric and concentric quadriceps contraction: Effects of resistance training. *Journal of Applied Physiology, 89*(6), 2249–2257.

Askling, C. M., Tengvar, M., & Thorstensson, A. (2013). Acute hamstring injuries in Swedish elite football: a prospective randomised controlled clinical trial comparing two rehabilitation protocols. *British Journal of Sports Medicine, 47*(15), 953–959.

Baar, K. (2017). Minimizing injury and maximizing return to play: lessons from engineered ligaments. *Sports Medicine, 47*(1), 5–11.

Barreto, R. V., de Lima, L. C. R., Greco, C. C., & Denadai, B. S. (2019). Protective effect conferred by isometric preconditioning against slow-and fast-velocity eccentric exercise-induced muscle damage. *Frontiers in Physiology, 10*, 1203.

Baumert, P. (2019). *The physiological and genetic factors underpinning the response to muscle damaging exercise (PhD).* Liverpool: John Moores University.

Bloomfield, J., Polman, R., & O'Donoghue, P. (2007). Physical demands of different positions in FA Premier League soccer. *Journal of Sports Science & Medicine, 6*(1), 63.

Channell, B. T., & Barfield, J. P. (2008). Effect of Olympic and traditional resistance training on vertical jump improvement in high school boys. *The Journal of Strength & Conditioning Research, 22*(5), 1522–1527.

Cometti, G., Maffiuletti, N. A., Pousson, M., Chatard, J.-C., & Maffulli, N. (2001). Isokinetic strength and anaerobic power of elite, subelite and amateur French soccer players. *International Journal of Sports Medicine, 22*(01), 45–51.

Daly, C., McCarthy Persson, U., Twycross-Lewis, R., Woledge, R. C., & Morrissey, D. (2016). The biomechanics of running in athletes with previous hamstring injury: a case-control study. *Scandinavian Journal of Medicine & Science in Sports, 26*(4), 413–420.

Doeven, S. H., Brink, M. S., Kosse, S. J., & Lemmink, K. A. P. M. (2018). Postmatch recovery of physical performance and biochemical markers in team ball sports: a systematic review. *BMJ Open Sport & Exercise Medicine, 4*(1), e000264.

Draganidis, D., Chatzinikolaou, A., Avloniti, A., Barbero-Álvarez, J. C., Mohr, M., Malliou, P., … Margonis, K. (2015). Recovery kinetics of knee flexor and extensor strength after a football match. *PLoS One, 10*(6), e0128072.

Draganidis, D., Chatzinikolaou, A., Jamurtas, A. Z., Carlos Barbero, J., Tsoukas, D., Theodorou, A. S., … Theodorou, A. (2013). The time-frame of acute resistance exercise effects on football skill performance: the impact of exercise intensity. *Journal of Sports Sciences, 31*(7), 714–722.

Duclay, J., Martin, A., Robbe, A., & Pousson, M. (2008). Spinal reflex plasticity during maximal dynamic contractions after eccentric training. *Medicine and Science in Sports and Exercise, 40*(4), 722–734.

Ekstrand, J., Waldén, M., & Hägglund, M. (2016). Hamstring injuries have increased by 4% annually in men's professional football, since 2001: a 13-year longitudinal analysis of the UEFA elite club injury study. *British Journal of Sports Medicine, 50*(12), 731–737.

Elumalai, G., Declaro, M., Sanyal, S., Bareng, M. B., & Mohammad, A. (2015). Soccer syndrome-2: common innominate malalignments and its manual diagnostic techniques in pelvic malalignments syndrome. *American Journal of Sports Science, 3*(6), 120–127.

Erskine, R. M., Fletcher, G., & Folland, J. P. (2014). The contribution of muscle hypertrophy to strength changes following resistance training. *European Journal of Applied Physiology, 114*(6), 1239–1249.

Erskine, R. M., Jones, D. A., Maffulli, N., Williams, A. G., Stewart, C. E., & Degens, H. (2011). What causes in vivo muscle specific tension to increase following resistance training? *Experimental Physiology, 96*(2), 145–155. https://doi.org/10.1113/expphysiol.2010.053975

Faude, O., Koch, T., & Meyer, T. (2012). Straight sprinting is the most frequent action in goal situations in professional football. *Journal of Sports Sciences, 30*(7), 625–631.

Goulart, K. N. de O., Duffield, R., Junior, G. O. C., Passos Ramos, G., Pimenta, E. M., & Couto, B. P. (2020). Recovery timeline following resistance training in professional female soccer players. *Science and Medicine in Football, 4*(3), 233–239.

Haugen, T. A., Tønnessen, E., & Seiler, S. (2013). Anaerobic performance testing of professional soccer players 1995–2010. *International Journal of Sports Physiology and Performance, 8*(2), 148–156.

Hegyi, A., Lahti, J., Giacomo, J.-P., Gerus, P., Cronin, N. J., & Morin, J.-B. (2019). Impact of hip flexion angle on unilateral and bilateral nordic hamstring exercise torque and high-density electromyography activity. *Journal of Orthopaedic & Sports Physical Therapy, 49*(8), 584–592.

Jakobsen, M. D., Sundstrup, E., Randers, M. B., Kjær, M., Andersen, L. L., Krustrup, P., & Aagaard, P. (2012). The effect of strength training, recreational soccer and running exercise on stretch–shortening cycle muscle performance during countermovement jumping. *Human Movement Science*, *31*(4), 970–986.

Jankowski, T. (2016). *Coaching soccer like Guardiola and Mourinho: the concept of tactical periodization*. Europe: Meyer & Meyer Sport.

Killen, N. M., Gabbett, T. J., & Jenkins, D. G. (2010). Training loads and incidence of injury during the preseason in professional rugby league players. *The Journal of Strength & Conditioning Research*, *24*(8), 2079–2084.

King, E., Franklyn-Miller, A., Richter, C., O'Reilly, E., Doolan, M., Moran, K., ... Falvey, É. (2018). Clinical and biomechanical outcomes of rehabilitation targeting intersegmental control in athletic groin pain: prospective cohort of 205 patients. *British Journal of Sports Medicine*, *52*(16), 1054–1062.

Krustrup, P., Ørtenblad, N., Nielsen, J., Nybo, L., Gunnarsson, T. P., Iaia, F. M., ... Bangsbo, J. (2011). Maximal voluntary contraction force, SR function and glycogen resynthesis during the first 72 h after a high-level competitive soccer game. *European Journal of Applied Physiology*, *111*(12), 2987–2995.

Lavender, A. P., & Nosaka, K. (2008). A light load eccentric exercise confers protection against a subsequent bout of more demanding eccentric exercise. *Journal of Science and Medicine in Sport*, *11*(3), 291–298.

Lima, L. C. R., & Denadai, B. S. (2015). Attenuation of eccentric exercise-induced muscle damage conferred by maximal isometric contractions: a mini review. *Frontiers in Physiology*, *6*, 300.

Loturco, I., Pereira, L. A., Kobal, R., Maldonado, T., Piazzi, A. F., Bottino, A., ... Nakamura, F. Y. (2016). Improving sprint performance in soccer: effectiveness of jump squat and Olympic push press exercises. *PloS One*, *11*(4), e0153958.

Mendiguchia, J., Castano-Zambudio, A., Jimenez-Reyes, P., Morin, J., Edouard, P., Conceicao, F., ... Colyer, S. (2021). Can we modify maximal speed running posture? Implications for performance and hamstring injuries management. *International Journal of Sports Physiology and Performance, 17*(3), 374–383.

Mendiguchia, J., Conceição, F., Edouard, P., Fonseca, M., Pereira, R., Lopes, H., ... Jiménez-Reyes, P. (2020). Sprint versus isolated eccentric training: comparative effects on hamstring architecture and performance in soccer players. *PLoS One*, *15*(2), e0228283.

Mendiguchia, J., Edouard, P., Samozino, P., Brughelli, M., Cross, M., Ross, A., ... Morin, J. B. (2016). Field monitoring of sprinting power–force–velocity profile before, during and after hamstring injury: two case reports. *Journal of Sports Sciences*, *34*(6), 535–541.

Mendiguchia, J., Gonzalez De la Flor, A., Mendez-Villanueva, A., Morin, J.-B., Edouard, P., & Garrues, M. A. (2021). Training-induced changes in anterior pelvic tilt: potential implications for hamstring strain injuries management. *Journal of Sports Sciences*, *39*(7), 760–767.

Morin, J.-B., Petrakos, G., Jiménez-Reyes, P., Brown, S. R., Samozino, P., & Cross, M. R. (2017). Very-heavy sled training for improving horizontal-force output in soccer players. *International Journal of Sports Physiology and Performance*, *12*(6), 840–844.

Murtagh, C. F., Brownlee, T. E., O'Boyle, A., Morgans, R., Drust, B., & Erskine, R. M. (2018). Importance of speed and power in elite youth soccer depends on maturation status. *Journal of Strength and Conditioning Research*, *32*(2), 297–303. https://doi.org/org/10.1519/JSC.0000000000002367

Murtagh, C. F., Naughton, R. J., McRobert, A. P., O'Boyle, A., Morgans, R., Drust, B., & Erskine, R. M. (2019). A coding system to quantify powerful actions in soccer match play: a pilot study. *Research Quarterly for Exercise and Sport*, *96*(2), 234-243. https://doi.org/10.1080/02701367.2019.1576838

Murtagh, C. F., Nulty, C., Vanrenterghem, J., O'Boyle, A., Morgans, R., Drust, B., & Erskine, R. M. (2018). The neuromuscular determinants of unilateral jump performance in soccer players are direction-specific. *International Journal of Sports Physiology and Performance*, *13*(5), 604–611. https://doi.org/10.1123/ijspp.2017-0589

Murtagh, C. F., Vanrenterghem, J., O'Boyle, A., Morgans, R., Drust, B., & Erskine, R. M. (2017). Unilateral jumps in different directions: a novel assessment of soccer-associated power? *Journal of Science and Medicine in Sport, 20*(11), 1018–1023. https://doi.org/10.1016/j.jsams.2017.03.016

Nedelec, M., McCall, A., Carling, C., Legall, F., Berthoin, S., & Dupont, G. (2014). The influence of soccer playing actions on the recovery kinetics after a soccer match. *The Journal of Strength & Conditioning Research, 28*(6), 1517–1523.

Newton, M. J., Morgan, G. T., Sacco, P., Chapman, D. W., & Nosaka, K. (2008). Comparison of responses to strenuous eccentric exercise of the elbow flexors between resistance-trained and untrained men. *The Journal of Strength & Conditioning Research, 22*(2), 597–607.

Nosaka, K., Sakamoto, K., Newton, M., & Sacco, P. (2001). The repeated bout effect of reduced-load eccentric exercise on elbow flexor muscle damage. *European Journal of Applied Physiology, 85*(1), 34–40.

Petersen, J., Thorborg, K., Nielsen, M. B., Budtz-Jørgensen, E., & Hölmich, P. (2011). Preventive effect of eccentric training on acute hamstring injuries in men's soccer: a cluster-randomized controlled trial. *The American Journal of Sports Medicine, 39*(11), 2296–2303.

Peterson, M. D., Rhea, M. R., & Alvar, B. A. (2004). Maximizing strength development in athletes: a meta-analysis to determine the dose-response relationship. *The Journal of Strength & Conditioning Research, 18*(2), 377–382.

Presland, J. D., Timmins, R. G., Bourne, M. N., Williams, M. D., & Opar, D. A. (2018). The effect of Nordic hamstring exercise training volume on biceps femoris long head architectural adaptation. *Scandinavian Journal of Medicine & Science in Sports, 28*(7), 1775–1783.

Roig, M., O'Brien, K., Kirk, G., Murray, R., McKinnon, P., Shadgan, B., & Reid, W. D. (2009). The effects of eccentric versus concentric resistance training on muscle strength and mass in healthy adults: a systematic review with meta-analysis. *British Journal of Sports Medicine, 43*(8), 556–568.

Schuermans, J., Van Tiggelen, D., Palmans, T., Danneels, L., & Witvrouw, E. (2017). Deviating running kinematics and hamstring injury susceptibility in male soccer players: Cause or consequence? *Gait & Posture, 57*, 270–277.

Timmins, R. G., Bourne, M. N., Shield, A. J., Williams, M. D., Lorenzen, C., & Opar, D. A. (2016). Short biceps femoris fascicles and eccentric knee flexor weakness increase the risk of hamstring injury in elite football (soccer): a prospective cohort study. *British Journal of Sports Medicine, 50*(24), 1524–1535.

Trecroci, A., Porcelli, S., Perri, E., Pedrali, M., Rasica, L., Alberti, G., ... Iaia, F. M. (2020). Effects of different training interventions on the recovery of physical and neuromuscular performance after a soccer match. *The Journal of Strength & Conditioning Research, 34*(8), 2189–2196.

Vanrenterghem, J., Nedergaard, N. J., Robinson, M. A., & Drust, B. (2017). Training load monitoring in team sports: a novel framework separating physiological and biomechanical load-adaptation pathways. *Sports Medicine, 47*(11), 2135–2142.

# 3 Aerobic and anaerobic training

*Liam Anderson and Barry Drust*

## Introduction

Soccer encompasses physiological, technical, tactical, and psychological/sociological contributions to performance. It is an intermittent sport consisting of short bouts of intense activity that are superimposed amongst longer periods of low-moderate-intensity activity (Reilly, 1997). This intermittent profile makes match demands highly contextual and complex, requiring players to perform varied actions such as walking, jogging, or sprinting during match play. Different actions are performed at varying intensities, altering the contributions from different energy systems. Understanding the match demands from a locomotion and physiological perspective provides the basis for a range of interventions, such as those targeted at physical development, talent identification, and nutrition. In this chapter, we discuss the demands of soccer match play, how these demands stress the two main energy systems; the aerobic and anaerobic energy systems and give some practical information relating to different training methods for energy system development within soccer.

## Demands of the game

The locomotive demands of soccer are well known, with players typically covering distances of 10–13 km (Dellal et al., 2011; Di Salvo et al., 2008). Relative to players overall distance, the vast majority (~80–90%) of this is performed at low-to-moderate intensities (speeds <19.8 km h$^{-1}$) (Bradley et al., 2009). These speeds correspond to various types of movement, such as standing, walking, jogging, and running. For example, in elite-level soccer players in Denmark, Mohr et al. (2003) observed that 19.5% of time was spent standing, 41.8% walking, 16.7% jogging, and 16.8% running. These actions can often consist of forward, backwards, and lateral movements both in possession (from an individual and team perspective) and out of possession. These data provide the basis of understanding that the aerobic energy system is stressed significantly during match play and can therefore play an important role in training strategies.

The remaining 10–20% of distance covered in soccer match play is accounted for with distances covered at high-intensity (speeds >19.8 km h$^{-1}$) and sprinting (speeds >25.2 km h$^{-1}$) (Bradley et al., 2009; Di Salvo et al., 2010). These distances are extremely variable from match-to-match in the English Premier League (EPL) with high coefficients of variation (~16–30%; Gregson et al., 2010), indicating that energy system contribution

DOI: 10.4324/9781003148418-4

can be highly variable from let's be consistent. Also, it appears that the distances covered within these high-intensity speed zones have increased over time across numerous leagues. Barnes et al. (2014) studied consecutive seasons from 2006–2007 to 2012–2013 in the EPL and found that distances covered at high-intensity speeds and high-intensity actions were ~30% and ~50% higher, respectively, in the later years. Similar data from the Spanish La-Liga between 2012 and 2019 has identified comparable trends (Lago-Penas et al., 2022). In addition to the distances covered, 90% of individual sprints are shorter than 5 s in duration, with the average number of sprints being ~11 per match (Andrzejewski et al., 2013) during match play. This finding has particular importance to soccer as high-intensity actions such as sprinting have been observed as the most common actions in goals scored (Faude et al., 2012; Martinez-Hernandez et al., 2022). Collectively, these Data provide an understanding of the anaerobic demands and the importance of these actions within the ever-evolving demands of soccer match play, outlining the requirement to train the anaerobic energy system.

In addition to the locomotive demands, there are instances when players are required to transition from low intensity to high-intensity activities and vice versa. For example, during an acceleration or deceleration, change of direction or change of velocity. Within match play, soccer players perform ~305 changes of direction with an average of 19.2 s between actions. The changes of direction are mostly <90° (77%), and peak demands over 15- and 5-min periods were 62 and 25 actions, respectively (Morgan et al., 2021). In addition, players perform ~1200 accelerations and decelerations during match play (Russell et al., 2016), with a change in activity every 4–6 s (Bangsbo, 1994; Mohr et al., 2003). These actions likely contribute to a significant proportion of the energy demands, although specific contributions from which energy system are less clear. This finding complicates the energy demands of soccer, and although no energy system dominates, there is a significant utilisation of varying amounts of energy sources from both the aerobic and anaerobic energy systems.

Given that soccer players play in different positions and strategic factors play a huge part in match performance, it is noteworthy that match demands are not always the same and can differ from let's be consistent. For example, players who play in central midfield cover the highest distances during a match and central defenders covering the least. This difference is likely due to a product of higher levels of fitness associated with such players and the role which they play in the team (i.e., central midfielders linking between defence and attack), a role which evidently requires more sustained running (Bangsbo, 1994; Bloomfield et al., 2007; Reilly & Thomas, 1976). Wide midfielders and full-backs have been reported to cover greater distances in high-intensity running and sprinting (Bradley et al., 2009). The greater high-intensity running distance covered is due to their tactical role in the team and their runs being the longest in distance (Bradley et al., 2009). In addition, soccer players have many different situational variables placed upon them, including match status (i.e., winning, drawing, or losing), match location (i.e., home or away), tactical strategy (i.e., playing formation and counterattacking), and standard of opposition can significantly influence the match demands (Lago-Penas, 2012). Moreover, soccer is played worldwide and in many different environmental climates, which can significantly influence match output and the physiological demands associated with match play (Mohr et al., 2012). These factors further complicate the energy demands of soccer players and highlights the importance of analysing match demands to design and implement training programmes.

## Physical capabilities of players

The aerobic energy system is significantly taxed within soccer match play (Stolen et al., 2005). Understanding the specific physical capacities of elite soccer players, compared to others at lower competitive standards, can provide insightful information to which energy systems are regularly stressed and adapted to meet their demands. This is evident in elite-level soccer players who typically possess high-aerobic test scores compared with non-elite players (see Table 3.1). Although soccer players' scores are high during such tests, the values are much lower than endurance athletes (i.e., ~70 ml kg$^{-1}$ $\dot{V}O_2$max), who rely on the aerobic energy system to a greater extent (Davies & Thompson, 1979). Soccer is multifactorial in nature, with other different physiological systems required to be trained to high levels and, therefore, limiting sole development of the aerobic energy system.

Physical assessments of the aerobic energy system show significant positive correlations with running performance in matches (Bradley et al., 2011). Additionally, aerobic training that subsequently improved $\dot{V}O_2$max and lactate threshold increased the total distance covered, and the number of sprints, which led to greater involvements with the ball during a match (Helgerud et al., 2001). The increased capacity for exercise and an improved recovery speed from high-intensity exercise during competition, leads to more repeated high-intensity efforts (Tomlin & Wenger, 2001). The higher frequency is likely due to increased aerobic contribution during match play itself, post-exercise $O_2$, lactate removal, and PCR restoration. Collectively, this evidence outlines the importance of the aerobic energy system for match play performance.

The anaerobic energy system has significant demands placed on it, with many intense actions being performed within match play. From a testing perspective, professional soccer players have high levels of anaerobic fitness (see Table 3.1). These physical attributes are typically greater in players who play at higher competitive standards, providing further clarification that the anaerobic energy system is frequently stressed and is adapted to meet the increasing match demands (Barnes et al., 2014; Lago-Penas et al., 2022). In addition, performing anaerobic training has shown increases in soccer-specific physical assessments such as Yo–Yo intermittent recovery tests, repeated sprint tests, and sprint tests (Ingebrigtsen et al., 2013; Mohr & Krustrup, 2016; Thomassen et al., 2010). These performance tests have been found to be good predictors for high-intensity performance within match play (Mohr et al., 2016).

*Table 3.1* Physical testing results of non-elite and elite soccer players

| Physical test | Non-elite | Elite |
| --- | --- | --- |
| $\dot{V}O_{2max}$ (ml·min$^{-1}$·kg$^{-1}$) | 50–60 | 60–70 |
| Velocity @ 4 mmol$^{-1}$ (km hr$^{-1}$) | 9.0–13.3 | 13.2–16.6 |
| Yo–Yo IR level 1 average (m) | 1810 | 2420 |
| Yo–Yo IR level 2 average (m) | 840 | 1260 |
| Mean repeated sprint time (s) | 4.5–4.9 | 4.3–4.5 |
| 5 m sprint time (s) | 1.01–1.1 | 0.80–0.90 |
| 30 m sprint time (s) | 4.11–4.31 | 3.92–4.21 |

IR = intermittent recovery, $\dot{V}O_2$max = maximal oxygen uptake

## Measurements during match play

In intermittent contact sports such as soccer, it is extremely difficult to determine the aerobic contribution due to a lack of methods to directly measure $\dot{V}O_2$ during match play. Therefore, indirect methods are required to estimate the energy systems contribution. Heart rate (HR) has emerged as a potential method to assess aerobic contribution within match play due to the HR-$\dot{V}O_2$ relationship (Bot & Hollander, 2000). Analysis into HR Anaerobic energy system and oxygen uptake utilising the K4 apparatus during soccer drills have observed similar HR for a given $\dot{V}O_2$ as found during treadmill running, validating this relationship (Esposito et al., 2004). Analysis into average and peak heart rates within match play were reported at around 85 and 98% of maximal, respectively (Krustrup et al., 2005; Suarez-Arrones et al., 2015; Torreno et al., 2016). Based on the individual relationships between heart rate and $\dot{V}O_2$ obtained in standardised tests in the laboratory, these values correspond to approximately 70% of $\dot{V}O_2$max (Bangsbo et al., 2006), highlighting via an indirect method the extent to of which the aerobic energy system is stressed during match play.

High-intensity actions in soccer require ATP resynthesis through the breakdown of creatine phosphate (CP) and the degradation of muscle glycogen via glycolysis to lactic acid (McCartney et al., 1986; Spriet et al., 1989; Withers et al., 1991). To assess anaerobic energy system contribution, muscle and blood metabolites can be analysed during different periods of match play (i.e., half-time or after an intense period).

One of the most direct methods for assessing anaerobic contribution is taking muscle biopsies from soccer players. Analysis of muscle samples indicated that CP was 30% below resting values after intense periods in the match (Bangsbo, Mohr, & Krustrup, 2006). In addition, blood lactate values of up to 10 mmol$^{-1}$ have been observed with individual values above 12 mmol$^{-1}$ (Bangsbo, 1994; Krustrup et al., 2006). These data clearly indicate that lactate production is high during match play but doesn't yet give a direct measurement of muscle lactate. In a friendly match between non-professional soccer players, muscle lactate values reached around 15 mmol kg dry weight$^{-1}$ compared with resting values after both halves, with the highest value being 35 mmol·kg dry weight$^{-1}$ (Krustrup et al., 2006). During high-intensity anaerobic activity, lactate is metabolised within active muscles (Brooks, 1987). Lactate that is released from active muscles to the blood is taken up by different tissues such as the heart, liver, kidney, and inactive muscles (Brooks, 1987). Therefore, when blood lactate is assessed, it represents the balance of production, release, and removal of lactate, being an appropriate indirect indicator of anaerobic energy production.

Muscle lactate values do not correlate with blood lactate in short-term intermittent exercise (Krustrup et al., 2003). Compared to continuous exercise, where blood lactate levels were lower but reflected the values observed within muscle, this is distinctly different (Bangsbo et al., 1993). Reasons for these differences are likely due to the turnover rates between both muscle and blood lactate, with the rate of clearance being higher in muscle than in blood. Given that muscle lactate can be low, and blood can be high, these values aren't linked to a single action in a game and rather represent an accumulated/balanced response to several high-intensity actions performed across the entirety of match-play. These data further support the complex nature of soccer match play and should be considered when interpreting physiological responses and during the design of training programmes of players.

## Practical considerations for training

Information around the aerobic and anaerobic demands of soccer has formed the basis of specific training methods. The importance of optimally preparing players to undertake individual and contextual match demands is greater than ever due to the ever-evolving match demands (Barnes et al., 2014; Lago-Penas et al., 2022). Players are now required to be able to meet these demands repeatedly, with often short recovery periods (<72 h) over an entire season. The multifactorial nature of soccer makes this complex and problematic, with training methods often required to develop multiple physiological systems and needs at once in addition to the technical, tactical, and physiological aspects of the sport (see Figure 3.1). Therefore, careful planning and delivery of training programmes to maximise both individual energy system and holistic soccer performance are required.

Soccer requires both the individual and simultaneous development of physiological, technical, tactical, and psychological characteristics (see Figure 3.1). A mixture of running drills (both with and without the ball) and soccer-specific drills (i.e., small-sided games (SSGs) and technical drills) can be used as a training stimulus for both energy systems. These methods require the manipulation of basic principles of training: frequency; intensity; time; type; specificity; progressive overload; and reversibility to

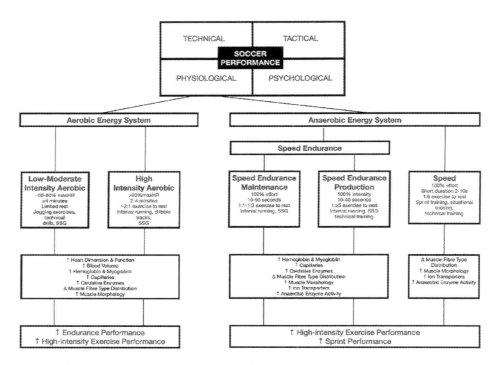

*Figure 3.1* An overview of energy system training guidelines, physiological adaptations, and performance changes for soccer players. SGG = small sided games

elicit specific physiological adaptations on energy systems. Training drills can therefore be manipulated to achieve the required physical outcome, although they must be planned into the overall physical loading.

## Aerobic training

Aerobic training consists of both low- and high-intensity training. It can be performed through traditional running exercises that can involve the ball and through soccer-specific training methods utilising SSGs and technical drills. Aerobic training elicits adaptations within cardiovascular parameters such as heart size (Ekblom, 1969), blood flow capacity (Laughlin & Roseguini, 2008), and artery distensibility (Rakobowchuk et al., 2009). These adaptations improve the capacity of the cardiovascular system to transport oxygen to working muscles, improving $\dot{V}O_2$ kinetics (Bailey et al., 2009), $\dot{V}O_2$max (Helgerud et al., 2001; Impellizzeri et al., 2006), and ventilation and lactate thresholds (Driller et al., 2009). Further metabolic adaptations include an upregulation of mitochondrial oxidative enzymes and increased muscular glycogen sparing through greater metabolism of fat (Iaia et al., 2009; Ross & Leveritt, 2001). These adaptations lead to players being able to sustain high-intensity exercise for longer and recover quicker after intense periods of the game (Tomlin & Wenger, 2001). Players are required to exercise at different intensities and durations to both stimulate and develop the aerobic energy system (see Figure 3.1).

## Low-moderate intensity aerobic training

Low-moderate intensity aerobic training can form an important component of programmes to help form part of the recovery process and maintain aerobic fitness (Mohr & Iaia, 2014). For this type of training, intensity should average ~60–80% of the maximum heart but can range between 50–90% due to intermittent and varied exercises being performed. A relatively high HR can be achieved with this type of training without the requirement to perform at high speeds or intense actions. Low-moderate intensity changes in speed and direction can be used, as well as the inclusion of technical aspects such as dribbling, passing, and ball control (Reilly & Ball, 1984). These movements likely limit muscle damage compared to high-intensity exercise and actions due to the damaging nature of eccentric muscle contractions (Clarkson et al., 1986). Therefore, low-moderate intensity aerobic training can be optimum during periods when players are required to maintain aerobic adaptation or when it is difficult to withstand high-intensity demands (i.e., as a recovery session, in the off-season, as a supplementary part of in-season loading or returning from an injury). Some examples of low-moderate intensity aerobic training are that of some SSGs and technical training (see Figure 3.2a).

## High-intensity aerobic training

High-intensity aerobic training can improve the aerobic contribution to high-intensity activities and improve the ability to recover from such actions within game (Bangsbo, 1994). It requires players to perform at exercise intensities of ~90% maximum HR (range = 80–100%), utilising an exercise-to-rest ratio of ~2:1 and for durations of 2–4 min (Bangsbo, Mohr, Poulsen, et al., 2006; Mohr & Iaia, 2014). When tracking and

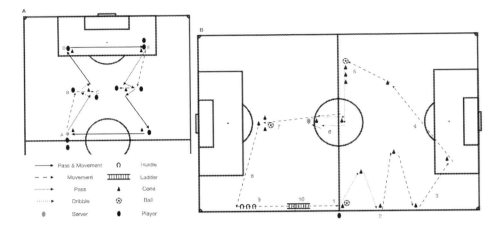

*Figure 3.2* Some typical training drills for the aerobic energy system. (a) low-intensity aerobic training in the form of a technical passing exercise and (b) a high-intensity aerobic training. (1) initiate the movement by dribbling around the cone to 2; (2) perform a high-intensity effort up to the cone and to the following one; (3) perform lateral shuffles/backwards jogging; (4) perform a high-intensity run at ~80% maximum speed and decelerate into 5; (5) dribble around the cones up to the centre circle before making a turn; (6) play a pass with a server/ bounce board and return to leave the ball on the centre circle; (7) perform a jog to the next ball and dribble around all three cones; (8) perform a 2–3 s sprint; (9) perform jumps over hurdles; and (10) complete fast feet through the ladders.

monitoring players physical load, this HR zone is typically called the 'red zone', as the cardiovascular system is significantly stressed during exercise. For optimal aerobic development, it is important to operate within this red zone from a training and match play perspective.

The addition of high-intensity aerobic training is commonplace within most professional soccer settings, but research on implementing it within the 'normal' training programme is limited. In high-level players in Scandinavian who performed an 8-week period of aerobic high-intensity training, in addition to their usual training load, improved $\dot{V}O_2$max, lactate threshold and running economy were reported (Helgerud et al., 2001). These aerobic adaptations led to a 20% increase in distance covered, 100% increase in number of sprints and 24% increase in number of involvements with the ball. However, in this study, training was performed on a treadmill, which is not typical for soccer players as they're required to undergo specific technical and tactical training as a team. Practitioners and researchers have overcome this shortcoming through the creation of soccer-specific dribble tracks and manipulation of SSG to elicit similar HR responses and likely aerobic adaptations (Hill-Haas et al., 2011; Hoff et al., 2002). Given the positive aerobic adaptations when operating at these high intensities, it seems important for soccer players to spend a significant amount of time within this red zone. Further evidence to support this concept is evident in Italian players, where the improved speeds attained at 2 and 4 mmol$^{-1}$ blood lactate concentrations was correlated to time spent >90% maximum HR across a preparatory period (Castagna et al., 2011). These data clearly indicate the requirement for high-intensity aerobic training, and it is important to consider when designing training programmes during different stages of the season (i.e., preparatory phase) and within the weekly in-season micro-cycle (i.e., middle of the week). It must be noted that there doesn't seem to be any difference in adaptions whether this type of training is performed as part of SSG or via traditional high-intensity interval training and should be left down to the individual coach's preference (Impellizzeri et al., 2006). An example of a dribble track that soccer players can use for aerobic development can be found in Figure 3.2b.

## Anaerobic training

Anaerobic training can be split into speed and speed endurance training (Bangsbo, 1994; see Figure 3.1). It can be performed in running drills (both with and without a ball) and in the form of SSG or technical drills. Key adaptations to anaerobic training include an increase in activity of anaerobic enzymes (Ross & Leveritt, 2001), improved $K^+$ handling (Bangsbo et al., 2009), lactate-$H^+$ transport capacity (Gunnarsson et al., 2013), $H^+$ regulation (Skovgaard et al., 2014) and muscle capillarisation (Jensen et al., 2004). Many of these adaptations improve the rate of anaerobic energy turnover during exercise and reduce the inhibitory effects of $H^+$ within the muscle cell. These factors may improve the ability to produce power rapidly, for longer periods and improve recovery after a high-intensity exercise bout allowing soccer players a greater ability to perform high-intensity actions for longer durations and repeat them, with less fatigue, over the duration of the match.

## Anaerobic speed training

Speed training specifically aims to improve the ability to produce a rapid force that improves acceleration and maintains a high force to obtain high peak velocities (Spinks et al., 2007; Tonnessen et al., 2011). It requires players to perform at their maximum for short periods of time (2–10 s) and sufficient rest. It is important to allow sufficient rest in between repetitions so that players can fully recover, and maximal force can be produced in the following repetition (Reilly & Bangsbo, 1998). Therefore, recovery between repetitions should be high (i.e., 1:6 exercise-to-rest ratio), repetitions should be low (<10) and should be performed early in the training session when players fatigue levels are low, but players are prepared with an adequate warm-up.

Given that sprinting is the most frequent mechanism associated with hamstring injuries (Ekstrand et al., 2011), careful consideration should be taken in making players familiar with this type of training through gradual increases in the intensity and volume, as well as appropriate management of training when administering. It is important for speed training to be integrated into the soccer-specific training to help maximise transfer into match play (i.e., counterattacking, crossing, and finishing). This also helps training efficiency by reducing overall training time and limiting unnecessary, low-quality exposures.

The addition of sprint training should occur in addition to (or carefully placed into the training design) other training load to which players are exposed. An examination into a short sprint training programme that was performed in addition to team sport athletes planned training load proved an effective method for improving short sprint durations (sprinting distance ≤30 m) (Spinks et al., 2007). Spinks and colleagues found improvements in short sprint durations when team sport athletes undertook sprint

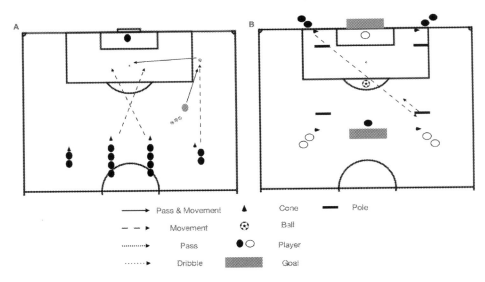

*Figure 3.3* Some typical training drills for the anaerobic energy system. Players perform both drills at maximum intensity. (a) Speed training, where three players perform maximal sprints by timing their run into the box. Wide player initiates the drill and performs an overlap of the server to receive the ball while two central players make a curved run into the penalty area (one to the front post and one to the back), the wide player delivers a ball into the area for one of the two central players to score. Alternate left and right wide players for each repetition. (b) Speed endurance training where players perform a diagonal run around the pole and into a 2v2. All four players perform a diagonal run prior to commencing the 2v2, with the winning team into the playing area receiving the ball first. Goalkeepers on both teams and points after each repetition being recorded to increase competition and intensity.

training consisting of 5, 10, 15, and 20 m sprints, 2× per week for 8 weeks. In addition, longer sprints (~40 m) seem to improve maximal sprinting velocity when performed as an addition to the training programme (Tonnessen et al., 2011). Given that soccer players typically sprint for <5 s in match play, these training modalities should account for a large proportion of sprints performed in match play (Andrzejewski et al., 2013). However, to prepare players for some worst-case scenarios (i.e., counterattacking from a corner kick, recovery runs), frequent speed training of 2–10 s in duration seems pertinent in eliciting an adaptive response. An example of a sprint training drill specific to soccer can be found in Figure 3.3.

## Anaerobic speed endurance training

Match demands are becoming more high-intensity, meaning players must perform at such intensities for longer and repeatedly to meet match demands (Barnes et al., 2014; Lago-Penas et al., 2022). Speed endurance training is a form of anaerobic training performed at maximal intensities with the aim to increase physical performance during the most intense periods of match play (Iaia et al., 2009; Mohr & Iaia, 2014). Training with a short exercise-to-rest ratio (1:1-1:3) with durations of 10-90 seconds is termed speed endurance maintenance (SEM), whereas reducing the exercise duration (10-40

s) and increasing the exercise-to-rest ratio (1:≥5) is termed speed endurance production (SEP) (Bangsbo, 2015; Mohr & Iaia, 2014; see Figure 3.1). Both training methods are designed to improve high-intensity performance. Specifically, SEM improves the ability to perform repeated high-intensity efforts, while SEP improves the ability to perform maximally for a relatively short period of time (Bangsbo, 2015)

Speed endurance training can be performed in SSG (Mohr & Krustrup, 2016), running without or minimal contact with the ball (Gunnarsson et al., 2012; Iaia et al., 2015) and in position-specific individual running drills (Ade et al., 2021). These studies examined the differences in physiological responses to SEM and SEP training. Due to the reduced rest periods, SEM training typically has a higher cardiovascular response, whereas SEP has a higher external output and blood lactate response due to being able to operate at higher intensities (Ade et al., 2014; Castagna et al., 2017; Iaia & Bangsbo, 2010). These data indicate that the anaerobic energy system has a greater involvement in SEP, and there is some crossover of the aerobic energy system in SEM (see Figure 3.1). In disagreement with these findings, Mohr and Krustrup (2016) performed 4 weeks of either individual running drills with balls to reflect game situations or 2v2 SSG for SEP and SEM, respectively. The SEP training protocol elicited greater peak and average running speeds as expected, however, this was accompanied by greater peak heart rate responses compared to the SEM protocol. These findings highlight the importance of the mode of exercise chosen in reflecting the training characteristics and the monitoring of training responses and adaptations.

Several researchers have identified high-intensity performance improvements with both SEM and SEP training (Iaia & Bangsbo, 2010; Iaia et al., 2015; Mohr & Krustrup, 2016; Vitale et al., 2018). Iaia et al. (2015) performed 3 weeks of either SEP or SEM training 3× per week as part of a reduced volume training programme at the conclusion of the competitive season. SEP improved repeated sprint and high-intensity exercise performance, whereas SEM increased the ability to maximise fatigue tolerance and maintain speed development during both repeated maximal and continuous short-duration maximal exercises. However, Mohr and Krustrup (2016) found that SEP training resulted in superior performance improvements in both high-intensity intermittent running capacity and during a repeated sprint test. Given that other research have found an enhanced ability to sustain exercise at high intensities in SEM training, these findings are conflicting (Iaia & Bangsbo, 2010; Iaia et al., 2015; Vitale et al., 2018). These conflicting findings further highlight the importance of eliciting the correct physiological response by altering the mode of training (i.e., running vs. SSG), whilst continuing monitoring physiological responses and adaptations to training. While there are many positives and negatives associated with each training method, for specific control of physiological responses during training, individual position-specific running drills that involve the ball may be a potential 'middle ground' training method (Ade et al., 2021). An example of a speed endurance drill can be found in Figure 3.3b.

## Training methods

Soccer is multifactorial, and there are often many different methods to improve both the aerobic and anaerobic energy systems. SSG (also known as small-sided and conditioned games) are manipulated to account for different aspects of a game to help achieve a specific tactical/technical objective while changing physiological, physical, and psychological demands (Bujalance-Moreno et al., 2019; Clemente et al., 2021; Davids et al., 2013). These training methods have been found to improve both aerobic (Impellizzeri et al., 2006) and anaerobic (Chaouachi et al., 2014) fitness. In addition, this type of training provides a stimulus for muscle groups that are actively engaged during match play (Bangsbo, 1994). They can be performed extensively across the entire season with specific focus on the preparatory period and manipulation of variables across the in-season training week to elicit a form of training periodisation (Anderson, Orme, Di Michele, Close, Morgans, et al., 2016; Martin-Garcia et al., 2018). These SSG offer exponential benefits for the development of holistic soccer performance (i.e., training technical, tactical, physiological, and psychological development) and have become a key tool to use for soccer training and conditioning programmes (Hill-Haas et al., 2011).

SSG, in brief can produce a wide range of physiological responses depending on their format. For example, reducing player numbers, increasing pitch sizes (higher individual playing area per player), a limited number of ball touches, man-to-man marking, or the use of small-goals or ball possession drills tend to increase the heart rate responses and blood lactate concentrations of players from different age groups (Bujalance-Moreno et al., 2019; Hill-Haas et al., 2011; Sarmento et al., 2018). To increase distances covered in high-intensity speed zones (and increasing the high-intensity aerobic training), SSGs can be played on large pitches (Clemente et al., 2021). Increasing player number and the pitch size can result in specific movement patterns that incorporate stretch-shortening-cycle (SSC) activities as well develop both the anaerobic and aerobic energy system and position-specific capabilities based around the team's tactical strategy (Morgans et al., 2014). Although SSGs seem an effective training strategy, the variability, and complex nature of soccer may not allow all players to reach desired intensities required for adaptation. Consequently, running-based drills (inclusive of drills with and without the ball) can be performed to ensure that players are obtaining the desired intensities.

Despite the clear advantages of SSGs to offer a potential 'all in one' solution to training, there are potential instances when running-based conditioning can be used to focus on specific adaptation or when desired intensities aren't able to be matched, such as the preparatory period (Faude et al., 2013), returning from an injury (Taberner et al., 2019) or when players are deemed not to have received enough match minutes (Anderson, Orme, Di Michele, Close, Milsom, et al., 2016; Hills et al., 2020). Typically, running-based conditioning is in the form of high-intensity interval training targeting aerobic (Buchheit & Laursen, 2013a) and anaerobic (Buchheit & Laursen, 2013b) systems. Clear advantages of this type of conditioning are that intensity can be based off current fitness levels (i.e., a percentage of $\dot{V}O_2$max, lactate threshold, or maximum speed) and coaches have a direct control over the volume and intensity of exercise. Aerobic and anaerobic training can be performed utilising singular or a hybrid of SSG and running-based conditioning within the training programme. It is down to coach preference and applicability of specific methods into other aspects of the training programme that may decide which method is chosen and when. Utilising monitoring techniques can allow coaches to understand the training stimulus, the physiological response, and adaptations better to gain awareness of when specific methods may be required.

## Monitoring soccer training

While understanding the demands of soccer and training prescription for the development of both aerobic and anaerobic energy systems, these physical training sessions have their own external (the nature of the exercise) and internal (anatomical, physiological, biochemical, and functional adaptations) load (Impellizzeri et al., 2004, 2005;

Viru & Viru, 2000). The external load is that which is prescribed by the coaches (i.e., the conditioning drill, technical drill, or SSG). The internal load is the consequence of the external load provided to players and its associated level of physiological stress that imposes on any given individual player (Viru & Viru, 2000). Internal training load is particularly important to assess (via multiple methods) as this is particularly important in stimulating adaptations and specific to different energy system development (Booth & Thomason, 1991; Viru & Viru, 2000). Monitoring can be used in an acute (i.e., drill by drill and session by session) and chronic (i.e., assessing longitudinal loading and adaptations) sense to provide feedback to coaches to help plan and implement improved training practices.

## Future directions and conclusions

The demands of soccer are continuing to increase with greater reliance on the anaerobic energy system during match play. These developments are likely due to numerous factors that are associated with improved training methods, greater adaptations, and improved talent identification. It is not clear yet where the training demands are in relation to the match demands and why these demands have increased. Future work into the training demands is anticipated to specifically examine how the manipulation of the training stimulus (i.e., increased volume) can elicit optimal adaptation and when different stimuli should be performed with regards to the overall training plan. This dose-response type research will aid the development of eliciting an effective training process by utilising adaptative measurements and assessing them against a desired outcome. In addition, molecular investigations to understanding specific signalling responses to different types of soccer training (i.e., high-intensity aerobic vs. SEP) are yet to be performed. Specific understanding of the signalling responses (and the energy cost) could allow for training and nutritional programmes to be tailored.

Soccer is a highly complex sport that requires multiple energy systems to be trained. Understanding the match demands and how they stress the aerobic and anaerobic energy system are important for implementing training strategies that are aimed at energy system development within soccer. Due to the complex nature of the sport, this training is formed of multiple concepts that elicit different physiological adaptations. Implementing training strategies into the overall periodised plan can allow for optimal physical development and improved performance. Caution should be taken when implementing training strategies due to the scheduling of other high-intensity training sessions or a congested fixture schedule where players are required to perform match-play every 2–3 days. Eliciting a significant training stimulus during these periods may lead to non-functional overreaching and injury occurrence. Monitoring strategies can be utilised to ensure players are training specific energy systems in the correct moments (i.e., high-intensity work when players are recovered from match play and still have significant time before the next competitive match), in the optimal form (i.e., SSG vs. running) and amount.

## References

Ade, J. D., Drust, B., Morgan, O. J., & Bradley, P. S. (2021). Physiological characteristics and acute fatigue associated with position-specific speed endurance soccer drills: production vs maintenance training. *Sci Med Footb*, 5(1), 6–17. https://doi.org/10.1080/24733938.2020.1789202

Ade, J. D., Harley, J. A., & Bradley, P. S. (2014). Physiological response, time-motion characteristics, and reproducibility of various speed-endurance drills in elite youth soccer players: small-sided games versus generic running. *Int J Sports Physiol Perform, 9*(3), 471–479. https://doi.org/10.1123/ijspp.2013-0390

Anderson, L., Orme, P., Di Michele, R., Close, G. L., Milsom, J., Morgans, R., Drust, B., & Morton, J. P. (2016). Quantification of seasonal-long physical load in soccer players with different starting status from the English premier league: implications for maintaining squad physical fitness. *Int J Sports Physiol Perform, 11*(8), 1038–1046. https://doi.org/10.1123/ijspp.2015-0672

Andrzejewski, M., Chmura, J., Pluta, B., Strzelczyk, R., & Kasprzak, A. (2013). Analysis of sprinting activities of professional soccer players. *J Strength Cond Res, 27*(8), 2134–2140. https://doi.org/10.1519/JSC.0b013e318279423e

Bailey, S. J., Wilkerson, D. P., Dimenna, F. J., & Jones, A. M. (2009). Influence of repeated sprint training on pulmonary O2 uptake and muscle deoxygenation kinetics in humans. *J Appl Physiol (1985), 106*(6), 1875–1887. https://doi.org/10.1152/japplphysiol.00144.2009

Bangsbo, J. (1994). The physiology of soccer–with special reference to intense intermittent exercise. *Acta Physiol Scand Suppl, 619*, 1–155. https://www.ncbi.nlm.nih.gov/pubmed/8059610

Bangsbo, J. (2015). Performance in sports–with specific emphasis on the effect of intensified training. *Scand J Med Sci Sports, 25*(Suppl 4), 88–99. https://doi.org/10.1111/sms.12605

Bangsbo, J., Gunnarsson, T. P., Wendell, J., Nybo, L., & Thomassen, M. (2009). Reduced volume and increased training intensity elevate muscle Na+-K+ pump alpha$^2$-subunit expression as well as short- and long-term work capacity in humans. *J Appl Physiol (1985), 107*(6), 1771–1780. https://doi.org/10.1152/japplphysiol.00358.2009

Bangsbo, J., Johansen, L., Graham, T., & Saltin, B. (1993). Lactate and H+ effluxes from human skeletal muscles during intense, dynamic exercise. *J Physiol, 462*, 115–133. https://doi.org/10.1113/jphysiol.1993.sp019546

Bangsbo, J., Mohr, M., & Krustrup, P. (2006). Physical and metabolic demands of training and match-play in the elite football player. *J Sports Sci, 24*(7), 665–674. https://doi.org/10.1080/02640410500482529

Barnes, C., Archer, D. T., Hogg, B., Bush, M., & Bradley, P. S. (2014). The evolution of physical and technical performance parameters in the English premier league. *Int J Sports Med, 35*(13), 1095–1100. https://doi.org/10.1055/s-0034-1375695

Bloomfield, J., Polman, R., & O'Donoghue, P. (2007). Physical demands of different positions in fa premier league soccer. *J Sports Sci Med, 6*(1), 63–70. https://www.ncbi.nlm.nih.gov/pubmed/24149226

Booth, F. W., & Thomason, D. B. (1991). Molecular and cellular adaptation of muscle in response to exercise: perspectives of various models. *Physiol Rev, 71*(2), 541–585. https://doi.org/10.1152/physrev.1991.71.2.541

Bot, S. D., & Hollander, A. P. (2000). The relationship between heart rate and oxygen uptake during non-steady state exercise. *Ergonomics, 43*(10), 1578–1592. https://doi.org/10.1080/001401300750004005

Bradley, P. S., Mohr, M., Bendiksen, M., Randers, M. B., Flindt, M., Barnes, C., Hood, P., Gomez, A., Andersen, J. L., Di Mascio, M., Bangsbo, J., & Krustrup, P. (2011). Submaximal and maximal Yo-Yo intermittent endurance test level 2: heart rate response, reproducibility and application to elite soccer. *Eur J Appl Physiol, 111*(6), 969–978. https://doi.org/10.1007/s00421-010-1721-2

Bradley, P. S., Sheldon, W., Wooster, B., Olsen, P., Boanas, P., & Krustrup, P. (2009). High-intensity running in English FA premier league soccer matches. *J Sports Sci, 27*(2), 159–168. https://doi.org/10.1080/02640410802512775

Brooks, G. A. (1987). Amino acid and protein metabolism during exercise and recovery. *Med Sci Sports Exe, 19*, 150–156.

Buchheit, M., & Laursen, P. B. (2013a). High-intensity interval training, solutions to the programming puzzle: Part I: cardiopulmonary emphasis. *Sports Med, 43*(5), 313–338. https://doi.org/10.1007/s40279-013-0029-x

Buchheit, M., & Laursen, P. B. (2013b). High-intensity interval training, solutions to the programming puzzle. Part II: anaerobic energy, neuromuscular load and practical applications. *Sports Med, 43*(10), 927–954. https://doi.org/10.1007/s40279-013-0066-5

Bujalance-Moreno, P., Latorre-Roman, P. A., & Garcia-Pinillos, F. (2019). A systematic review on small-sided games in football players: acute and chronic adaptations. *J Sports Sci, 37*(8), 921–949. https://doi.org/10.1080/02640414.2018.1535821

Castagna, C., Francini, L., Povoas, S. C. A., & D'Ottavio, S. (2017). Long-sprint abilities in soccer: ball versus running drills. *Int J Sports Physiol Perform, 12*(9), 1256–1263. https://doi.org/10.1123/ijspp.2016-0565

Castagna, C., Impellizzeri, F. M., Chaouachi, A., Bordon, C., & Manzi, V. (2011). Effect of training intensity distribution on aerobic fitness variables in elite soccer players: a case study. *J Strength Cond Res, 25*(1), 66–71. https://doi.org/10.1519/JSC.0b013e3181fef3d3

Chaouachi, A., Chtara, M., Hammami, R., Chtara, H., Turki, O., & Castagna, C. (2014). Multidirectional sprints and small-sided games training effect on agility and change of direction abilities in youth soccer. *J Strength Cond Res, 28*(11), 3121–3127. https://doi.org/10.1519/JSC.0000000000000505

Clarkson, P. M., Byrnes, W. C., McCormick, K. M., Turcotte, L. P., & White, J. S. (1986). Muscle soreness and serum creatine kinase activity following isometric, eccentric, and concentric exercise. *Int J Sports Med, 7*(3), 152–155. https://doi.org/10.1055/s-2008-1025753

Clemente, F. M., Ramirez-Campillo, R., Sarmento, H., Praca, G. M., Afonso, J., Silva, A. F., Rosemann, T., & Knechtle, B. (2021). Effects of small-sided game interventions on the technical execution and tactical behaviors of young and youth team sports players: a systematic review and meta-analysis. *Front Psychol, 12*, 667041. https://doi.org/10.3389/fpsyg.2021.667041

Davids, K., Araujo, D., Correia, V., & Vilar, L. (2013). How small-sided and conditioned games enhance acquisition of movement and decision-making skills. *Exerc Sport Sci Rev, 41*(3), 154–161. https://doi.org/10.1097/JES.0b013e318292f3ec

Davies, C. T., & Thompson, M. W. (1979). Aerobic performance of female marathon and male ultramarathon athletes. *Eur J Appl Physiol Occup Physiol, 41*(4), 233–245. https://doi.org/10.1007/BF00429740

Dellal, A., Chamari, K., Wong del, P., Ahmaidi, S., Keller, D., Barros, R., Bisciotti, G. N., & Carling, C. (2011). Comparison of physical and technical performance in European soccer match-play: FA Premier League and La Liga. *Eur J Sports Sci, 11*(1), 51–59. https://doi.org/10.1080/17461391.2010.481334

Di Salvo, V., Baron, R., Gonzalez-Haro, C., Gormasz, C., Pigozzi, F., & Bachl, N. (2010). Sprinting analysis of elite soccer players during European Champions League and UEFA Cup matches. *J Sports Sci, 28*(14), 1489–1494. https://doi.org/10.1080/02640414.2010.521166

Di Salvo, V., Benito, P. J., Calderon, F. J., Di Salvo, M., & Pigozzi, F. (2008). Activity profile of elite goalkeepers during football match-play. *J Sports Med Phys Fitness, 48*(4), 443–446. https://www.ncbi.nlm.nih.gov/pubmed/18997646

Driller, M. W., Fell, J. W., Gregory, J. R., Shing, C. M., & Williams, A. D. (2009). The effects of high-intensity interval training in well-trained rowers. *Int J Sports Physiol Perform, 4*(1), 110–121. https://doi.org/10.1123/ijspp.4.1.110

Ekblom, B. (1969). Effect of physical training in adolescent boys. *J Appl Physiol, 27*(3), 350–355. https://doi.org/10.1152/jappl.1969.27.3.350

Ekstrand, J., Hagglund, M., & Walden, M. (2011). Epidemiology of muscle injuries in professional football (soccer). *Am J Sports Med, 39*(6), 1226–1232. https://doi.org/10.1177/0363546510395879

Esposito, F., Impellizzeri, F. M., Margonato, V., Vanni, R., Pizzini, G., & Veicsteinas, A. (2004). Validity of heart rate as an indicator of aerobic demand during soccer activities in amateur soccer players. *Eur J Appl Physiol, 93*(1–2), 167–172. https://doi.org/10.1007/s00421-004-1192-4

Faude, O., Koch, T., & Meyer, T. (2012). Straight sprinting is the most frequent action in goal situations in professional football. *J Sports Sci, 30*(7), 625–631. https://doi.org/10.1080/02640414.2012.665940

Faude, O., Schnittker, R., Schulte-Zurhausen, R., Muller, F., & Meyer, T. (2013). High intensity interval training vs. high-volume running training during pre-season conditioning in high-level youth football: a cross-over trial. *J Sports Sci, 31*(13), 1441–1450. https://doi.org/10.1080/02640414.2013.792953

Gregson, W., Drust, B., Atkinson, G., & Salvo, V. D. (2010). Match-to-match variability of high-speed activities in premier league soccer. *Int J Sports Med, 31*(4), 237–242. https://doi.org/10.1055/s-0030-1247546

Gunnarsson, T. P., Christensen, P. M., Holse, K., Christiansen, D., & Bangsbo, J. (2012). Effect of additional speed endurance training on performance and muscle adaptations. *Med Sci Sports Exerc, 44*(10), 1942–1948. https://doi.org/10.1249/MSS.0b013e31825ca446

Gunnarsson, T. P., Christensen, P. M., Thomassen, M., Nielsen, L. R., & Bangsbo, J. (2013). Effect of intensified training on muscle ion kinetics, fatigue development, and repeated short-term performance in endurance-trained cyclists. *Am J Physiol Regul Integr Comp Physiol, 305*(7), R811–821. https://doi.org/10.1152/ajpregu.00467.2012

Helgerud, J., Engen, L. C., Wisloff, U., & Hoff, J. (2001). Aerobic endurance training improves soccer performance. *Med Sci Sports Exerc, 33*(11), 1925–1931. https://doi.org/10.1097/00005768-200111000-00019

Hill-Haas, S. V., Dawson, B., Impellizzeri, F. M., & Coutts, A. J. (2011). Physiology of small-sided games training in football: a systematic review. *Sports Med, 41*(3), 199–220. https://doi.org/10.2165/11539740-000000000-00000

Hills, S. P., Barrett, S., Busby, M., Kilduff, L. P., Barwood, M. J., Radcliffe, J. N., Cooke, C. B., & Russell, M. (2020). Profiling the post-match top-up conditioning practices of professional soccer substitutes: an analysis of contextual influences. *J Strength Cond Res, 34*(10), 2805–2814. https://doi.org/10.1519/JSC.0000000000003721

Hoff, J., Wisloff, U., Engen, L. C., Kemi, O. J., & Helgerud, J. (2002). Soccer specific aerobic endurance training. *Br J Sports Med, 36*(3), 218–221. https://doi.org/10.1136/bjsm.36.3.218

Iaia, F. M., & Bangsbo, J. (2010). Speed endurance training is a powerful stimulus for physiological adaptations and performance improvements of athletes. *Scand J Med Sci Sports, 20*(Suppl 2), 11–23. https://doi.org/10.1111/j.1600-0838.2010.01193.x

Iaia, F. M., Fiorenza, M., Perri, E., Alberti, G., Millet, G. P., & Bangsbo, J. (2015). The effect of two speed endurance training regimes on performance of soccer players. *PLoS One, 10*(9), e0138096. https://doi.org/10.1371/journal.pone.0138096

Iaia, F. M., Hellsten, Y., Nielsen, J. J., Fernstrom, M., Sahlin, K., & Bangsbo, J. (2009). Four weeks of speed endurance training reduces energy expenditure during exercise and maintains muscle oxidative capacity despite a reduction in training volume. *J Appl Physiol (1985), 106*(1), 73–80. https://doi.org/10.1152/japplphysiol.90676.2008

Impellizzeri, F. M., Marcora, S. M., Castagna, C., Reilly, T., Sassi, A., Iaia, F. M., & Rampinini, E. (2006). Physiological and performance effects of generic versus specific aerobic training in soccer players. *Int J Sports Med, 27*(6), 483–492. https://doi.org/10.1055/s-2005-865839

Impellizzeri, F. M., Rampinini, E., Coutts, A. J., Sassi, A., & Marcora, S. M. (2004). Use of RPE-based training load in soccer. *Med Sci Sports Exerc, 36*(6), 1042–1047. https://doi.org/10.1249/01.mss.0000128199.23901.2f

Impellizzeri, F. M., Rampinini, E., & Marcora, S. M. (2005). Physiological assessment of aerobic training in soccer. *J Sports Sci, 23*(6), 583–592. https://doi.org/10.1080/02640410400021278

Ingebrigtsen, J., Shalfawi, S. A., Tonnessen, E., Krustrup, P., & Holtermann, A. (2013). Performance effects of 6 weeks of aerobic production training in junior elite soccer players. *J Strength Cond Res, 27*(7), 1861–1867. https://doi.org/10.1519/JSC.0b013e31827647bd

Jensen, L., Bangsbo, J., & Hellsten, Y. (2004). Effect of high intensity training on capillarization and presence of angiogenic factors in human skeletal muscle. *J Physiol, 557*(Pt 2), 571–582. https://doi.org/10.1113/jphysiol.2003.057711

Krustrup, P., Mohr, M., Amstrup, T., Rysgaard, T., Johansen, J., Steensberg, A., Pedersen, P. K., & Bangsbo, J. (2003). The yo-yo intermittent recovery test: physiological response, reliability, and validity. *Med Sci Sports Exerc, 35*(4), 697–705. https://doi.org/10.1249/01.MSS.0000058441.94520.32

Krustrup, P., Mohr, M., Ellingsgaard, H., & Bangsbo, J. (2005). Physical demands during an elite female soccer game: importance of training status. *Med Sci Sports Exerc, 37*(7), 1242–1248. https://doi.org/10.1249/01.mss.0000170062.73981.94

Krustrup, P., Mohr, M., Steensberg, A., Bencke, J., Kjaer, M., & Bangsbo, J. (2006). Muscle and blood metabolites during a soccer game: implications for sprint performance. *Med Sci Sports Exerc, 38*(6), 1165–1174. https://doi.org/10.1249/01.mss.0000222845.89262.cd

Lago-Penas, C. (2012). The role of situational variables in analysing physical performance in soccer. *J Hum Kinet, 35*, 89–95. https://doi.org/10.2478/v10078-012-0082-9

Lago-Penas, C., Lorenzo-Martinez, M., Lopez-Del Campo, R., Resta, R., & Rey, E. (2022). Evolution of physical and technical parameters in the Spanish LaLiga 2012–2019. *Sci Med Footb, 7*, 1–6. https://doi.org/10.1080/24733938.2022.2049980

Laughlin, M. H., & Roseguini, B. (2008). Mechanisms for exercise training-induced increases in skeletal muscle blood flow capacity: differences with interval sprint training versus aerobic endurance training. *J Physiol Pharmacol, 59*(Suppl 7), 71–88. https://www.ncbi.nlm.nih.gov/pubmed/19258658

Martin-Garcia, A., Gomez Diaz, A., Bradley, P. S., Morera, F., & Casamichana, D. (2018). Quantification of a professional football team's external load using a microcycle structure. *J Strength Cond Res, 32*(12), 3511–3518. https://doi.org/10.1519/JSC.0000000000002816

Martinez-Hernandez, D., Quinn, M., & Jones, P. (2022). Linear advancing actions followed by deceleration and turn are the most common movements preceding goals in male professional soccer. *Sci Med Footb, 7*, 1–9. https://doi.org/10.1080/24733938.2022.2030064

McCartney, N., Spriet, L. L., Heigenhauser, G. J., Kowalchuk, J. M., Sutton, J. R., & Jones, N. L. (1986). Muscle power and metabolism in maximal intermittent exercise. *J Appl Physiol (1985), 60*(4), 1164–1169. https://doi.org/10.1152/jappl.1986.60.4.1164

Mohr, M., & Iaia, F. M. (2014). Physiological basis of fatigue resistance training in competitive football. *Sports Sci Exchange, 27*, 1–9.

Mohr, M., & Krustrup, P. (2016). Comparison between two types of anaerobic speed endurance training in competitive soccer players. *J Hum Kinet, 51*, 183–192. https://doi.org/10.1515/hukin-2015-0181

Mohr, M., Krustrup, P., & Bangsbo, J. (2003). Match performance of high-standard soccer players with special reference to development of fatigue. *J Sports Sci, 21*(7), 519–528. https://doi.org/10.1080/0264041031000071182

Mohr, M., Nybo, L., Grantham, J., & Racinais, S. (2012). Physiological responses and physical performance during football in the heat. *PLoS One, 7*(6), e39202. https://doi.org/10.1371/journal.pone.0039202

Mohr, M., Thomassen, M., Girard, O., Racinais, S., & Nybo, L. (2016). Muscle variables of importance for physiological performance in competitive football. *Eur J Appl Physiol, 116*(2), 251–262. https://doi.org/10.1007/s00421-015-3274-x

Morgan, O. J., Drust, B., Ade, J. D., & Robinson, M. A. (2021). Change of direction frequency off the ball: new perspectives in elite youth soccer. *Sci Med Footb. 6*, 473–482 https://doi.org/10.1080/24733938.2021.1986635

Morgans, R., Orme, P., Anderson, L., & Drust, B. (2014). Principles and practices of training for soccer. *J Sport Health Sci, 3*, 251–257.

Rakobowchuk, M., Stuckey, M. I., Millar, P. J., Gurr, L., & Macdonald, M. J. (2009). Effect of acute sprint interval exercise on central and peripheral artery distensibility in young healthy males. *Eur J Appl Physiol, 105*(5), 787–795. https://doi.org/10.1007/s00421-008-0964-7

Reilly, T. (1997). Energetics of high-intensity exercise (soccer) with particular reference to fatigue. *J Sports Sci, 15*(3), 257–263. https://doi.org/10.1080/026404197367263

Reilly, T., & Ball, D. (1984). The net physiological cost of dribbling a soccer ball. *Res Quart Exe Sport, 55*(3), 267–271. https://doi.org/10.1080/02701367.1984.10609363

Reilly, T., & Bangsbo, J. (1998). *Anaeroibc and aerobic training*. Chichester: Wiley.

Reilly, T., & Thomas, V. (1976). A motion analysis of work-rate in different positional roles in professional football match-play. *J Human Movem Studies, 2*, 87–97.

Ross, A., & Leveritt, M. (2001). Long-term metabolic and skeletal muscle adaptations to short-sprint training: implications for sprint training and tapering. *Sports Med, 31*(15), 1063–1082. https://doi.org/10.2165/00007256-200131150-00003

Russell, M., Sparkes, W., Northeast, J., Cook, C. J., Love, T. D., Bracken, R. M., & Kilduff, L. P. (2016). Changes in acceleration and deceleration capacity throughout professional soccer match-play. *J Strength Cond Res, 30*(10), 2839–2844. https://doi.org/10.1519/JSC.0000000000000805

Sarmento, H., Clemente, F. M., Harper, L. D., da Costa, I. T., Owen, A., & Figueiredo, A. J. (2018). Small sided games in soccer: a systematic review. *Intl J Perf Anal Sport, 18*(5), 693–749.

Skovgaard, C., Christensen, P. M., Larsen, S., Andersen, T. R., Thomassen, M., & Bangsbo, J. (2014). Concurrent speed endurance and resistance training improves performance, running economy, and muscle NHE1 in moderately trained runners. *J Appl Physiol (1985), 117*(10), 1097–1109. https://doi.org/10.1152/japplphysiol.01226.2013

Spinks, C. D., Murphy, A. J., Spinks, W. L., & Lockie, R. G. (2007). The effects of resisted sprint training on acceleration performance and kinematics in soccer, rugby union, and Australian football players. *J Strength Cond Res, 21*(1), 77–85. https://doi.org/10.1519/00124278-200702000-00015

Spriet, L. L., Lindinger, M. I., McKelvie, R. S., Heigenhauser, G. J., & Jones, N. L. (1989). Muscle glycogenolysis and H+ concentration during maximal intermittent cycling. *J Appl Physiol (1985), 66*(1), 8–13. https://doi.org/10.1152/jappl.1989.66.1.8

Stolen, T., Chamari, K., Castagna, C., & Wisloff, U. (2005). Physiology of soccer: an update. *Sports Med, 35*(6), 501–536. https://doi.org/10.2165/00007256-200535060-00004

Suarez-Arrones, L., Torreno, N., Requena, B., Saez De Villarreal, E., Casamichana, D., Barbero-Alvarez, J. C., & Munguia-Izquierdo, D. (2015). Match-play activity profile in professional soccer players during official games and the relationship between external and internal load. *J Sports Med Phys Fitness, 55*(12), 1417–1422. https://www.ncbi.nlm.nih.gov/pubmed/25289717

Taberner, M., Allen, T., & Cohen, D. D. (2019). Progressing rehabilitation after injury: consider the 'control-chaos continuum'. *Br J Sports Med, 53*(18), 1132–1136. https://doi.org/10.1136/bjsports-2018-100157

Thomassen, M., Christensen, P. M., Gunnarsson, T. P., Nybo, L., & Bangsbo, J. (2010). Effect of 2-wk intensified training and inactivity on muscle Na+-K+ pump expression, phospholemman (FXYD1) phosphorylation, and performance in soccer players. *J Appl Physiol (1985), 108*(4), 898–905. https://doi.org/10.1152/japplphysiol.01015.2009

Tomlin, D. L., & Wenger, H. A. (2001). The relationship between aerobic fitness and recovery from high-intensity intermittent exercise. *Sports Med, 31*(1), 1–11. https://doi.org/10.2165/00007256-200131010-00001

Tonnessen, E., Shalfawi, S. A., Haugen, T., & Enoksen, E. (2011). The effect of 40-m repeated sprint training on maximum sprinting speed, repeated sprint speed endurance, vertical jump, and aerobic capacity in young elite male soccer players. *J Strength Cond Res, 25*(9), 2364–2370. https://doi.org/10.1519/JSC.0b013e3182023a65

Torreno, N., Munguia-Izquierdo, D., Coutts, A., de Villarreal, E. S., Asian-Clemente, J., & Suarez-Arrones, L. (2016). Relationship between external and internal loads of professional soccer players during full matches in official games using global positioning systems and heart-rate technology. *Int J Sports Physiol Perform*, *11*(7), 940–946. https://doi.org/10.1123/ijspp.2015-0252

Viru, A., & Viru, M. (2000). Nature of training effects. In W. Garret & D. Kirkendall (Eds.), *Exercise and Sport Science* (pp. 67–95). Lippincott: Williams & Williams.

Vitale, J. A., Povia, V., Vitale, N. D., Bassani, T., Lombardi, G., Giacomelli, L., Banfi, G., & La Torre, A. (2018). The effect of two different speed endurance training protocols on a multiple shuttle run performance in young elite male soccer players. *Res Sports Med*, *26*(4), 436–449. https://doi.org/10.1080/15438627.2018.1492402

Withers, R. T., Sherman, W. M., Clark, D. G., Esselbach, P. C., Nolan, S. R., Mackay, M. H., & Brinkman, M. (1991). Muscle metabolism during 30, 60 and 90 s of maximal cycling on an air-braked ergometer. *Eur J Appl Physiol Occup Physiol*, *63*(5), 354–362. https://doi.org/10.1007/BF00364462

# 4 Soccer in the heat

## Performance and mitigation

*Caroline Sunderland, Stacey Cowe and,*
*Rachel Malcolm*

### Introduction

Soccer is one of the world's most popular sports and is played across all seven continents, resulting in highly variable environmental conditions across competitions. This phenomenon is becoming increasingly important due to global warming. Although understanding of thermoregulation has improved, the complexities of team sports, specifically soccer, makes understanding the influence of heat on different components extremely difficult. In recent years, a number of competitions have taken place in extreme environments, such as the Tokyo Olympics and the FIFA World Cup in Qatar (anticipated 29°C and 59% relative humidity; Chodor et al., 2021). As a result, it is imperative that coaches, players, governing bodies, and medical staff have an adequate awareness of the risks associated with hyperthermia and the potential influences on performance.

Performance incorporates a combination of factors, including tactical, technical, physical, and psychological (Slattery & Coutts, 2019). Few researchers have investigated how heat effects a combination of these components, however, a number of studies have assessed the individual effects of heat on each of these components. These studies have shown that a range of these elements can be negatively influenced by heat stress, including cognitive function (Bandelow et al., 2010), the ability to perform repeated sprints (Maxwell, Aitchison, & Nimmo, 1996), and the perception of effort (Duffield, Coutts, & Quinn, 2009). This emphasises the need for well-designed strategies to cool and acclimate athletes to minimise the effect on performance. Considerations must also be made with regards to the timing of matches, whereby in extreme environmental conditions, match times will need to avoid peak day-time temperatures to protect athletes against hyperthermia. A significant amount of individual variation occurs with regards to thermoregulation, often influenced by sex, age, body composition, and disability status, all of which must be considered when planning for performance.

In this chapter, we examine the influence of high external temperatures on different components of soccer performance. These will include the effects on physical output and cognitive function, whilst detailing the effects on different populations, including female players, youth players, referees, and disabled athletes. Also, we aim to detail some the strategies utilised to counteract these effects and help optimise soccer performance.

DOI: 10.4324/9781003148418-5

## Physical performance

Performance in soccer tends to be divided into tactical aspects and physical elements, with power, speed, and endurance being instrumental to success (Figueira, Goncalves, Masiulis, & Sampaio, 2018; Rösch et al., 2000). In research related to soccer, these physical elements are a common measurement used to quantify how certain variables may affect performance, such as hot environmental conditions.

One of the main concerns when exercising in the heat is the negative effect it could have on an athlete's performance. A potential reason for these performance decrements is that an increase in core body temperature causes a reduction in exercise capacity (Nybo, Rasmussen, & Sawka, 2014). In a study carried out by Aldous et al. (2015), which utilised an intermittent soccer performance test in a control (18°C) and hot environment (30°C), participant's total and sprint distance covered was significantly less when completing the test in the heat (see Figures 4.1 and 4.2). Similarly, Mohr, Nybo, Grantham, and Racinais (2012) found that participants completed less high-speed running when playing soccer in the heat (43°C) in comparison to a control environment (21°C) (Figure 4.3). These findings highlight the negative effect increases in core body temperature may have on performance.

As well as increases in core body temperature and dehydration causing an individual to become fatigued resulting in poorer performance (Shirreffs, Sawka, & Stone, 2006), perceptual responses, such as thermal sensation, can play a role. Previously, researchers have demonstrated that ratings of thermal sensation are significantly higher when exercising in a hot environment (34°C), which is accompanied by a rise in skin temperature (Periard et al., 2014). Due to perceptual measures being heightened when exercising in the heat, it can result in physiological and perceptual strain as well as

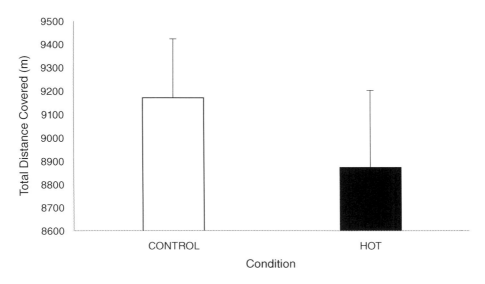

*Figure 4.1* The total distance covered in a simulated soccer match in control (18°C) and hot (30°C) environmental conditions (control vs hot: $P < 0.05$). Redrawn from Aldous et al. (2015).

54  *Caroline Sunderland et al.*

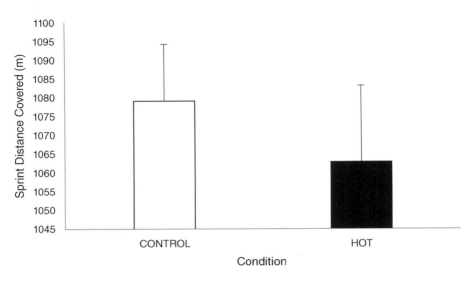

*Figure 4.2* The sprint distance covered in a simulated soccer match in control (18°C) and hot (30°C) environmental conditions (control vs hot: $P < 0.05$). Redrawn from Aldous et al. (2015).

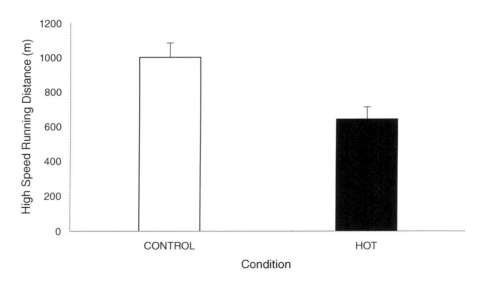

*Figure 4.3* The high-speed running distance completed during a soccer match in control (21°C) and hot (43°C) environmental conditions (control vs hot: $P < 0.05$). Redrawn from Mohr et al. (2012).

heat-related illnesses, such as heat exhaustion (Sawka et al., 2007). In addition, an increase in thermal sensation ratings causes individuals to adjust their physical activity patterns to ensure core temperature is kept within safe levels and minimise discomfort (Duffield et al., 2009; Periard et al., 2014). This finance indicates that an individual's performance may worsen when exercising in the heat due to increased thermal/perceptual strain. Therefore, because of this potential effect perceptual responses to exercise in the heat may have on performance, it is imperative to understand how to attenuate the rise in subjective perceptual ratings.

The influence of heat stress on soccer players is not only important for our understanding of performance, but it is essential for preventing heat-related illness. Heat-related illness can be life-threatening if not treated promptly. During a soccer tournament played in the heat, in total, 34 players collapsed due to heat exhaustion, highlighting the serious consequences of hyperthermia (Kirkendall, 1993). Knowledge of at-risk players and signs of heat-related illness is essential.

## Cognitive function and decision-making

Performance in team sport is dictated by the ability to produce skilful actions consistently across a prolonged period, whilst under significant physical stress. The ability to produce skilful actions depends upon optimal functioning of various cognitive domains, controlled by different regions of the brain (Schmitt, Benton, & Kallus, 2005). Due to heat influencing different brain regions variably, this becomes a complex aspect of performance to assess and optimise.

Cognitive performance has previously been linked with changes in stress and arousal, whereby the different domains of cognitive function each have an optimal zone of functioning in terms of the level of arousal experienced in response to a specific stressor. Optimising arousal levels allows athletes to narrow their attention to focus on task-relevant cues and process that information more efficiently (Lee et al., 2014; Schlader et al., 2015; Simmons, Saxby, McGlone, & Jones, 2008). Whereas when arousal is too low, the focus of the athlete may be too broad, taking in too many stimuli and reducing their ability to process and act quickly enough. Similarly, if arousal is too high, and attention narrows too much, then an athlete may miss task relevant information (Gaoua, Racinais, Grantham, & El Massioui, 2011; Liu et al., 2013; Racinais, Gaoua, & Grantham, 2008). Practically speaking, this may be the difference between a pass being completed or intercepted by a defender. Therefore, due to the influence of various domains of cognition on the overall performance in sport, it is imperative to understand the effects of heat on these domains (Malcolm, Cooper, Folland, Tyler, & Sunderland, 2018), to provide adequate advice for soccer players and referees competing in hot environments.

Specific domains of cognitive function have greater relevance to soccer than others. Visual perception is a player's ability to pick up cues in their visual field, for example, the ability to pick up and react to a defender or ball quickly. Executive function refers to higher-level functioning, which requires an athlete to suppress an automatic response to select the correct one when faced with conflicting stimuli, for example suppressing the desire to dribble when the correct option is to pass to a teammate. Working memory refers to the ability to store information, which is beneficial when recalling tactical information and previous experience from within a game. Finally, sustained attention is relevant due to the length of time required for soccer players to produce skilful actions within a game.

In further research by Malcolm (2018), which examined soccer-specific exercise in the heat, response times on a visual search test (representing a player's ability to pick up visual cues) slowed across a match in the heat (Figure 4.4). Similarly, accuracy got worse across the match in the heat, whilst improving throughout the trial in moderate conditions (Figure 4.5). Bandelow et al. (2010) also found that soccer in the heat negatively influenced response times across cognitive domains. Cognition is influenced by several factors, such as rise in core temperature, negative subjective feelings towards the heat as well as substantial increases in skin temperature (Gaoua, Grantham,

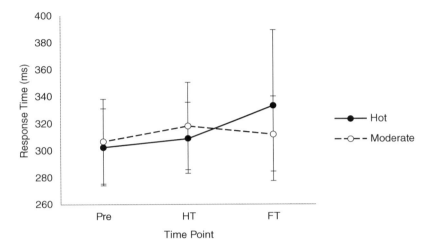

*Figure 4.4* The baseline level response times for visual search.
Data are mean ± SD. Pre, prior to the match simulation; HT, half time; FT, full time. Main effect of trial $P<0.01$; and trial time interaction $P<0.01$. Redrawn from Malcolm (2018).

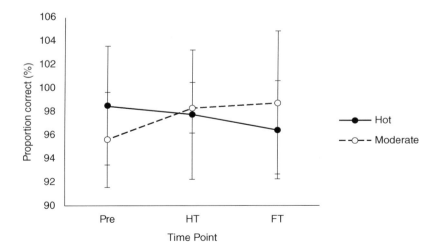

*Figure 4.5* The proportion correct on the baseline level of the visual search test.
Data are mean ± SD. Pre, prior to the match simulation; HT, half time; FT, full time. Main effect of trial $P<0.01$; main effect of time $P<0.01$. Trial time interaction, $P<0.01$. Redrawn from Malcolm (2018).

Racinais, & El Massioui, 2012; Lieberman et al., 2005; Morley et al., 2012). Negative perceptual feeling and rises in skin temperature can detrimentally impact cognition, in the absence of changes in core temperature, due to providing a distracting influence on athletes and limiting their ability to process task relevant cues (Gaoua et al., 2012; Malcolm et al., 2018). Introducing cooling methods (such as neck cooling), can positively influence cognition and resulting performance by improving thermal comfort, whereas changes in core temperature require more extreme intervention such as pre-cooling and acclimation to be altered. These interventions will be discussed in greater detail in future sections.

The research to date examining soccer in the heat and cognitive function has employed task generic cognitive function assessments due to their reliability in repeated measure designs, ease of use during and immediately after soccer simulations or matches, and their extensive use in sport and physical activity research across the age range. In contrast, task-specific measures, which may include videos of soccer players with areas occluded or videos stopped at pertinent moments and then asking players to decide how to react, have not been used and should be explored. Further, studying skills during matches in the heat versus temperate conditions is warranted, but the variation between matches and the limited control must be considered from the research perspective. However, from an applied perspective, employing performance analysts to record player skill success and decision-making during matches in different climatic conditions will provide the coach with important information about how players perform in the heat.

## Female players

Due to the hormonal changes that occur during the menstrual cycle and with oral contraceptive use, deep body temperature fluctuates across an approximately monthly cycle. Thus, when playing or training in a hot environment, performance, and thermoregulatory responses may be at risk of being affected due to these cyclic variations in deep body temperature.

Due to the large inter-match variation in performance, research relating to the effects of the menstrual cycle and oral contraceptive use has focussed on laboratory-based studies. During simulated soccer-specific running in the heat (31°C), there was no difference in distance ran by unacclimatised players between the follicular and luteal phases of the menstrual cycle, however in monophasic oral contraceptive users, distance ran was greater by 21% in the quasi-luteal phase (Sunderland & Nevill, 2003). It was postulated that this related to the change in hormonal milieu observed when in the first couple of days of starting to re-take the oral contraceptive following the pill-free week. For both eumenorrheic players and those take oral contraceptives, there were no differences in sprint performance, heart rate or plasma lactate, or ammonia across the menstrual cycle (Sunderland & Nevill, 2003). To date, there is no research relating to changes in soccer-specific performance across the menstrual cycle in acclimatised players, and this clearly warrants further investigation.

Although there is limited research relating to heat acclimation, the data have shown that females adapt efficiently to improve performance (Sunderland, Morris, & Nevill, 2008). However, compared with their male counterparts, adaptation rate has been shown to differ (Mee, Gibson, Doust, & Maxwell, 2015; Wickham, Wallace, & Cheung, 2021) (see Acclimation and Acclimatisation section for further details).

58   *Caroline Sunderland et al.*

In summary, for eumenorrheic females, the stress of the heat appears to override any potential differences in performance across the menstrual cycle. However, in oral contraceptive users, consideration should be given relating to the initial days following the pill-free week. Whether menstrual cycle or oral contraceptive hormonal changes will impact upon soccer performance in acclimatised players remains to be elucidated. However, changes across the menstrual cycle and during different phases of oral contraceptive use should be considered on an individual player basis. Symptoms, whether physical or psychological, differ, considerably between players, so this should be discussed with the players as the additional stress from playing in the heat may further exacerbate these symptoms (e.g., nausea and feeling flushed). A suitable individual player strategy can then be put in place to optimise their performance.

## Disability players

Since the start of the Paralympic Games in 1948, the competition has experienced rapid growth, with over 4,000 athletes participating at the Games in Rio, Brazil, in 2016 (International Paralympic Committee, 2016). As a result of this growth, and the importance of preparing para-athletes for challenging environmental conditions, there has been an increased pressure placed on coaches and support staff to understand disability sports in the heat (Griggs, Stephenson, Price, & Goosey-Tolfrey, 2020; O'Brien, Lunt, Stephenson, & Goosey-Tolfrey, 2022). The physiological characteristics of various disabilities pose a risk when exercising in a hot environment. Therefore, to recognise and lessen the risk of heat injury in an effective manner, an increased awareness and the educating of support staff is imperative for athletes who are physically and/or visually impaired (Webborn, 1996).

Para-athletes who suffer from spinal cord injuries may be at greater risk of heat injury because of a loss of autonomic function (Webborn, 2004), which also causes problems relating to temperature regulation. The reason for this is due to a reduction in the heat loss mechanisms and working peripheral receptors that are responsible for sweating (Webborn, 1996). As a result, spinal cord injury athletes may experience complications with heat dissipation whilst exercising in hot environmental conditions. This, however, is dependent on the severity of the injury. Generally, the worse the injury or, the higher the level of lesion, the greater the problems are regarding temperature control (Dawson, Bridle, & Lockwood, 1994; Fitzgerald, Sedlock, & Knowlton, 1990; Petrofsky, 1992).

Another disability that poses a risk when exercising in the heat is amputation. Following a bilateral leg amputation, there is a reduced surface area that leads to a reduction in evaporative cooling during exercise in the heat. In other words, bilateral amputees sweat and lose heat less due to a reduced surface area following their injury (Webborn, 1996). In addition to a reduced surface area posing problems related to evaporative heat loss, gait asymmetry present in these individuals also cause elevations in heat production (Ghoseiri & Safari, 2014). Another aspect of this injury that could worsen the risks of exercising in the heat is the use of prosthetics. The effects of friction and compression when using a prosthetic have been said to result in possible risks to the residual limb (Webborn, 2004). Elements, such as a rise in skin temperature, that are present when exercising in a hot environment could worsen these risks, posing more danger for the athletes. As a result, considerations must be made regarding cooling strategies for disability athletes.

## Youth

Young players thermoregulate differently to their adult counterparts, having lower sweat rates and are therefore less able to use evaporative heat loss, however, they have an increased skin blood flow and a higher surface area to mass ratio. In addition, young players have less experience, respond to thermal strain differently and cognitively are still developing (Falk & Dotan, 2011). These factors make them more susceptible to heat illness and injury, and therefore it is imperative that coaches, monitor young players very closely in hot environments, providing frequent cooling and fluid breaks, training in the cooler parts of the day and in shade, ensuring sun cream is applied, and hats are worn whenever possible.

Young players acclimatise successfully but at a slower rate than adults, so this should be considered by increasing the period for acclimation and the number of sessions completed prior to match or tournament play in the heat.

## Strategies to improve performance

### *Acclimation and acclimatisation*

Heat acclimation which takes place in an artificial environment, or acclimatisation outside is the recommended preparation strategy prior to any soccer match or tournament in the heat. This process is essential for those players who have not recently regularly trained or competed in similar environmental conditions, specifically temperature and humidity. Heat acclimation or acclimatisation involves repeated exposures to heat stress which increase core and skin temperature and results in high sweat rates. Consecutive day and intermittent day are both beneficial for performance (Duvnjak-Zaknich, Wallman, Dawson, & Peeling, 2019). In addition, acclimatisation can reduce the chance of heat-related illness.

Short-term heat acclimation of 5–7 days of both intermittent running mimicking soccer and steady-state cycling have been shown to improve performance in the heat. The completion of four 30- to 45-min sessions of soccer-specific running in the heat (30°C, 27% RH) in a 10-day period increased running capacity by 33% in female team sport athletes, due to a lower rectal temperature and improved thermal comfort and an ability to tolerate a higher end core temperature (Sunderland et al., 2008). This heat acclimation protocol has been shown to improve field hockey skill performance in the heat and is, therefore, likely to help with the maintenance of soccer skill (unpublished observations). Similarly, five consecutive days of heat acclimation of 90-min cycling using the controlled hyperthermia technique (maintaining a rectal temperature of 38.5°C) resulted in performance improvements in repeated cycle sprinting interspersed with intermittent running, and reduced rectal, skin, and body temperature, and heart rate (Garrett et al., 2019). The controlled hyperthermia method requires continuous monitoring and therefore is most suited to players who can only acclimate in laboratory conditions or those players who are rehabilitating from injury prior to a tournament in the heat. Acclimation can take the form of passive heating through sauna use and hot baths following training sessions in moderate conditions if players don't have access to environmental chambers (Zurawlew, Mee, & Walsh, 2019).

Recently, researchers have examined how players acclimatise to the heat prior to international tournaments providing evidence of its efficacy in elite players. International

## 60  *Caroline Sunderland et al.*

female players completed 6 days of heat acclimatisation (34.5°C), which compromised of their normal soccer training prior to the World Cup in France. Core temperature, via ingestible telemetric pills, was monitored to ensure that it was maintained >38.5°C throughout the acclimatisation sessions. The acclimatisation induced thermoregulatory and cardiovascular benefits that lasted for at least 2 weeks and enhanced performance. Both male and female players benefit from heat acclimatisation, however, there is evidence they adapt at different rates. Mee and colleagues (2015) demonstrated that after 5 days of heat acclimation, rectal temperature and heart rate were decreased in men and not women, whereas sweat rate increased in females and not males. Following a further 5 days heat acclimation, rectal temperature and heart rate decreased for the females but remained unchanged in the males, for whom sweat rate did increase. This difference between the sexes may relate to differences in the thermal load experienced by males and females during acclimation (Wickham et al., 2021).

In summary, heat acclimation and acclimatisation should be specific to the environmental conditions where the players are competing as well as being soccer-specific. Where possible, acclimatisation should take place so that technical as well as physical training, in the heat can take place. This should consist of high-intensity soccer-specific training drills and small-sided games that last 30–45 min for at least four sessions in the 7–10 days prior to the first match in the heat. Where acclimatisation can't take place, acclimation in environmental chambers will be very beneficial for physiological adaptation and should compromise of high-intensity intermittent running, rather than cycling whenever possible, as this results in a greater acclimation stimulus. For female soccer players, you should try to complete additional acclimatisation sessions compared with their male counterparts to maximise performance benefits. Females could also increase the thermal load by increasing session length or completing passive heating before or after sessions. Whether undertaking acclimatisation or acclimation, monitor core temperature and heart rate whenever possible, watch closely for signs of heat-related illness and ensure hydration replaces all fluid losses after sessions. If acclimatisation occurs in sunny environments, then it is imperative to apply sports-specific sun lotion to prevent burning.

## Cooling strategies

### *Pre-cooling*

During intermittent-sprint exercise completed in hot conditions, it has been reported that pre-cooling can be beneficial at slowing the elevation in core temperature as well as perceptual stress (Duffield & Marino, 2007; Price, Boyd, & Goosey-Tolfrey, 2009). Researchers tend to highlight both the physiological and performance benefits of pre-cooling before intermittent-sprint exercise (Duffield & Marino, 2007). For example, pre-cooling has been found to reduce core and skin temperatures during a simulated soccer match (Price et al., 2009). As discussed previously, elevated skin temperature can lead to negative perceptual feelings and a distracting influence for players, whereas elevated core temperature can result in early onset of fatigue and decreased drive to the muscle.

Examples of pre-cooling include muscle and torso cooling, cold water immersion and systemic pre-cooling. In a study investigating the effects of pre-cooling on leg muscle on intermittent sprint performance in hot, humid conditions, it was reported that peak power output was negatively affected only when completing exercise in the heat without pre-cooling (control) (Castle et al., 2006). It was also found that heat strain and muscle temperature were reduced when utilising a combination of local muscle cooling through ice packs and cold-water immersion for 20 min (Castle et al., 2006). Internal cooling through ice slurry or cold drink ingestion (5–15°C) can also decrease core temperature prior to exercise and increase thermal comfort, though may result in increased heat storage through altered sweating responses (Gibson et al., 2020).

### Cooling/drinks breaks

In recent years, cooling/drink breaks have been introduced when temperatures are at least 32°C. These occur approximately mid-way through each half and can last between 2 and 5 min depending on league rules and regulations. These allow for the intake of additional fluid as well as an opportunity to reduce core temperature and/or thermal sensation and comfort (Chalmers et al., 2019). Researchers have demonstrated that cooling breaks coupled with various methods of cooling (cold water and cold towels) during a simulated match reduced thermal strain in comparison to when they weren't included (Chalmers et al., 2019). However, it was also found that no one method was more successful at reducing core body temperature than another. During breaks, ice slurry or cold fluids should be drunk, neck collars/ice towels should be applied, and fans with misting sprays can be used, with the further addition of ice vests at half-time (Gibson et al., 2020). During matches, substitutes should ensure they remain cool through both internal and external cooling as required.

In summary, when incorporating pre-cooling or mid-match cooling strategies, it is important to apply these techniques within training settings prior to completing during matches. Cold water or ice slurry ingestion can be uncomfortable or cause gastrointestinal problems for some players, menthol spray can be a skin irritant, and ice towels placed around the neck can cause players to suffer from 'brain freeze'. In addition, players will have highly variable sweat rates and core temperature responses to matches, and therefore hydration and cooling strategies must be individualised. An important consideration is also the warm-up period which should be modified for hot environmental conditions to maintain a low core temperature prior to match onset.

## Disability players

As mentioned above, cooling strategies have great benefits when performing intermittent exercise in the heat, and a lot of research has focused on able-bodied athletes. As a result, there are limited amounts of research on cooling strategies for disability athletes, and in particular, a vast majority of investigations conducted focus on cooling methods for spinal cord injury athletes as they experience both motor and neurological difficulties (Price, 2015). This lack of research leads to a hindrance in the development of guidelines for athletes competing in competitions with difficult environmental conditions, such as the Paralympic Games (Goosey-Tolfrey, Swainson, Boyd, Atkinson, & Tolfrey, 2008). Nevertheless, it has been found that, overall, cooling reduced spinal cord injury athlete's core temperature as well as thermal sensation during exercise (O'Brien et al., 2022). More specifically, pre-cooling strategies were seen to reduce athlete's core temperature to a greater extent in comparison to cooling during exercise, as well as the greatest benefits of cooling mainly being seen in individuals with a more severe spinal cord injury (O'Brien et al., 2022).

Griggs, Price, and Goosey-Tolfrey (2015), highlighted that wearing an ice vest during intermittent exercise led to a reduction in thermal strain and improvements in performance in spinal cord injury athletes. The reduction witnessed in thermal strain is beneficial as this could lead to a reduction in the psychological stress of exercising in a hot environment (Goosey-Tolfrey et al., 2008), thus potentially improving performance. It has been found that the use of an ice vest before and during exercise increased spinal cord injury athlete's ability to perform repeated sprints and total exercise capacity, which was indicated through an increase in the number of sprints completed (Webborn, Price, Castle, & Goosey-Tolfrey, 2010).

Whilst these findings demonstrate the benefits of cooling garments on intermittent exercise and sprint performance, the fit of these garments has been a cause for concern within the sporting world. Many of these garments tend to be made for able-bodied athletes, therefore, in the future, there needs to be considerations of how these garments will fit disability athletes (Griggs et al., 2020). In addition to the future considerations regarding the fit of cooling garments, more research must be conducted to aid the direction of guidelines provided to disability athletes and their support staff. Due to the nature of differing physiological characteristics of various disabilities, it is imperative that research is carried out to investigate the use of different cooling strategies on different disabilities.

## Future directions and conclusions

As the global temperature continues to rise and soccer competitions continue to be scheduled in hot environments, it is more important than ever for care to be taken in the planning of strategies to optimise the health and performance of athletes. Due to the known variability in individual responses of athletes to heat stress, future directions will look at the most appropriate means to test and monitor athletes. Although heat tolerance testing is currently used in many elite settings, the application of the data is limited. Coaches should endeavour to use substitutions more strategically when competing in the heat, specifically altering strategies for athletes more susceptible to heat stress. In line with this, due to the known effects of passive heat stress on cognitive function (Malcolm et al., 2018), practitioners should look at specific interventions for substitutes to prevent them entering the pitch in a below optimal state.

The use of telemetric pills to get live feedback on temperature status of competing athletes may be the next step in health and performance optimisation (Gosselin et al., 2019). This approach will enable coaches to remove individuals who are at risk of hyperthermia or underperformance.

Further development of intervention strategies to improve the various aspects of soccer performance is required. One of these, which is currently in its infancy, is the use of 'cooling breaks' (Chalmers et al., 2019). At present, UEFA rules state that these breaks are only allowed when pitch side temperatures reach 32°C, at which point a 90-s break is permitted 25 min into each half. Research must be done to assess the efficacy of the current strategy in promoting the health and performance of athletes, and improvements must be researched and implemented.

In conclusion, soccer performance in hot environmental conditions is impaired, both in terms of physical and cognitive performance. This performance decrease can be reduced by the completion of soccer-specific acclimation or acclimatisation prior to competing in heat, and this should be tailored specifically to the needs of the playing group as well as the individual. On match days, acute cooling strategies should be applied before and during matches, and these should be practised during the acclimation period to determine player tolerance and response. During recovery, fluid and electrolyte replacement should be closely monitored, and this is particularly important when matches are in close proximity. Whether training or playing matches in hot environmental conditions, players' heart rates and core temperatures should be monitored whenever possible, along with signs of heat illness.

## References

Aldous, J. W., Chrismas, B. C., Akubat, I., Dascombe, B., Abt, G., & Taylor, L. (2015). Hot and hypoxic environments inhibit simulated soccer performance and exacerbate performance decrements when combined. *Front Physiol, 6*, 421. doi:10.3389/fphys.2015.00421

Bandelow, S., Maughan, R., Shirreffs, S., Ozgunen, K., Kurdak, S., Ersoz, G., ... Dvorak, J. (2010). The effects of exercise, heat, cooling and rehydration strategies on cognitive function in football players. *Scand J Med Sci Sports, 20*(Suppl 3), 148–160. doi:10.1111/j.1600–0838.2010.01220.x

Castle, P. C., Macdonald, A. L., Philp, A., Webborn, A., Watt, P. W., & Maxwell, N. S. (2006). Precooling leg muscle improves intermittent sprint exercise performance in hot, humid conditions. *J Appl Physiol, 100*(4), 1377–1384.

Chalmers, S., Siegler, J., Lovell, R., Lynch, G., Gregson, W., Marshall, P., & Jay, O. (2019). Brief in-play cooling breaks reduce thermal strain during football in hot conditions. *J Sci Med Sport, 22*(8), 912–917. doi:10.1016/j.jsams.2019.04.009

Chodor, W., Chmura, P., Chmura, J., Andrzejewski, M., Jowko, E., Buraczewski, T., ... Konefal, M. (2021). Impact of climatic conditions projected at the World Cup in Qatar 2022 on repeated maximal efforts in soccer players. *Peer J, 9*, e12658. doi:10.7717/peerj.12658

Dawson, B., Bridle, J., & Lockwood, R. J. (1994). Thermoregulation of paraplegic and able bodied men during prolonged exercise in hot and cool climates. *Paraplegia, 32*(12), 860–870. doi:10.1038/sc.1994.132

Duffield, R., Coutts, A. J., & Quinn, J. (2009). Core temperature responses and match running performance during intermittent-sprint exercise competition in warm conditions. *J Strength Cond Res, 23*(4), 1238–1244. doi:10.1519/JSC.0b013e318194e0b1

Duffield, R., & Marino, F. E. (2007). Effects of pre-cooling procedures on intermittent-sprint exercise performance in warm conditions. *Eur J Appl Physiol, 100*(6), 727–735. doi:10.1007/s00421-007-0468-x

Duvnjak-Zaknich, D. M., Wallman, K. E., Dawson, B. T., & Peeling, P. (2019). Continuous and intermittent heat acclimation and decay in team sport athletes. *Eur J Sport Sci, 19*(3), 295–304. doi:10.1080/17461391.2018.1512653

Falk, B., & Dotan, R. (2011). Temperature regulation and elite young athletes. *Med Sport Sci, 56*, 126–149. doi:10.1159/000320645

Figueira, B., Goncalves, B., Masiulis, N., & Sampaio, J. (2018). Exploring how playing football with different age groups affects tactical behaviour and physical performance. *Biol Sport, 35*(2), 145–153. doi:10.5114/biolsport.2018.71603

Fitzgerald, P. I., Sedlock, D. A., & Knowlton, R. G. (1990). Circulatory and thermal adjustments to prolonged exercise in paraplegic women. *Med Sci Sports Exerc, 22*(5), 629–635. doi:10.1249/00005768–199010000-00014

64    *Caroline Sunderland et al.*

Gaoua, N., Grantham, J., Racinais, S., & El Massioui, F. (2012). Sensory displeasure reduces complex cognitive performance in the heat. *J Environ Psychol, 32*(2), 158–163. doi:10.1016/j.jenvp.2012.01.002

Gaoua, N., Racinais, S., Grantham, J., & El Massioui, F. (2011). Alterations in cognitive performance during passive hyperthermia are task dependent. *Int J Hyperthermia, 27*(1), 1–9. doi:10.3109/02656736.2010.516305

Garrett, A. T., Dodd, E., Biddlecombe, V., Gleadall-Siddall, D., Burke, R., Shaw, J., ... Gritt, J. (2019). Effectiveness of short-term heat acclimation on intermittent sprint performance with moderately trained females controlling for menstrual cycle phase. *Front Physiol, 10*, 1458. doi:10.3389/fphys.2019.01458

Ghoseiri, K., & Safari, M. R. (2014). Prevalence of heat and perspiration discomfort inside prostheses: literature review. *J Rehabil Res Dev, 51*(6), 855–868. doi:10.1682/JRRD.2013.06.0133

Gibson, O. R., James, C. A., Mee, J. A., Willmott, A. G. B., Turner, G., Hayes, M., & Maxwell, N. S. (2020). Heat alleviation strategies for athletic performance: a review and practitioner guidelines. *Temperature (Austin), 7*(1), 3–36. doi:10.1080/23328940.2019.1666624

Goosey-Tolfrey, V., Swainson, M., Boyd, C., Atkinson, G., & Tolfrey, K. (2008). The effectiveness of hand cooling at reducing exercise-induced hyperthermia and improving distance-race performance in wheelchair and able-bodied athletes. *J Appl Physiol (1985), 105*(1), 37–43. doi:10.1152/japplphysiol.01084.2007

Gosselin, J., Beliveau, J., Hamel, M., Casa, D., Hosokawa, Y., Morais, J. A., & Goulet, E. D. B. (2019). Wireless measurement of rectal temperature during exercise: comparing an ingestible thermometric telemetric pill used as a suppository against a conventional rectal probe. *J Therm Biol, 83*, 112–118. doi:10.1016/j.jtherbio.2019.05.010

Griggs, K. E., Price, M. J., & Goosey-Tolfrey, V. L. (2015). Cooling athletes with a spinal cord injury. *Sports Med, 45*(1), 9–21. doi:10.1007/s40279-014-0241-3

Griggs, K. E., Stephenson, B. T., Price, M. J., & Goosey-Tolfrey, V. L. (2020). Heat-related issues and practical applications for paralympic athletes at Tokyo 2020. *Temperature (Austin), 7*(1), 37–57. doi:10.1080/23328940.2019.1617030

International Paralympic Committee. (2016). Rio 2016 paralympic games. Retrieved from https://www.paralympic.org/rio-2016. Accessed 2/3/22.

Kirkendall, D. T. (1993). Effects of nutrition on performance in soccer. *Med Sci Sports Exerc, 25*(12), 1370–1374.

Lee, J. K., Koh, A. C., Koh, S. X., Liu, G. J., Nio, A. Q., & Fan, P. W. (2014). Neck cooling and cognitive performance following exercise-induced hyperthermia. *Eur J Appl Physiol, 114*(2), 375–384. doi:10.1007/s00421-013-2774-9

Lieberman, H. R., Bathalon, G. P., Falco, C. M., Kramer, F. M., Morgan, C. A., 3rd, & Niro, P. (2005). Severe decrements in cognition function and mood induced by sleep loss, heat, dehydration, and undernutrition during simulated combat. *Biol Psychiatry, 57*(4), 422–429. doi:10.1016/j.biopsych.2004.11.014

Liu, K., Sun, G., Li, B., Jiang, Q., Yang, X., Li, M., ... Liu, Y. (2013). The impact of passive hyperthermia on human attention networks: an fMRI study. *Behav Brain Res, 243*, 220–230. doi:10.1016/j.bbr.2013.01.013

Malcolm, R. (2018). *The influence of intermittent exercise and heat exposure on neuromuscular and cognitive function.* (PhD), Nottingham Trent University, UK.

Malcolm, R. A., Cooper, S., Folland, J. P., Tyler, C. J., & Sunderland, C. (2018). Passive Heat Exposure Alters Perception and Executive Function. *Front Physiol, 9*, 585. doi:10.3389/fphys.2018.00585

Maxwell, N. S., Aitchison, T. C., & Nimmo, M. A. (1996). The effect of climatic heat stress on intermittent supramaximal running performance in humans. *Exper Physiol, 81*(5), 833–845.

Mee, J. A., Gibson, O. R., Doust, J., & Maxwell, N. S. (2015). A comparison of males and females' temporal patterning to short- and long-term heat acclimation. *Scand J Med Sci Sports, 25*(Suppl 1), 250–258. doi:10.1111/sms.12417

Mohr, M., Nybo, L., Grantham, J., & Racinais, S. (2012). Physiological responses and physical performance during football in the heat. *PLoS ONE, 7*(6), e39202. doi:10.1371/journal.pone.0039202

Morley, J., Beauchamp, G., Suyama, J., Guyette, F. X., Reis, S. E., Callaway, C. W., & Hostler, D. (2012). Cognitive function following treadmill exercise in thermal protective clothing. *Eur J Appl Physiol, 112*(5), 1733–1740. doi:10.1007/s00421-011-2144-4

Nybo, L., Rasmussen, P., & Sawka, M. N. (2014). Performance in the heat-physiological factors of importance for hyperthermia-induced fatigue. *Compr Physiol, 4*(2), 657–689. doi:10.1002/cphy.c130012

O'Brien, T. J., Lunt, K. M., Stephenson, B. T., & Goosey-Tolfrey, V. L. (2022). The effect of pre-cooling or per-cooling in athletes with a spinal cord injury: a systematic review and meta-analysis. *J Sci Med Sport. 25(7)*, 606–614. doi:10.1016/j.jsams.2022.02.005

Periard, J. D., Racinais, S., Knez, W. L., Herrera, C. P., Christian, R. J., & Girard, O. (2014). Thermal, physiological and perceptual strain mediate alterations in match-play tennis under heat stress. *Br J Sports Med, 48*(Suppl 1), i32–i38. doi:10.1136/bjsports-2013–093063

Petrofsky, J. S. (1992). Thermoregulatory stress during rest and exercise in heat in patients with a spinal cord injury. *Eur J Appl Physiol Occup Physiol, 64*(6), 503–507. doi:10.1007/BF00843758

Price, M. J. (2015). Preparation of paralympic athletes; environmental concerns and heat acclimation. *Front Physiol, 6*, 415. doi:10.3389/fphys.2015.00415

Price, M. J., Boyd, C., & Goosey-Tolfrey, V. L. (2009). The physiological effects of pre-event and midevent cooling during intermittent running in the heat in elite female soccer players. *Appl Physiol Nutr Metab, 34*(5), 942–949. doi:10.1139/H09–078

Racinais, S., Gaoua, N., & Grantham, J. (2008). Hyperthermia impairs short-term memory and peripheral motor drive transmission. *J Physiol, 586*(19), 4751–4762. doi:10.1113/jphysiol.2008.157420

Rösch, D., Hodgson, R., Peterson, L., Graf-Baumann, T., Junge, A., Chomiak, J., & Dvorak, J. (2000). Assessment and evaluation of football performance. *Amer J Sports Medi, 28*(5 S29–S39).

Sawka, M. N., Burke, L. M., Eichner, E. R., Maughan, R. J., Montain, S. J., & Stachenfeld, N. S. (2007). American college of sports medicine position stand: exercise and fluid replacement. *Med Sci Sports Exerc, 39*(2), 377–390. doi:10.1249/mss.0b013e31802ca597

Schlader, Z. J., Gagnon, D., Adams, A., Rivas, E., Cullum, C. M., & Crandall, C. G. (2015). Cognitive and perceptual responses during passive heat stress in younger and older adults. *Am J Physiol Regul Integr Comp Physiol, 308*(10), R847–854. doi:10.1152/ajpregu.00010.2015

Schmitt, J. A., Benton, D., & Kallus, K. W. (2005). General methodological considerations for the assessment of nutritional influences on human cognitive functions. *Eur J Nutr, 44*(8), 459–464. doi:10.1007/s00394-005-0585-4

Shirreffs, S. M., Sawka, M. N., & Stone, M. (2006). Water and electrolyte needs for football training and match-play. *J Sports Sci, 24*(7), 699–707.

Simmons, S. E., Saxby, B. K., McGlone, F. P., & Jones, D. A. (2008). The effect of passive heating and head cooling on perception, cardiovascular function and cognitive performance in the heat. *Eur J Appl Physiol, 104*(2), 271–280. doi:10.1007/s00421-008-0677-y

Slattery, K., & Coutts, A. J. (2019). The application of heat stress to team sports: football/soccer, Australian football and rugby. In J. D. Periard & S. Racinais (Eds.), *Heat Stress in Sport and Exercise: Thermophysiology of Health and Performance* (pp. 181–202). Switzerland: Springer.

Sunderland, C., Morris, J. G., & Nevill, M. E. (2008). A heat acclimation protocol for team sports. *Br J Sports Med, 42*(5), 327–333. doi:10.1136/bjsm.2007.034207

Sunderland, C., & Nevill, M. (2003). Effect of the menstrual cycle on performance of intermittent, high-intensity shuttle running in a hot environment. *Eur J Appl Physiol, 88*(4–5), 345–352.

Webborn, A. D. J. (1996). Heat-related problems for the Paralympic Games, Atlanta 1996. *Br J Ther Rehab, 3*(8), 429–435.

Webborn, N. (2004). Sport and disability. *Br Med J, 12*(329), 0407275.

Webborn, N., Price, M. J., Castle, P., & Goosey-Tolfrey, V. L. (2010). Cooling strategies improve intermittent sprint performance in the heat of athletes with tetraplegia. *Br J Sports Med,* *44*(6), 455–460. doi:10.1136/bjsm.2007.043687

Wickham, K. A., Wallace, P. J., & Cheung, S. S. (2021). Sex differences in the physiological adaptations to heat acclimation: a state-of-the-art review. *Eur J Appl Physiol, 121*(2), 353–367. doi:10.1007/s00421-020-04550-y

Zurawlew, M. J., Mee, J. A., & Walsh, N. P. (2019). Post-exercise hot water immersion elicits heat acclimation adaptations that are retained for at least two weeks. *Front Physiol, 10*, 1080. doi:10.3389/fphys.2019.01080

# 5 Nutrition for match play and training

*James P. Morton, Liam Anderson, Hannah Sheridan and Graeme L. Close*

## Introduction

The importance of nutrition is now widely recognised by professional soccer players, support staff, and coaches. In 2021, UEFA published an expert group statement on nutrition in elite football (Collins et al., 2021). A specific call was made for clubs to adopt an integrated and evidence-based nutrition support programme that positively affects the performance, health, and well-being of players (Wenger, 2021). In the coming decade, it is likely that professional soccer clubs worldwide will employ accredited sports nutritionists and dieticians on a full-time basis, with the remit of delivering an evidence-based nutrition service to adult and academy soccer players.

The primary focus of the performance nutritionist should be to formulate nutritional strategies that ensure that players' daily energy requirements are being met by sufficient energy and macronutrient intake. Using the gold standard technique of doubly labelled water, the energy expenditures of adult players have been quantified as 40–60 kcal kg$^{-1}$ fat-free mass (FFM), whereas players undergoing growth and maturation tend to exhibit higher relative energy expenditures of 60–80 kcal kg$^{-1}$ FFM (see Figure 5.1). In accordance with changes in loading patterns as well as individual player training objectives, a player's nutritional requirements are not static and likely change throughout the micro-, meso-, and macro-cycles. For this reason, the concept of nutritional periodisation is gaining increased popularity amongst academics and practitioners (Stellingwerff et al., 2019; Anderson et al., 2022).

In this chapter, we provide an overview of the scientific basis of performance nutrition in terms of the key macronutrient (i.e., carbohydrates (CHOs) and protein), micronutrient (i.e., iron, vitamin D, and calcium), and fluid requirements for professional players. Additionally, we discuss nutritional considerations for female and adolescent players before outlining some evidence-based ergogenic aids (i.e., caffeine, creatine, beta-alanine, and nitrate) that may enhance aspects of physical performance. We close by offering critical reflections from applied practice.

## Carbohydrate (CHO) requirements

The importance of CHO and muscle glycogen availability for soccer-specific physical performance was recognised in the 1970s (Saltin, 1973). It was demonstrated that commencing match play with low versus high muscle glycogen (<200 versus >400 mmol kg$^{-1}$ dw) reduced the total distance covered by 20% (9.7 km versus 12 km, respectively). Krustrup et al. (2006) observed that match play decreases muscle glycogen by approximately

DOI: 10.4324/9781003148418-6

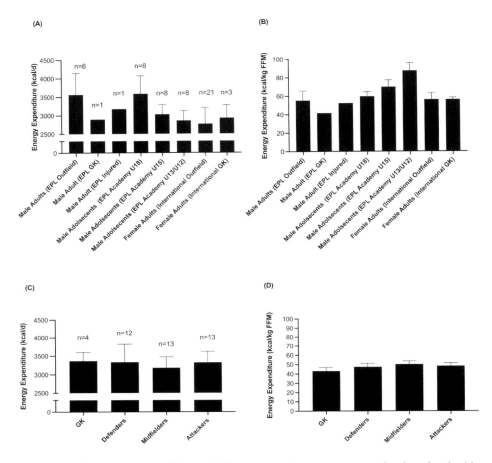

*Figure 5.1* The energy expenditure of elite soccer players, as assessed using the doubly labelled water method. Data presented in panels A and B represent male adult and adolescent players from the English Premier League (EPL) and are redrawn from Anderson et al. (2017a, 2018, 2019) and Hannon et al. (2021). Adult female players are representative of international standard (Morehen et al., 2022). Data presented in panels C and D represent adult male players from the Dutch Premier League (data redrawn from Brinkmans et al., 2019).

50%, with pre-game values decreasing from 449 ± 23 mmol kg$^{-1}$ dw to 225 ± 23 mmol kg$^{-1}$ dw immediately after match play. Although post-game glycogen values suggest sufficient availability to continue exercising, analysis of individual muscle fibre types revealed that 50% of fibres are classified as *empty* or *almost empty*. This pattern of depletion or near depletion was evident in type IIa and IIx fibres, the fibres responsible for sprinting and high-intensity activity. As such, glycogen depletion is cited as a contributing factor for the progressive reduction in high-intensity running and sprinting that occurs throughout the course of a game (Mohr et al., 2003). For this reason, CHO is considered the most important macronutrient to promote soccer-specific physical performance. An overview of CHO recommendations is presented in Table 5.1.

*Table 5.1* An overview of CHO recommendations for soccer match play and training

| Scenario | Nutritional and physiological objectives | Suggested CHO range | Practical considerations |
|---|---|---|---|
| **CHO recommendations for match play** | | | |
| MD-1 | • To facilitate muscle glycogen storage | 6–8 g kg$^{-1}$ BM | Emphasise low-fibre foods that are moderate to high glycaemic in nature so as to promote digestion, absorption, and glycogen storage. CHO-containing fluids and snacks are a practical approach to achieving daily CHO intakes. |
| Breakfast/pre-match meal | • To facilitate liver and muscle glycogen storage | 1–3 g kg$^{-1}$ BM | Emphasise low-fibre foods that are moderate to high glycaemic in nature so as to promote digestion, absorption, and glycogen storage. CHO-containing fluids and snacks are a practical approach to achieving CHO intakes at this time. |
| In-game | • To maintain plasma glucose concentration<br>• To reduce liver glycogen utilization<br>• To maintain whole-body rates of CHO oxidation | 30–60 g h$^{-1}$ | Total CHO intake for a 90–95 min match may equate to 60–120 g. Consider distributing CHO intake in equal 20–30 g doses before the warm-up, end of warm-up, half-time, and mid-second half. Consider using a combination of isotonic gels and fluids to achieve these targets. Practice and refine each player's individual strategy during training. |
| Post-game | • To facilitate muscle and liver glycogen resynthesis | 1.2 g kg$^{-1}$ h$^{-1}$ for 3–4 h | Emphasise low-fibre foods and fluids that are highly glycaemic in nature so as to promote digestion, absorption, and short-term glycogen storage. The provision of fructose may also promote liver glycogen storage. |
| **Daily CHO recommendations for training** | | | |
| Pre-season training | • Increase aerobic and anaerobic fitness<br>• Increase/maximise strength, speed, power for performance, and injury prevention<br>• Increase lean mass/reduce fat mass | 4–8 g kg$^{-1}$ BM | Suggested range accommodates likely variations in loads (e.g., potential twice per day sessions, recovery days) as well as individual training goals (e.g., manipulation of body composition to accommodate weight loss and fat loss or weight gain and lean mass gain). For example, twice per day training structures would likely require higher CHO intakes (e.g., 6–8 g kg$^{-1}$ BM/day) whereas lower absolute intakes may be required where players are aiming for body fat loss or training intensity and duration are reduced (e.g., 4–6 g kg$^{-1}$ BM/day). |

(*Continued*)

| Scenario | Nutritional and physiological objectives | Suggested CHO range | Practical considerations |
|---|---|---|---|
| In-season training (one game per week) | • Maintain (or increase) aerobic and anaerobic fitness<br>• Maintain (or increase) strength, power, and speed<br>• Maintain (or increase) lean body mass | 3–8 g kg$^{-1}$ BM | Suggested range accommodates likely variations in loads across the micro-cycle (e.g., low load days and MD-1 CHO loading protocols) as well as individual training goals (e.g., manipulation of body composition). For example, MD-1 and MD+1 would require higher CHO intakes (e.g., 6–8 g kg$^{-1}$ BM/day) whereas lower absolute intakes may be required on other days of the week (e.g., 3–6 g kg$^{-1}$ BM/day) depending on training intensity, duration, and player-specific goals. |
| In-season training (congested fixture periods) | • Restore muscle function as quickly as possible<br>• Promote glycogen resynthesis<br>• Rehydration<br>• Alleviate mental fatigue | 6–8 g kg$^{-1}$ BM | Suggested range accommodates the requirement to replenish muscle glycogen stores in the 48–72 h period between games. During this time, it is suggested that players consistently consume CHO within this range so as to promote glycogen availability. |
| Off-season training | • Minimise the loss of aerobic and anaerobic capacity<br>• Minimise decrements in strength, power, and speed<br>• Minimise decreases in lean mass and increases in fat mass | <4 g kg$^{-1}$ BM | Suggested intake accommodates the cessation of normal training loads, to avoid gains in fat mass. Note, for players who may be undergoing higher training loads (e.g., off-season training programmes) CHO intake should be increased accordingly. |

## CHO requirements on match day minus 1 (MD-1)

In accordance with the role of muscle glycogen in promoting high-intensity intermittent exercise performance (Saltin, 1973; Bangsbo et al., 1992; Balsom et al., 1999), the major goal of nutritional interventions in the day prior to the game (often referred to MD-1) should be to ensure sufficient pre-game muscle and liver glycogen stores. Professional players are likely to achieve high glycogen stores with as little as 24–36 h of a CHO-rich diet (Bussau et al., 2002) providing that training intensity and duration are significantly reduced on MD-1 (Anderson et al., 2015). To help promote muscle glycogen storage, it is recommended players consume larger portion sizes and frequency of high glycaemic index foods and drinks (Burke et al., 1993), where daily intakes should at least equate to 6–8 g.kg$^{-1}$ BM. It is noteworthy, however, that professional players from the English Premier League (EPL) are reported to consume as little as 4 g.kg$^{-1}$ BM on MD-1, values that may reduce the total distance covered on match day when compared with 8 g.kg$^{-1}$ (Souglis et al., 2013). Further research is required to verify the glycogen cost of match play in elite professional players and the associated effects of muscle glycogen availability on physical and technical performance during match play.

## CHO requirements for the pre-match meal

In contrast to increasing muscle glycogen storage, the pre-match meal is important for augmenting liver glycogen storage, a goal that becomes particularly relevant for late morning or lunch-time kick-offs (Nicholas et al. 1995 and Foskett et al. 2008). Liver glycogen may be depleted by as much as 50% after an overnight fast and may not fully recover until early evening, depending on the frequency and dose of CHO consumed (Iwayma et al., 2020). Although the ergogenic effects of pre-exercise CHO availability on endurance performance are documented, the topic has been largely under-researched in team sport athletes. Nonetheless, research from academy EPL soccer demonstrates improved dribbling performance during the second half of a 90-min soccer match play simulation when a breakfast containing 80 g versus 40 g of CHO was consumed (Briggs et al., 2017). It is recommended that this meal be consumed approximately 3 h before kick-off and contains at least 1–3 g.kg$^{-1}$ BM. Professional players from the EPL have been reported to consume CHO intakes equating to 1–1.5 g.kg$^{-1}$ BM in the pre-match meal, values that could be sub-optimal for performance when considered with insufficient CHO intakes on MD-1 (Anderson et al., 2017a).

### In-game CHO requirements

There is sufficient evidence to demonstrate that CHO feeding during exercise is likely to improve elements of match-day performance (Baker et al., 2015; Russell & Kingsley, 2014) when fed at a rate of 30–60 g h$^{-1}$. Such ingestion rates have been shown to improve physical aspects of performance such as total distance (Rodriguez-Giustiniani et al., 2019) and sprint distance (Harper et al., 2017) covered as well as the technical actions of passing (Currell et al., 2009), dribbling (Currell et al., 2009), and shooting (Russell et al., 2012). When considering the duration of the warm-up (e.g., 20–30 min) and match play itself (e.g., 90–95 min), this ingestion rate is likely to correspond to an absolute dose of CHO equating to 60–120 g. We suggest that players may benefit from

72    *James P. Morton et al.*

CHO intake at the beginning (e.g., 20–30 g) and end of the warm-up period (20–30 g) as well as the half-time period (30–40 g) and if possible, during the second half (20–30 g). We acknowledge, however, that larger boluses of 30 g before the match itself and at half-time may facilitate performance (Harper et al., 2017). The provision of CHO gels, as opposed to fluids, may prove advantageous owing to the flexibility of achieving CHO targets in those instances where players may not tolerate or require such large volumes of fluid from sports drinks. Like MD-1 and pre-match meal, we observed that professional players from the EPL do not readily achieve in-game CHO guidelines (Anderson et al., 2017a), with most players consuming <30 g $h^{-1}$.

### *Post-game CHO requirements*

In relation to acute muscle glycogen re-synthesis, the consensus is that consuming 1.2 g.$kg^{-1}$ $h^{-1}$ of high glycaemic CHO for 3–4 h is optimal to facilitate short-term glycogen re-synthesis (Burke et al., 2016). Post-match feeding should begin immediately after match play (i.e., in the changing room) as this is when the muscle is most receptive to glucose uptake and the enzymes responsible for glycogen synthesis are most active (Ivy et al., 1988). Post-match intake of CHO has also been identified as an area where players may not adhere to best practice guidelines, especially in recovery from evening games. For example, in recovery from a match commenced at 8:15 pm, EPL players reported consuming <1 g.$kg^{-1}$ $h^{-1}$ in the initial 2-h recovery period whereas CHO intake in recovery from a 4:15 pm kick-off increased to 1–1.5 g.$kg^{-1}$ $h^{-1}$ (Anderson et al., 2017b). Such differences between kick-off times may be because players do not feel like eating or drinking after late-night games and/or the logistical challenges of ensuring food availability, especially where recovery corresponds with late-night travel schedules.

Given the time course required to fully replenish muscle glycogen (i.e., 24–72 h), there is a requirement to consume adequate CHO on the day(s) after the match, often referred to as MD+1. In the previously cited study, the EPL players were required to compete in another competitive game 72 h later and yet, daily CHO intake in the 48-h period between games was only 4 g.$kg^{-1}$ (Anderson et al., 2017a). These intakes are considerably less than the range of 6–9 g.$kg^{-1}$ that has been documented to facilitate glycogen re-synthesis in a cohort of Danish players within 2–3 days of match play (Krustrup et al., 2011; Gunnarsson et al., 2013). Nonetheless, while recovery of glycogen appeared complete when assessed in whole muscle homogenate and type I fibres at 48 h post-match play, complete restoration of type II fibres was still not apparent (Gunnarrson et al., 2013). Such data clearly highlight the need for high daily CHO intakes in recovery from match play, especially in those situations of two and three games per week micro-cycles.

## CHO requirements for training

Based on different physical loads associated with training and match play (see Table 5.2), daily CHO and within-day CHO distribution patterns should differ accordingly. Professional players report consuming less CHO on training days versus match days. Brinkmans et al. (2019) reported daily CHO intakes of <4 g.$kg^{-1}$ in professional players from the Dutch Premier League on training and rest days. Additionally, we observed comparable CHO intakes of 4 g.$kg^{-1}$ in EPL players during training days (Anderson et al., 2017a).

Table 5.2 A suggested practical model of the "fuel for the work required" CHO periodisation paradigm as applied to professional soccer players during a one-game-per-week schedule with match day on Saturday. Representative loads are taken from Anderson et al. (2015)

| | Typical external load | Breakfast | During training | Lunch | Snack(s) | Dinner |
|---|---|---|---|---|---|---|
| Monday (MD+2) | No training | Medium CHO 0.5–1 g kg$^{-1}$ | No training | Medium CHO 1 g kg$^{-1}$ | Medium CHO 0.5–1 g kg$^{-1}$ | Medium CHO 1 g kg$^{-1}$ |
| Tuesday (MD-4) | Duration = 70–80 min TD = ~5000 m HSR = <100 m | Medium CHO 1 g kg$^{-1}$ | No CHO | High CHO 1.5–2 g kg$^{-1}$ | Medium CHO 0.5–1 g kg$^{-1}$ | Medium CHO 1 g kg$^{-1}$ |
| Wednesday (MD-3) | Duration = 80–90 min TD = 6500 m HSR = 300–600 m | High CHO 1.5–2 g kg$^{-1}$ | No CHO | High CHO 1.5–2 g kg$^{-1}$ | Medium CHO 0.5–1 g kg$^{-1}$ | Medium CHO 0.5–1 g kg$^{-1}$ |
| Thursday (MD-2) | Duration = <70 min TD = <4500 m HSR = <100 m | Low CHO 0.5 g kg$^{-1}$ | No CHO | High CHO 1.5–2 g kg$^{-1}$ | Medium CHO 0.5–1 g kg$^{-1}$ | Medium CHO 0.5–1 g kg$^{-1}$ |
| Friday (MD-1) | Duration = <60 min TD = <3000 m HSR = <50 m | High CHO 2 g kg$^{-1}$ | High CHO 60 g hr$^{-1}$ | High CHO 2 g kg$^{-1}$ | High CHO 1.5 g kg$^{-1}$ | High CHO 2 g kg$^{-1}$ |
| Saturday (MD) | Duration = 90–95 min TD ~11 km HSR = ~1000 m | Breakfast High CHO 2 g kg$^{-1}$ | Pre-match meal High CHO 2 g kg$^{-1}$ | During game High CHO 30–60 g hr$^{-1}$ | Post-match High CHO 1.2 g kg hr$^{-1}$ for 3 h | |
| Sunday (MD+1) | Recovery session | Breakfast High CHO 2 g kg$^{-1}$ | During training High CHO 60 g hr$^{-1}$ | Lunch High CHO 2 g kg$^{-1}$ | Snack High CHO 1.5 g kg$^{-1}$ | Dinner High CHO 2 g kg$^{-1}$ |

MD = Match day, TD = Total distance, HSR = High-speed running, CHO = Carbohydrate.

The assessment of energy expenditure in these studies (i.e., approximately 3000–3500 kcal $d^{-1}$, equivalent to ~47–55 kcal $kg^{-1}$ FFM) provides a basis from which to formulate daily CHO requirements (Anderson et al. 2017a; Brinkmans et al. 2019). Since daily protein recommendations range from 1.6 to 2.2 g $kg^{-1}$, and that recommended fat intakes are equivalent to 30% of total energy intake (Collins et al., 2021), an average daily CHO intake of 3–6 g $kg^{-1}$ would be sufficient to meet the daily energy requirements that encompass the typical range in training intensity and duration associated with in-season training schedules. When considered in combination with the requirement to promote glycogen storage on MD-1 and MD+1, we suggest that daily CHO requirements for training should operate on a sliding scale of 3–8 g $kg^{-1}$ body mass per day depending on the specific training scenario, fixture schedule, and player-specific training goals (see Table 5.1).

## Practical CHO periodisation strategies

In addition to simply matching energy intake to energy demands, the rationale for practical application of CHO periodisation strategies has been developed on the premise that commencing and/or recovering from exercise with reduced CHO availability up-regulates cell signalling pathways that regulate oxidative adaptations of human skeletal muscle. While research has largely been explored using protocols relevant to endurance athletes (see Impey et al., 2018), such adaptations may manifest in high-intensity intermittent exercise protocols. Commencing high-intensity intermittent running with reduced pre-exercise muscle glycogen (and without provision of CHO during exercise) augments training-induced up-regulation of oxidative enzyme activity in both the gastrocnemius and vastus lateralis muscle, as compared with conditions of normal muscle glycogen and consumption of CHO during training (Morton et al., 2009). The principle of "fueling for the work required" is a practical framework to adjust CHO intake day-by-day and meal-by-meal according to the metabolic demands and training goals of the upcoming training sessions (Impey et al., 2018). On this basis, we provide a theoretical overview of day-by-day and meal-by-meal CHO intakes in Table 5.2. In this scenario, a one-game-per-week micro-cycle is presented, whereby daily CHO intake on training days is equivalent to 4 g $kg^{-1}$ but increased to 8 g $kg^{-1}$ on MD-1, MD, and MD+1. In accordance with the lower physical loading on training days, CHO intake is reduced at breakfast and no CHO is consumed during training. On such days, the largest portion of CHO is consumed in the post-training meal (i.e., lunch) to facilitate glycogen re-synthesis (Ivy et al., 1988). Finally, CHO intake is reduced in the evening meal because the upcoming physical load on the subsequent day does not likely require high CHO availability to complete the desired training demands. In contrast to a one-game-per-week micro-cycle, daily CHO intake should be increased to at least 6–8 g $kg^{-1}$ during those instances where consecutive games are interspersed with only 2–3 days of recovery. A critical discussion of CHO periodisation for soccer is also provided by Anderson et al. (2022).

## Protein requirements

Protein does not provide a substantial contribution towards energy production during exercise. The amino acids we obtain from dietary protein sources are used to support whole body and muscle protein synthesis throughout the day. In this way, protein plays an important modulatory role in remodelling of musculoskeletal and tendinous structures in response to training. Although exercise itself stimulates muscle protein synthesis,

*Nutrition for match play and training* 75

when completed in the fasted state muscle protein degradation occurs such that a net negative protein balance is present. In the presence of adequate protein feeding, however, the combined effects of exercise and protein ingestion augment muscle protein synthesis such that a net protein balance occurs. It is these repeated changes in protein turnover (in favour of protein synthesis to yield a positive protein balance) which form the molecular basis of how skeletal muscle and related tissues adapt to the demands of training.

## Daily protein requirements

A daily intake of 1.6–2.2 g kg$^{-1}$ per day is recommended for endurance and strength athletes (Morton et al., 2018); a value twice that of the RDA for Europeans. Professional players from the EPL habitually exceed these daily targets with intakes of 2.5 g kg$^{-1}$ reported during a two-game-per-week micro-cycle (Anderson et al., 2017a). The reported absolute daily protein intakes (205 ± 30 g) are like those reported (150–200 g) in adult professional players from the Dutch Premier League (Bettonviel et al., 2016), but are higher than that reported over two decades ago (Maughan, 1997) in British professional players (108 ± 26 g). Such differences between eras are potentially driven by the increased practitioner, player, and coach awareness of the role of protein in facilitating training adaptations and recovery from both aerobic and strength training (MacNaughton et al., 2016). Additionally, the higher daily protein intakes reported may be driven by the increased use of protein supplements, a practice that seems to be commonplace amongst players. This is especially the case in acute recovery from training and match play where 20–30 g boluses are often consumed (Anderson et al., 2017b).

## Daily protein distribution

The pattern of daily protein distribution may be important in modulating protein synthesis. A total of 20 g boluses consumed every 3 h is superior to larger boluses consumed less frequently, as is the case for both whole body (Moore et al., 2012) and muscle protein synthesis (Areta et al., 2013). It is recommended that daily protein intakes be distributed across four meals each containing 0.4 g kg$^{-1}$ per meal (Collins et al., 2021). Such a pattern of intake would readily achieve the lower end of the total daily requirement cited above and is likely to align with traditional meal timings of breakfast, lunch, and dinner. In relation to exercise, protein should be consumed near the cessation of the training session or match so as to stimulate remodelling of tissues. Dose-response studies demonstrate that 30 g (0.49 g kg$^{-1}$) is optimal in stimulating muscle protein synthesis (Churchward-Venne et al., 2020). In practice, post-exercise ingestion of protein in the immediate recovery period is often achieved by protein supplements in the form of drinks or bars. Given its higher leucine content and rapid digestion, whey protein supplements are superior to casein and soy-based formulations for activating muscle protein synthesis (Tang et al., 2009). Liquid forms of protein induce a more rapid rise in plasma amino acids than solid foods and may therefore be considered a superior strategy in the post-exercise period (Burke et al., 2012).

## Additional considerations

Given that sleep is effectively a period of prolonged fasting (e.g., 6–10 h) which induces muscle protein degradation, there is a rationale to ingest a suitable quantity of protein prior to bed. Ingestion of 0.4 g kg$^{-1}$ of protein within 1–2 h before sleep stimulates muscle protein synthesis and improves overnight protein balance when compared with no protein feeding (Trommelen et al., 2018; Snijders et al., 2015). Consuming protein prior to sleep augments training-induced increases in muscle mass and strength (Snijders et al., 2015). Professional EPL players reported an intake of only 0.1 g kg$^{-1}$ at this time-point (Anderson et al., 2017b), thus highlighting an important feeding opportunity for those players aiming to gain and/or maintain muscle mass. In relation to the latter, the requirement to manipulate body composition (i.e., reduce fat mass in tandem with maintaining or increasing muscle mass) is often a fundamental training objective, especially during the pre-season period. To offset the effects of energy restriction on protein catabolism, increasing daily protein intake to 3 × RDA (i.e., 2.4 g kg$^{-1}$), alongside a resistance training programme, can maintain or increase muscle mass despite a reduction in daily energy intake (Longland et al., 2016). Increased daily protein intake may prove beneficial in reducing muscle atrophy (Anderson et al., 2019) that can occur during times of prolonged injury. In such conditions, the absolute loading of skeletal muscle is significantly reduced, and players are prone to reducing their total daily energy intake in the belief that it will prevent gains in fat mass during a time of reduced training load (Milsom et al., 2014).

## Fluid requirements

### *Dehydration and performance*

Metabolic heat production can increase rectal and muscle temperature to >39°C during match play (Mohr et al., 2004). Sweat losses of 2 L have been observed during both match play and training (Rollo et al., 2021), even when ambient temperature is <10°C (Maughan et al., 2007). Dehydration >2% body mass loss reduces repeated sprint capacity (Mohr et al., 2010) as well as dribbling performance (McGregor et al., 1999). Potential mechanisms underpinning dehydration-induced decrements in physical and mental performance include increased core temperature, cardiovascular strain, muscle glycogen depletion, and impaired brain function (Gonzalez-Alonso, 2007). From observations of players during training and match play, sweat loss appears to be lower in temperate (<15°C) compared with warm environments (25–35°C) (Kurdak et al., 2010; Rollo et al., 2021). To compensate for the warmer conditions, players consume significantly more fluid during training (Rollo et al., 2021). The development of fatigue during match play is more pronounced during high ambient temperatures (Mohr et al., 2010). In addition to fluid loss, sweat contains electrolytes such as sodium, chloride, potassium, calcium, and magnesium. Loss of sodium is the most significant for athletes (given its role in promoting fluid retention) and players can lose between 2 and 3 g during training or match play (Kurdak et al., 2010; Maughan et al., 2007). It is, therefore, important to identify players who are *salty sweaters* to develop individually tailored hydration strategies.

## Practical assessment of hydration status

Pre-training or pre-match assessments of urine osmolality and colour provides reasonably inexpensive and informative measures. Osmolality values <700 m Osmol kg$^{-1}$

*Nutrition for match play and training*   77

are suggestive of euhydration as is a urine colour that is pale yellow. Urine indices of hydration are sensitive to changes in posture, food intake, and body water content and for these reasons, a urine sample passed upon waking is often advised as the criterion sample. However, values indicative of dehydration at this time (e.g., 7:00 am) may not mean the player is dehydrated upon commencing training at 10:30 am, assuming that appropriate fluid intake has been consumed upon waking and with breakfast. The same can be said for match day in that samples suggestive of dehydration collected prior to the pre-match meal may not mean players are dehydrated at kick-off. Players should be assessed at both the former and latter time-points to initially identify players who are causes for concern and to verify that any subsequent hydration strategies implemented are effective to ensure euhydration prior to competition. Soccer players studied prior to an evening kick-off have exhibited pre-game osmolality values >900 m Osmol kg$^{-1}$ (Maughan et al., 2007), despite the fact that they would have had the morning and afternoon to hydrate. Such values are indicative of 2% dehydration and effectively mean that players are commencing the game dehydrated thereby running the risk of impaired physical and mental performance.

## Fluid requirements

It is difficult to provide fixed prescriptive fluid recommendations for soccer players due to differences in workload, heat acclimatisation, training status, and match-to-match variations in ambient temperatures. The American College of Sports Medicine advises fluid ingestion at a rate that limits body mass loss to <2% of pre-exercise values (Thomas et al., 2016). Players should not aim to drink to gain mass during exercise as this can lead to water intoxification, a condition known as hyponatremia (a serum sodium concentration <135 mmol L$^{-1}$) which in extreme cases is fatal. It is recommended that 5–7 ml kg$^{-1}$ of fluid is consumed at least 3–4 h prior to the game. Additionally, if the individual does not produce urine or the urine remains dark in colour, a further 3–5 ml kg$^{-1}$ could be consumed 2 h before kick-off. Consumption of sports drinks, as opposed to water, is beneficial given that they contain electrolytes and CHO. For training days, fluid intake should be consumed upon waking (before travelling to training) and with breakfast, where the latter is often consumed at the training ground.

To promote a drinking strategy which prevents weight losses >2%, players should routinely weigh themselves nude before and after exercise to ascertain if their habitual drinking patterns are effective. Cold beverages (10°C as opposed to 37°C or 50°C) are beneficial to attenuate the rise in body temperature during exercise (Lee & Shirreffs, 2007). It is important that players practice with different fluid intake strategies during training so as to develop individually suited approaches which maximise gastric emptying, fluid absorption, and CHO delivery but yet are suited for taste and do not cause gastrointestinal discomfort during match-play. Finally, there is likely no need for aggressive re-hydration strategies post-training (unless there is an afternoon training session and ambient temperature is high) or match play as the normal schedule would allow for appropriate re-hydration within several hours post-exercise. Nevertheless, those players identified as salty sweaters may benefit

## Nutritional considerations for female players

Based on current evidence (Moore et al., 2021), it is premature to substantiate that a female player requires specific guidelines in relation to the macronutrient requirements described previously. The primary focus is to ensure female players consume sufficient energy, macronutrient, and micronutrient intake to reduce the risk of negative symptoms associated with the Female Athlete Triad or Relative Energy Deficiency in Sport (RED-S) syndrome (Mountjoy et al., 2014). Low energy availability (LEA) is one of three inter-related components of the Female Athlete Triad and is purported to be the contributory cause of impaired menstrual function and bone health (Loucks et al., 2011). Energy availability (EA) is expressed relative to FFM and is defined as the amount of energy that is available to support body functions after subtracting the amount of energy that is expended during exercise. In considering the RED-S model (Mountjoy et al., 2014), the consequence of LEA is thought to extend to multiple health (e.g., reduced immune function, cardiovascular function, and protein synthesis) and performance (e.g., reduced strength, power, and endurance), indices beyond that of menstrual function and bone health.

When classifying values >45, 30–45, and <30 kcal $kg^{-1}$ FFM as optimal, reduced, and LEA (Loucks et al., 2011), it was recently identified that only 15% of professional players from a Women's Super League team were deemed optimal (Moss et al., 2020). It was observed that players did not adjust daily energy or CHO intake on harder training or match days (i.e., exercise energy expenditure >700 kcal) when compared with lighter training (i.e., exercise energy expenditure <400 kcal) or complete rest days. As such, the prevalence of players presenting with LEA increased from 40% on light training days to 70% on harder training days. In studying a cohort of adult female players of international standard, Morehen et al. (2022) reported that only one player (from a sample of 23) consumed CHO on MD-1 that was greater than 6 g $kg^{-1}$ body mass. Such data clearly highlight the necessity for practitioners to emphasise appropriate "fuelling" in female players. In using the doubly labelled water technique, these researchers also observed a relative energy expenditure (40-60 kcal $kg^{-1}$ FFM) that was comparable to male players (Morehen et al., 2022).

Given that exercise performance may be trivially impaired in the early follicular phase (McNulty et al., 2020), and that negative physical symptoms are often reported at the onset or during menses (Findlay et al., 2020), specific attention should be given to CHO availability during this phase of the cycle. This is especially relevant in congested fixture schedules or intense training periods where glycogen availability may be limiting to performance. At present, practitioners should adopt an individualised approach that considers player-specific training and match schedules whilst considering personal symptoms associated with the menstrual cycle. Further assessments of the energetic requirements of adult and academy female players (alongside prevalence of RED-S) is a recommended area for future research. When assessing the efficacy of any novel nutritional strategy, researchers should also adopt soccer-specific competition and training-related exercise protocols that rigorously control for prior exercise, CHO/energy intake, contraceptive use, and phase of menstrual cycle.

## Nutritional considerations for adolescent players

In the adolescent player, prolonged periods of insufficient energy intake can compromise growth and maturation as well as affect the ability to tolerate daily loading. An increase in resting metabolic rate (RMR) of ~400 kcal day$^{-1}$ occurs between ages 12 and 16, thus highlighting the requirement to adjust daily energy intake to support growth and maturation (see Figure 5.2). In addition, daily total energy expenditure (TEE) progressively increases as players transition through the academy pathway (see Figure 5.1). For example, U18 players presented with a TEE (3586 ± 487 kcal day$^{-1}$) that was approximately 600 and 700 kcal day$^{-1}$ higher than both the U15 (3029 ± 262 kcal day$^{-1}$) and U12/13 players (2859 ± 265 kcal day$^{-1}$), respectively (Hannon et al., 2021). Such differences in TEE are likely due to differences in anthropometric profile, RMR, and physical loading between squads. Some individuals (in all age groups) have presented a TEE that is comparable to, or exceeds that, previously reported in adult Premier League soccer players. Clearly, the practice of nutritional periodisation and reduced periods of energy intake (to reduce fat mass) is not recommended for players who are not yet fully mature. The principle of ensuring consistent daily energy, CHO,

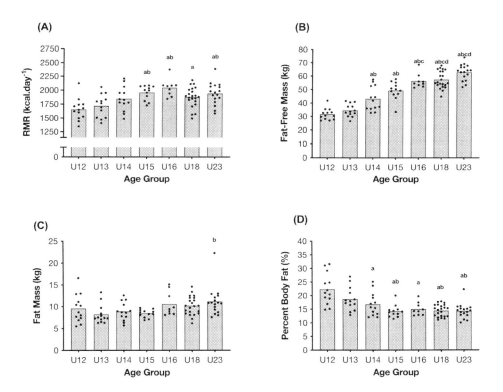

*Figure 5.2* (a) Resting metabolic rate (RMR), (b) fat-free mass, (c) fat mass, and (d) percent body fat between in adolescent male soccer players (U12–U23 age groups; n = 99) from an English Premier League academy.

a significant difference from the U12 age group, [b]significant difference from the U13 age group, [c]significant difference from the U14 age group, [d]significant difference from the U15 age group, all $P < 0.05$. Data redrawn from Hannon et al. (2020). Black dots represent individual players.

80 *James P. Morton et al.*

and protein availability should be practised. From observations of academy players who did not display any loss in body mass over a 2-week period, daily CHO, protein, and fat intakes ranging from 5 to 8, 1.6 to 2.2, and 1.5 to 2.5 g kg$^{-1}$ body mass, respectively, appear appropriate to meet daily energy requirements (Hannon et al., 2021).

## Micronutrient considerations

Micronutrients (typically classified as vitamins and minerals) are compounds that are required in small quantities (<1 g) to maintain normal physiological function. Although they do not directly supply energy, micronutrients play essential roles in several metabolic pathways. Most micronutrients will be obtained comfortably in a player's everyday diet without the need for supplementation. However, there may be specific situations that could contribute to a player presenting with micronutrient deficiency. These include players who consciously eliminate food groups (because of food dislikes, allergies, or moral/ethical and religious reasons), LEA (may occur when players are attempting to reduce body fat or during intense training and/or fixture schedules), a lack of variety in the diet or a lack of sunlight exposure (including constant use of sunscreens or protective clothing).

It has been suggested that soccer players should pay specific attention to vitamin D, calcium, and iron status (Collins et al., 2021). Vitamin D is a unique vitamin given that it is predominantly synthesised in the skin *via* sunlight exposure, with only around 10% of our daily needs coming from the diet (Owens et al., 2018). Given that many countries have low sunlight exposure (especially in the winter months), it is not surprising that players present with vitamin D deficiencies. EPL players exhibit a 50% decline in vitamin D between August and December (Morton et al., 2012). Inadequate vitamin D concentrations can impair muscle function and recovery (Owens et al., 2015) as well as compromise immune health (He et al., 2013). Vitamin D is assessed by measuring serum 25(OH)D and whilst there is controversy as to what defines a true vitamin D deficiency, it is generally accepted that <50 nmol L$^{-1}$ is deficient with emerging research suggesting that 75 nmol L$^{-1}$ may be a suitable target concentration for players.

Iron is the functional component of haemoglobin and myoglobin as well as being an essential constituent of mitochondrial enzymes. Iron deficiencies, even without anaemia, can have major effects on aerobic performance (DellaValle & Haas, 2011). Although iron deficiency is common in many athletes (Clenin et al., 2015) (with a prevalence of 15–35% in female athletes and 5–11% in male athletes), the iron status of professional soccer players at various stages of the season is not well characterised. Iron deficiencies present as lethargy and reduce athletic performance and, like vitamin D, are usually identified through routine blood screening. It has been suggested that female athletes should be assessed for iron deficiency at least biannually and even quarterly if there are any suspicions of factors that could indicate low iron status such as LEA, irregular menses, and high training loads (Sim et al., 2019).

Calcium status is somewhat difficult to assess since serum calcium concentration is tightly regulated regardless of acute calcium intake. The largest store of calcium is in skeleton, and it is this store that is utilised as an immediate supply of calcium when dietary intake is inadequate. The consequence of this mobilisation of calcium is demineralisation of bone tissue through the action of parathyroid hormone which long term could lead to numerous health problems including stress fractures. Specific attention should be given to those players who eliminate food sources such as dairy products and those presenting with LEA. The function, recommended nutrient intake (RNI), food sources, and potential supplement strategy for vitamin D, calcium, and iron are displayed in Table 5.3.

## Supplement considerations

There are hundreds of commercially available supplements that are purported to improve muscle strength, power, speed, and endurance as well as prevent (and promote recovery from) illness and injury. It is unsurprising that elite players, coaches, and sport science staff are often overwhelmed when faced with the challenge of developing a practical and evidence-based supplement strategy that is ergogenic for soccer match play and training. Additionally, many of the sports supplements commonly used by professional players are commercially driven (as opposed to evidence-based) and based on lucrative sponsorship deals to the individual player, club, and/or the governing body of the professional league in question. Most importantly, the chosen approach to supplementation should adhere to the World Anti-Doping Association (WADA) code of conduct in that all supplements are free from contamination with prohibited substances. Table 5.4 provides an overview of those supplements that we consider suitable for practical use for match play and training (for further reading, see Collins et al., 2021).

## Practitioner reflections

### Critical reflections on the soccer environment

Translating the relevant science into a practical performance nutrition program should, in principle, be a relatively straightforward process. In practice, however, there are many cultural, organisational, financial, and political factors that occur in the day-to-day running of a professional soccer club which greatly affect the quality and extent of the service provided. The initial challenge is to establish sound working relationships with the wider multi-disciplinary sports science and medical team (e.g., club doctors, fitness and conditioning staff, and physiotherapists), club catering staff and of course, those influential players who can act as positive role models (e.g., team captain and senior professionals). It is common for many individuals to have prior beliefs and biases as to what constitutes the "best" diet for a soccer player. The performance nutritionist will often be challenged by the unqualified opinions of others, some of which can be greatly impacted by the "Twitter" and "Netflix" culture of changing rooms. Getting everyone "on the same page" as to the performance benefits of evidence-based nutrition is therefore an essential element of the role. Unlike traditional endurance sports (e.g., cycling and running), however, demonstrating a measurable impact of the performance nutrition programme is not always easy. Commencing match play with optimal muscle glycogen concentration may not necessarily translate to more passes completed or games won. Rationalising the financial investment required to deliver a high-quality nutrition programme can therefore be hard to justify to those key stakeholders above

*Table 5.3* An overview of specific vitamin and minerals that have been highlighted as a potential cause for concern for soccer players (Collins et al., 2021), including their physiological function, recommended nutrient intake (RNI), typical food sources, and potential supplement strategy if required. Note that RNIs vary for different countries, and for differing ages, therefore, the numbers provided here may not be precise for all countries and all situations

| | RNI | | Food sources | Supplement strategy (if required) |
|---|---|---|---|---|
| | **Male** | **Female** | | |
| **Vitamin D** | NO DRVs because of sun-related synthesis | | Oily fish, eggs, and fortified foods. | Studies have suggested 2000 iU will safely correct deficiencies. Safe upper limit is 4000 iU per day. |
| **Calcium***  | 11–18 years (1000 mg) 19+ years (700 mg) | 11–18 years (800 mg) 19+ years (700 mg) | Dairy products including milk, cheese, and yoghurt. Small fish with bones (e.g., sardines), beans, and broccoli. | Approximately 1350 mg of calcium consumed 90 min prior to exercise has been shown to attenuate the deleterious changes in bone turnover (Haakonssen et al., 2015) |
| **Iron** | 11–18 years (11.3 mg) 19–49 years (8.7 mg) | 11 18 years (14.8**) 19–49 years (14.8 mg**) | Red meat, liver broccoli, spinach, fortified cereals, eggs, dried fruits, nuts, and seeds. | If a deficiency has been identified, iron supplements may be considered, following consultation with a dietician or doctor. These supplements should be the most bioavailable forms including iron sulphate, iron gluconate, and iron fumarate. Routine iron supplementation without deficiency is not recommended and can induce toxicity. |

*   Suggested that an athlete's diet should contain 1500 mg per day (Collins et al., 2021).
** Approximately 10% of females with high menstrual losses may need more iron than the RNI. These athletes should seek appropriate advice and may need to consider iron supplements.

*Nutrition for match play and training* 83

*Table 5.4* An overview of supplements that may be ergogenic to soccer-specific physical performance

| Supplement | Suggested dosing strategy | Reported physiological and ergogenic benefits |
|---|---|---|
| Caffeine | 2–4 mg kg$^{-1}$ BM at 45–60 min before match play or training. Usually consumed in capsule, concentrated drink, or CHO gel format. May reduce sleep quality when consumed prior to night games. | Central nervous stimulant which acts as an adenosine antagonist thereby reducing perception of effort. Reported to improve repeated sprint performance on the Yo–Yo intermittent recovery test 2, agility, jump performance, and passing accuracy. |
| Creatine | 4–5 days of loading dose of 20 g (4 × 5 g per day) followed by maintenance dose of 3–5 g daily. Should be consumed with CHO so as to enhance muscle creatine uptake. Usually consumed in powder format mixed with CHO and/or protein beverages. | Increases the creatine stores of skeletal muscle which enhances capacity to generate ATP through the ATP-PCr system. Reported to enhance power output during single and repeated sprints and promotes PCr resynthesis between sprints. May also augment increases in fat-free mass, strength, and power when combined with an appropriate strength training programme. |
| β-alanine | 4 weeks of loading dose of 3–6 g per day (3–6 × 1 g servings) followed by maintenance dose of 3 g per day. Usually consumed in capsule format although powder can also be mixed with CHO and/or protein beverages. Side effects often include "tingling" of the skin. | Increases carnosine stores of skeletal muscle which acts an intracellular buffer to protect against the fatiguing effects associated with metabolic acidosis induced by high-intensity exercise. Reported to improve repeated sprint performance on the Yo–Yo intermittent recovery test 2 and may also improve the capacity to perform high-intensity training thus augmenting training adaptations. |
| Nitrate | 1 g on MD-1 (e.g., 2 × 500 mg servings served with breakfast and dinner) followed by 500 mg with pre-match meal and 250 mg at start of warm-up period. Often consumed in the form of beetroot juice, concentrated drinks or gels. | Improves exercise efficiency by reducing the oxygen cost to perform a given workload. Reported to improve repeated sprint performance on the Yo–Yo intermittent recovery test 1 as well as 5, 10, and 20 m sprint times. |

and below your position in the organizational hierarchy. With the inevitable high turnover of club staff and players, the process of education and stakeholder management is never-ending. The ability to adapt and adopt a personalised approach when dealing with individual players and staff (i.e., coaching and leadership skills) is a prerequisite for success for the applied practitioner specialising in performance nutrition.

## Practical reflections on critical performance priorities

With the intense competitive and travel schedule inherent to elite soccer, the professional player is required to possess optimal body composition whilst simultaneously

84 *James P. Morton et al.*

adhering to best practice fuelling and recovery strategies for 10 months of the year. An essential role of the performance nutritionist is to, therefore, ensure that players are nutritionally prepared for match play, especially in those instances with short turn-around (e.g., 48–72 h) between games. As such, the practical challenge of ensuring players consume sufficient CHO intake (without the fear of consuming excessive calories) is a critical performance priority. The performance nutritionist should "bring this to life" by ensuring that MD-1 is accompanied by a plentiful and varied supply of CHO-rich foods, snacks, and drinks such that the boredom of mundane food offerings does not retract from what remains the most fundamental nutrition priority. Similarly, given the role of CHO intake in promoting post-match muscle glycogen resynthesis, the provision of such foods in the changing room environment and when travelling home from games (especially after night games) is also a critical element of practice. Where possible, it is encouraged that practitioners collect detailed and individual dietary intake data over the course of MD-1, MD, and MD+1.

## Critical reflections on the role of the performance chef

The club catering staff play an essential role in "activating" the performance nutrition programme by creating a positive eating and dining environment for players. From a practical perspective, this includes support with menu innovation, trialling of new performance foods and service of appropriate macronutrient portions to achieve some of the performance priorities described above. For this reason, building strong relationships with club chefs and catering personnel is perhaps one of the most critical working relationships. This process can often be challenging in scenarios where clubs employ long-standing chefs who may lack enthusiasm for "performance" nutrition and are resistant to change. It is now common for teams to have the luxury of travelling to away games with their own chef. This approach helps to create a consistent dining experience to that of the training ground environment and instils a sense of trust and familiarity amongst the players and coaching staff. Away games present an additional opportunity to work collaboratively with the performance chef by assisting with logistical challenges of working in an unfamiliar kitchen environment as well as assisting with food service provision on the coach home from games. The latter scenario presents an opportunity to align the chef on elements of performance nutrition by assisting with recovery in action. If the performance nutritionist is the "architect" of evidence-based nutritional strategies, it is the performance chef who "builds" the plates.

## Future directions and conclusions

In relation to soccer match play, it is well documented that CHO availability can promote components of both physical and technical performance. Additionally, sufficient energy and macronutrient intake in the hours and days after match play is necessary to promote recovery between games. Although our understanding of nutrition for training is less advanced than nutrition for match play, it is recognised that manipulation of energy, macronutrient and micronutrient availability can readily affect training adaptations associated with strength, power, and endurance. It is noteworthy that much of our current understanding is based on laboratory trials and field-based studies largely conducted on recreationally active male players. It is hoped that the coming decade will see a growth of studies specifically conducted on adult and adolescent players from both the men's and women's professional game. The energetic and substrate demands of match play and the typical training sessions completed by these players remain to be accurately quantified. Where possible, randomised control trials should be completed (e.g., short-term manipulation of macronutrient and micronutrient availability, utilisation of supplements and ergogenic aids) to ascertain the effects of nutrition more accurately on modulating training adaptation. Significant attention should also be given to the adolescent and female soccer player to provide evidence-based strategies that promote growth and maturation and reduce the risk of negative consequences associated with LEA.

## References

Anderson, L., Close, G. L., Konopinski, M., Rydings, D., Milsom, J., Hambly, C., ... Morton, J. P. (2019). Case study: muscle atrophy, hypertrophy, and energy expenditure of a premier league soccer player during rehabilitation from anterior cruciate ligament injury. *International Journal of Sports Nutrition and Exercise Metabolism, 29,* 559–566.

Anderson, L., Close, G. L., Morgans, R., Hambly, C., Speakman, J. R., Drust, B., & Morton, J. P. (2018). Assessment of energy expenditure of a professional goalkeeper from the English premier league using the doubly labeled water method. *International Journal of Sports Physiology and Performance, 14*(5), 681–684.

Anderson, L., Drust, B., Close, G. L., & Morton, J. P. (2022). Physical loading in professional soccer players: implications for contemporary guidelines to encompass carbohydrate periodization. *Journal of Sports Sciences, 40*(9), 1000–1019.

Anderson, L., Orme, P., Di Michele, R., Close, G. L., Morgans, R., Drust, B., & Morton, J. P. (2015). Quantification of training load during one-, two- and three-game week schedules in professional soccer players from the English premier league: implications for carbohydrate periodization. *Journal of Sports Sciences, 4,* 1–10.

Anderson, L., Orme, P., Naughton, R. J., Close, G. L., Milsom, J., Rydings, D., ... Morton, J. P. (2017a). Energy intake and expenditure of professional soccer players of the English premier league: evidence of carbohydrate periodization. *International Journal of Sports Nutrition and Exercise Metabolism, 27,* 228–238.

Anderson, L., Naughton, R. J., Close, G. L., Di Michele, R., Morgans, R., Drust, B., & Morton, J. P. (2017b). Daily distribution of macronutrient intakes of professional soccer players from the English premier league. *International Journal of Sports Nutrition and Exercise Metabolism, 27,* 491–498.

Areta, J. L., Burke, L. M., Ross, M. L., Camera, D. M., West, D. W., Broad, E. M., Coffey, V. G. (2013). Timing and distribution of protein ingestion during prolonged recovery from resistance exercise alters myofibrillar protein synthesis. *The Journal of Physiology, 591,* 2319–2331.

Baker, L. B., Rollo, I., Stein, K. W., & Jeukendrup, A. E. (2015). Acute effects of carbohydrate supplementation on intermittent sports performance. *Nutrients, 7,* 5733–5763.

Balsom, P. D., Wood, K., Olsson, P., & Ekblom, B. (1999). Carbohydrate intake and multiple sprint sports: with special reference to football (soccer). *International Journal of Sports Medicine, 20,* 48–52.

Bangsbo, J., Nørregaard, L., & Thorsøe, F. (1992). The effect of carbohydrate diet on intermittent exercise performance. *International Journal of Sports Medicine, 13,* 152–157.

Bettonviel, A. E. O., Brinkmans, N. Y. J., Russcher, K., Wardenaar, F. C., & Witard, O. C. (2016). Nutritional status and daytime pattern of protein intake on match, post-match, rest and training days in senior professional and youth elite soccer players. *International Journal of Sports Nutrition and Exercise Metabolism, 26*(3), 285–293.

Briggs, M. A., Harper, L. D., McNamee, G., Cockburn, E., Rumbold, P. L. S., Stevenson, E. J., & Russell, M. (2017). The effects of an increased calorie breakfast consumed prior to simulated match-play in academy soccer players. *European Journal of Sport Science, 17,* 858–866.

Brinkmans, N. Y. J., Iedema, N., Plasqui, G., Wouters, L., Saris, W. H. M., van Loon L. J. C., & van Dijk, J. W. (2019). Energy expenditure and dietary intake in professional football players in the Dutch premier league: implications for nutritional counselling. *Journal of Sports Sciences, 16,* 1–9.

Burke, L. M., Collier, G. R., & Hargreaves, M. (1993). Muscle glycogen storage after prolonged exercise: effect of the glycemic index of carbohydrate. *Journal of Applied Physiology, 75,* 1019–1023.

Burke, L. M., van Loon, L. J. C., & Hawley, J. A. (2016). Postexercise muscle glycogen resynthesis in humans. *Journal of Applied Physiology, 122,* 1055–1067.

Burke, L. M., Winter, J. A., Cameron-Smith, D., Enslen, M., Farnfield, M., & Decombaz, J. (2012). Effects of different dietary protein sources on plasma amino acid profiles at rest and after exercise. *International Journal of Sports Nutrition and Exercise Metabolism, 22*(6), 452–462.

Bussau, V. A., Fairchild, T. J., Rao, A., Steele, P., & Fournier, P. A. (2002). Carbohydrate loading in human muscle: an improved 1 day protocol. *European Journal of Applied Physiology, 87*(3), 290–295.

Churchward-Venne, T. A., Pinckaers, P. J. M., Smeets, J. S. J., Betz, M. W., Senden, J. M., Goessens, J. P. B., Gijsen, A. P., Rollo, I., Verdijk, L. B., & van Loon, L. J. C. (2020). Dose-response effects of dietary protein on muscle protein synthesis during recovery from endurance exercise in young men: a double-blind randomized trial. *American Journal of Clin Nutrition, 112*(2), 303–317.

Clenin, G., Cordes, M., Huber, A., Schumacher, Y. O., Noack, P., Scales, J., & Kriemier, S. (2015). Iron deficiency in sports: definition, influence on performance and therapy. *Swiss Medical Weekly, 145,* w14196.

Collins, J., Maughan, R. J., Gleeson, M., Bilsborough, J. C., Jeukendrup, J. E., Morton, J. P., … McCall, A. (2021). UEFA Expert group statement on nutrition in elite football. Part 1: current evidence to inform practical recommendations and future directions. *British Journal of Sports Medicine.* 55(8), 416.

Currell, K., Conway, S., & Jeukendrup, A. E. (2009). Carbohydrate ingestion improves performance of a new reliable test of soccer performance. *International Journal of Sports Nutrition and Exercise Metabolism, 19,* 34–46.

DellaValle, D. M., & Haas, J. D. (2011). Impact of iron depletion without anemia on performance in trained endurance athletes at the beginning of a training season: a study of female collegiate rowers. *International Journal of Sports Nutrition and Exercise Metabolism, 21*(6), 501–506.

Findlay, R. J., Macrae, E. H. R., Whyte, I. Y., Easton, C., & Forrest Née Whyte, L. J (2020). How the menstrual cycle and menstruation affect sporting performance: experiences and perceptions of elite female rugby players. *Br J Sports Med, 54*(18), 1108–1113.

Foskett, A., Williams, C., Boobis, L., & Tsintzas, K. (2008). Carbohydrate availability and muscle energy metabolism during intermittent running. *Medicine & Science in Sport & Exercise, 40*(1), 96–103.

Gonzalez-Alonso, J. (2007). Hyperthermia impairs brain, heart and muscle function in exercising humans. *Sports Medicine, 37*(4–5), 371–373.

Gunnarsson, T. P., Bendiksen, M., Bischoff, R., Christensen, P. M., Lesivig, B., Madsen, K., … Bangsbo, J. (2013). Effect of whey protein- and carbohydrate-enriched diet on glycogen resynthesis during the first 48 h after a soccer game. *Scandinavian Journal of Medicine & Science in Sports, 23,* 508–515.

Haakonssen, E. C., Ross, M. L., Knight, E. J., Cato, L. E., Nana, A., Wluka, A. E., Cicuttini, F. M., Wang, B. H., Jenkins, D. G., & Burke, L. M. (2015). The effects of a calcium-rich pre-exercise meal on biomarkers of calcium homeostasis in competitive female cyclists: a randomised crossover trial. *PLoS One, 10*(5), e0123302.

Hannon, M. P., Parker, L. J. F., Carney, D. J., McKeown, J., Speakman, J. R., Hambly, C., Drust, B., Unnithan, V. B., Close, G. L., & Morton, J. P. (2021). Energy requirements of male academy soccer players from the English premier league. *Medicine & Science in Sport & Exercise, 53*(1), 200–210.

Hannon, M. P., Carney, D. J., Floyd, S., McKeown, J., Drust, B., Unnithan, V. B., Close, G. L., & Morton, J. P. (2020). Cross-sectional comparison of body composition and resting metabolic rate in premier league academy soccer players: implications for growth and maturation. *Journal of Sports Science, 38*(11–12), 1326–1334.

Harper, L. D., Stevenson, E. J., Rollo, I., & Russell, M. (2017). The influence of a 12% carbohydrate-electrolyte beverage on self-paced soccer-specific exercise performance. *Journal of Science and Medicine in Sport, 20*(12), 1123–1129.

He, C. S., Handzlik, M., Fraswer, W. D., Muhamad, A., Preston, H., Richardson, A., & Gleeson, M. (2013). Influence of vitamin D status on respiratory infection incidence and immune function during 4 months of winter training in endurance sport athletes. *Exercise Immunology Review, 19*, 86–101.

Impey, S. G., Hearris, M. A., Hammond, K. M., Bartlett, J. D., Louis, J., Close, G. G., & Morton, J. P. (2018). Fuel for the work required: a theoretical framework for carbohydrate periodization and the glycogen threshold hypothesis. *Sports Medicine, 48*, 1031–1048.

Ivy, J. L., Katz, A. L., Cutler, C. L., Sherman, W. M., & Coyle, E. F. (1988). Muscle glycogen synthesis after exercise: effect of time of carbohydrate ingestion. *Journal of Applied Physiology, 64*, 1480–1485.

Iwayma, K., Onishi, T., Maruyama, K., & Takahashi, H. (2020). Diurnal variation in the glycogen content of human liver using 13C MRS. *NMR in Biomedicine, 33*(6), e4289.

Krustrup, P., Mohr, M., Steensberg, A., Bencke, J., Kjer, M., & Bangsbo, J. (2006). Muscle and blood metabolites during a soccer game: implications for sprint performance. *Physical Fitness and Performance, 38*, 1165–1174.

Krustrup, P., Ørtenblad, N., Nielsen, J., Nybo, L., Gunnarsson, T. P., Iaia, F. M., … Bangsbo, J. (2011). Maximal voluntary contraction force, SR function and glycogen resynthesis during the first 72 h after a high-level competitive soccer game. *European Journal of Applied Physiology, 111*, 2987–2995.

Kurdak, S. S., Shirreffs, S. M., Maughan, R. J., Ozgunen, K. T., Zeren, C., Korkmaz, S., … Dvorak, J. (2010). Hydration and sweating responses to hot-weather football competition. *Scandinavian Journal of Medicine & Science in Sports, 20*(3), 133–139.

Lee, J. K., & Shirreffs, S. M. (2007). The influence of drink temperature on thermoregulatory responses during prolonged exercise in a moderate environment. *Journal of Sports Science, 25*(9), 975–985.

Longland, T. M., Oikawa, S. Y., Mitchell, C. J., Devries, M. C., & Phillips, S. M. (2016). Higher compared with lower dietary protein during an energy deficit combined with intense exercise promotes greater lean mass gain and fat mass loss: a randomized trial. *American Journal of Clinical Nutrition, 103*(3), 738–746.

Loucks, A. B., Kiens, B., & Wright, H. H. (2011). Energy availability in athletes. *Journal of Sports Sciences, 29*(1), S7–15.

MacNaughton, L. S., Wardle, S., Witard, O. C., McGlory, C., Hamilton, D. L., Jeromson, S., Lawrence, C. E., Walls, G. A., & Tipton, K. D. (2016). The response of muscle protein synthesis following whole-body resistance exercise is greater following 40 g than 20 g of ingested whey protein. *Physiological Reports, 4*(15), e12893.

Maughan, R. J. (1997). Energy and macronutrient intakes of professional football (soccer) players. *Br Journal of Sports Medicine, 31*, 45–47.

Maughan, R. J., Watson, P., Evans, G. H., Broad, N., & Shirreffs, S. M. (2007). Water balance and salt losses in competitive football. *International Journal of Sports Nutrition and Exercise Metabolism, 17*(6), 583–594.

McGregor, S. J., Nicholas, C. W., Lakomy, H. K., & Williams, C. (1999). The influence of intermittent high-intensity shuttle running and fluid ingestion on the performance of a soccer skill. *Journal of Sports Science, 17*(11), 895–903.

McNulty, K. L., Elliott-Sale, K. J., Dolan, E., Swinton, P. A., Ansdell, P., Goodall, S., ... Hicks, K. M. (2020). The effects of menstrual cycle phase on exercise performance in eumenorrheic women: a systematic review and meta-analysis. *Sports Medicine, 50*(10), 1813–1827. doi: 10.1007/s40279-020-01319-3

Milsom, J., Barreira, P., Burgess, D. J., Iqbal, Z., & Morton, J. P. (2014). Case study: muscle atrophy and hypertrophy in a premier league soccer player during rehabilitation from ACL injury. *International Journal of Sports Nutrition and Exercise Metabolism, 24*, 543–552.

Mohr, M., Krustrup, P., & Bangsbo, J. (2003). Match performance of high-standard soccer players with special reference to development of fatigue. *Journal of Sports Sciences, 21*, 439–449.

Mohr, M., Krustrup, P., Nybo, L., Nielsen, J. J., & Bangsbo, J. (2004). Muscle temperature and sprint performance during soccer matches--beneficial effect of re-warm-up at half-time. *Scandinavian Journal of Medicine & Science in Sports, 14*(3), 156–162.

Mohr, M., Mujika, I., Santisteban, J., Randers, M. B., Bischoff, R., Solano, R., ... Krustrup, P. (2010). Examination of fatigue development in elite soccer in a hot environment: a multi-experimental approach. *Scandinavian Journal of Medicine & Science in Sports, 20*(3), 125–132.

Moore, D. R., Sygo, J. & Morton, J. P. (2021). Fuelling the female athlete: carbohydrate and protein considerations. *European Journal of Sports Sciences, 22*(5), 684-696.

Moore, D. R., Areta, J., Coffey, V. G., Stellingwerff, T., Phillips, S. M., Burke, L. M., Cléroux, M., Godin, J. P., & Hawley, J. A. (2012). Daytime of post-exercise protein intake affects whole-body protein turnover in resistance-trained males. *Nutrition & Metabolism, 9*(1), 91.

Morehen, J. C., Rosimus, C., Cavanagh, B. P., Hambly, C., Speakman, J. R., Elliot-Sale, K. J., Hannon, M. P., & Morton, J. P. (2022). Energy expenditure of female international standard soccer players: a doubly labeled water investigation. *Medicine Science, Sports, & Exercise, 54*(5), 769–779.

Morton, J. P., Croft, L., Bartlett, J. D., Maclaren, D. P. M., Reilly, T., Evens, L., ... Drust, B. (2009). Reduced carbohydrate availability does not modulate training-induced heat shock protein adaptations but does up regulate oxidative enzyme activity in human skeletal muscle. *Journal of Applied Physiology, 106*, 1513–1521.

Morton, J. P., Iqbal, Z., Drust, B., Burgess, D., Close, G. L., & Brukner, P. D. (2012). Seasonal variation in vitamin D status in professional soccer players of the English premier league. *Applied Physiology Nutrition, and Metabolism, 37*(4), 798–802.

Morton, R. W., Murphy, K. T., McKellar, S. R., Schoenfeld, B. J., Henselmans, M., Helms, E., ... Phillips, S. M. (2018). A systematic review, meta-analysis and meta-regression of the effect of protein supplementation on resistance training-induced gains in muscle mass and strength in healthy adults. *British Journal of Sports Medicine, 52*(6), 376–384.

Moss, S. L., Randell, R. K., Burgess, D., Ridley, S., ÓCairealláin, C., Allison, R., & Rollo, I. (2020). Assessment of energy availability and associated risk factors in professional female soccer players. *European Journal of Sports Sciences, 6*, 1–10.

Mountjoy, M., Sundgot-Borgen, J., Burke, L., Carter. S., Constantini, N., Lebrun, C., Meyer, N., Sherman, R., Steffen, K., Budgett, R., & Ljungqvist, A. (2014). The IOC consensus statement: beyond the female athlete triad-relative energy deficiency in sport (RED-S). *British Journal of Sports Medicine, 48*, 491–497.

Nicholas, C. W., Williams, C., Lakomy, H. K., Phillips, G., & Nowitz, A. (1995). Influence of ingesting a carbohydrate-electrolyte solution on endurance capacity during intermittent, high-intensity shuttle running. *Journal of Sports Sciences, 13*(4), 283–290.

Owens, D. J., Allison, R., & Close, G. L. (2018). Vitamin D and the athlete: current perspectives and new challenges. *Sports Medicine, 48*(1), 3–16.

Owens, D. J., Sharples, A. P., Polydorou, I., Alwan, N., Donovan, T., Tang, J., Fraser, W., Cooper, R. G., Morton, J. P., Stewart, C., & Close, G. L. (2015). A systems based investigation into vitamin d and skeletal muscle repair, regeneration and hypertrophy. *American Journal of Physiology Endocrinology and Metabolism, 309*(12), E1019–1031.

Rodriguez-Giustiniani, P., Rollo, I., Witard, O. C., & Galloway, S. D. R. (2019). Ingesting a 12% carbohydrate-electrolyte beverage before each half of a soccer match simulation facilitates retention of passing performance and improves high-intensity running capacity in academy players. *International Journal of Sports Nutrition and Exercise Metabolism, 29*, 397–405.

Rollo, I., Randell, R. K., Baker, L., Leyes, J. Y., Leal, D. M., Lizarraga, A., Mesalles, J., Jeukendrup, A. E., James, L. J., & Carter, J. M. (2021). Fluid balance, sweat Na+ losses, and carbohydrate intake of elite male soccer players in response to low and high training intensities in cool and hot environments. *Nutrients, 13*, 401.

Russell, M., Benton, D., & Kingsley, M. (2012). Influence of carbohydrate supplementation on skill performance during a soccer match simulation. *Journal of Science and Medicine in Sport, 15*, 348–354.

Russell, M., & Kingsley, M. (2014). The efficacy of acute nutritional interventions on soccer skill performance. *Sports Medicine, 44*, 957–970.

Saltin, B. (1973). Metabolic fundamentals in exercise. *Medicine and Science in Sports, 5*, 137–146.

Sim, M., Garvican-Lewis, L. A., Cox, G. R., Govus, A., McKay, A. K. A., Stellingwerff, T., & Peeling, P. (2019). Iron considerations for the athlete: a narrative review. *European Journal of Applied Physiology, 119*(7), 1463–1478.

Snijders, T., Res, P. T., Smeets, J. S. J., van Vliet, S., van Kranenburg, J., Maase, K., Kies, A. K., Verdijk, L. B., & van Loon, L. J. C. (2015). Protein ingestion before sleep increases muscle mass and strength gains during prolonged resistance-type exercise training in healthy young men. *The Journal of Nutrition, 145*(6), 1178–1184.

Souglis, A. G., Chryssanthopoulos, C. I., Travlos, A. K., Zorzou, A. E., Gissis, I. T., Papadopoulos, C. N., & Sotiropoulos, A. A. (2013). The effect of high vs. low carbohydrate diets on distances covered in soccer. *Journal of Strength and Conditioning Research*, 27, 2235–2247.

Stellingwerff, T., Morton J. P., & Burke, L. M. (2019). A framework for periodized nutrition for athletes. *International Journal of Sports Nutrition and Exercise Metabolism, 29*(2), 141–151.

Tang, J. E., Moore, D. R., Kujbida, G. W., Tarnopolsky, M. A., & Phillips, S. M. (2009). Ingestion of whey hydrolysate, casein, or soy protein isolate: effects on mixed muscle protein synthesis at rest and following resistance exercise in young men. *Journal of Applied Physiology, 107*(3), 987–992.

Thomas, D. T., Erdman, K. A., & Burke, L. M. (2016). Position of the academy of nutrition and dietetics, dieticians of Canada, and the American college of sports medicine: nutrition and athletic performance. *Journal of the Academy of Nutrition Dietetics, 116*(3), 501–528.

Trommelen, J., Kouw, I. W. K., Holwerda, A. M., Snijders, T., Halson, S. L., Rollo, I., Verdijk, L. B., & van Loon, L. J. C. (2018). Presleep dietary protein-derived amino acids are incorporated in myofibrillar protein during post exercise overnight recovery. *American Journal of Physiology Endocrinology & Metabolism, 314*(5), 457–467.

Wenger, A. (2021). Importance of nutrition in football: the coach's perspective. *British Journal of Sports Medicine, 55*(8), 409.

# 6 Recovery strategies

*Warren Gregson, Gregory Dupont,*
*Abd-Elbasset Abaidia and Robin Thorpe*

## Introduction

In this chapter, we bring together the latest scientific research as well as real-world experience of implementing recovery strategies in elite soccer to provide a contemporary overview of the key concepts. The initial section serves to contextualise the growing importance of recovery for elite players. Next, we provide an overview of the key physiological mechanisms which underpin the recovery process which serve as the targets for strategies which aim to optimise the recovery process. The final section examines the important recovery strategies employed in the elite game. We focus on the scientific basis of recovery interventions rather than monitoring strategies used to evaluate whether the player is adapting positively or negatively to the collective stresses of training and competition. Information on the latter can be found in several excellent previous reviews (e.g., Thorpe et al., 2017).

## The rising importance of recovery in the modern elite game

The typical season is structured around a short preparation period (~6 weeks) followed by a long competitive season lasting approximately 40 weeks. Players are, therefore, exposed to extended time periods where the combined demands of training and match-play can induce a high degree of physical and mental stress. In the modern game, the increasing physical demands of competition (Barnes et al., 2014), together with a high frequency of competition, particularly in those players representing the most successful teams, has further accentuated the physical and mental load incurred by players. Players are now routinely exposed to two to three games per week with leading players often competing 70 matches per season interspersed with 4–5 days of recovery between matches. These demands are further increased in those players competing in leagues such as the English Premier League due to the absence of a winter break (Ekstrand et al., 2018). Similarly, international competitions taking place during the off-season period, which typically reduces the rest period available to players, further increasing the cumulative load experienced by players.

Soccer involves many high-intensity activities such as high-speed running, sprinting, changing direction, jumping, and shooting which can lead to fatigue. Fatigue is defined as an inability to complete a task that was once achievable within a recent time frame (Pyne & Martin, 2011; Halson, 2014). During a match, fatigue can arise temporarily at any time following a short-term intense period, towards the end of the match and following the match (Nedelec et al., 2012). Many non-contact injuries occur

DOI: 10.4324/9781003148418-7

during the latter stages of each half (Ekstrand et al., 2011), suggesting that fatigue may be a risk factor for injury.

In recent years, increasing evidence has highlighted the potential impact of match-related fatigue on injury risk. During periods where the match schedule is congested (e.g., two to three matches per week over several weeks), recovery time between successive matches (2–3 days) may be insufficient to allow the player to fully regenerate (Dupont et al., 2010). Under such conditions, injury rates in elite-level players participating in the UEFA Champions League were more than six times higher when players played two matches per week compared to one match per week despite similar physical performance levels (Dupont et al., 2010). In a large cohort of elite players, total injury rates and muscle injury rates were increased in matches where the recovery time was less than or equal to 4 days compared with matches where the recovery time was more than or equal to 6 days (Bengtsson et al., 2013). The absence of a winter break in leagues such as the English Premier League increases the risk of injury. For example, elite European club teams without a winter break (English clubs) lost on average 303 days more per season due to injuries across the entire season compared with teams with a winter break (Ekstrand et al., 2018).

Increased availability of players for selection, because of a reduction in injuries, substantially increases a team's chance of success (Hagglund et al., 2013). Changes in injury occurrence have a significant impact on the financial performance of the club. During the 2016–2017 season, the average English Premier League team lost approximately £45 million per season due to injury-related (team underachievement and player salaries) decrements in performance (Eliakim et al., 2020). Consequently, the importance of managing player loading with respect to fatigue and subsequent injury risk has increased attention on the area of recovery both in the form of academic research together with attempts in the field to develop strategies which optimise player recovery.

## Overview of the physiological and psychological mechanisms underpinning recovery

Recovery is regarded as a multifaceted (e.g., physiological and psychological) restorative process relative to time (Kellmann et al., 2018). Under conditions where a player's recovery status is disturbed by external or internal factors, fatigue as a condition of augmented tiredness arises due to physical and mental effort (Halson, 2014; Kellmann et al., 2018). A certain degree of fatigue resulting in functional overreaching is required to mediate adaptations to training which drive performance enhancement (Pyne & Martin, 2011). On the contrary, excessive fatigue through under-recovery may increase the players' susceptibility to non-functional over-reaching, injury, and illness (Nimmo et al., 2007). Fatigue can be compensated with recovery strategies which serve to re-establish the invested resources on a physiological and psychological level (Kellmann et al., 2018).

Due to the nature of the eccentric actions performed during a match, soccer is a sport inducing a high level of muscle damage (Nédélec et al., 2013). This impact is characterised by a decrease in neuromuscular function, an increase in the blood concentrations of intramuscular proteins and an increase in muscle soreness (Warren et al., 1999). In this context, following a game, a period of rest is needed to return to a homeostatic state (Nédélec et al., 2013). Scientists have analysed the time needed to recover following a match. The results have been compiled in a systematic review with

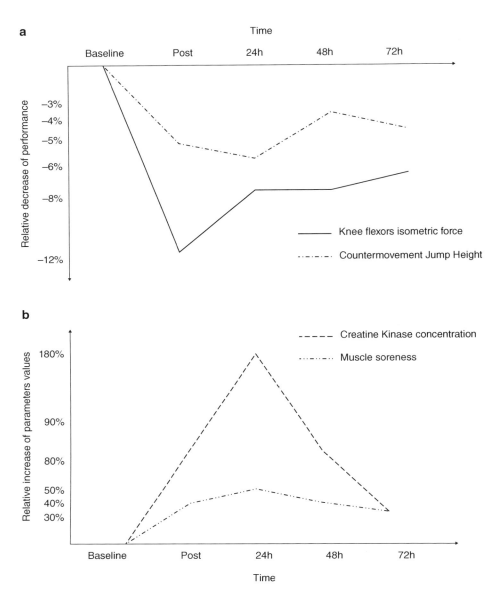

*Figure 6.1a and 6.1b* Recovery of knee flexor isometric force, counter-movement jump height (1a) and ratings of subjective muscle soreness and creatine kinase concentrations (1b) throughout the 72-h period following match-play. Redrawn from Silva et al. (2018).

meta-analysis and showed that a period of 72 h is insufficient for performance parameters to return to baseline values (Figure 6.1a and b; Silva et al., 2018). Some perceptual or physiological parameters may recover faster. However, contrary to neuromuscular performance, these parameters are not sensitive nor representative enough to be considered as good markers of muscle damage (Warren et al., 1999).

Post-exercise recovery is a complex process which involves several phenomena. Some mechanisms of the recovery process have been observed and described in the scientific literature. These mechanisms centre on the role of muscle damage, inflammation, and regeneration, the repeated bout effect, energetic substrates, and psychological aspects.

### The role of muscle damage, inflammation, and regeneration

The mechanical stress induced by eccentric actions is considered one of the dominant factors mediating muscle damage (Tee et al., 2007). The ultrastructure of the muscle, the extracellular matrix and probably the capillaries are damaged (Clarkson & Hubal, 2002). This muscle damage constitutes a stimulus for an acute inflammatory response that may last for several days (Cannon & St Pierre, 1998; Malm, 2001; Smith et al., 2000; Suzuki et al., 2002). The inflammation process is mediated by proteins such as interleukins, tumour necrosis factor-α (TNF-α), and C-reactive protein (CRP). The role of these proteins is to regulate the migration of immune cells (neutrophils and macrophages) into the injured area of the muscle and to initiate the repair (Cannon & St Pierre, 1998; Suzuki et al., 2002; Peake et al., 2005).

In soccer, match participation is characterised by an increase in interleukine-6 (IL-6), TNF-α, and CRP concentrations (Silva et al., 2018). While IL-6 and TNF-α peak immediately after the match, CRP peaks 24 h after the match. In addition, the immunological response is characterised by a substantial increase of leucocytes, monocytes, macrophages, and lymphocytes 24 and 48 h following the match (Silva et al., 2018). This process stimulates muscle regeneration in coordination with hormonal aspects. Some hormones such as testosterone, growth hormone, and insulin-like growth factor-1 directly stimulate the satellite cells involved in the process of muscle repair (Hawke & Garry, 2001; Chakravarthy et al., 2000; Sinha-Hikim et al., 2013; Schoenfeld, 2013). Muscle regeneration is accelerated in the presence of these hormones. Inducing an increase in these hormones may accelerate recovery kinetics following exercise-induced muscle damage (Abaïdia et al., 2017; Crewther & Cook, 2012).

### The repeated bout effects

The repetition of an exercise has a protective effect which can be influenced by several variables including intensity, velocity of contraction, number of damaging contractions, muscle length, muscle group, age, and sex (Hyldahl et al., 2017). Potential mechanisms underpinning the repeated bout effect include neural adaptations, alterations to muscle mechanical properties, structural remodelling of the extracellular matrix and biochemical signalling (Hyldahl et al., 2017; McHugh et al., 1999; McHugh, 2003). From a practical point of view, athletes previously exposed to an exercise modality are likely to recover faster than athletes who have not been previously exposed.

For global activities such as soccer, researchers have reported conflicting results as to whether match exposure provides a protective effect. Although data on the repeated bout effect after a match are sparse, scientists have analysed the influence of the repeated bout effect on recovery kinetics following other team sports and global activities. Following a repeated intermittent sprint exercise, Leeder et al. (2014) observed lower muscle soreness following the second bout of exercise but no significant difference in recovery kinetics of muscle function and blood creatine kinase concentrations between the two bouts. These results differ from those obtained by Verma et al. (2016), who reported accelerated recovery kinetics following the second bout compared with the first for strength, soreness, blood creatine kinase, and lactate dehydrogenase concentrations.

The repeated bout effect may also be associated with the player's experience and the aptitude to cope with a given level of load during a season. Sterczala et al. (2014) evaluated the recovery response of ten American Football players after two games separated by one season. Blood creatine kinase and myoglobin concentrations were assessed, and the authors found no difference at any time point between the two matches. The ability to recover may also be different between young players acceding to elite level and players having years of experience. During an entire season of Australian Football Rules, Hunkin et al. (2014) showed higher levels of blood creatine kinase concentrations in less experienced players. This finding may be associated with residual muscle damage resulting from an intense training period.

### Energetic substrates

Post-match fatigue in soccer is also associated with a decrease in glycogen stores. Match participation may induce up to a 50% decrease in muscular glycogen concentrations (Krustrup et al., 2006). Furthermore, muscle glycogen stores may not be fully replenished at 48–72 h following a soccer match (Jacob et al., 1982). The decline in muscle glycogen may impact recovery kinetics following exercise-induced muscle damage (Gavin et al., 2016). For example, a reduced maximal voluntary contraction has been observed 48 h following eccentric exercise in a reduced glycogen state (Gavin et al., 2016). To counteract the deleterious effects of muscle glycogen depletion, it has been observed that an elevated muscle glycogen content through a carbohydrate diet may enhance the replenishment of glycogen stores 48 h post-match (Krustrup et al., 2011).

### Psychologic aspects

Psychological factors may also influence post-match recovery kinetics. Stults-Kolehmainen et al. (2014) studied the effects of chronic stress on recovery kinetics following exercise-induced muscle damage. After answering a questionnaire to evaluate their level of stress, 31 participants were divided into high-stress and low-stress groups. The level of force was assessed every 24 h over a period of 96 h following exercise-induced muscle damage with the high-stress group demonstrating slower recovery of their muscle force.

## Key interventions to drive the recovery process

Researchers and practitioners alike have investigated the efficacy of commonly used interventions to combat the physical and mental stress associated with training and match-play (Nédélec et al., 2012). A recent investigation reviewing commonly used recovery strategies in the Spanish top Division (Spanish La Liga) reported that all teams utilised at least one recovery strategy following match-play, however, the range of interventions adopted was substantially different between teams with water immersion (cold and hot), massage, and foam rolling accounting for 74%, 70%, and 57%, respectively (Altarriba-Bartes et al., 2020). Nedelec and colleagues (2013) reported that active recovery, stretching, compression garments, and cold-water immersion were the

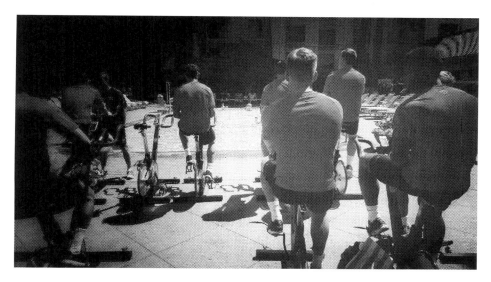

*Figure 6.2* An example of an active recovery strategy.

most prevalent recovery interventions used by practitioners working in the top French League (France Ligue 1). The following section will briefly review the efficacy of such interventions.

### *Active recovery*

Active recovery can be performed via multiple modalities including sub-maximal cycling and running including exercising in water (Figure 6.2; Nédélec et al., 2013; Pooley et al., 2020). In France, 81% of professional teams reported that they prescribed active recovery modalities immediately following games (Nédélec et al., 2013). The purported mechanism associated with aerobic-based active recovery is centred on the removal of disruptive metabolites from areas of muscular exertion via an increase in circulation (Nédélec et al., 2013; Pooley et al., 2020). The majority of data have shown active recovery to accelerate the removal of blood lactate (Fairchild et al., 2003), however, in a study of professional female players, no improvements in physical performance (countermovement jump, sprint time, maximal isokinetic knee flexion, and extension) or blood markers (creatine kinase, uric acid, and inflammatory) was observed when comparing active recovery and passive recovery following match-play (Andersson et al., 2008).

A more recent study in younger players showed that active recovery improved perceptual recovery and reduced creatine kinase compared to static stretching post-match and for 48 h thereafter (Pooley et al., 2020). Other forms of active recovery such as hydrotherapy and resistance training of the upper limbs have become popular with practitioners. It is thought the associated hormonal and anabolic response alongside a global increase in blood flow may be favourable to recovery in soccer players (Yarrow et al., 2007). Overall, active recovery may have beneficial effects on perceptual recovery and has clear mechanistic effects on blood flow and circulation. Therefore,

## 96 *Warren Gregson et al.*

during periods of high metabolic cost/fatigue, active recovery is a suitable modality. Active recovery utilisation in the immediate timeframe post-exercise, particularly, in the event of mechanical disruption is still unclear.

### Stretching

Stretching has been practised by players for decades as a method perceived to improve flexibility and recovery and prevent injury (Nédélec et al., 2013). The proposed mechanisms include an increase in joint range of motion and a reduction in musculotendinous stiffness (Nédélec et al., 2013). In the English Premier League, players reportedly spend 40% of training time stretching, while in France in Ligue 1 50% of the time is spent using stretching for recovery purposes (Dadebo et al., 2004). In England, static stretching was the most prevalent form of stretching consisting of typically 30 s per muscle group for 2–5 sets per session (Nédélec et al., 2013). Although the use of stretching and in particular static stretching is widespread, there is no evidence to date to support the use of stretching in enhancing the recovery process in elite soccer (Herbert et al., 2011; Kinugasa & Kilding, 2009). A recent investigation of professional youth soccer players from a Premier League team found no differences in muscle damage markers 24–48 h following match-play when static stretching was performed (Pooley et al., 2020). In a similar cohort, and similar study design, active recovery, and cold water immersion improved recovery markers significantly greater than static stretching (Pooley et al., 2020). Lund and colleagues (1998) suggested that static stretching may even hinder the recovery process following eccentric muscle damage. In summary, despite the widespread use of stretching across all levels of professional soccer, there is little evidence to support its effect on recovery and under certain conditions (e.g., muscle damage) caution should be taken.

### Self-myofascial release – foam rolling

Self-myofascial release or foam rolling is performed as a recovery strategy by 91% of clubs in La Liga (Altarriba-Bartes et al., 2020). Self-myofascial release has been likened to traditional massage, however, many investigations have shown greater improvements in joint range of motion following self-myofascial release compared to a limited number studying traditional massage techniques (Cheatham et al., 2015). Recent investigations have found that short bouts of foam rolling (30 s per muscle group) on soft-tissue areas may lead to a significant increase in the joint range of movement (MacDonald et al., 2013). Furthermore, the use of foam rolling as a means of self-myofascial release has shown positive effects on perceived muscle soreness following exercise (Cheatham et al., 2015). Although mainly adopted in the training process as a recovery strategy, the use of self-myofascial release largely serves to improve joint range of motion and in some cases perceptions of recovery; hence, it is advantageous during all periods of the training process especially following games and intense strenuous training sessions (Figure 6.3).

### Massage

Massage, including its various forms, such as effleurage, petrissage, tapotement, friction, and vibration, was used by 78% of players in France's Ligue 1 teams with handheld percussion devices increasingly used (Nédélec et al., 2013). A common belief

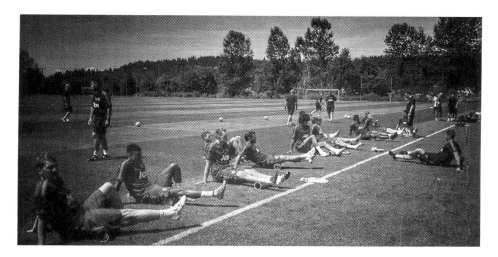

*Figure 6.3* An example of a foam rolling exercise.

among practitioners and players alike has been that massage enhances muscle blood flow and, therefore, the removal of disruptive metabolites from fatigued muscle regions. However, researches have shown that massage has a limited effect on blood flow or the removal of waste products from the muscle (Massage et al., 2010; Fuller et al., 2015; Thomson et al., 2015). Furthermore, Wiltshire and Colleagues (2010) showed a detrimental effect of massage on blood flow by reducing the mechanical processes of muscle fibres, glycogen re-synthesis and in turn reducing recovery. Additionally, Viitasaslo et al. (1995) observed a potentially debilitating rise in muscle damage proteins following strength exercise with the addition of immediate massage (Viitasalo et al., 1995). Small positive psychological and perceptual effects have been shown in nontrained individuals following tissue massage (Viitasalo et al., 1995). There seems to be a small positive subjective response to massage; however, the physiological effect of massage remains unclear and lacks strong support.

## Cryotherapy

Cold-water immersion has been shown to be the most common cryotherapy-based recovery strategy amongst the top tier of Ligue 1 in France with 88% of teams using cold-water immersion in an attempt to enhance recovery (Nédélec et al., 2013). Athletes use cold-water immersion immediately following games and throughout the recovery process. Similarly, short durations (30 s to 1 min) of cold-water immersion interspersed with short durations of hot-water immersion, known as contrast water therapy, is popular among athletes (Altarriba-Bartes et al., 2020). The literature has shown cold-water immersion alone to be more effective for accelerating surrogate markers of recovery (Elias et al., 2013), therefore, this chapter will only discuss cold-water immersion as a standalone strategy.

A cascade of mechanisms starting with a reduction in tissue temperature, metabolism, and blood flow has been shown following cold-water immersion (Bleakley & Davison, 2010; Mawhinney et al., 2020). Protocols differ substantially both in the literature and in the field, ranging from 5 to 20 min and temperatures of 6–22°C, however, recent data suggest that a dose of 10–11 min at 12–15°C may be most effective for reducing muscle tissue temperature and muscle blood flow (Vromans et al., 2019; Mawhinney et al., 2020). Cold-water immersion has been shown to be more effective in enhancing physical performance markers (maximal strength, sprint time, and countermovement jump) and biological metrics of muscle damage (creatine kinase and myoglobin) compared to other common strategies such as contrast water therapy and passive recovery in individual athletes (Ingram et al., 2009; Vaile et al., 2008). Similar improvements in physical performance assessments, as well as self-reported ratings and objective markers of muscle damage, have also been observed when comparing cold-water immersion to static stretching and passive recovery in soccer players (Elias et al., 2013; Pooley et al., 2020). Recently, cold-water immersion has been shown as an effective and safe method to improve autonomic modulation by improving parasympathetic reactivation, which in theory, may be seen as advantageous for the global recovery of athletes (Almeida et al., 2015; Buchheit et al., 2009; Douglas et al., 2015). However, more data are required to fully understand the role of cold-water immersion in the inflammatory cascade following soccer (Peake et al., 2020).

Whole-body cryotherapy has attracted a lot of interest regarding athlete recovery in recent years, with athletes normally exposed to 1–3 min durations of –110 to –160°C air temperatures (Costello et al., 2016). Costello et al. (2016) concluded there was insufficient evidence to support the use of whole-body cryotherapy in alleviating muscle damage in athletes (Costello et al., 2016). The majority of positive effects have been solely related to the players' perceptions of recovery (Wilson et al., 2018). Moreover, greater reductions in tissue temperatures and blood flow are promoted by alternative cooling strategies such as cold-water immersion (Costello et al., 2012; Abaïdia et al., 2017; Mawhinney et al., 2017; Wilson et al., 2018). Whole-body cryotherapy has also been shown to effect hormonal alterations (steroid hormone and testosterone) and shift autonomic nervous system function to a more parasympathetic status (Louis et al., 2020). However, no data currently exist showing these promising biological fluctuations influence recovery markers in soccer players (Grasso et al., 2014; Russell et al., 2017). Overall, there is a lack of support for whole-body cryotherapy as a recovery modality in soccer players. Alternative cryotherapy methods such as cold-water immersion demonstrate greater efficacy for improving recovery. Potential positive endocrine and immune alterations following whole-body cryotherapy require further investigation (Figure 6.4).

### Hot-water immersion

Hot-water immersion typically involves shoulder depth submergence in 36°C or more and is commonly used by 71% of La Liga teams in Spain as a recovery strategy (Altarriba-Bartes et al., 2020). Practically, hot or thermoneutral water immersion recovery may be used to increase the range of movement at specific joints whilst reducing load and utilising the hydrostatic pressure to increase blood flow (Ménétrier et al., 2013). To date, there is a lack of data on athletes, particularly, team sports in relation to the performance recovery outcomes of hot-water immersion. Versey et al. (2013) observed no beneficial effects on recovery compared to other more commonly used variations of water immersion (cold, thermoneutral, and contrast). The theory underpinning the possible beneficial effects of hot-water immersion is plausible. The

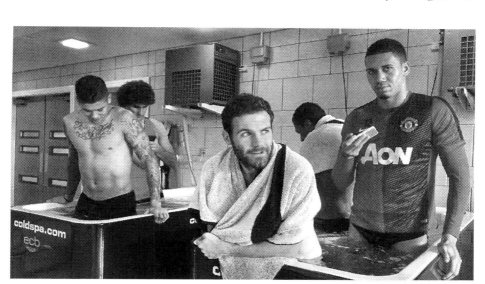

*Figure 6.4* Cold-water immersion.

combination of the hydrostatic pressure of water and increased temperatures have been shown to substantially improve tissue temperature and blood flow, which may provide an unloaded method through which to remove disruptive metabolites following strenuous exercise/match-play (Ménétrier et al., 2013). Furthermore, promising data exist showing the accelerative healing effects of heat application to exercised muscle alongside systemic pro-inflammatory and haemodynamic properties of hot-water immersion in non-athletic populations (Hoekstra et al., 2008; Cheng et al., 2017; Francisco et al., 2021). Similarly, increasing in popularity among athletes, sauna bathing, performed for decades and with positive associations with cardiovascular and mental health in the general population, worsened performance in elite swimmers when used as a recovery strategy between races (Skorski et al., 2020). On the contrary, sauna bathing improved neuromuscular performance in trained men following resistance exercise (Mero et al., 2015). Although there is currently a lack of supporting evidence for enhanced recovery in soccer, augmented circulatory, perceptual, and healing responses following post-exercise heating remains plausible.

## *Compression garments*

Compression garments have been used for decades in the clinical setting and have become increasingly popular in athletic environments. Around 25% of teams in France and 74% of teams in Spain's top divisions use compression garments for recovery purposes (Nédélec et al., 2013; Altarriba-Bartes et al., 2020). Compression garments apply external mechanical pressure to the skin, thereby, providing tissue structural support and possibly stabilisation (MacRae et al., 2011). Other potential mechanisms include enhanced venous return through superficial veins and improved capillary filtration which may reduce venous pooling in the lower limbs following exercise (Partsch & Mosti, 2008). This effect is achieved by applying a pressure gradient which is the highest

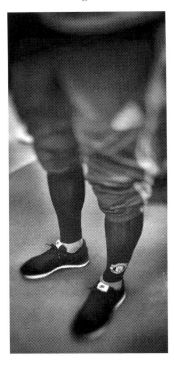

*Figure 6.5* Compression garments.

in the foot/ankle region and lowest in the upper calf (stockings) and quad (tights). As a result, the increase in venous return is thought to aid in the removal of waste products promoting a quicker return to blood gas homeostasis (Davies et al., 2009). Moreover, advantageous hemodynamic mechanisms have been observed following the use of compression garments after physically exerting exercise (Lee et al., 2018).

Recent reviews have shown a positive effect of compression garments on recovery in elite athletes (Hill et al., 2014). In particular, custom-fitted compression garments improved the recovery of perceptual and muscle damage markers in team sports athletes (Upton et al., 2017). Moreover, the efficacy of pneumatic sequential compression for increased blood flow has been demonstrated in clinical populations (Feldman et al., 2012). In athlete populations, pneumatic sequential compression has been seen to increase circulating lactate post-exercise, however, there is a lack of evidence supporting improved recovery or reduced muscle damage markers (Zelikovski et al., 1993). Overall, there is sufficient evidence to support the use of compression garments for accelerating recovery in soccer (Figure 6.5).

### *Sleep*

In a survey performed in a soccer team participating in the UEFA Europa League, 95% of the players highlighted poor sleep following night matches (Nédélec et al., 2015). This may be a consequence of the heightened physical and mental load involved during match-play (Nédélec et al., 2015). The recovery process may be affected, and recovery kinetics slowed, following a perturbed sleep at night (Nédélec et al., 2015). In addition, poor sleep at night may accentuate muscle damage or limit muscle repair, which slows muscle performance recovery kinetics (Skein et al., 2013; Nédélec et al., 2015). Central function plays a key role in fatigue perception but also in muscle function. It has been hypothesised that this cognitive aspect may be negatively affected when the period of sleep is insufficient or when the quality of sleep is bad (Nédélec et al., 2015).

Scientists have shown a possible negative effect of a lack of sleep on glycogen resynthesis (Skein et al., 2011). A poor night's sleep may be compensated by a short post-lunch nap. Waterhouse et al. (2007) found that a nap, followed by a 30-min recovery period, improved alertness and aspects of mental and physical performance following partial sleep loss. The ability to nap for short periods during the day may be a useful skill for players to acquire especially during a congested fixture schedule. Recommendations for sleep induction include adopting a dark and quiet environment using eyeshades and earplugs, listening to relaxing music, and adopting regular sleep-wake schedules. Conversely, consumption of caffeine prior to the match for performance enhancement, alcohol as a means of celebrating after the match, and hyper-hydration could lead to sleep disturbance.

### Psychological aspects

Psychological aspects are an important consideration in the process of recovery. It is important to consider these aspects by individually monitoring the factors leading to detrimental effects on recovery. A high level of stress impairs the recovery process (Stults-Kolehmainen et al., 2014). The speech delivered by the coach may also influence the psychobiological response of the players. Comparing positive and negative feedback of the coach showed different physiological responses the day after a match (Crewther & Cook, 2012). More specifically, the use of video feedback from the previous match alongside positive coach feedback leads to beneficial effects on testosterone secretions (Crewther & Cook, 2012). Psychological aspects are also involved when applying recovery strategies. Players' perceptions of recovery are linked to psychological and social aspects (Venter, 2014). For instance, prayer, relaxation strategies, and discussions with teammates and friends are considered as important recovery strategies by elite soccer players (Venter, 2014). Removing a recovery strategy perceived as effective by a player could also impair the recovery process. Beliefs and expectations from a strategy may have a beneficial or deleterious effect on recovery (Abaïdia et al., 2017). These placebo and nocebo effects are individual processes that should be known when applying a recovery strategy. From a practical point of view, questioning the players about their habits and beliefs at the beginning of the season may be an interesting approach to educate and individualise the recovery protocol.

An array of different strategies are used by professional teams and players in an attempt to alleviate the deleterious symptoms associated with training and games (Nédélec et al., 2013; Altarriba-Bartes et al., 2020). However, there is currently a lack of efficacy for several strategies in improving the multifactorial systems which underpin recovery. Cold-water immersion, compression garments, self-myofascial release, and active or hot-water recovery appear able to promote specific physiological changes at various time points to accelerate the players' return towards their pre-training/match state. These include a reduction in tissue temperature and blood flow together with an increase in joint range of motion, blood flow, and venous return.

## Future directions and conclusions

The physical and mental stress induced by match-play and training lead to increased levels of fatigue in the player. Recovery is a complex and multifaceted process involving physiological and psychological parameters which need to be regenerated at certain time points to reduce susceptibility to non-functional overreaching, injury, and illness. A recovery intervention strategy should serve to match a given stress with the most effective intervention at a given time point on the recovery continuum. A plethora of recovery strategies are commonly applied in the field despite limited scientific evidence to support their efficacy. The foundation of any intervention strategy should be based on quality sleep and rest along with nutrition and hydration. Beyond this, there is sufficient scientific evidence to advocate the use of cold-water immersion and compression garments to further accelerate the recovery process. Self-myo-fascial release and heating modalities may support specific physiological processes at various time points though more research is needed to fully support their efficacy. Finally, an optimal recovery intervention strategy likely reflects a balance between evidence-based prescription and individual athlete preferences.

In future, research is needed to better understand the efficacy of different recovery modalities in isolation together with the interaction between various interventions at relevant time points on the recovery continuum. This integrated focus should centre on the influence of different interventions on the restoration of physical performance alongside studies using advanced laboratory techniques (e.g., assessment of muscle perfusion and cellular and molecular responses) to foster a better understanding of the mechanisms which mediate their effects. Finally, recovery remains one of the least understood aspects of the exercise-adaptation cycle (Peake & Gandevia, 2017). More work is, therefore, needed to better understand the impact of the varied intervention strategies on the balance between accelerating recovery and mediating long-term adaptation.

## References

Abaïdia, A. E., Lamblin, J., Delecroix, B., Leduc, C., McCall, A., Nédélec, M., Dawson, B., Baquet, G., & Dupont, G. (2017). Recovery from exercise-induced muscle damage: cold-water immersion versus whole-body cryotherapy. *Int J Sports Physiol Perform, 12*(3), 402–409. https://doi.org/10.1123/ijspp.2016-0186.

Almeida, A. C., Machado, A. F., Albuquerque, M. C., Netto, L. M., Vanderlei, F. M., Vanderlei, L. C. M., Junior, J. N., & Pastre, C. M. (2015). The effects of cold water immersion with different dosages (duration and temperature variations) on heart rate variability post-exercise recovery: a randomized controlled trial. *J Sci Med Sport, 19*(8), 676–81. doi: 10.1016/j.jsams.2015.10.003.

Altarriba-Bartes, A., Peña, J., Vicens-Bordas, J., Casals, M., Peirau, X., & Calleja-González, J. (2020). The use of recovery strategies by Spanish first division soccer teams: a cross-sectional survey. *Physician Sports Med, 15*, 1–11. https://doi.org/10.1080/00913847.2020.1819150.

Andersson, H., Raastad, T., Nilsson, J., Paulsen, G., Garthe, I., & Kadi, F. (2008). Neuromuscular fatigue and recovery in elite female soccer: effects of active recovery. *Med Sci Sports Exerc, 40*(2), 372–380. https://doi.org/10.1249/mss.0b013e31815b8497.

Bengtsson, H., Ekstrand, J., & Hägglund, M.(2013). Muscle injury rates in professional football increase with fixture congestion: an 11-year follow-up of the UEFA champions league injury study. *Br J Sports Med*, *47*(12), 743–747. doi: 10.1136/bjsports-2013-092383.

Barnes, C., Archer, D., Hogg, B., Bush, M. & Bradley, P. S. The evolution of physical and technical performance parameters in the English Premier League. International journal of sports medicine 35, 1095–1100 (2014).

Bleakley, C. M., & Davison, G. W. (2010). What is the biochemical and physiological rationale for using cold-water immersion in sports recovery? A systematic review. *Br J Sports Med*, *44*(3), 179–187. https://doi.org/10.1136/bjsm.2009.065565

Buchheit, M., Peiffer, J. J., Abbiss, C. R., & Laursen, P. B. (2009). Effect of cold water immersion on postexercise parasympathetic reactivation. *Am J Physiol Heart Circ Physiol*, *296*(2), H421–H427. https://doi.org/10.1152/ajpheart.01017.2008.

Cannon, J. G., & St Pierre, B. A. (1998). Cytokines in exertion-induced skeletal muscle injury. *Mol Cell Biochem*, *179*(1–2), 159–167. https://doi.org/10.1023/a:1006828425418.

Chakravarthy, M. V., Davis, B. S., & Booth, F. W. (2000). IGF-1 restores satellite cell proliferative potential in immobilized old skeletal muscle. *J Appl Physiol*, *89*, 1365–1379. https://doi.org/10.1152/jappl.2000.89.4.1365.

Cheatham, S. W., Kolber, M. J., Cain, M., & Lee, M. (2015). The effects of self-myofascial release using a foam roll or roller massager on joint range of motion, muscle recovery, and performance: a systematic review. *Int J Sports Phys Ther*, *10*(6), 827–838.

Cheng, A. J., Willis, S. J., Zinner, C., Chaillou, T., Ivarsson, N., Ørtenblad, N., Lanner, J. T., Holmberg, H. C., & Westerblad, H. (2017). Post-exercise recovery of contractile function and endurance in humans and mice is accelerated by heating and slowed by cooling skeletal muscle. *J Physiol*, *595*(24), 7413–7426. https://doi.org/10.1113/JP274870.

Clarkson, P. M., & Hubal, M. J. (2002). Exercise-induced muscle damage in humans. *Am J of Phys Med Rehab*, *81*(11 Suppl), S52–S69. https://doi.org/ 10.1097/00002060-200211001-00007

Costello, J. T., Algar, L. A., & Donnelly, A. E. (2012). Effects of whole-body cryotherapy (–110 °C) on proprioception and indices of muscle damage. *Scand J Med Science Sports*, *22*(2), 190–198. https://doi.org/10.1111/j.1600-0838.2011.01292.x

Costello, J. T., Baker, P. R., Minett, G. M., Bieuzen, F., Stewart, I. B., & Bleakley, C. (2016). Cochrane review: whole-body cryotherapy (extreme cold air exposure) for preventing and treating muscle soreness after exercise in adults. *J Evid Med*, *9*(1), 43–44. https://doi.org/10.1111/jebm.12187.

Crewther, B. T., & Cook, C. J. (2012). Effects of different post-match recovery interventions on subsequent athlete hormonal state and game performance. *Physiol Behav*, *106*(4), 471–475. doi: 10.1016/j.physbeh.2012.03.015.

Dadebo, B., White, J., & George K. P. (2004). A survey of flexibility training protocols and hamstring strains in professional football clubs in England. *Br J Sports Med*, *38*(4), 388–394. doi: 10.1136/bjsm.2002.000044.

Davies, V., Thompson, K. G., & Cooper, S.-M. (2009). The effects of compression garments on recovery. *J Strength Cond Res*, *23*(6), 1786–1794. https://doi.org/10.1519/JSC.0b013e3181b42589

Douglas J, Plews DJ, Handcock PJ, Rehrer NJ. The Beneficial Effect of Parasympathetic Reactivation on Sympathetic Drive During Simulated Rugby Sevens. Int J Sports Physiol Perform. 2016 May;11(4):480-8. doi: 10.1123/ijspp.2015-0317. Epub 2015 Sep 10. PMID: 26356254.

Dupont, G., Nedelec, M., McCall, A., McCormack, D., Berthoin, S., & Wisløff, U. (2010). Effect of 2 soccer matches in a week on physical performance and injury rate. *Am J Sports Med*, *38*(9), 1752–1758. doi: 10.1177/0363546510361236.

Ekstrand J, Hägglund M, Fuller CW. Scand J Med Sci Sports. 2011 Dec;21(6):824–32. doi: 10.1111/j.1600-0838.2010.01118.x

Ekstrand, J., Spreco, A., & Davison, M. (2018). Elite football teams that do not have a winter break lose on average 303 player-days more per season to injuries than those teams that do: a comparison among 35 professional European teams. *Br J Sports Med*, *53*(19), 1231–1235. doi: 10.1136/bjsports-2018-099506.

Eliakim, T., Morgulev, E., & Lidor, R. and Meckel, M. (2020). Estimation of injury costs: financial damage of English Premier League teams' underachievement due to injuries. *BMJ Open Sport Exerc Med*, *6*(1), e000675. doi: 10.1136/bmjsem-2019-000675corrl.

Elias, G. P., Wyckelsma, V. L., Varley, M. C., Mckenna, M. J., & Aughey, R. J. (2013).Effectiveness of water immersion on postmatch recovery in elite professional footballers. *Int J Sports Physiol Perform*, *8*(3), 243–254. doi: 10.1123/ijspp.8.3.243.

Fairchild, T. J., Armstrong, A. A., Rao, A., Liu, H., Lawrence, S., & Fournier, P. A. (2003). Glycogen synthesis in muscle fibers during active recovery from intense exercise. *Med Sci Sports Exerc*, *35*(4), 595–602. https://doi.org/10.1249/01.MSS.0000058436.46584.8E

Feldman, J. L., Stout, N. L., Wanchai, A., Stewart, B. R., Cormier, J. N., & Armer, J. M. (2012). Intermittent pneumatic compression therapy: a systematic review. *Lymphology*, *45*(1), 13–25.

Francisco, M. A., Colbert, C., Larson, E. A., Sieck, D. C., Halliwill, J. R., & Minson, C. T. (2021). Hemodynamics of post-exercise vs. post hot water immersion recovery. *J Appl Physiol.*, *30*, 1362–1372. https://doi.org/10.1152/japplphysiol.00260.2020. Online ahead of print.

Fuller, J. T., Thomson, R. L., Howe, P. R. C., & Buckley, J. D. (2015). Vibration therapy is no more effective than the standard practice of massage and stretching for promoting recovery from muscle damage after eccentric exercise. *Clin J Sport Med*, *25*(4), 332–337. https://doi.org/10.1097/JSM.0000000000000149.

Gavin, J. P., Myers, S. D., & Willems, M. E. (2016). Effect of eccentric exercise with reduced muscle glycogen on plasma interleukin-6 and neuromuscular responses of musculus quadriceps femoris. *J Appl Physiol* (1985), *121*(1), 173–184. https://doi.org/10.1152/japplphysiol.00383.2015.

Grasso, D., Lanteri, P., Di Bernardo, C., Mauri, C., Porcelli, S., Colombini, A., Zani, V., Bonomi, F. G., Melegati, G., Banfi, G. & Lombardi, G. (2014). Salivary steroid hormone response to whole-body cryotherapy in elite rugby players. *J Biol Regul Homeost Agents*, *28*(2), 291–300.

Hägglund, M., Waldén, M., Magnusson, H., Kristenson, K., Bengtsson, H., & Ekstrand, J. (2013). Injuries affect team performance negatively in professional football: an 11-year follow-up of the UEFA Champions League injury study. *Br J Sports Med*, *47*(12), 738–742. doi: 10.1136/bjsports-2013-092215. Epub 2013 May 3.

Halson, S. L. (2014). Monitoring training load to understand fatigue in athletes. *Sports Med*, *44*(Suppl 2), S139–S147.

Hawke, T. J., & Garry, D. J. (2001). Myogenic satellite cells: physiology to molecular biology. *J Appl Physiol*, *91*, 534–551. https://doi.org/10.1152/jappl.2001.91.2.534.

Herbert, R. D., de Noronha, M., & Kamper, S. J. (2011). Stretching to prevent or reduce muscle soreness after exercise. *Coch Datab System Rev*, *7*, CD004577. https://doi.org/10.1002/14651858.CD004577.

Hill, J., Howatson, G., van Someren, K., Leeder, J., & Pedlar, C. (2014). Compression garments and recovery from exercise-induced muscle damage: a meta-analysis. *Br J Sports Med*, *48*(18), 1340–1346. https://doi.org/10.1136/bjsports-2013-092456

Hoekstra, S. P., Bishop, N. C., Faulkner, S. H., Bailey, S. J., & Leicht, C. A. (2008–2018). Acute and chronic effects of hot water immersion on inflammation and metabolism in sedentary, overweight adults. *J Appl Physiol*, *125*. https://doi.org/10.1152/japplphysiol.00407.2018.-Regular.

Hunkin, S. L., Fahrner, B., & Gastin, P. B. (2014). Creatine kinase and its relationship with match performance in elite Australian Rules football. *J Sci Med Sport*, *17*(3), 332–336. doi: 10.1016/j.jsams.2013.05.005.

Hyldahl, R. D., Chen, T. C., & Nosaka, K. (2017). Mechanisms and mediators of the skeletal muscle repeated bout effect. *Exerc Sport Sci Rev*, *45*(1), 24–33. https://doi.org/10.1249/JES.0000000000000095.

Ingram, J., Dawson, B., Goodman, C., Wallman, K., & Beilby, J. (2009). Effect of water immersion methods on post-exercise recovery from simulated team sport exercise. *J Sci Med Sport*, *12*(3), 417–421. https://doi.org/10.1016/j.jsams.2007.12.011.

Jacobs, I., Westlin, N., Karlsson, J., Rasmusson, M., & Houghton, B. (1982). Muscle glycogen and diet in elite soccer players. *Eur J Appl Physiol, 48*(3), 297–302. https://doi.org/10.1007/BF00430219.

Kellmann, M., Bertollo, M., Bosquet, L., Brink, M., Coutts, A. J., Dufffield, R., Erlacher, D., Halson, S. L., Hecksteden, A., Heidari, J., Kallus, W., Meeusen, R., Mujika, I., Robazz, C., Skorski, S., Venter, R., and Beckmann, J. (2018). Recovery and performance in sport: consensus statement. *Int J Sports Physiol Perform, 13*(2), 240–245.

Kinugasa, T., & Kilding, A. E. (2009). A comparison of post-match recovery strategies in youth soccer players. *J Strength Cond Res, 23*(5), 1402–1407. https://doi.org/10.1519/JSC.0b013e3181a0226a.

Krustrup, P., Mohr, M., Steensberg, A., Bencke, J., Kjaer, M., & Bangsbo, J. (2006) Muscle and blood metabolites during a soccer game: implications for sprint performance. *Med Sci Sports Exerc, 38*(6), 1165–1174. https://doi.org/10.1249/01.mss.0000222845.89262.cd

Krustrup, P., Ortenblad, N., Nielsen, J., Nybo, L., Gunnarsson, T.P., Iaia, F.M., Madsen, K., Stephens, F., Greenhaff, P., & Bangsbo, J. (2011). Maximal voluntary contraction force, SR function and glycogen resynthesis during the first 72 h after a high-level competitive soccer game. *Eur J Appl Physiol, 111*(12), 2987–2995. https://doi.org/10.1007/s00421-011-1919-y

Lee, D. C. W., Lee, S. W. Y., Khaw, K., Ali, A., Sheridan, S. E., & Wong, S. H. S. (2018). Haemodynamic responses of wearing low-pressure sports compression tights during an orthostatic challenge in healthy individuals. *J Sci Med Sport, 21*(10), 1062–1067. https://doi.org/10.1016/j.jsams.2017.12.004

Leeder, J., van Someren, K. A., Gaze, D., Jewell, A., Deshmukh, N. I. K., Shah, I., Barker, J., & Howatson, G. (2014). Recovery and adaptation from repeated intermittent-sprint exercise. *Int J Sports Physiol Perform, 9*(3), 489–496. doi: 10.1123/ijspp.2012-0316.

Louis, J., Theurot, D., Filliard, J. R., Volondat, M., Dugué, B., & Dupuy, O. (2020). The use of whole-body cryotherapy: time- and dose-response investigation on circulating blood catecholamines and heart rate variability. *Eur J Appl Physiol, 120*(8), 1733–1743. https://doi.org/10.1007/s00421-020-04406-5

Lund, H., Vestergaard-Poulsen, P., Kanstrup, I. L., & Sejrsen, P. (1998). The effect of passive stretching on delayed onset muscle soreness, and other detrimental effects following eccentric exercise. *Scand J Med Sci Sports, 8*(4), 216–221.

MacDonald, G. Z., Penney, M. D. H., Mullaley, M. E., Cuconato, A. L., Drake, C. D. J., Behm, D. G., & Button, D. C. (2013). An acute bout of self-myofascial release increases range of motion without a subsequent decrease in muscle activation or force. *J Strength Cond Res, 27*(3), 812–821. https://doi.org/10.1519/JSC.0b013e31825c2bc1

MacRae, B. A., Cotter, J. D., & Laing, R. M. (2011). Compression garments and exercise: garment considerations, physiology and performance. *Sports Med, 41*(10), 815–884. https://doi.org/10.2165/11591420-000000000-00000.

Malm, C. (2001). Exercise-induced muscle damage and inflammation: fact or fiction? *Acta Physiol Scand, 171*(3), 233–239. https://doi.org/ 10.1046/j.1365-201x.2001.00825.

Massage, I., Water, C., Herrera, E., Sandoval, M. C., Camargo, D. M., & Salvini, T. F. (2010). Motor and sensory nerve conduction are affected differently by ice pack. *Phys Therap, 90*(4), 581–591. doi: 10.2522/ptj.20090131.

Mawhinney, C., Heinonen, I., Low, D. A., Han, C., Jones, H., Kalliokoski, K. K., Kirjavainen, A., Kemppainen, J., Di Salvo, V., Weston, M., Cable, T., & Gregson, W. (2020). Changes in quadriceps femoris muscle perfusion following different degrees of cold-water immersion. *J Appl Physiol, 128*(5), 1392–1401. https://doi.org/10.1152/JAPPLPHYSIOL.00833.2019

Mawhinney, C., Low, D. A., Jones, H., Green, D. J., Costello, J. T., & Gregson, W. (2017). Cold water mediates greater reductions in limb blood flow than whole body cryotherapy. *Med Sci Sports Exerc, 49*(6), 1252–1260. https://doi.org/10.1249/MSS.0000000000001223.

McHugh, M. P. (2003). Recent advances in the understanding of the repeated bout effect: the protective effect against muscle damage from a single bout of eccentric exercise. *Scand J Med Sci Sports, 13*(2), 88–97. https://doi.org/10.1034/j.1600-0838.2003.02477.x.

McHugh, M. P., Connolly, D. A., Eston, R. G., Gleim, G. W. (1999). Exercise-induced muscle damage and potential mechanisms for the repeated bout effect. *Sports Med*, *27*(3), 157–170. https://doi.org/10.2165/00007256-199927030-00002.

Ménétrier, A., Béliard, S., Ravier, G., Mourot, L., Bouhaddi, M., Regnard, J., & Tordi, N. (2013). Changes in femoral artery blood flow during thermoneutral, cold, and contrast-water therapy. *J Sports Med Phys Fit*, *55*(7–8), 768–775.

Mero, A., Tornberg, J., Mäntykoski, M., & Puurtinen, R. (2015). Effects of far-infrared sauna bathing on recovery from strength and endurance training sessions in men. *SpringerPlus*, *4*(1), 1–7. https://doi.org/10.1186/s40064-015-1093-5.

Nimmo MA, Ekblom B; International Association of Athletics Federations. J Sports Sci. 2007;25 Suppl 1:S93-102. doi: 10.1080/02640410701607379.

Nédélec, M., Halson, S., Delecroix, B., Abaidia, A. E., Ahmaidi, S., & Dupont G. (2015). Sleep hygiene and recovery strategies in elite soccer players. *Sports Med*, *45*(11), 1547–1559. doi: 10.1007/s40279-015-0377-9.

Nédélec, M., McCall, A., Carling, C., Legall, F., Berthoin, S., & Dupont, G. (2012). Recovery in soccer: part I - post-match fatigue and time course of recovery. *Sports Med*, *42*(12), 997–1015. https://doi.org/10.2165/11635270-000000000-00000.

Nédélec, M., McCall, A., Carling, C., Legall, F., Berthoin, S., & Dupont, G. (2013). Recovery in soccer : part ii-recovery strategies. *Sports Med*, *43*(1), 9–22. https://doi.org/10.1007/s40279-012-0002-0

Partsch, H., & Mosti, G. (2008). Thigh compression. *Phlebol Ven Forum Royal Soc Med*, *23*(6), 252–258. doi.org/10.1258/phleb.2008.008053.

Peake, J. M., & Gandevia, S. C.(2017). Replace, restore, revive: the keys to recovery after exercise. *J Appl Physiol*, *122*(3), 531–532. doi: 10.1152/japplphysiol.00086.2017.

Peake, J. M., Markworth, J. F., Cumming, K. T., Aas, S. N., Roberts, L. A., Raastad, T., Cameron-Smith, D., & Figueiredo, V. C. (2020). The effects of cold water immersion and active recovery on molecular factors that regulate growth and remodeling of skeletal muscle after resistance exercise. *Front Physiol*, *11*. https://doi.org/10.3389/fphys.2020.00737.

Peake, J., Nosaka, K., & Suzuki, K. (2005). Characterization of inflammatory responses to eccentric exercise in humans. *Exer Immunol Rev*, *11*, 64–85.

Pooley, S., Spendiff, O., Allen, M., & Moir, H. J. (2020). Comparative efficacy of active recovery and cold water immersion as post-match recovery interventions in elite youth soccer. *J Sports Sci*, *38*(11–12), 1423–1431. https://doi.org/10.1080/02640414.2019.1660448

Pyne, D. B., & Martin, D. T. (2011). Fatigue insights from individual and team sports. In Marino, F. E. (ed.), *Regulation of Fatigue in Exercise*, pp. 177–185. New York: Nova Science.

Russell, M., Birch, J., Love, T., Cook, C. J., Bracken, R. M., Taylor, T., Swift, E., Cockburn, E., Finn, C., Cunningham, D., Wilson, L., & Kilduff, L. P. (2017). The effects of a single whole-body cryotherapy exposure on physiological, performance, and perceptual responses of professional academy soccer players after repeated sprint exercise. *J Strength Cond Res*, *31*(2), 415–421. doi: 10.1519/JSC.0000000000001505.

Schoenfeld, B. J. (2013). Post-exercise hypertrophic adaptations: a re-examination of the hormone hypothesis and its applicability to resistance training program design. *J Strength Cond Res*, *27*(6), 1720–1730. https://doi.org/10.1519/JSC.0b013e31828ddd53.

Silva, J. R., Rumpf, M. C., Hertzog, M., Castagna, C., Farooq, A., Girard, O., Hader, K. (2018). Acute and residual soccer match-related fatigue: a systematic review and meta-analysis. *Sports Med*, *48*(3), 539–583. https://doi.org/10.1007/s40279-017-0798-8.

Sinha-Hikim, I., Roth, S. M., Lee, M. I., & Bhasin, S. (2013). Testosterone-induced muscle hypertrophy is associated with an increase in satellite cell number in healthy, young men. *Am J Physiol-Endocrinol Metab*, *285*, E197–E205. https://doi.org/10.1152/ajpendo.00370.2002.

Skein, M., Duffield, R., Edge, J., Short, M. J., & Mündel, T. (2011). Intermittent-sprint performance and muscle glycogen after 30 h of sleep deprivation. *Med Sci Sports Exerc*, *43*(7), 1301–1311. doi: 10.1249/MSS.0b013e31820abc5a.

Skein, M., Duffield, R., Minett, G. M., Snape, A., & Murphy, A. (2013). The effect of overnight sleep deprivation after competitive rugby league matches on postmatch physiological and perceptual recovery. *Int J Sports Physiol Perform*, 8(5), 556–564. doi: 10.1123/ijspp.8.5.556.

Skorski, S., Schimpchen, J., Pfeiffer, M., Ferrauti, A., Kellmann, M., & Meyer, T. (2020). Effects of postexercise sauna bathing on recovery of swim performance. *Int J Sports Physiol Perform*, 15(7), 934–940. https://doi.org/10.1123/ijspp.2019-0333.

Smith, L. L., Anwar, A., Fragen, M., Rananto, C., Johnson, R., & Holbert, D. (2000). Cytokines and cell adhesion molecules associated with high-intensity eccentric exercise. *Eur J Appl Physiol*, 82(1–2), 61–67. https://doi.org/10.1007/s004210050652.

Sterczala, A. J., Flanagan, S. D., Looney, D. P., Hooper, D. R., Szivak, T. K., Comstock, B. A., DuPont, W. H., Martin, G. J., Volek, J. S., Maresh, C. M., & Kraemer, W. J. (2014). Similar hormonal stress and tissue damage in response to National Collegiate Athletic Association Division I football games played in two consecutive seasons. *J Strength Cond Res*, 28(11), 3234–3238. https://doi.org/10.1519/JSC.0000000000000467.

Stults-Kolehmainen, M. A., Bartholomew, J. B., & Sinha, R. (2014). Chronic psychological stress impairs recovery of muscular function and somatic sensations over a 96-hour period. *J Strength Cond Res*, 28(7), 2007–2017. doi: 10.1519/JSC.0000000000000335.

Suzuki, K., Nakaji, S., Yamada, M., Totsuka, M., Sato, K., & Sugawara, K. (2002). Systemic inflammatory response to exhaustive exercise: cytokine kinetics. *Exer Immunol Rev*, 8, 6–48.

Tee, J. C., Bosch, A. N., & Lambert, M. I. (2007). Metabolic consequences of exercise-induced muscle damage. *Sports Med*, 37(10), 827–836. https://doi.org/10.2165/00007256-200737100-00001

Thomson, D., Gupta, A., Arundell, J., & Crosbie, J. (2015). Deep soft-tissue massage applied to healthy calf muscle has no effect on passive mechanical properties: a randomized, single-blind, cross-over study. *BMC Sports Science, Med Rehab*, 7, 21. https://doi.org/10.1186/s13102-015-0015-8

Thorpe, R. T., Atkinson, G., Drust, B., & Gregson, W. (2017). Monitoring fatigue status in elite team sport athletes: implications for practice. *Int J Sports Physiol Perform*, 12(Suppl 2), S227–S234. doi: 10.1123/ijspp.2016-0434.

Upton, C. M., Brown, F. C. W., & Hill, J. A. (2017). Efficacy of compression garments on recovery from a simulated rugby protocol. *J Strength Cond Res*, 31(11), 2977–2982. https://doi.org/10.1519/JSC.0000000000002145.

Vaile, J., Halson, S., Gill, N., & Dawson, B. (2008). Effect of hydrotherapy on the signs and symptoms of delayed onset muscle soreness. *Eur J Appl Physiol*, 102(4), 447–455. https://doi.org/10.1007/s00421-007-0605-6.

Venter, R. E. (2014). Perceptions of team athletes on the importance of recovery modalities. *Eur J Sport Sci*, 14(Suppl 1), S69–S76. doi: 10.1080/17461391.2011.643924.

Verma, S., Moiz, J. A., Shareef, M. Y., & Husain, M. E. (2016). Physical performance and markers of muscle damage following sport-specific sprints in male collegiate soccer players: repeated bout effect. *J Sports Med Phys Fitness*, 56(6), 765–774.

Versey, N. G., Halson, S. L., & Dawson, B. T. (2013). Water immersion recovery for athletes: effect on exercise performance and practical recommendations. *Sports Med*, 43(11), 1101–1130. https://doi.org/10.1007/s40279-013-0063-8

Viitasaslo, J. T., Niemelä, K., Kaappola, R., Korjus, T., Levola, M., Mononen, H. V, Rusko, H. K., & Takala, T. E. (1995). Warm underwater water-jet massage improves recovery from intense physical exercise. *Eur J Appl Physiol*, 71(5), 431–438.

Vromans, B. A., Thorpe, R. T., Viroux, P. J., & Tiemessen, I. J. (2019). Cold water immersion settings for reducing muscle tissue temperature: a linear dose-response relationship. *J Sports Med Phys Fitness*, 59(11), 1861–1869. https://doi.org/10.23736/S0022-4707.19.09398-8.

Warren, G. L., Lowe, D. A., & Armstrong, R. B. (1999). Measurement tools used in the study of eccentric contraction-induced injury. *Sports Med*, 27(1), 43–59. https://doi.org/10.2165/00007256-199927010-00004.

Waterhouse, J., Atkinson, G., Edwards, B., Reilly, T. (2007). The role of a short post-lunch nap in improving cognitive, motor, and sprint performance in participants with partial sleep deprivation. *J Sports Sci*, *25*(14), 1557–1566. doi: 10.1080/02640410701244983.

Wilson, L. J., Cockburn, E., Paice, K., Sinclair, S., Faki, T., Hills, F. A., Gondek, M. B., Wood, A., & Dimitriou, L. (2018). Recovery following a marathon: a comparison of cold water immersion, whole body cryotherapy and a placebo control. *Eur J Appl Physiol*, *118*(1), 153–163. https://doi.org/10.1007/s00421-017-3757-z.

Wiltshire, E. V., Poitras, V., Pak, M., Hong, T., Rayner, J., & Tschakovsky, M. E. (2010). Massage impairs postexercise muscle blood flow and "lactic acid" removal. *Med Sci Sports Exerc*, *42*(6), 1062–1071. doi: 10.1249/MSS.0b013e3181c9214f.

Yarrow, J. F., Borsa, P. A., Borst, S. E., Sitren, H. S., Stevens, B. R., & White, L. J. (2007). Neuroendocrine responses to an acute bout of eccentric-enhanced resistance exercise. *Med Sci Sports Exerc*, *39*(6), 941–947. https://doi.org/10.1097/mss.0b013e318043a249.

Zelikovski, A., Kaye, C. L., Fink, G., Spitzer, S. A., & Shapiro, Y. (1993). The effects of the modified intermittent sequential pneumatic device (MISPD) on exercise performance following an exhaustive exercise bout. *Br J Sports Med*, *27*(4), 255–259.

# Section B

# Social and Behavioural Sciences

# 7 Psychological characteristics of players

*Geir Jordet and Tynke Toering*

## Introduction

In 1958, Brazil wins the World Cup, and a spectacular 17-year-old named Pele scores six goals, including two in the final. Brazil had a team psychologist on staff, Dr Joao Carvalhaes (for full story, see FIFA, 2016). Ahead of departure to the tournament in Sweden, he strongly advised against Pele featuring, saying: "He is too young to feel aggression and respond with appropriate force. In addition to that, he does not possess the sense of responsibility necessary for a team game." However, Brazil coach Feola rejected the psychologist's advice with these words: "You may be right. The thing is you don't know anything about football. If Pele's knee is ready, he plays." Since this historical encounter between a psychologist and a soccer coach, the integration of psychology and soccer knowledge may still be an "Achilles heel" for psychologists. However, the field has made substantial strides, and in this chapter, we attempt to point this out.

In a survey of soccer coaches in the Netherlands about what they want from sports science, the area that most identified as of interest was "mental skills" and the area that they had the least knowledge of was "mental skills" (Brink et al., 2018). Furthermore, in the previous edition of this book, Pain and Harwood (2013) pointed out that the research and general interest in the mental side of the game had increased a lot over the past decade. This growth has continued since then. A search for peer-reviewed articles in the database Sport Discus (in February 2021) with keywords "soccer" and "psychology" generated 2,538 publications. This reflects a doubling of outputs in only 7 years (from the 1,167 hits that were found in the same search in May 2014, Jordet, 2016) (for an overview of the year-by-year development in published articles on soccer and psychology, see Figure 7.1).

In this chapter, we primarily review and discuss research published over the last 5–8 years (since Jordet, 2016; Pain & Harwood, 2013). We will not be able to review everything, but we cover a selection of topics that will have an impact on the field for the years to come. Our major distinction is between performance and development. Where possible, we aim to move beyond the traditional self-report research in sport psychology (i.e., questionnaires and interviews) to report more observation and experimental research.

DOI: 10.4324/9781003148418-9

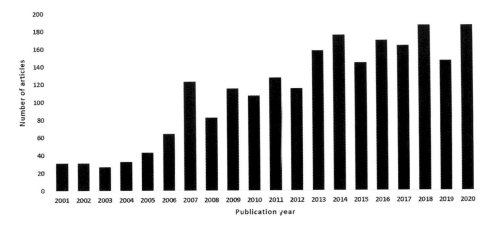

*Figure 7.1* The number of peer review articles from a search with keywords "psychology" and "soccer", registered in the bibliographic database SPORT Discus between 2001 and 2020.

## Performance

In this section, we examine some of the recent knowledge that has emerged about the psychology of game performance, presenting what we know about skilled players' responses to game events, location, confidence, and emotions.

### *Game events*

Soccer players' decision-making is reported to be highly influenced by transient and dynamic aspects of the game that they play, such as their own performance, the score, and the momentum in the game, which makes them vulnerable to external factors beyond their own control (Levi & Jackson, 2018). Psychological momentum can be described as a state of mind where a performer senses that events are going his or her way, and the accompanied perceived competitive superiority, attribution of success to oneself, and increased confidence contributes to an experience of a psychological force that enables a performer to achieve levels ordinarily not possible (Iso-Ahola & Dotson, 2014). Whether momentum in sport is a real phenomenon has been heavily debated by scientists, with cases being made for this simply being an illusion (e.g., Avugos, Köppen, Czienskowski, Raab, & Bar-Eli, 2013). However, in a relatively recent and thorough review, it is argued that methodological and statistical problems have tended to preclude what probably is a real effect, and that psychological momentum exists as a powerful empirical phenomenon, yet one that is occurring occasionally and temporarily (Iso-Ahola & Dotson, 2014).

With that said, there are few comprehensive and well-designed empirical tests of momentum and individual or team performance in or across soccer games. However, in a study of all soccer penalty shootouts in the World Cup and European Championships between 1976 and 2006 (Jordet, Hartman, & Vuijk, 2011), there was evidence of historical dependency, where players on teams who had lost their preceding shootout in one of these tournaments performed worse than players on teams with a preceding win. Although this effect took place over years, sometimes even decades, it is possible that the emotional magnitude of these events (penalty shootouts) would constitute a type of momentum. In another recent study, an analysis of a vast number of games ($N$ = 72,426) shows that scoring right before half-time increases the chances of the scoring team to win (Greve, Nesbø, Rudi, & Salikhov, 2020). This is not evidence of momentum per se, but it is an indication that certain game events carry particularly high importance for future game events and the outcome.

Recently, researchers obtained the perceptions of psychological momentum from a total of 85 professional soccer players (Redwood-Brown, Sunderland, Minniti, & O'Donoghue, 2018). They found that goals were the game events most frequently associated with momentum. Confidence, positive attitude, and team cohesion were important for positive momentum, whereas low confidence and high anxiety were important for negative momentum. Moreover, an experiment with 40 experienced French soccer coaches (with UEFA A or Pro licenses) showed that momentum was a strong influential factor in strategic game decisions (Briki & Zoudji, 2019). Specifically, the study documented that changes in ball possession affected the coaches' perception of momentum, and this again influenced their strategic decisions, with the interesting observation that negative events had a stronger affective effect than positive events.

From these studies, it seems certain game events carry the potential to influence psychological factors, which in turn will influence performance. However, it is surprising that more research has not been conducted to identify specific game events and conditions that might affect the outcome of soccer games via psychological processes.

### Game location

Another focus of research has been on the home advantage. This can be defined as the tendency that the home team is taking more points than the away team, which is well-known and documented in soccer (at the top level, Pollard & Gomez, 2014; and at the youth level, Staufenbiel, Riedl, & Strauss, 2018). Some of the reasons hypothesized to produce home advantage have received empirical support in soccer, such as crowd support (Ponzo & Scoppa, 2018), venue familiarity (van Ours, 2019), travel fatigue (Oberhofer, Philippovich, & Winner, 2010), and territoriality (Neave & Wolfson, 2003). These reasons were all supported in interviews with professional-level soccer players and coaches, from which also, notably, there was a united agreement that crowd support was very important (Forthergill, Wolfson, & Little, 2014).

In perhaps the most comprehensive study to date, Pollard and Gomez (2014) analysed a total of 157 national soccer leagues in the period 2006–2012 (spanning about 170,000 games). The results showed a robust home advantage across the world. Among the most contributing factors were the FIFA ranking (proxy for crowd size), distance between game locations, altitude difference between game locations, the occurrence of a civil war, and perception of corruption. The five countries with the highest home advantage in the world (i.e., #1 Nigeria, #2 Bosnia-Herzegovina, #3 Guatemala, #4 Indonesia, and #5 Algeria) all have regional ethnic division and/or a history of civil wars, which supports a view that territoriality is an influential factor for home advantage. This adds to the findings by Neave and Wolfson (2003) that players for home teams (in the United Kingdom) have increased testosterone levels compared to away team players (indicating that territoriality or an intention to protect the home turf is a factor). Recently, this was elaborated on in a study where observers were asked to assess whether randomly collected photos taken prior to UEFA Champions League (and amateur) games showed home or away players (Furley, Schweizer, & Memmert, 2018). The observers were indeed able to identify the players who played home or away, and home players were perceived to have a more dominant body language (significantly more assertive, confident, and aggressive) than the away-players.

Covid-19 made it possible for researchers to conduct natural experiments on the effects of playing without crowds. In certain leagues, the home advantage without crowds dropped significantly, and occasionally turned into a home disadvantage (e.g., in the German Bundesliga, where teams took 54% of the points with crowds and 44% without crowds, Tilp & Thaller, 2020). A report comparing 63 major soccer leagues on the number of home-wins with normal crowds (January 2015–March 2020) and without crowds (April–August 2020) shows more variation across leagues, but with home-wins dropping in 65% of the leagues (41 of 63) and a total of 2.1% drop in home-wins when playing without crowd (CIES Football Observatory, 2020). This finding suggests that crowd support is a considerable factor to explain the home advantage. Moreover, a study of Red Bull Salzburg players' behaviours with and without crowds, showed that the players were involved in about 20% fewer emotional situations in games without crowd, than with crowd (e.g., self-reproaching, protesting, and discussions, Leitner & Richlan, 2021). The researchers argue that without the impact of supporters, players, and staff behaved less emotionally.

### Confidence

There seems to be a robust link between self-confidence and performance in soccer players (e.g., Bray, Balaguer, & Duda, 2003). Interviews show that players' confidence in a game is most impacted by a player's own game performance, the result in that game, and game momentum, with positive events leading players to more risky decisions and negative events to more conservative decisions (Levi & Jackson, 2018). Academy soccer players (12–15 years of age) were most confident about aspects of their skill execution, compared to physical and psychological aspects, whereas confidence-debilitative factors cited were lack of social support, weak performances, bad preparation, pressure and expectations, and injury/illness (Thomas, Thrower, Lane, & Thomas, 2019).

Most research on confidence has relied on self-report measures, and we now turn to a perspective focusing on on-pitch behaviours. In major soccer penalty shootouts, it has been shown that players taking so-called positive shots (where a potential goal immediately would secure the win) score considerably more goals than players with negative shots (where a miss immediately would cement a loss) (Jordet & Hartman, 2008). This says something quite powerful about the indirect and likely influence of pre-performance hopes, fears, and/or expectations on performance in high-pressure moments. In addition, in the leadup to their shots, players with positive shots showed significantly more approach behaviours (maintained their gaze looking forward and took time after the referee's whistle to start the run-up), than did the players with negative shots (who showed more avoidance behaviours – diverted their gaze and rushed their shot preparations).

Furley, Dicks, Stendke, and Memmert (2012) exposed 20 experienced goalkeepers to point-light video clips of penalty shooters exhibiting these exact approach and avoidance behaviours. The results supported and added to the results from the field studies,

_Psychological characteristics of players_    115

as the goalkeepers' impressions of the shooters were less favourable, and they were more confident in saving penalties, against shooters that turned their back towards them and rushed through their preparation. In further studies, it is well-documented that soccer players with a dominant body language (e.g., erect posture, limbs slightly spread to occupy space, eyes looking directly at the viewer, and maintaining that gaze) are viewed more positively, are expected to perform better (Furley, Dicks, & Memmert, 2012; Bijlstra, Furley, & Nieuwenhuys, 2020), and inspire more confidence in teammates – even when additional (and even contradictory) information is introduced about teammates' performance capability (Seiler, Schweizer, & Seiler, 2018) than those with a submissive body language. Moreover, additional experiments showed that those feeling confident displayed a more dominant, confident, and composed body language compared to those feeling more under threat (task demands exceeded their coping resources) (Brimmel, Parker, Furley, & Moore, 2018) and professional Bundesliga soccer referees who made decisions on ambiguous situations showed a less confident body language than referees making decisions about less ambiguous situations (Furley & Schweizer, 2016). These studies strongly document the impact of soccer players' confidence on performance, one's own and that of others (both teammates and opponents) and the behavioural signs that one can look for when assessing confidence.

### Emotions

Emotional expressions in soccer have been studied in different ways, some quite creative. For example, researchers found that displays of anger and happiness in 4,318 portrait pictures of players from 304 participating teams in all the FIFA World Cup tournaments between 1970 and 2014 were positively correlated with team performance in the World Cup (Hopfensitz & Mantilla, 2019). Specifically, teams whose players displayed more anger conceded significantly fewer goals, and teams whose players displayed more happiness scored significantly more goals. Furthermore, teams whose players' national anthem singing ($N = 102$ anthems) were rated by observers as more passionate and intense were less likely to concede goals, and more likely to win their subsequent game (in the knockout stage) in the 2016 European Championships (Slater, Haslam, & Steffens, 2018). The researchers argue that these effects may have occurred as a result of increased social identity in the teams whose national anthems are delivered with a strong passion.

Focusing on the impact of post-performance behaviours, it was shown that players celebrating a goal increase their chance of ultimately ending up on the winning team in major penalty shootouts (Moll, Pepping, & Jordet, 2010). Certain celebratory gestures significantly reduced the chance that the subsequent opponent would score a goal, and there was a non-significant trend that the next teammate's probability of scoring a goal would go up. These results were supported across four experiments, where observing opponents and teammates showing pride after their shots had the expected effect on stress, confidence, and focus (Furley, Moll, & Memmert, 2015). For example, observing teammates displaying pride made players expect to be more confident and perform better on upcoming shots than when observing teammates displaying a neutral expression. Recent studies extend these findings by showing that coach expressions of emotions influence their players' emotions, and the coach's expressions of pride and happiness were associated with increased player performance (Moll & Davies, 2021; van Kleef, Chesin, Koning, & Wolf, 2019). The practical implication

116  *Geir Jordet and Tynke Toering*

of these studies is that soccer players, teams, and coaches can benefit from showing happiness and pride, as these expressions are likely to affect performance positively.

## Development

Researchers have identified many psychological characteristics potentially related to talent development (TD) in soccer; and a recent review revealed 22 psychological factors: "discipline, self-control, self-awareness, adaptive perfectionism, self-acceptance, task/mastery orientation, commitment, determination, intrinsic motivation, self-regulation, resilience, grit, non-verbal intelligence, fear of failure, psychological wellbeing, reflective skills, enjoyment, perceived competence, anticipatory skills, decision-making skills, delaying gratification and coping strategies" (Gledhill, Harwood, & Forsdyke, 2017, p. 105). However, it remains largely unknown how these psychological factors eventually relate to adult performance.

### *Lack of knowledge about underlying mechanisms*

Being aware that psychological factors are just one part of the puzzle, important reasons for the limited knowledge about the psychology of development seem to be that the majority of studies have been conducted solely with youth participants (e.g., Erikstad, Høigaard, Johansen, Kandala, & Haugen, 2018; Zuber, Zibung, & Conzelmann, 2015), have based their predictions of eventual adult performance on players' score as an academy player years ago (e.g., Forsman, Blomqvist, Davids, Liukkonen & Konttinen, 2016; Van Yperen, 2009), and have primarily focused on the success stories rather than the "failures" (exceptions are Holt & Mitchell, 2006; Taylor & Collins, 2019). Longitudinal studies about the exact relationship between psychological factors and the outcomes of transitions along the talent pathway to first-team soccer are lacking, as confirmed by a recent meta-analysis based on 11 prospective studies, 10 of which were conducted solely with youth players (three studies predicted adult performance based on academy scores; Ivarsson, Kilhage-Persson, Martindale, Priestley, Huijgen, Ardern, & McCall, 2020). The lack of knowledge about mechanisms underpinning successful transition into the senior professional context warrants questions, such as whether a specific combination of predictors is equally important throughout development and across individuals and contexts. Alternatively, we agree with several other researchers that a broad range of psychological attributes is needed to face these transitions regardless (cf., Collins, MacNamara & Cruickshank, 2019; Jordet, 2016).

### *Transition to professional soccer*

It has been pointed out before that the context of professional soccer is very different from academy soccer (e.g., Røynesdal, Toering, & Gustafsson, 2018; Swainston, Wilson, & Jones, 2020); young players move from a relatively supportive, development-focused environment in the academy to the brutal, short-term success-driven environment of professional soccer. The chances of succeeding and becoming a professional soccer player are small, knowing that only 0.04% of all people playing soccer are professional players (Haugaasen & Jordet, 2012). To further complicate the process, the age range in which the transition to professional soccer takes place comes

*Psychological characteristics of players* 117

around the same time as several other developmental challenges, such as growing from adolescence into young adulthood and dual career demands, while pressure from parents, coaches, and support staff to continuously perform well may impact on players' performance and wellbeing (e.g., Morris, Tod, & Eubank, 2017; Morris, Tod & Oliver, 2016). In line with this, a meta-study on factors positively associated with a successful junior-to-senior transition in sports included a long list of psychological aspects (Drew, Morris, Tod, & Eubank, 2019).

Specifically, soccer research has shown that, while male youth players tend to be aware that men's soccer is going to be completely different than academy soccer in terms of physical demands, playing style, decision-making demands, and fitting in socially (e.g., Morris et al., 2017; Swainston et al., 2020), dealing with several of these challenges for real often turns out to be difficult (e.g., Champ, Nesti, Ronkainen, Tod, & Littlewood, 2020). Players' experiences being part of the first squad for a while are characterized by frustration related to being on the bottom of the pile, as well as motivation to improve as a player (e.g., Mitchell, Gledhill, Nesti, Richardson, & Littlewood, 2020; Swainston et al., 2020). To not be prioritized as challenging and can affect player confidence. They try to find out what the first-team coach wants from players in their position. Being sent on loan could be a good or bad experience, largely dependent on the received amount of playing time and availability of psychological skills to handle switching clubs (Champ et al., 2020; Mitchell et al., 2020; Swainston et al., 2020). If a club is happy to have you and you get to play, it boosts your confidence; if not, being a soccer player can be very lonely. Furthermore, impression management could be essential; young players must make sure that senior professionals perceive them as credible cases (Røynesdal et al., 2018). Other challenges could be dealing with the fact that you have to grasp an opportunity once you get it, pressure from parents and friends, living away from home, and dealing with success (new status, media attention, friends/girlfriends; e.g., Champ et al., 2020; Mitchell et al., 2020; Morris et al., 2017).

Social support seems particularly important for successful transitions to professional. For example, being on a U23 team may help, given that others in the team are in the same situation (transitioning) and talking about experiences is experienced as helpful (e.g., Swainston et al., 2020). Some players seem hesitant to speak with first-team players or the first-team coach for fear of being regarded as weak. Support from coaches seems to become more important later in the process (Morris et al., 2017) and it has been suggested that organizational support by clubs should be improved (e.g., Champ et al., 2020; Morris et al., 2017; Røynesdal et al., 2018). Although female players transitioning to the professional level report similar factors affecting their transition as their male counterparts, one difference seems to be that they do seek social support from senior players (McGreary, Morris, & Eubank, 2021). The latter could be related to a less masculine culture within women's football, with different key values. Another key aspect is that dual career issues were pertinent due to the recent professionalization of women's soccer, meaning that young players could spend less time on their education given that more time was devoted to their sport (McGreary et al., 2021).

### *Behavioural outcomes*

It is clear then that the development of a broad range of psychological attributes is necessary to help players develop throughout the academy pathway and transition

118  *Geir Jordet and Tynke Toering*

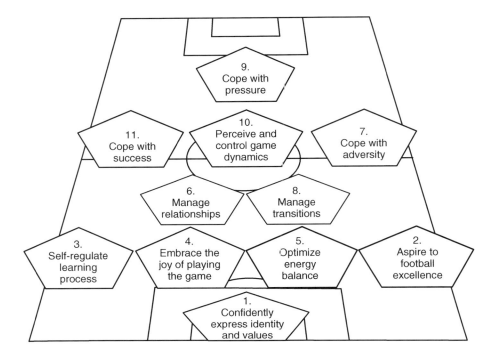

*Figure 7.2* The 11-model. Behavioural outcomes that are important to successfully transition from youth academy to professional first team. Adapted from Jordet, 2016.

into professional soccer. Figure 7.2 presents an updated model with behavioural outcomes we suggest is important to successfully traverse the bumpy path from youth academy to professional soccer (cf., Jordet, 2016). These behavioural outcomes are underpinned by a broad range of psychological attributes. Researchers have indicated the importance of confidence, its relationship with body language, and expressing one's identity and values (e.g., Brimmel et al., 2018; Champ et al., 2020), as well as optimally balancing one's energy (e.g., McLoughlin, Fletcher, Slavich, Arnold, & Moore, 2021). Together with embracing the joy of playing the game (e.g., Zuber, Zibung, & Conzelmann, 2015), taking care of and resonating optimal mental and physical fitness, and a healthy sense of self are essential building blocks for both performance and well-being. Additionally, players must aspire to excellence, which sometimes means sacrificing short-term comfort (e.g., Toering & Jordet, 2015), self-regulate their learning (e.g., Toering, in press), manage transitions (e.g., Roynesdal et al., 2018), manage relationships (e.g., Taylor & Collins, 2019), perceive and control game dynamics (e.g., Jordet et al., 2020), cope with adversity (e.g., Ivarsson et al., 2020), cope with pressure (e.g., Furley, Dicks, & Jordet, 2020), and cope with success (e.g., Taylor & Collins, 2019). Academy players need to be educated and supported in developing all these behavioural outcomes to flexibly deal with transitions and key events on their pathway to professional soccer.

The capacity to display the behavioural outcomes in Figure 7.2 is expected to increase players' ability to self-regulate their behaviour, in that the increased cognitive-behavioural flexibility frees up resources that now can be used to optimally perform or pick up the lessons to be learned (Toering, in press). One specific way to work on the latter is video-feedback which coaches and youth players reported to regard as beneficial for several psychological processes previously highlighted in the literature (Middlemas & Harwood, 2018), such as imagery and self-regulation (Collins et al., 2019; Toering, Elferink-Gemser, Jordet, & Visscher, 2009), as well as contribute to the encouragement of self-regulatory skills. Reflective thinking was specifically identified as a key process in coping with setbacks and learning from mistakes (Middlemas & Harwood, 2018, 2020).

## Future directions and conclusions

There has been a considerable growth in research on psychology in soccer this past decade, but some biases are still at play though – with substantially more research on male players compared to women, and as this review reflects, there is a lot of research from the United Kingdom, Germany, the Netherlands, and Scandinavia, and less from many other parts of the world. Recently, a case was made that in the future psychology research will be more soccer-specific, explore more the integration with analytics, and rely more on technology (Jordet, 2019). Here, we will elaborate and add some nuance to some of these points.

Generally, there is still too little research on psychology in soccer where the game itself is the centre of attention. Traditionally, sport psychology researchers are more interested in the psychological process in question, rather than how the process relates to the game itself (for more on this issue, see Jordet & Pepping, 2019). This is one of the reasons that the penalty kick has been researched quite extensively; it is a closed skill executed under relatively controlled conditions, lending itself well to psychological experiments and analyses. Going forward, we hope to see more research on the ways that psychological aspects support and facilitate performance in dynamic, open play games. To achieve this, researchers need to embrace the game and ask research questions that originate from people in soccer. Game location and momentum are good examples of areas where the game can drive research questions, because those involved in the sport will easily recognize the impact of these areas on performance and results. However, there is still very limited knowledge about both the specific behavioural mechanisms at play, and ways to address this in practice for players, teams, and coaches. In this chapter, we have presented some studies that have started to close this gap (e.g., Furley et al. 2018).

We have also shown how analyses of behaviours have become more popular, including some impressive work on non-verbal communication. However, much more research is needed on physical manifestations of psychology, observable, and measurable, which can enable and support on-field observations and measurements (Shiperd et al., 2018). It is long overdue that psychology meets game analytics, to give analyses of individual and team behaviours in soccer games, combining psychological constructs with the methodological precision and rigour from analytics, which would be useful for both performance and development. A recent example is our own study on visual perception in a Premier League team, where videos of real games were filmed and a behavioural indication of perception prior to receiving the ball (i.e., scanning, where the face and eyes are moved away from the ball to detect information relevant for engaging with the ball) was analysed with the help of game analysts and data analysts at the club (Jordet et al., 2020). This research produced a detailed understanding of how scanning systematically varies in games and how it is linked to performance.

Finally, we are likely to see much more sophisticated use of technology to better understand and affect players' psychology. Computer vision (to automatically code behaviours), artificial intelligence (to more effectively interpret patterns in behavioural data), and virtual/augmented reality (to more effectively simulate and train game situations) are all technologies that not only belong to the future, but they are also currently used now. More research is needed into the effective use of this technology, to benefit the research and applied field.

In conclusion, all these points stress the increasing importance of the context. It also indicates that more interdisciplinary research is necessary to enable a useful translation of findings to the practice field because only then we will be able to capture enough of the complexity of the context. This will help advance the psychological side of the game as well as the psychological development of soccer players from the academy to professional environments.

## References

Avugos, S., Koppen, J., Csienskowski, U., Raab, M., & Bar-Eli, M. (2013). The "hot hand" reconsidered: a meta-analytic approach. *Psychology of Sport and Exercise, 14*, 21–27. doi:10.1016/j.psychsport.2012.07.005

Bijlstra, G., Furley, P., & Nieuwenhuys, A. (2020). The power of nonverbal behavior: penalty-takers' body language influences impression formation and anticipation performance in goalkeepers in a simulated soccer penalty task. *Psychology of Sport and Exercise, 46*, 1.

Bray, S. R., Balaguer, I., & Duda, J. (2003). The relationship of task self-efficacy and role efficacy beliefs to role performance in Spanish youth soccer. *Journal of Sports Sciences, 22*, 429–437.

Briki, W., & Zoudji, B. (2019). Gaining or losing team ball possession: the dynamics of momentum perception and strategic choice in football coaches. *Frontiers in Psychology, 10*, 1019.

Brimmell, J., Parker, J. K., Furley, P., & Moore, L. J. (2018). Nonverbal behavior accompanying challenge and threat states under pressure. *Psychology of Sport and Exercise, 39*, 90–94.

Brink, M., Kuyvenhoven, Toering, T. T., Jordet, G., & Frencken, W. (2018). What do football coaches want from sport science? *Kinesiology, 50*(Suppl 1), 150–154.

Champ, F. M., Nesti, M. S., Ronkainen, N. J., Tod, D. A., & Littlewood, M. A. (2020). An exploration of the experiences of elite youth footballers: the impact of organizational culture. *Journal of Applied Sport Psychology, 32*(2), 146–167.

CIES Football Observatory (2020). *What About the Home Advantage After the COVID-19 Pandemic?* Switzerland: International Centre for Sports Studies (CIES) https://football-observatory.com/IMG/sites/b5wp/2020/wp304/en/

Collins, D., MacNamara, Á., & Cruickshank, A. (2019). Research and practice in talent identification and development—Some thoughts on the state of play. *Journal of Applied Sport Psychology, 31*(3), 340–351.

Drew, K., Morris, R., Tod, D., & Eubank, M. (2019). A meta-study of qualitative research on the junior-to-senior transition in sport. *Psychology of Sport and Exercise, 45*, 101556.

Erikstad, M. K., Høigaard, R., Johansen, B. T., Kandala, N. B., & Haugen, T. (2018). Childhood football play and practice in relation to self-regulation and national team selection; a study of Norwegian elite youth players. *Journal of sports sciences, 36*(20), 2304–2310.

FIFA (2016). *Behind the World Cup record: Pele.* Switzerland: FIFA. https://www.fifa.com/worldcup/news/behind-the-world-cup-record-pele-2852661

Forsman, H., Blomqvist, M., Davids, K., Liukkonen, J., & Konttinen, N. (2016). Identifying technical, physiological, tactical and psychological characteristics that contribute to career progression in soccer. *International Journal of Sports Science & Coaching, 11*, 505–513.

Fothergill, M., Wolfson, S., & Little, L. (2014). A qualitative analysis of perceptions of venue: do professional soccer players and managers concur with the conceptual home advantage framework? *International Journal of Sport and Exercise Psychology, 12*(4), 316–332.

Furley, P., Dicks, M., & Jordet, G. (2020). The influence of emotions on penalty taker and goalkeeper performance. In J. G. Dixon, J. B. Barker, R. C. Thelwell, & I. Mitchell (eds.), *The Psychology of Soccer* (pp. 29–43). New York: Routledge.

Furley, P., Dicks, M., Stendke, F., & Memmert, D. (2012). 'Get it out the way. The wait's killing me' hastening and hiding during soccer penalty kicks. *Psychology of Sport and Exercise, 13*(4), 454–465.

Furley, P., Moll, T., & Memmert, D. (2015). Put your hands up in the air'? the interpersonal effects of pride and shame expressions on opponents and teammates. *Frontiers in Psychology, 6*, 1361.

Furley, P., & Schweizer, G. (2016). Nonverbal communication of confidence in soccer referees: an experimental test of Darwin's leakage hypothesis. *Journal of Sport & Exercise Psychol, 38*(6), 590–597.

Furley, P., Schweizer, G., & Memmert, D. (2018). Thin slices of athletes' nonverbal behavior give away game location: testing the territoriality hypothesis of the home game advantage. *Evolutionary Psychology, 16*(2). ArtID: 1474704918776456

Gledhill, A., Harwood, C., & Forsdyke, D. (2017). Psychosocial factors associated with talent development in football: a systematic review. *Psychology of Sport and Exercise, 31*, 93–112.

Greve, H. R., Nesbø, J., Rudi, N., & Salikhov, M. (2020). Are goals scored just before half-time worth more? An old soccer wisdom statistically tested. *PLoS One, 15*(10), e0240438. doi:10.1371/journal.pone.0240438. eCollection 2020.

Haugaasen, M., & Jordet, G. (2012). Developing football expertise: a football-specific research review. *International Review Sport Exercise Psychology, 5*(2), 177–201.

Holt, N. L., & Mitchell, T. (2006). Talent development in English professional soccer. *International Journal of Sport Psychology, 37*(2/3), 77.

Hopfensitz, A., & Mantilla, C. (2019). Emotional expressions by sports teams: An analysis of World Cup soccer player portraits. *Journal of Economic Psychology, 75*, 102071.

Iso-Ahola, S. E., Dotson, C. O. (2014). Psychological momentum: why success breeds success. *Rev Gen Psychol, 18*(1), 19–33. doi:10.1037/a0036406

Ivarsson, A., Kilhage-Persson, A., Martindale, R., Priestley, D., Huijgen, B., Ardern, C., & McCall, A. (2020). Psychological factors and future performance of football players: a systematic review with meta-analysis. *Journal of Science and Medicine in Sport, 23*, 415–420.

Jordet, G. (2016). Psychology and elite soccer performance. In T. Strudwick (Ed.), *Soccer Science: Using Science to Develop Players and Teams* (pp. 367–388). Champaign, IL: Human Kinetics

Jordet, G. (2019). Working with psychology in professional football. In D. Collins, A. Cruickshank, & G. Jordet (Eds.), *Routledge Handbook of Elite Sport Development* (pp. 114–132). London: Routledge

Jordet, G., Aksum, K. M., Pedersen, D. N., Walvekar, A., Trivedi, A., McCall, A., Ivarsson, A., & Priestley, D. (2020). Scanning, contextual factors, and association with performance in English Premier League footballers: an investigation across a season. *Frontiers in Psychology, 11*, 2399.

Jordet, G., & Hartman, E. (2008). Avoidance motivation and choking under pressure in soccer penalty shootouts. *Journal of Sport andExercise Psychology, 30*, 450–457.

Jordet, G., Hartman, E., & Jelle Vuijk, P. (2011). Team history and choking under pressure in major soccer penalty shootouts. *British Journal of Psychology, 103*, 268–283.

Jordet, G., & Pepping, G. J. (2019). Flipping sport psychology theory into practice: a context- and behaviour-centered approach. In M. L. Cappuccio (Ed.), *Handbook of Embodied Cognition and Sport Psychology*. Boston, MA: MIT Press

Leitner, M. C., & Richlan, F. (2021). Analysis system for emotional behavior in football (aseb-f): matches of fc red bull salzburg without supporters during the COVID-19 pandemic. *Humanities and Social Sciences Communications, 8*, 14. https://doi.org/10.1057/s41599-020-00699-1

Levi, H. R., & Jackson, R. C. (2018). Contextual factors influencing decision making: perceptions of professional soccer players. *Psychology of Sport &Exercise, 37,* 19–25.

McGreary, M., Morris, R., & Eubank, M. (2021). Retrospective and concurrent perspectives of the transition into senior professional female football within the United Kingdom. *Psychology of Sport andExercise, 53,* 101855.

McLoughlin, E., Fletcher, D., Slavich, G. M., Arnold, R., & Moore, L. J. (2021). Cumulative lifetime stress exposure, depression, anxiety, and well-being in elite athletes: a mixed-method study. *Psychology of Sport and Exercise, 52,* 101823.

Middlemas, S., & Harwood, C. (2018). No place to hide: football players' and coaches' perceptions of the psychological factors influencing video feedback. *Journal of Applied Sport Psychology, 30*(1), 23–44.

Middlemas, S., & Harwood, C. (2020). A pre-match video self-modeling intervention in elite youth football. *Journal of Applied Sport Psychology, 32*(5), 450–475.

Mitchell, T., Gledhill, A., Nesti, M., Richardson, D., & Littlewood, M. (2020). Practitioner perspectives on the barriers associated with youth-to-senior transition in elite youth soccer academy players. *International Sport Coaching Journal, 7*(3), 273–282.

Moll, T., & Davies, G. L. (2021). The effects of coaches' emotional expressions on players' performance: experimental evidence in a football context. *Psychology of Sport andExercise, 54.*

Moll, T., Jordet, G., & Pepping, G.-J. (2010). Emotional contagion in soccer penalty shootouts: celebration of individual success is associated with ultimate team success. *Journal of Sports Sciences, 28,* 983–992. doi:10.1080/02640414.2010.484068

Morris, R., Tod, D., & Eubank, M. (2017). From youth team to first team: an investigation into the transition experiences of young professional athletes in soccer. *International Journal of Sport andExercise Psychology, 15*(5), 523–539.

Morris, R., Tod, D., & Oliver, E. (2016). An investigation into stakeholders' perceptions of the youth-to-senior transition in professional soccer in the United Kingdom. *Journal of Applied Sport Psychology, 28*(4), 375–391.

Neave, N., & Wolfson, S. (2003). Testosterone, territoriality and the 'home advantage'. *Physiology and Behavior, 78,* 269–275.

Oberhofer, H., Philippovich, T., & Winner, H. (2010). Distance matters in away games: evidence from German football league. *Journal of Economic Psychology, 31,* 200–211.

Pain, M., & Harwood, C. (2013). Stress, coping and the mental qualities of elite players. In: M. Williams (Ed.), *Science and Soccer: Developing Elite Performers* (pp. 154–169). London: Routledge.

Pollard, R., & Gomez, M.A. (2014). Components of home advantage in 157 national soccer leagues worldwide. *International Journal of Sport and Exercise Psychology, 12*(3), 218–233.

Ponzo, M., & Scoppa, V. (2018). Does the home advantage depend on crowd support? Evidence from same-stadium derbies. *Journal of Sports Economics, 19*(4), 562–582. doi:10.1177/1527002516665794

Redwood-Brown, A. J., Sunderland, C. A., Minniti, A. M., & O'Donoghue, P. G. (2018). Perceptions of psychological momentum of elite soccer players. *International Journal of Sport and Exercise Psychology, 16*(6), 590–606.

Røynesdal, Ø., Toering, T., & Gustafsson, H. (2018). Understanding players' transition from youth to senior professional football environments: a coach perspective. *International Journal of Sports Science & Coaching, 13*(1), 26–37.

Seiler, K., Schweizer, G., & Seiler, R. (2018). Do the effects of nonverbal behaviour on team outcome confidence in team sports depend on the availability of additional performance information? *Psychology of Sport and Exercise, 36,* 29–40.

Shipherd, A. M., Basevitch, I., Filho, E., & Gershgoren, L. (2018). A scientist-practitioner approach to an on-field assessment of mental skills in collegiate soccer student-athletes. *Journal of Sport Psychology in Action, 9*(3), 196–205.

Slater, M. J., Haslam, S. A., & Steffens, N. K. (2018). Singing it for 'us': team passion displayed during national anthems is associated with subsequent success. *European Journal of Sport Science, 18*(4), 541–549.

Staufenbiel, K., Riedl, D., & Strauss, B. (2018). Learning to be advantaged: the development of home advantage in high-level youth soccer. *International Journal of Sport and Exercise Psychology, 16*(1), 36–50.

Swainston, S. C., Wilson, M. R., & Jones, M. I. (2020). Player experience during the junior to senior transition in professional football: a longitudinal case study. *Frontiers in Psychology, 11*, 1672.

Taylor, J., & Collins, D. (2019). Shoulda, coulda, didnae—Why don't high-potential players make it? *The Sport Psychologist, 33*(2), 85–96.

Thomas, O., Thrower, S. N., Lane, A., & Thomas, J. (2019). Types, sources, and debilitating factors of sport confidence in elite early adolescent academy soccer players. *Journal of Applied Sport Psychology, 33*, 192-217. doi:10.1080/10413200.2019.1630863

Tilp, M., & Thaller, S. (2020). Covid-19 has turned home advantage into home disadvantage in the German soccer Bundesliga. *Frontiers in Psychology, 2*. https://doi.org/10.3389/fspor.2020.593499

Toering, T. (in press). Self-regulation. In D. Collins & A. Cruickshank (Eds.), *Sport Psychology Essentials*. Champaign, IL: Human Kinetics.

Toering, T. T., Elferink-Gemser, M. T., Jordet, G., & Visscher, C. (2009). Self-regulation and performance level of elite and non-elite youth soccer players. *Journal of Sports Sciences, 27*(14), 1509–1517.

Toering, T., & Jordet, G. (2015). Self-control in professional soccer players. *Journal of Applied Sport Psychology, 27*(3), 335–350.

Van Kleef, G. A., Cheshin, A., Koning, L. F., & Wolf, S. A. (2019). Emotional games: how coaches' emotional expressions shape players' emotions, inferences, and team performance. *Psychology of Sport and Exercise, 41*, 1–11.

Van Ours, J. C. (2019). A note on artificial pitches and home advantage in Dutch professional football. *De Economist, 167*, 89–103. https://doi.org/10.1007/s10645-019-09332-2

Van Yperen, N. W. (2009). Why some make it and others do not: identifying psychological factors that predict career success in professional adult soccer. *The Sport Psychologist, 23*(3), 317–329.

Zuber, C., Zibung, M., & Conzelmann, A. (2015). Motivational patterns as an instrument for predicting success in promising young football players. *Journal of Sports Sciences, 33*(2), 160–168.

# 8 Anticipation and decision-making

*A. Mark Williams, Joseph L. Thomas, Geir Jordet, and Paul R. Ford*

## Introduction

The ability to anticipate what opponents will do next and to make the most appropriate decision as to how to respond are important components of performance in soccer (Williams & Jackson, 2020). These attributes become more important to performance at the highest level in soccer when compared with anthropometric or physiological characteristics (e.g., Reilly et al., 2000). Tactical ability (e.g., anticipation and decision-making), in conjunction with the technical ability (e.g., ball control and passing skill) and psychological characteristics (e.g., mental toughness, resilience, and grit), are the factors that most likely discriminate players at the very highest level.

In this chapter, we focus on anticipation and decision-making. In colloquial or lay terms, coaches, and pundits often refer to these attributes using phrases such as 'game intelligence' or 'the ability to read the game'. Anticipation necessitates players to perceive ahead of the event itself what opponents and teammates are likely to do in any situation. Decision-making is the ability to select and execute the appropriate action based on the current circumstances on the field of play, as well as the demands of the game strategically and tactically. Scientists have consistently shown that skilled soccer players are quicker and more accurate in anticipation and decision-making when compared to their lesser-skilled counterparts (e.g., Roca, Ford, McRobert, & Williams, 2011; Williams & Davids, 1998). We have two main aims. First, we identify how players anticipate and make decisions in soccer and in so doing, illustrate how these attributes are measured. Second, we assess how players develop superior anticipation and decision-making and how interventions can be developed to create more 'game-intelligent' players.

## Anticipation and decision-making

Over the last 50 years, researchers have successfully identified several perceptual-cognitive skills that underpin successful anticipation and decision-making (Williams & Jackson, 2020). Although there is a substantive research base involving other sports (Williams & Ericsson, 2005; Williams, Ford, Eccles, & Ward, 2010), we focus solely on research involving adult and youth male soccer players. Unfortunately, there remains relatively limited research on female players and special population groups. However, while these remain important gaps in understanding, it is likely that the specific nature of the skills identified does not differ greatly, if at all, due to differences in gender, ethnicity, or disability, over and beyond the accumulation of experience/practice in

DOI: 10.4324/9781003148418-10

*Anticipation and decision-making* 125

soccer. In the opening part of the first section, we review research that has highlighted the processes and skills underpinning superior anticipation in soccer. In the second part, we review how skilled players are better than their lesser-skilled counterparts at making correct and timely decisions.

## 'Reading the game': anticipation

### *The importance of looking and seeing*

When observing a soccer match, one can witness skilled players consistently moving their eyes and heads to 'look around' the pitch, at the ball, the movements of opponents and teammates, and areas of space that may be exploited or exposed. Scientists have demonstrated that skilled soccer players use the visual system in a systematically different manner when compared to lesser-skilled players. The earliest studies examining visual search or gaze behaviours in soccer focused on goalkeepers attempting to predict the direction of a penalty-kicks (e.g., Tyldesley, Bootsma, & Bomhoff, 1982; for subsequent work on this theme, see Dicks, Button, & Davids, 2010a, b; Savelsbergh, Williams, van der Kamp, & Ward, 2002; Savelsbergh, van der Kamp, Williams, & Ward, 2005). However, advances in technology have led to progressive improvements in the methods employed to measure such behaviours, enabling data capture in increasingly more realistic scenarios. Gaze behaviours have been evaluated as soccer players attempt to anticipate the actions of opponents in outfield scenarios involving 1 *vs.* 1 situations, in various micro phases of defensive play involving 3 *vs.* 3 simulations, and in more macro phases involving larger groups of outfield players (Roca et al., 2011, 2013; Williams & Davids, 1998; Williams, Davids, Burwitz, & Williams, 1994). Similarly, scientists have measured gaze in situations that require players to make decisions during various phases of play, in offensive situations involving set-plays, and in sequences of play that traverse the length of the playing field and involve numerous interactions between players (Helsen & Starkes, 1999; Roca et al., 2011; Vaeyens, Lenoir, Williams, Mazyn, & Philippaerts, 2007a, b). The broad conclusion is that skilled players generally look at different areas of the display, for varying periods of time, using different search strategies when compared with less-skilled counterparts.

As an illustration, Roca et al. (2011) recorded the gaze behaviours of skilled and less-skilled soccer players while moving and interacting with life-size video sequences of 11 *vs.* 11 soccer situations filmed from the perspective of a central defender. The video clips were occluded just prior to the main offensive action (e.g., final pass). Participants were required to anticipate the action of the player in possession of the ball and to decide what course of action they should take (e.g., maintain position or move right or left). Skilled defenders were more accurate in anticipating what the opponent was going to do next and in deciding what action to take when compared to less-skilled players. Skilled players employed more fixations of shorter duration and oriented gaze on significantly more locations in the display compared with less skilled players. They spent more time fixating on the opposing team players and areas of space compared to less skilled players who, in contrast, spent more time fixating the player in possession and ball (i.e., ball watching). Skilled players use vision in a fundamentally different manner compared to lesser-skilled players to pick-up the key information needed to guide anticipation and decision-making. Yet, in some studies, no specific differences in gaze characteristics have been reported across skill groups. In these latter instances, variations in performance between skilled and less-skilled players are likely due to more effective pick up of information using peripheral vision or differences in the amount or quality of information extracted per fixation (Williams & Davids, 1998).

Scientists have examined how stressors such as anxiety and fatigue influence gaze behaviours (Causer, Holmes, Smith, & Williams, 2011; Vickers & Williams, 2007; Wilson, Wood, & Vine, 2009). Wilson et al. (2009; see also Wood & Wilson, 2011) examined the gaze behaviours of players as they completed penalty kicks under low- and high-threat conditions. In the high-threat condition, the penalty-takers made faster first fixations and fixated for longer periods on the goalkeeper, with these changes in gaze leading to reductions in shooting accuracy and an increased likelihood of placing the ball nearer the goalkeeper when compared to the low-threat condition. In similar vein, Casanova and colleagues (2013) reported that workload/fatigue built up over the course of a match negatively impacted the information processed by outfield players in the early and late stages of each half in a soccer match. The current evidence suggests that skilled athletes are more robust to the negative effects of stressors such as anxiety and fatigue.

While technology has improved significantly over recent decades, it has historically been difficult to record accurate gaze data during actual match situations. An alternative approach has been to record player head movements in matches as a rough proxy for visual search and scanning. When closely observing individual players in a soccer game, one can observe players turning their heads to look around, especially prior to receiving the ball. Scientists have measured the active head movements of players where the face (and hence, the eyes) is temporarily directed away from the ball, with the assumed intention of gathering information about teammates and/or opponents, to prepare for subsequently engaging with the ball (e.g., Jordet, 2005b; Jordet et al., 2020). Figure 8.1 presents an illustration of this scanning behaviour.

Jordet (2005a, b) started filming soccer players in matches to generate close-shot videos for analysis. Several published reports have subsequently presented data gathered using these video recordings of players (e.g., Eldridge et al., 2013; Jordet, Heijmerikx, & Bloomfield, 2013). In the largest study to date, 27 players in the English Premier League (EPL) were filmed across a total of 21 games, which produced an analysis of almost 10,000 individual ball possessions (Jordet et al., 2020). A statistical model that accounted for context, pass difficulty, and player differences showed that scanning plays a robust and positive, albeit small, role in performance. Furthermore,

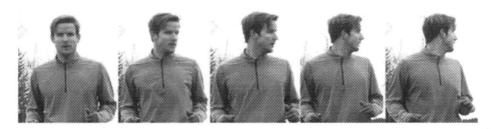

*Figure 8.1* A scan (filmed from the position of the ball), where a player's face is temporarily directed away from the ball.

Photo credit: Karl Marius Aksum and Lars Brotangen.

player scanning varied with different contextual conditions (i.e., playing position, pitch location, opponent pressure, and state of the game). Midfielders scanned the most, followed by central defenders, full backs, wingers, and forwards. Similar findings emerged for players during the U17 and U19 European Championships (Aksum, Pokolm, Bjørndal, Rein, Memmert, & Jordet, 2021). Aksum and colleagues (2021) report a significant positive relationship between scanning frequency and pass completion rates. Moreover, the U19 players scanned significantly more frequently than the U17 players.

Another innovative approach has been to use a headband containing an inertial measurement unit to examine the links between head-turning frequency or excursion (i.e., extent of head-turning and measured in degrees) and turning with ball, as well as switching play from one side of the pitch to the other (McGuckian, Cole, Jordet, Chalkley, & Pepping, 2018). In a study of U13 and U23 players performing at a German Bundesliga club, the U23 players had a significantly higher head turn frequency prior to ball possession and a lower frequency during ball possession, when compared to the U13 players (McGuckian, Beavan, Mayer, Chalkley, & Pepping, 2020). Higher head turn frequency (for the U13 players) and higher excursion (for the U23 players) were related to turning and switching performance.

Most recently, gaze tracking data have been gathered during actual matches. In one such study, players fixated most often around the ball, and fixation duration to any type of information increased when more information sources (i.e., ball, teammates, and opponents) were available (Aksum, Magnaguagno, Bjørndal, & Jordet, 2020). Figure 8.2 illustrates the approach employed. The average fixation durations were considerably shorter than previously reported in laboratory studies, which could be because field conditions place different constraints on visual behaviours compared to laboratory settings. Another study focused on the scan itself, showing that

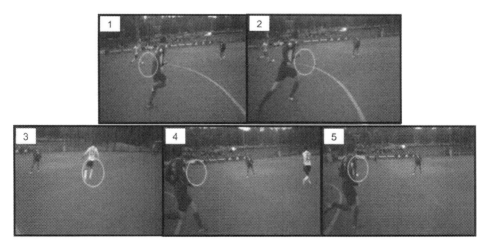

*Figure 8.2* Some images from eye-tracking goggles worn by a central midfielder in an 11 vs. 11 match, with the small circle indicating the player's foveal gaze location in a scan (scan starting at 1, ending at 5).

Photo credit: Karl Marius Aksum and Geir Jordet.

approximately 2% of scans contained visual fixations, suggesting that a scan does not typically result in the recognition of detailed information, but blurred impressions of positions, movements, and colours (Aksum, Brotangen, Bjørndal, Magnaguagno, & Jordet, 2021). Findings support other research showing that when vision is blurred skilled players are still able to anticipate accurately based on very course and global (i.e., spread across the display) information rather than local sources (e.g., a single cue; Ryu, Mann, Abernethy, & Poolton, 2016; Ryu, Abernethy, Park, & Mann, 2018).

### Picking-up postural cues

A related body of research exists to suggest that skilled soccer players extract early arising information from the postural movements of opponents (and probably teammates) before they execute a pass or shot. This body of work has not recorded gaze behaviours per se, but rather has used an alternative approach based on manipulating the information in the display to identify the information used during skilled anticipation. Williams and Burwitz (1993) used the so-called 'temporal occlusion approach' to measure the ability of skilled and less-skilled goalkeepers to predict penalty-kick direction. Several players were filmed from the perspective of a goalkeeper facing the penalty. These action sequences were then selectively edited to present varying extents of early and late information relative to foot-ball contact; the video sequences were occluded 120 ms before ball contact, 80 ms before ball contact, at foot-ball contact, and 120 ms after foot-ball contact. Figure 8.3 presents an illustration of the film sequences

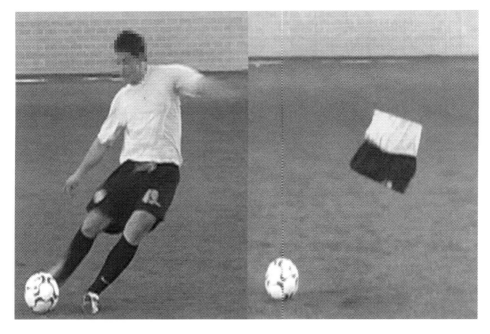

*Figure 8.3* The penalty-taker as presented in a temporal-occlusion condition where information is available up to foot-ball contact (left side) and a spatial occlusion condition where only the hips are presented (right side) (from Causer & Williams, 2015).

Anticipation and decision-making    129

presented when using temporal occlusion techniques. Players viewed the action sequences on a near life-size screen and were required to indicate which corners of the goal the penalty-kicks were directed towards using a pen-and-paper response. Skilled players recorded response accuracy scores above chance levels even in the pre-foot-to-ball contact conditions, illustrating their ability to process advanced information from the penalty taker during the run-up and kicking action. The accuracy of predicting ball height increased significantly after viewing the first portion of the ball flight.

Some researchers have simultaneously recorded gaze data as players view these film-based simulations (Dicks et al., 2010a; Savelsbergh et al., 2002, 2005) or as they perform the task *in situ* (Dicks et al., 2010a; Piras & Vickers, 2011). Moreover, there have been efforts to describe biomechanically the kinematic information available to the goalkeeper (Dicks et al., 2010b; Lees & Owens, 2011). Savelsbergh et al. (2002) used a very similar temporal occlusion methodology to Williams and Burwitz (1993), but in addition, they recorded eye movement data. Skilled goalkeepers were more accurate at anticipating penalty direction, making fewer visual fixations of longer duration to a smaller number of locations when compared with the less-skilled goalkeepers. During the early stages of the penalty kick, the skilled goalkeepers spent more time fixating on the face of the kicker (which may give them early information as to the direction of the kick) compared to less-skilled keepers who fixated on 'unclassified' regions. In the moments before foot-ball contact, the skilled keepers fixated on the kicking leg, non-kicking leg, and ball regions, whereas less skilled keepers fixated on the trunk, arm, and hip regions. The search strategies used by the skilled goalkeepers, and their ability to recognise advanced postural cues emanating from the movements of the taker, led to them being more successful at saving penalties.

### Recognising patterns and detecting familiarity in sequences of play

Another perceptual-cognitive skill that appears to be important when 'reading the game' is the ability to recognise familiarity or patterns in evolving sequences of play. Skilled players identify familiarity through structures or patterns in play as sequences unfold (e.g., 2 *vs.* 1 situation, triangle or diamond shape forming between players in possession) and this ability enables them to anticipate the likely outcome ahead of time. Players are typically presented with filmed clips from competitive matches lasting 3–10 s involving either structured (i.e., footage involving a typical offensive move) or unstructured sequences (e.g., players warming up before a match). In a subsequent recognition phase, players are presented with a combination of clips that were presented in the earlier viewing phase and some that were novel. Skilled players are more accurate than less-skilled players in recognising previously viewed structured sequences, but not unstructured sequences. Several published studies illustrate this ability in soccer (e.g., North, Williams, Ward, Hodges, & Ericsson, 2009; North, Ward, Ericsson, & Williams, 2011; Williams, Hodges, North, & Barton, 2006). A combination of visual search recording, think-aloud verbal reports, and different manipulations of the film displays (e.g., occlusion of players and removal of superficial display features) has been used to identify the specific sources of information used when making these judgements (see Williams & North, 2009).

One proposal is that skilled players initially extract relational information from the positions and movements of players and the ball and match these stimulus

130  *A. Mark Williams et al.*

characteristics with their previous knowledge and experience (Dittrich, 1999). Skilled players recognise familiar patterns of play based upon structural relations between features (e.g., teammates, opponents, and the ball), as well as the tactical and strategic significance of these relations. In contrast, lesser-skilled players are unable to pick up important relational information and have less knowledge constraining them to employ more distinctive surface or background features (e.g., pitch condition and colour of playing uniforms) when making such decisions.

### Predicting likely event occurrences

Another perceptual-cognitive skill that has received attention over the past decade has been the use of situational probabilities or more broadly, contextual information or priors in anticipation. It has been reported that players assign a hierarchy of probabilities to potential events as the action unfolds (i.e., they weigh up the likely options and their potential of occurring). These probabilities could exist across a broad range of situations, as well as being task, player/opponent, and context-specific (Williams, 2000). In recent studies, different sources of contextual information have been identified that can influence perception of the most likely situational occurrence. These sources include the positions of players (Roca, Ford, McRobert, & Williams, 2013), the score of the game (Runswick, Roca, Williams, Bezodis & North, 2018), and prior knowledge of opponent action tendencies (Gredin, Bishop, Broadbent, Tucker & Williams, 2018). Navia, van der Kemp, and Ruiz (2013) assessed goalkeepers during on-field penalty-kick scenarios under distinct situational information conditions that differed on the strength of the probabilistic information. When goalkeepers are informed that the penalty taker has a high probability of shooting to the left or right, performance with respect to diving to the correct side is significantly enhanced, whereas this is not the case when taker preferences are ambiguous.

Another emphasis has been on measuring how the possession of *a priori* information related to the most likely behaviours of opponents influences anticipation. These investigations have manipulated how this *contextual prior* information is provided either by explicit instruction – as a performance analyst might do in a tactical report – or more implicitly by providing access to this information through exposure to previous actions of the opponent. Gredin et al. (2018) examined the ability of skilled and novice soccer players to anticipate a final action from videos of dynamic 2 *vs.* 2 counterattacks. The players were provided stable contextual prior information about the action tendencies of the attacker in possession of the ball that were dependent on the positioning of the secondary attacker. Thus, the final prediction necessitated integrating the previously acquired situational knowledge with the visual information from the unfolding movement of the secondary attacker. The provision of explicit contextual priors altered how the expert players allocated visual attention towards more situationally relevant information (i.e., the secondary attacker off the ball). As such, trials in which the final action was congruent, or aligned, with opponent action tendencies led to enhanced performance. When the outcome was incongruent with the contextual prior information, anticipation performance in novices suffered, whereas experts maintained their performance. However, this was an unexpected finding considering evidence in other sporting domains has reported expert performance often suffers when action outcomes do not align with contextual prior information.

## 'Making the right choices': decision-making

An equally important challenge for players is to select and execute the correct response to positively influence the current and evolving situation in the match. In this section, we review current understanding of decision-making in soccer. We separate action selection and execution for descriptive purposes, with the former providing description of the choice made and the latter whether the decision selected is successfully executed; in reality, these are a single variable during performance in matches.

Scientists have used representative video-based tasks (e.g., Roca et al., 2011; Vaeyens et al., 2007a; b) to provide empirical evidence supporting the observation that expert players make more successful decisions in a variety of representative soccer situations compared to lesser-skilled players. More recently, other researchers using performance analysis techniques have assessed the selection and execution of decisions by players in match-play. Serrano et al. (2017) used the Game Performance Evaluation Tool (GPET) to assess success in both the selection and execution of passing, dribbling, and shooting skills across 30 matches involving skilled Spanish youth soccer players aged U10–U19. The GPET requires observers to assign a single value to each decision selection deemed appropriate across a game and separately for a successful execution, with zero allocated for each inappropriate and unsuccessful decision. They found an average of 69% of ball possessions involved appropriate selections and 47% were successfully executed. In comparison, players in the EPL have higher success rates for executing ball possessions, although to our knowledge selections have not been assessed in this cohort. An analysis of matches demonstrated that the proportion of successful executions of ball possessions for 15 players across 9 matches was 75% (Whelan, 2021), whereas the success of passing executions for 570 players across 376 EPL matches was 74%, with higher values when the score line for the team was ahead or behind compared to drawing (Redwood-Brown et al., 2019). It is likely that the percentage of appropriate *action selections* in EPL players on the ball exceeds the 75% found for executions (e.g., Serrano et al., 2017). Moreover, it may be that successful ball possession executions of 75% and above demonstrates skilled performance in the game. In the future, researchers should test these hypotheses and assess the appropriateness and success of decisions 'off the ball'.

The data gathered on the success of action executions and appropriateness of action selections by players in matches provide us with important descriptive information, but unfortunately, such an approach does not explain how decision-making occurs in matches. Gallivan et al. (2018) describe the basic nature of decision-making as involving 'a sequence of sub-actions that are performed to achieve a high-level goal' (p. 519). Certainly, observations of players in matches confirm this idea, in that players select and execute actions to achieve a higher-level goal or intention, such as shooting to score, pressing an opponent to regain possession, or manipulating the ball to avoid a tackle to maintain possession. Moreover, often, a few sub-actions or changes of action occur in service of achieving that higher-level goal or intention, for example, a jog to a sideways curved cruise to a backward sidestep to achieve the goal of pressing an opponent and channelling them toward a teammate (Whelan, 2021).

Several contextual factors influence how actions are selected and executed during matches. Levi and Jackson (2018) conducted semi-structured interviews to identify the contextual factors affecting decision-making with eight professional soccer players. Players revealed that during a match their decisions were influenced by the dynamic contextual variables or self-perceptions of their own current performance, match score, team momentum (e.g., periods of attacking play by their team), and concurrent instruction from coaches. Moreover, their decision-making in the match was influenced by static variables related to match importance, personal pressures (e.g., gaining a new contract), and preparation from coaches and in training (e.g., tactical plans). These findings support those reported by McPherson and colleagues (e.g., McPherson & Kernodle, 2003) who showed 'in-game' decision-making is influenced by contextual factors that are situational (e.g., score or time in a match), player characteristics (e.g., age and skill level), phase of play (e.g., team in possession), opponent characteristics (e.g., shot tendencies), and environmental characteristics (e.g., pitch, weather) (McPherson & Kernodle, 2003).

Overall, there remains a paucity of research relating to how players make decisions in matches and the factors that impact these processes. The work is largely descriptive highlighting the frequency and type of decisions made rather than attempting to explain and predict how skilled players make these judgments during matches. In the future, more controlled and systematic research is needed using process-tracing measures such as verbal reports and semi-structured interviews to improve understanding of the mechanisms underlying decision-making (Williams & Jackson, 2020).

## The acquisition of anticipation and decision-making

### *The activities engaged in during development*

Scientists have examined whether players who exhibit varying levels of anticipation and decision-making ability differ in the amount and type of activity they have engaged in during development. Although initial attempts focused on sports such as field-hockey, netball, basketball, Australian rules football, and cricket (Baker, Côté, & Abernethy, 2003a, b; Berry, Abernethy, & Côté, 2008; Ford, Low, McRobert, & Williams, 2010a), there are reports involving soccer. Williams Ward, Bell-Walker, and Ford (2012) categorised skilled soccer players aged 18 years into 'high-performing' and 'low-performing' based on their performance on established tests of perceptual-cognitive expertise involving anticipation and situational assessment tasks. A group of non-elite soccer players acted as controls. A Career Practice Questionnaire was completed by all players to elicit information about their participation history profiles (Ward, Hodges, Starkes, & Williams, 2007). The 'high-performing group' had accumulated more hours in soccer-specific play activity over their last 6 years of engagement in the sport compared to their low-performing counterparts and the non-elite controls. No differences were reported for hours accumulated in soccer-specific practice or competition. The mean hours in each type of activity for the different groups and across each age category are presented

*Table 8.1* The average hours per year in three soccer activities for soccer players aged 18 years in the six years prior to the perceptual-cognitive test (Williams et al., 2012)

| Group | Match-play | Practice | Play |
|---|---|---|---|
| Elite high-performing | 47.6 | 270.6 | 245.9 |
| Elite low-performing | 1.0 | 285.9 | 172.5 |
| Recreational | 78.5 | 222.1 | 92.2 |

*Anticipation and decision-making* 133

in Table 6.1. Players who had superior 'game intelligence' had accumulated significantly more hours in soccer-specific, peer-led play activity (i.e., street soccer).

In a follow-up study, Roca, Williams, and Ford (2012) categorised skilled adult soccer players into 'high-performing' and 'low-performing' groups based on their performance on an interactive test that measured the ability of players to anticipate and make decisions. A group of recreational players acted as controls. The Participation History Questionnaire (Ford et al., 2010b) was used to collect retrospectively recalled developmental activity data across participants. During childhood (6–12 years), the high-performing skilled group averaged more hours per year in soccer-specific, peer-led play compared to the other two groups. During adolescence (13–18 years), both skilled groups engaged in more hours of soccer-specific practice and competition compared to the recreational group. Statistical analysis showed that 21.8% of the variance in performance on the test was accounted for by the average hours per year accumulated in soccer-specific play activity during childhood, with a further 13.2% of the variance being due to the hours spent in soccer-specific practice during adolescence.

A key question is why soccer-specific play would facilitate game intelligence more so than practice. An argument might be that during play, players recreate realistic practice conditions that mimic what they see during matches. The absence of overly prescriptive coaching, in conjunction with challenging and realistic scenarios, may create more opportunities for match-like perceptions and decisions. In contrast, there is evidence to suggest that during coach-led practice, too much time may be spent in drill and grid-based practices that might not mimic the scenarios that exist in match-play, coupled also with more prescriptive instructional approaches (Ford et al., 2010b).

Skill-based differences in 'game intelligence' and in hours accumulated in soccer activity arise as early as 8 years of age in soccer (Ward & Williams, 2003). The structure and conditions of soccer-specific peer-led play create the opportunity for players to experiment with different skills and tactics against opponents and with teammates, which likely leads to the acquisition of superior anticipation and decision-making. No evidence exists to suggest that engagement in sports other than soccer during the developmental years may lead to perceptual-cognitive expertise in the sport (e.g., players in Roca et al., in prep, engaged in two other sports to a minimal degree). However, some support exists for the notion that perceptual-cognitive skills transfer across sports of a similar nature (Rosalie & Müller, 2014; Christopher & Müller, 2014), yet, in contrast, research exists to suggest that skills may be specific to a particular position (Williams, Ward, Smeeton, & Ward, 2008) or role (Catteeuw, Helsen, Gilis, & Wagemans, 2009) within a sport.

### Simulation training

An important issue for coaches and practitioners is how to develop structured training interventions to improve anticipation and decision-making. Certainly, coaches can structure practice in a manner that facilitates the acquisition of these attributes (see Ford & O'Connor, 2019). In this section, we discuss how simulation-based training in its various guises (e.g., video-based, virtual reality (VR)) can be used to facilitate the acquisition of anticipation and decision-making. A detailed review of this broad field of research is available elsewhere (e.g., see Miles, Pop, Watt, Lawrence, & John, 2012; Neumann et al., 2017; Gray, 2019).

Most researchers have focused on using simulation to train goalkeepers in the penalty-kick. Williams and Burwitz (1993) used video training to develop anticipation in a group

134  *A. Mark Williams et al.*

of inexperienced goalkeepers. Penalty-takers were filmed from the perspective of the goalkeeper and the footage presented in conjunction with instruction and feedback. The instruction highlighted key postural cues (e.g., orientation of the lower leg in penalty kicks), as well as critical relationships between these display features and subsequent performance. Significant improvements in performance were observed following 90 min of video training. Savelsbergh, Van Gastel, and Van Kampen (2010) modified the visual search behaviours employed by inexperienced soccer goalkeepers using video training. An intervention group viewed clips where key information from the run-up was highlighted, whereas a training group watched unedited sequences and a control group only completed the pre- and post-tests. The visual search behaviours of participants in the intervention group changed significantly from pre- to post-test, leading to earlier initiation of movement and significant improvements in anticipation when compared with the training and control groups.

Williams, Heron, Ward, and Smeeton (2005) attempted to improve the ability of players to use situational probabilities when attempting to predict pass destination in soccer. Players were assessed, pre- and post-training, on their ability to identify the passing options available to the player in possession of the ball, and then to determine the relative threat posed to the participant's team for each highlighted option. An intervention group received 45 min of video training in which they received instruction regarding the passing options facing a specific player in possession of the ball, areas of space that could be exploited or exposed, runs made by forward players, and the importance of defensive shape and organization in the specific context. Participants in a placebo group were instructed on standard defensive soccer techniques using the video simulation. The training group improved their ability to highlight key passing options over and above that of the placebo group, implying that these context-specific skills may be amenable to simulation training and instruction.

Although such training interventions have significant potential, there are many unanswered questions and considerable scope exists for further empirical work (Carling, Reilly, & Williams, 2009). The key question is whether improvements found in these simulation training studies transfer to enhanced performance on the pitch (Williams, Ward, Knowles, & Smeeton, 2002). Thus far, there have been no reported attempts to improve the ability of players to recognise sequences or patterns of play in soccer or to change the visual search behaviours or thought processes that may be engaged during performance using simulation-based training. However, simulation training has potential to improve the performance of players.

A major advantage of simulation training is that players can engage when injured or resting and recovering from physical activity. Moreover, players can experience multiple soccer situations in a short space of time compared to when physically playing the game. Advances in technology enable performance to be captured relatively easily offering varied opportunities to use simulation in all its various guises for performance enhancement (e.g., cave-based VR, smartphones, and web-based applications). Published reports (e.g., Wulf, Raupach, & Pfeiffer, 2005) show the learning that occurs from observational practice provides strong support for the use of simulation training with players.

### *Training with feedback (computer-aided and VR)*

With modern technology becoming increasingly prevalent in professional sports, many practitioners have turned to use performance analysis and augmented, or VR to gain a cutting edge (see McRobert & Williams, 2019). Wright, Atkins, Jones, and Todd (2013) surveyed 48 performance analysts working in elite soccer and found that 88% of the clubs used self-coded platforms for performance analysis. These tools allow coaches and support staff to provide players with feedback post-match, feed-forward information pre-match, live analysis, and practice opportunities. Video-based feedback is a useful tool for both coaches and players. For coaches, video-based performance analysis is seen as a support tool that can assist in learning (i.e., anticipation/decision-making) and towards developing a mutual understanding between coaches and players (Groom, Cushion, & Nelson, 2011). Elite youth academy players were interviewed on their perceived impact performance analysis stating that video-based feedback was useful for identifying discrepancies between positive and negative performances (Reeves & Robert, 2013).

Video-based feedback has also been used as a training intervention to develop perceptual-cognitive skills. Nimmerichter, Weber, Wirth, and Haller (2015) assigned 34 youth players from a national academy to either a training group or a control group. The training group underwent a 6-week intervention during which they used video feedback to draw their attention to the most informative stimulus during 1 *vs.* 1 situations, in order to identify opponent actions quickly and accurately. The video training group significantly improved both the accuracy and speed of their decision-making over the 6-week period, and demonstrated superior performance compared to the control group, which did not show a significant improvement after 6 weeks. Moreover, the relative effectiveness of self-controlled, tactical video-based feedback has been tested using on-field performances via 3 *vs.* 2 small-sided games. Van Maarseveen, Oudejans, and Savelsbergh (2018) examined whether elite youth soccer players who had autonomy when feedback was provided benefited compared to a control group that was tethered to the feedback frequency of another player. The self-controlled group requested more feedback after good trials (e.g., after a goal was scored) and demonstrated higher levels of perceived performance. Self-regulated video feedback increased involvement in the learning process and, subsequently, improved performance.

VR simulations can augment training environments by allowing adaptive difficulty levels (Lammfromm & Gopher, 2011) and controlling feedback (Sigrist et al., 2015). Professional clubs are known to use systems, such as Rezzil, Beyond Sports, and Be Your Best to practice VR scenario drills, for player and match analysis, and for pressure testing (Thatcher, Ivanov, Szerovay, & Mills, 2020). Thatcher et al. (2020) interviewed elite coaches and performance analysts about barriers and opportunities when implementing VR. The interviewees reported that VR could serve as a useful tool for demonstrating models of gameplay representative of team tactics; a factor that could be helpful for individual player development and during rehabilitation. However, the practicality of using VR and the lack of empirical evidence highlighting its usefulness were seen as potential barriers. However, Wood et al. (2020) have reported that a soccer-specific VR platform was successfully able to differentiate between professional, academy, and novice players, providing a modicum of construct validity. With an increasing number of VR soccer platforms entering the market, it suggests that simulations will continue to improve potentially providing increasing realism that better replicates the actual demands of actual match-play.

## Future directions and conclusions

We reviewed research that has focused on anticipation and decision-making in soccer. We highlighted the key perceptual-cognitive skills and processes that differentiate

## 136  *A. Mark Williams et al.*

those with exceptional levels of these attributes compared to those with less exceptional ability. Those with superior levels of anticipation and decision-making are better able to pick up postural information from the orientation of opponents and teammates, identify structure and familiarity in sequences of play, and predict more accurately the likely opportunities available during play. These skills are underpinned by more refined gaze strategies and more forward-thinking rather than reactive thought processes. The ability to anticipate and to make decisions develops progressively through extensive engagement in soccer-specific practice and play activities. Thus far, no predictors of progression on these attributes have been identified, beyond specific practice on related tasks and playing experience. Physical and simulation training interventions to facilitate the acquisition of anticipation and decision-making skill were discussed with the overall aim being to develop players with superior abilities. This area of work appears to offer considerable scope for performance enhancement in coming years.

## References

Aksum, K. M., Pokolm, M., Bjørndal, C. T., Rein, R., Memmert, D., & Jordet, G. (2021). Visual exploratory scanning activity in elite youth football players. *Journal of Sports Sciences,* Advanced online publication.

Aksum, K. M., Magnaguagno, L., Bjørndal, C. T., & Jordet, G. (2020). What do football players look at? An eye-tracking analysis of the visual fixations of players in 11 v 11 elite football match play. *Frontiers in Psychology,* Advanced online publication.

Baker, J., Côté., J., & Abernethy, B. (2003a). Learning from the experts: practice activities of expert decision makers in sport. *Research Quarterly for Exercise and Sport, 74,* 342–347.

Baker, J., Côté., J., & Abernethy, B. (2003b). Sport-specific practice and the development of expert decision making in team ball sports. *Journal of Applied Sport Psychology, 15,* 12–25.

Berry, J., Abernethy, B., & Côté., J. (2008). The contribution of structured activity and deliberate play to the development of expert perceptual and decision-making skill. *Journal of Sport & Exercise Psychology, 30,* 685–708.

Carling, C., Reilly, T. P., & Williams, A. M. (2009). *Performance Assessment in Field Sports.* London: Routledge.

Casanova, F., Garganta, J., Silva, G., Alves, A., Oliveira, J., & Williams, A. M. (2013). Effects of prolonged intermittent exercise on perceptual-cognitive processes. *Medicine and Science in Sports and Exercise, 45*(8), 1610–1617.

Catteeuw, P., Helsen, W. F., Gilis, B., & Wagemans, J. (2009). Decision-making skills, role specificity, and deliberate practice in association football refereeing. *Journal of Sports Sciences, 27,* 1125–1136.

Causer, J., & Williams, A. (2015). The use of patterns to disguise environmental cues during an anticipatory judgment task. *Journal of Sport & Exercise Psychology, 37,* 74–82.

Causer, J., Holmes, P. S., Smith, N. J., & Williams, A. M. (2011). Anxiety, visual attention, and movement kinematics in elite-level performers. *Emotion, 11,* 595–602.

Christopher, G. M., & Müller, S. (2014). Transfer of expert visual anticipation to a similar domain. *Quarterly Journal of Experimental Psychology, 67,* 186–196.

Dicks, M., Button, C., & Davids K. (2010a). Examination of gaze behaviours under in situ and video simulation task constraints reveals differences in information pickup for perception and action. *Attention Perception & Psychophysics, 72* 706–720.

Dicks, M., Davids, K., & Button, C., (2010b). Individual differences in the visual control of intercepting a penalty kick in association football. *Human Movement Science, 29,* 401–411.

Dittrich, W. H. (1999). Seeing biological motion: Is there a role for cognitive strategies? In A. Braffort, R. Gherbi, S. Gibet, J. Richardson, & D. Teil (Eds.), *Gesture-based Communication in Human-computer Interaction* (pp. 3–22). Berlin, Germany: Springer-Verlag.

Eldridge, D., Pulling, C., & Robins, M. T. (2013). Visual exploratory activity and resultant behavioural analysis of youth midfield soccer players. *Journal of Human Sport and Exercise, 8*, 560–577.

Ford, P. R., Low, J., McRobert, A. P., & Williams, A. M. (2010a). Developmental activities that contribute to high or low performance by elite cricket batters at recognizing type of delivery from advanced postural cues. *Journal of Sport and Exercise Psychology, 32*, 638–654.

Ford P. R., & O'Connor D. (2019). Practice and sports activities in the acquisition of anticipation and decision making. In: A. M. Williams & R. C. Jackson (Eds.), *Anticipation and Decision Making in Sport* (pp. 269–285). London: Routledge.

Ford, P. R., Yates, I. & Williams, A.M. (2010b). An analysis of practice activities and instructional behaviours used by youth soccer coaches during practice: exploring the link between science and application. *Journal of Sports Sciences, 28*, 483–495.

Gallivan, J. P., Chapman, C. S., Wolpert, D. M., & Randall Flanagan, J. (2018). Decision-making in sensorimotor control. *Nature Reviews: Neuroscience, 19*, 219–534.

Gray, R. (2019). Sports training technologies. In A. M. Williams & N. J. Hodges (Eds.), *Skill Acquisition in Sport: Research, Theory and Practice*. London: Routledge.

Gredin, V. G., Bishop, D. T., Broadbent, D. P., Tucker, A., & Williams, A. M. (2018). Experts integrate contextual priors and environmental information to improve anticipation efficiency. *Journal of Experimental Psychology, 24*, 509–520.

Groom, R., Cushion, C., & Nelson, L. (2011) The delivery of video-based performance analysis by England youth soccer coaches: towards a grounded theory. *Journal of Applied Sport Psychology, 23*, 16–30.

Helsen, W. F., & Starkes, J. L. (1999). A multidimensional approach to skilled perception and performance in sport. *Applied Cognitive Psychology, 13*, 1–27.

Jordet, G. (2005a). Applied cognitive sport psychology in team ball sports: an ecological approach. In R. Stelter & K. K. Roessler (Eds.), *New Approaches to Sport and Exercise Psychology* (pp. 147–174). Europe: Meyer & Meyer Sport.

Jordet, G. (2005b). Perceptual training in soccer: An imagery intervention study with elite players. *Journal of Applied Sport Psychology, 17*, 140–156.

Jordet, G., Aksum, K. M., Pedersen, D. N., Walvekar, A., Trivedi, A., McCall, A., Ivarsson, A., & Priestley, D. (2020). Scanning, contextual factors, and association with performance in English Premier League footballers: an investigation across a season. *Frontiers in Psychology, 11*, 2399.

Jordet, G., Bloomfield, J., & Heijmerikx, J. (2013). The hidden foundation of field vision in English Premier League (EPL) soccer players. In *Proceedings of the MIT Sloan Sports Analytics Conference* London: Routledge.

Lammfromm, R., & Gopher, D. (2011). Transfer of skill from a virtual reality trainer to real juggling. *Bio Web Conf, 1*, 0054.

Lees, A., & Owens, L. (2011). Early visual cues associated with a directional place kick in soccer. *Sports Biomechanics, 10*, 125–134.

Levi, H. R., & Jackson, R. C. (2018). Contextual factors influencing decision making: perceptions of professional soccer players. *Psychology of Sport & Exercise, 37*, 19–25.

McGuckian, T. B., Beavan, A., Mayer, J., Chalkley, D., & Pepping, G. J. (2020). The association between visual exploration and passing performance in high-level U13 and U23 football players. *Science and Medicine in Football, 4(4)*, 278-284.

McGuckian, T. B., Cole, M. H., Jordet, G., Chalkley, D., & Pepping, G.-J. (2018). Don't turn
blind! The relationship between exploration before ball possession and on-ball performance in association football. *Frontiers in Psychology, 9*, 1–13

McPherson, S. L., & Kernodle, M. W. (2003). Tactics, the neglected attribute of expertise: problem representations and performance skills in tennis. In J. Starkes & K.A. Ericsson (Eds.), *Expert Performance in Sport: Recent Advances in Research on Sport Expertise* (pp. 137–168). Champaign, IL: Human Kinetics.

McRobert, A. P., & Williams, A. M. (2019). Integrating performance analysis and perceptual-cognitive training research. In A. M. Williams & R. C. Jackson (Eds.) *Anticipation and Decision Making in Sport*. Abingdon, Oxon: Routledge.

Miles, H. C., Pop, S. R., Watt, S. J., Lawrence, G. P., & John, N. W. (2012). A review of virtual environments for training in ball sports. *Computers and Graphics, 36*(6), 714–726.

Navia, J. A., van der Kamp, J., & Ruiz, L. M. (2013). On the use of situational and body information in goalkeeper actions during a soccer penalty kick. *International Journal of Sport Psychology, 44*, 234–251.

Neumann, D. L., Moffitt, R. L., Thomas, P., Loveday, K., Watling, D., Lombard, C. L., Antonova, S., & Tremeer, M. A. (2017). A systematic review of the application of interactive virtual reality to sport. *Virtual Reality, 22*, 183–198.

Nimmerichter, A., Weber, N. J., Wirth, K., & Haller, A. (2015). Effects of video-based visual training on decision-making and reactive agility in adolescent football players. *Sports, 4(1)*, 1.

North, J. S., Ward, P., Ericsson, K. A., & Williams, A. M. (2011). Mechanisms underlying skilled anticipation and recognition in a dynamic and temporally constrained domain. *Memory, 19*, 155–168.

North, J. S., Williams, A. M., Ward, P., Hodges, N. J., & Ericsson, K. A. (2009). Perceiving patterns in dynamic action sequences: the relationship between anticipation and pattern recognition skill. *Applied Cognitive Psychology, 23*, 1–17.

Piras, A., & Vickers, J. N. (2011). The effect of fixation transitions on quiet eye duration and performance in the soccer penalty kick: instep versus inside kicks. *Cognitive Processing, 12*, 245–255

Redwood-Brown A. J., O'Donoghue, P. G., Nevill, A. M., Saward, C., & Sunderland, C. (2019). Effects of playing position, pitch location, opposition ability and team ability on the technical performance of elite soccer players in different score line states. *PLoS ONE, 14*(2), e021170.

Reeves, M. J., & Roberts, S. J. (2013) Perceptions of performance analysis in elite youth football. *International Journal of Performance Analysis in Sport, 13*, 200–211.

Reilly, T., Williams, A. M., Nevill, A., & Franks, A. (2000). A multidisciplinary approach to talent identification in soccer. *Journal of Sports Sciences, 18*, 668–676.

Roca, A., Ford, P. R., McRobert, A., & Williams, A. M. (2011). Identifying the processes underpinning anticipation and decision-making in a dynamic time- constrained task. *Cognitive Processing, 12,* 301–310.

Roca, A., Ford, P. R., McRobert, A. P., & Williams, A. M. (2013). Perceptual-cognitive skills and their interaction as a function of task constraints in soccer. *Journal of Sport & Exercise Psychology, 35*, 144–155.

Roca, A., Williams, A. M., & Ford, P. R. (2012). Developmental activities and the acquisition of superior anticipation and decision making in soccer players. *Journal of Sports Sciences, 30*, 1643–1652.

Rosalie, S. M., & Müller, S. (2014). A model for the transfer of perceptual motor skill learning in human behaviors. *Research Quarterly for Exercise and Sport, 83*, 413– 421.

Runswick, O. R., Roca, A., Williams, A. M., Bezodis, N. E., & North, J. S. (2018). The effects of anxiety and situation-specific context on perceptual-motor skill: a multi-level investigation. *Psychological Research, 82*, 708–719.

Ryu, D., Mann, D. L., Abernethy, B., & Poolton, J. M. (2016). Gaze-contingent training enhances perceptual skill acquisition. *Journal of Vision, 16*, 2.

Ryu, D., Abernethy, B., Park, S. H., & Mann, D. L. (2018). The perception of deceptive information can be enhanced by training that removes superficial visual information. *Frontiers in Psychology, 9*, 1132.

Savelsbergh, G. J. P., Van Gastel, P. J., & Van Kampen, P. M. (2010). Anticipation of penalty kicking direction can be improved by directing attention through perceptual learning. *International Journal of Sport Psychology, 41*, 24–41.

Savelsbergh, G. J. P., Williams, A. M., van der Kamp, J., & Ward, P. (2002). Visual search, anticipation and expertise in soccer goalkeepers. *J Sports Sci, 20*, 279–287.

Savelsbergh, G. J. P., van der Kamp, J. Williams, A.M., & Ward, P. (2005). Anticipation and visual search behaviour in expert soccer goalkeepers: a within-group comparison. *Ergonomics, 48*, 11–14.

Serrano, J. S., Pizarro, A. P., García-González, L., Domínguez, A. M. & del Villar Álvarez, F. (2017). Evolution of tactical behavior of soccer players across their development. *International Journal of Performance Analysis in Sport, 17*, 885–901.

Sigrist, R., Rauter, G., Marchal-Crespo, L., Riener, R., Wolf, P. (2015). Sonification and haptic feedback in addition to visual feedback enhances complex motor task learning. *Experimental Brain Research, 233*, 909–925.

Thatcher, B., Ivanov, G., Szerovay, M., & Mills, G. (2020). Virtual reality technology in football coaching: barriers and opportunities. *International Sport Coaching Journal*, (1–9), *8(2)*, 234-243.

Tyldesley, D. A., Bootsma, R. J., & Bomhoff, G. (1982). Skill level and eye movement patterns in a sport orientated reaction time task. In H. Rieder, K. Mechling, & K. Reischle (Eds.), *Proceedings of an International Symposium on Motor Behaviour: Contribution to Learning in Sport* (pp. 290–296). Cologne: Hofmann.

Vaeyens, R., Lenoir, M., Williams, A. M., Mazyn, L., & Philippaerts, R. M. (2007a). The effects of task constraints on visual search behavior and decision-making skill in youth soccer players. *Journal of Sport & Exercise Psychology, 29*, 156–175.

Vaeyens, R., Lenoir, M., Williams, A. M., Mazyn, L., & Philippaerts, R. M. (2007b) Visual search behavior and decision-making skill in soccer. *Journal of Motor Behavior, 39* (5), 395–408.

Van Maarseveen, M., Oudejans, R., & Savelsbergh, G. (2018). Self-controlled video feedback on tactical skills for soccer teams results in more active involvement of players. *Human Movement Science, 57*, 194–204

Vickers, J. N., & Williams, A. M. (2007). Why some choke and others don't! *Journal of Motor Behavior, 39*, 381–394.

Ward, P., & Williams, A. M. (2003). Perceptual and cognitive skill development in soccer: the multidimensional nature of expert performance. *Journal of Sport & Exercise Psychology, 25*, 93–111.

Ward, P., Hodges, N. J., Starkes, J., & Williams, A. M. (2007). The road to excellence: deliberate practice and the development of expertise. *High Ability Studies, 18*, 119–153.

Whelan, J. (2021). Decision making in soccer (Doctoral dissertation, Liverpool John Moores University, UK). Unpublished.

Williams, A. M. (2000). Perceptual skill in soccer: implications for talent identification and development. *Journal of Sports Sciences, 18*, 737–740.

Williams, A. M., & Burwitz, K. (1993). Advance cue utilization in soccer. In T. P. Reilly, J. Clarys, & A. Stibbe (Eds.), *Science and Football II* (pp. 239–244). London: E. & F.N. Spon.

Williams, A. M., & Davids, K. (1998). Visual search strategy, selective attention, and expertise in soccer. *Research Quarterly for Exercise and Sport, 69*, 111–128.

Williams, A. M., & Ericsson, K. A. (2005). Some considerations when applying the expert performance approach in sport. *Human Movement Science, 24*, 283–307.

Williams, A. M., & North, J. S. (2009). Identifying the minimal essential information underlying pattern recognition. In D. Arajuo, H. Ripoll, & M. Raab (Eds), *Perspectives on Cognition and Action* (pp. 95–107). New York: Nova Science Publishing Inc.

Williams, A. M., Ward, P., Bell-Walker, J., & Ford, P. R. (2012). Perceptual-cognitive expertise, practice history profiles and recall performance in soccer. *British Journal of Psychology, 103, 393–411.*

Williams, A. M., Davids, K., Burwitz, L. & Williams, J. G. (1994). Visual search strategies of experienced and inexperienced soccer players. *Research Quarterly for Exercise and Sport, 5*, 127–135.

Williams, A. M., Ford., P. R., Eccles, D., & Ward, P. (2010) Perceptual-cognitive expertise in sport and its acquisition: implications for applied cognitive psychology. *Applied Cognitive Psychology, 25*, 432–442.

Williams, A. M., Heron, K., Ward, P., & Smeeton, N. J. (2005) Using situational probabilities to train perceptual and cognitive skill in novice soccer players. In T. P. Reilly, J. Cabri, & D. Araujo (Eds.), *Science and Football V* (pp. 337–340). London: Taylor and Francis.

Williams, A. M., Hodges, N. J., North, J. S., & Barton, G. (2006). Perceiving patterns of play in dynamic sport tasks: identifying the essential information underlying skilled performance. *Perception, 35*, 317–332.

Williams, A. M., & Jackson, R. C. (2020). Psychology of sport & exercise anticipation in sport: fifty years on, what have we learned and what research still needs to be undertaken? *Psychology of Sport and Exercise, 42* (August), 16–24.

Williams, A. M., Ward, P., Smeeton, N. J., & Ward, J. (2008). Task specificity, role, and anticipation skill in soccer. *Research Quarterly for Exercise and Sport, 79*, 429–433.

Williams, A. M., Ward, P., Knowles, J. M., & Smeeton, N. J. (2002). Anticipation skill in a real-world task: measurement, training, and transfer in tennis. *Journal of Experimental Psychology, 8*, 259–270.

Wilson, M. R., Wood, G., & Vine, S. J. (2009). Anxiety, attentional control, and performance impairment in penalty kicks. *Journal of Sport and Exercise Psychology, 31*, 761–775.

Wood, G., & Wilson, M. R. (2011). Quiet-eye training for soccer penalty kicks. *Cognitive Processing, 12(3),* 257–266. doi:10.1007/s10339-011-0393-0.

Wood, G., Wright, D. J., Harris, D., Pal, A., Franklin, Z. C., & Vine, S. J. (2020). Testing the construct validity of a soccer-specific virtual reality simulator using novice, academy, and professional soccer players. *Virtual Reality, 25,* 43–51.

Wright, C., Atkins, S., Jones, B., & Todd, J. (2013). The role of an elite match analysts within football. *International Journal of Performance Analysis, 22*, 240–261.

Wulf, G., Raupach, M., & Pfeiffer, F. (2005). Self-controlled observational practice enhances learning. *Research Quarterly for Exercise and Sport, 76*, 107–111.

# 9 Skill acquisition

## Player pathways and effective practice

*Paul R. Ford and A. Mark Williams*

## Introduction

Skill is an essential component of soccer at all levels of the game. A key challenge is how best to develop skilled young players who can potentially become successful professionals. While several factors must combine across an extended period for youths to progress to professional status (see Rees et al., 2016), the activities that they engage in during development contribute significantly to the attainment of expertise. In this chapter, we provide a review of the various types of sporting activities that players engage in during development. We review research assessing the role of practice, play, and competition in soccer (see Table 9.1). In soccer, coach-led team practice is the activity in which players spend most time, so this activity will form the focus of the chapter. We separate the chapter into sections based on three main areas of research and theory. First, we review studies where researchers have had professional players retrospectively recall the amount of time spent in practice and other *developmental activities* since starting in the sport. Second, we synthesise studies in which researchers have conducted a *systematic observation* of coach-led practice sessions in soccer. Third, we review theoretical accounts of how practice and other activities can be designed to *optimally* improve the performances of players. We conclude by presenting future directions on this topic.

## Developmental activcties and pathways

Most professional players start playing soccer in childhood, typically at around 5 or 6 years of age, with some variation (Güllich, 2019; Hendry et al., 2019; Hornig et al., 2016; Ford et al., 2020). Start age in formal coach-led soccer practice often occurs 1 or 2 years after the initial start age in the sport, with relatively small variation across most countries (e.g., Ford et al., 2012). No researchers have longitudinally tracked the activities of players from early childhood into adulthood and professional status. The problem is identifying from the large playing population base those children who will eventually progress to professional status. Consequently, researchers have assessed developmental activities and pathways by asking adult professional players to retrospectively recall the activities they engaged in since starting the sport, usually using questionnaires to collect the data (Güllich, 2019; Hendry et al., 2019; Hornig et al., 2016; Ford et al., 2020).

Hornig et al. (2016) recorded the developmental activities of 52 Bundesliga and 50 fourth- to sixth-league *male* players in Germany. Players reported starting soccer through peer-led play at an average age of 4–5 years, with their start in formal coach-led

DOI: 10.4324/9781003148418-11

142  *Paul R. Ford and A. Mark Williams*

*Table 9.1* The main soccer activities in which players participate. Nb. The main intentions of a small set of individual players within the activity might differ compared to the main intention

| Activity | Main intention of participants | Main setting |
| --- | --- | --- |
| Practice | To improve performance | Formal |
| Play | Fun and enjoyment | Informal |
| Competition | Winning | Formal |

soccer practice occurring 1 or 2 years later. The 52 Bundesliga players participated more frequently in soccer peer-led play compared to coach-led practice up to the age of 10 years. The frequency of coach-led soccer practice increased as they aged, becoming significantly greater than soccer peer-led play sometime in mid- to late-adolescence, with peer-led play decreasing across adolescence. The time spent in coach-led soccer practice increased linearly from an approximate average of 2.5 h per week over a 40-week season up to 10 years of age to 13.5 h per week over a 40-week season in adulthood. Players ended significant engagement in other sports at an average age of 12–13 years and first played for a representative team at 14 years of age. Players accumulated an average of 4,264 h ($SD$ = 1,631) in coach-led soccer practice prior to making their debut in the first Bundesliga at age 21–22 years. Half of the players engaged in one to two other sports across their youth at a significantly lower frequency of sessions when compared to soccer. The data are comparable to those reported for players in other nations (e.g., Ford et al., 2012).

The first Bundesliga players engaged in significantly greater amounts of soccer peer-led play up to 10 years of age when compared to fourth- to sixth-league players, as well as reporting a significantly earlier start age in junior representative teams (approximate average of 14 years of age *vs.* 16 years). The first Bundesliga players who subsequently represented the national team ended their significant engagement in other sports later (approximate average of 14 years of age *vs.* 12 years) and made their first Bundesliga debut earlier (approximate average of 15 years of age *vs.* 16 years), when compared to the other first Bundesliga players. Moreover, national team players differed from other first Bundesliga players and fourth- to sixth-league players by engaging in significantly more coach-led practice sessions in other sports during adolescence. However, the frequency of these sessions was significantly lower than that reported for coach-led soccer practice. The first Bundesliga players engaged in a greater amount and frequency of coach-led soccer practice in early adulthood (19–21 years of age) when compared to the other two groups, but from 22 years of age onwards, there was no difference between national team and other first Bundesliga players. There were no other between-group differences reported. It is worth noting that relatively large variations existed across many of the measured variables.

Professional *female* players have been participants in three studies. The developmental activities of 29 female first Bundesliga players from one of the leading clubs in Germany, half of whom were national team players, were assessed by Güllich (2019). Similarly, Hendry et al. (2019) assessed the developmental activities of 21 national team and 24 university-level female players in Canada. Finally, the developmental activities of 86 players across the female national teams of Australia, Canada, England, Sweden, and the United States of America were recorded by Ford et al. (2020). The average

*Skill acquisition* 143

start age in soccer in these studies was around 5 years of age, with start age in coach-led soccer practice occurring approximately a year later. Professional female players in the three studies engaged in significantly more soccer activity than other sports during childhood and adolescence. The relative amounts of play/practice in soccer during this period differed between the three studies. Güllich (2019) reported that the first Bundesliga players engaged in more sessions and amounts of peer-led play in soccer compared to coach-led soccer practice during childhood and early adolescence (see

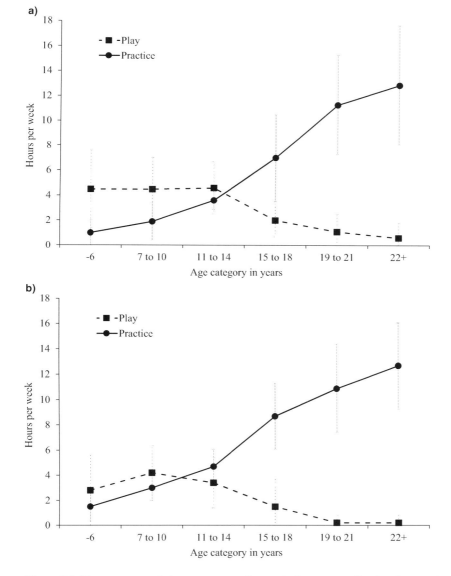

*Figure 9.1* Hours per week in soccer practice and play across the development of (a) 14 national team and (b) 15 Bundesliga players in Germany.

Figure 9.1), whereas in the other two studies there was either no difference in hours accumulated between these two activities for this period (Ford et al., 2020) or less play than practice (Hendry et al., 2019). Two studies report the start age for playing mixed-gender soccer as 6–7 years, whereas the end age for this activity was earlier for players in Canada (11 years of age, Hendry et al. 2019) compared to players in Germany (17 years of age, Güllich, 2019). The engagement in other sports did not differ between studies in childhood, albeit not all players engaged in other sports. The players who participated accumulated around an average of 1,000 h in an average of four other sports between 6 and 12 years of age in two of the studies (Ford et al., 2020; Hendry et al., 2019), which equates to around 2–3 h week$^{-1}$ over 7 × 50-week years, similar to that found for the players in Germany (Güllich, 2019). Overall, these studies show early engagement in soccer as the predominant approach with some diversification into other sports during childhood and early adolescence.

Published reports suggest that professional soccer players should engage in meaningful amounts of soccer-specific peer-led play during childhood (Ford et al., 2020; Güllich, 2019; Hornig et al., 2016). A concern is that children in some countries do not engage in as much soccer-specific peer-led play activity compared to previous generations. Moreover, children in some countries may be engaging in too much formal practice and competition at a young age, which might lead to negative consequences later in life (e.g., Baker et al., 2009). Therefore, there is a need for adults to provide more opportunities for children to engage in meaningful amounts of soccer-specific peer-led play. Some practical solutions include scheduling more soccer-specific play in formal physical education classes and coach-led practice sessions; designing and creating school playgrounds, parks, and areas that enable children to safely engage in this activity; encouraging child players to engage in this activity; and changing the formal match or games programme so that it becomes more play-oriented (e.g., Fenoglio, 2003).

In all three studies (Ford et al., 2020; Güllich, 2019; Hendry et al., 2019), the time spent in coach-led soccer practice increased across adolescence when compared to childhood, whereas time spent in peer-led soccer play and other sports decreased from mid-adolescence. The average time spent in coach-led soccer practice during adolescence was slightly higher in Canadian national team players (greater than 10 h week$^{-1}$ across 7 × 50-week years, Hendry et al., 2019) when compared to players in the other two studies. The start age in senior professional soccer was 17–18 years and with the national teams, it was 19–20 years (Ford et al., 2020; Güllich, 2019). In early adulthood, the time spent in coach-led soccer practice was greater when compared to adolescence, equating to around 12–13 h week$^{-1}$ over 50-week years in the two studies that reported this variable (Ford et al., 2020; Güllich, 2019), plus at least one match per week over a 40-week season (Ford et al., 2020). The time spent in other sports decreased to negligible amounts in adulthood compared to adolescence (Ford et al., 2020; Güllich, 2019). Overall, these three studies show specialisation in soccer occurring in adolescence and an intensification of participation in the sport occurring across this period and into adulthood, as evidenced by increasing amounts of coach-led soccer practice and promotions to higher-level teams.

Two of the studies reported comparisons of national team players to other professional players (Güllich, 2019) or university-level players (Hendry et al., 2019). Güllich (2019) reported that national team players had an earlier start age in peer-led soccer play, more hours in peer-led play in soccer and coach-led practice in other sports through childhood and early adolescence, fewer hours in coach-led soccer practice across that period, and a later start age in soccer competition and national youth teams, when compared with the other professional players. Hendry et al. (2019) reported that national team players had a later start age in formal soccer activities and in an academy, more hours in peer-led play in soccer through childhood and early adolescence, and fewer other sports, when compared with university-level players. Some *differentiating* variables were the same in the two studies (Güllich, 2019; Hendry et al., 2019). First, later start ages in some formal soccer activities and in joining higher-level teams were found in both studies for national team players. Second, more hours in soccer-specific peer-led play compared to other activities through childhood and early adolescence were found in both studies. Other researchers have found more hours in peer-led soccer play through childhood for male youth players in English academies who received a professional contract compared to those who did not (Ford et al., 2009; Ford & Williams, 2012) and in first Bundesliga male players compared to fourth- to sixth-league players (Hornig et al., 2016).

In three out of the four studies, the authors explicitly noted that there was large variability in their data (Hendry et al., 2019; Hornig et al., 2016; Ford et al., 2020). In other words, there were professional players in the studies whose developmental activities notably *differed* to the reported averages for their group (for detail, see Ford et al., 2020). Moreover, there was no measure in these four studies of the effects on current or future player performance of each different bout, block, or phase of activity. Therefore, these studies do not show that any of the activities *caused* the attainment of professional status and performance (Ford & Williams, 2017). Furthermore, there is no measurement of player soccer performance in these studies, so the relationship between activities engaged in and performance cannot be tested. Of course, it is obvious that different bouts, blocks, or phases of activity could have very different effects on improving current or future player performance. Finally, these studies assess practice, play, and competition at a macro-level and provide no information on what the players did during those activities. In the next section, we review studies that assess the microstructure of these soccer activities to reveal what players are doing.

## Microstructure of practice

Researchers have filmed coach-led soccer practice sessions and analysed the microstructure of the activities engaged in by youth players. In two separate studies (Ford et al., 2010; Partington & Cushion, 2011) youth players engaged in drill-based activities for approximately two-thirds of coach-led team practice time, with the remaining third of the time being spent in games-based activities. Coaches are thought to use drill-based activities to lessen the demands of the game for learners and because performance appears to be successful during this type of activity (Patterson & Lee, 2008). Although the use of these types of activities is well-intended, and broadly speaking repetition is an important part of practice, such widespread use has been questioned (Ford et al., 2010; Partington & Cushion, 2011). A suggestion is that drill-based activities present a reduced opportunity for players to develop the perceptual-cognitive skills that are important during match-play at higher levels of the sport, particularly visual search, anticipation, and decision-making. It was suggested that games-based activities present a better way to engage and develop the perceptual-cognitive skills required in match-play (Ford et al., 2010; Partington & Cushion, 2011).

More recently, in three other studies (Ford & Whelan, 2016; O'Connor et al., 2018; Roca & Ford, 2020) researchers filmed coach-led youth soccer practice sessions and analysed the microstructure of the activities. In these studies, youth players spent more time in *games-based practice activities* compared with drill-based activities. Ford and Whelan (2016) analysed 108 coaching sessions involving child and adolescent teams from the academies of three Premier League clubs, three Football League clubs, and three amateur clubs in England. Three in-season sessions were filmed per team and the video was analysed for the relative amounts of drill- or games-based activities. The sessions contained 59% games-based activity, 20% drill-based activity, and 21% time transitioning between activities. More time was spent in games-based activities for the child compared with adolescent teams, but there were no differences between skill levels. Most practice sessions were held in small- or medium-sized areas on artificial grass. The increase in games-based activity in these later compared to earlier studies may be due to recent changes to coach education and national guidelines (e.g., The Football Association). However, coaches should consider training more often than currently on natural compared to artificial grass to increase realism, representativeness, variability, and specificity (e.g., Andersson et al., 2008).

There are a few limitations with studies in which the microstructure of coach-led soccer practice has been recorded and analysed. First, there is a lack of studies on adult professional and female soccer teams. Second, some key contextual factors surrounding the sessions are missing in that the intentions of the coaches have not been recorded; we do not know why they used a particular activity at that specific time point in player or team development. Third, soccer is a complex sport and there are multiple aspects of performance that one can choose to practice with the ball in training or coaching sessions at any given time (i.e., various technical skills and tactics or strategies), but this has not been considered in this research. Fourth, although it is assumed that peer-led soccer play involves mostly games-based activities, there are no studies published in which researchers have assessed what players do in this activity, unlike for coach-led youth soccer practice. Finally, the binary differentiation between drill- and games-based activities was a heuristic used to ease understanding and help change coach behaviour. In reality, common practice activities with the ball in soccer lie on a continuum of representativeness when compared to match-play, as is shown in Figure 9.2. Moreover, the activity categories themselves in Figure 9.2 are continuous and potentially mixable. For example, some phases of play activities in soccer can be very similar to small-sided games and decision-making drills and others can be more like the target context of match-play. Coaches are encouraged to work with specialists in skill acquisition to design these types of activity and practice environments (Williams & Ford, 2009). In the next section, we review the theory that details how to optimise these practice activities.

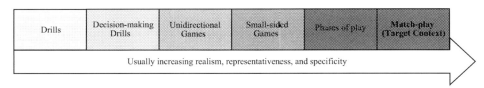

*Figure 9.2* The continuum of representativeness for common practice activities with the ball in soccer.

## Theoretical accounts

### Deliberate practice

Deliberate practice theory has been outlined in detail in several publications by Ericsson (1996; 1998; 2003; 2006; 2007; 2013; 2017; 2020; Ericsson & Pool, 2016; Ericsson et al., 1993; Ericsson & Towne, 2010) and there has been a debate between researchers about its content, including in sport (Macnamara et al., 2016a, b; Ericsson, 2016). The activity of deliberate practice differs according to Ericsson (2020; Ericsson & Pool, 2016) from other forms of practice, such as maintenance practice. Two recent publications have used acronyms to clarify the definition of deliberate practice (Eccles et al., 2020) and demonstrate how it can be administered in sport (Ford & Coughlan, 2019).

Eccles et al. (2020) forwarded the acronym EXPERTS to clarify the definition of deliberate practice. They state that deliberate practice occurs in domains and for skills where established (E) and effective training techniques exist. Moreover, it involves improving existing (X) individual skills in a step-by-step process and attempts at skills beyond the current ability level of the performer, termed 'pushing (P) the envelope'. Deliberate practice enhances (E) mental representations making them more sophisticated. Furthermore, improvement occurs by obtaining and responding (R) to individualised feedback from instructors during the activity. It requires total (T) application from the performer in terms of giving their full attention and involves setting and focusing on specific (S) goals for improvement.

Second, Ford and Coughlan (2019) use the acronym ASPIRE (Analyse, Select, Practice, Individualise, Repetition, Evaluate) to detail how deliberate practice can be administered in sport. First, player or team performance is analysed (A) to select (S) the key aspect of performance requiring improvement at that time. Second, practice (P) bouts occur to improve the selected key aspect of performance involving individualisation (I) of processes and feedback, along with repetition (R) of the aspect in a representative environment. Finally, player or team performance is evaluated (E) to determine the amount of improvement in the key aspect, with further practice bouts required when there is no or little improvement or a new aspect of performance selected from analysis if there is. Researchers have not assessed these hypotheses (Eccles et al., 2020; Ford & Coughlan, 2019) or those from deliberate practice theory in relation to their effect on performance improvement in soccer players.

The 'power law of practice' holds that in the earlier stages of learning a new task or domain, performance improvement is rapid, whereas later in the process the rate begins to slow or plateau (Newell & Rosenbloom, 1981). For many performers, the plateau occurs because they are competent at the task and are satisfied to remain at that level of performance. However, Ericsson (2003, 2007) has termed this plateau in performance 'arrested development'. He holds that expert performers are not satisfied with being merely competent, rather they begin to repetitively engage in bouts of deliberate practice with the intention of improving performance beyond its current level. Almost certainly, adolescent players desiring to be professionals should engage in deliberate practice to avoid a plateau in performance and 'arrested development'. In addition, deliberate practice can focus on aspects of performance for the team, unit, and/or player, focusing on enhancing strengths and improving weaknesses, but this process should be *individualised* to each player. Therefore, the aspect of performance that is chosen to practice very much depends on the current strengths and weaknesses

148 *Paul R. Ford and A. Mark Williams*

of the team, unit, or individual under consideration. Of course, there are multiple physical, psychological, anthropometrical, skill, and social aspects of performance that require improvement. In soccer, the difficulty comes when trying to individualise this process to each player as is required in theory because there are usually too few coaches available. We recommend the ASPIRE process (Ford & Coughlan, 2019) is used as the framework for these decisions and for the practice itself which should also match the characteristics outlined in the EXPERTS acronym (Eccles et al., 2020).

A key part of deliberate practice theory is that it is an effortful activity that can only be maintained for short periods, such that rest and recovery are required (Ericsson et al., 1993). Therefore, rest and recovery processes should be optimised for adolescents and adult players who not only engage in deliberate practice but also frequently play in professional soccer matches. We would expect to see this activity occurring in what we term a *deliberate environment* (Ford et al., 2013; 2015; Ford & Coughlan, 2019). A deliberate environment exists where the decisions, behaviours, and activities of the players in their sporting and home life are optimally goal-directed toward improving or maintaining their competitive performance (Ford et al., 2015).

### Challenge point hypothesis

The *challenge point framework* presented by Guadagnoli and Lee (2004; see also Hodges & Lohse, 2022) holds that practice activities present different levels of difficulty depending on the skill level of the performer and the practice conditions. *Nominal task difficulty* is the constant difficulty of the task, irrespective of the person performing the task. In contrast, *functional task difficulty* includes the task and how challenging it is to the individual. The *optimal challenge point* occurs around the point of functional task difficulty that a performer at a specific skill level would need to optimise perceptual, cognitive, and motor learning. When a practice task is too easy or too difficult for a performer either no or minimal learning may occur. A related concept is *task simplification* (Renshaw, Chow, Davids, & Hammond, 2010; Davids et al., 2008) which involves lowering the difficulty of the task to an appropriate level for the learner while maintaining the natural performance conditions of the task (e.g., small-sided games in soccer). There are several methods that coaches can use to reduce the functional task difficulty of small-sided games for the skill level of the learners participating (e.g., Table 9.2).

*Table 9.2* Some examples of manipulations to the rules of small-sided games (e.g., 3 vs. 3) that may reduce the difficulty of the sport for learners

| |
|---|
| (1)  Increase the size of the pitches (e.g, Clemente & Sarmento, 2020) |
| (2)  Reduce the number of players on each team (e.g., Clemente & Sarmento, 2020) |
| (3)  Include extra players who play for whichever team is in possession of the ball during the game (e.g., Clemente & Sarmento, 2020) |
| (4)  Ban tackling only allowing blocks of passes and pressure |
| (5)  Ban tackling in the middle half of the pitch only – only allowing blocks of passes and pressure in that area |
| (6)  Use unidirectional games in which there are more teammates than opposition (e.g., 2 *vs.* 1; 3 *vs.* 1; 4 *vs.* 2) |
| (7)  Have the coach join in the play |
| (8)  Ban running – have the players walk only |

When an aspect of an activity is too demanding for learners, this is known as a *rate limiter*. Rate limiters are most often thought of as an individual characteristic, such as height or muscle strength, that is holding back the progression of learning and development (Haywood & Getchell, 2001; Horn & Williams, 2004). However, rate limiters can exist within characteristics of the task or environment that can hold back the progression of learning. For example, in soccer, opponents tackling the player in possession of the ball and reducing time/space make the game very difficult for relatively novice players and acts as a key rate limiter reducing the opportunity for them to learn how to manipulate the ball and move around opponents. By identifying and changing the task or environmental rate limiters, the difficulty of the task can be lowered to the optimal challenge point for the learners (see Table 9.2).

### Constraints-led approach

The constraints-led approach has been fully outlined in detail in several books (e.g., Button et al., 2020; Chow et al., 2015; Davids et al., 2008; Renshaw et al., 2019) and review articles (e.g., Otte et al., 2021; Renshaw et al.; 2016; Renshaw & Chow, 2019). Constraints are defined as interacting boundaries that shape and bring order to behaviour and its emergence in humans (Newell, 1986). Three types of interacting constraints exist that operate at differing timescales: (i) individual constraints, such as leg strength, current ability, or aerobic capacity; (ii) environment constraints, such as the ground surface and light; and (iii) task constraints, such as the rules, goals, and conditions of soccer. The performer generates movement solutions through a self-organisation process that is bound by these constraints in their current environment (Newell, 1986). Learning and acquisition occurs through the performer becoming better attuned to key information and intentions in that environment (Renshaw & Chow, 2019). Of course, information in the match-play environment includes the movements, actions, intentions, patterns, and tactics of teammates and opponents upon a pitch that has its markings and a goal at either end. A key aspect of this approach is that information, intentions, and actions from the target context should be represented during practice so that performers can search, discover, and exploit its use (Otte et al., 2021). Furthermore, coaches can manipulate constraints during practice so that behaviour emerges and learning occurs that is relevant for the later target context of match-play. Task constraints are perhaps the easiest for coaches to manipulate and many coaches already do this intuitively. For example, Table 9.3 shows practice activities in which the rules of the game (or task constraints) have been changed to bring about a greater frequency of desired actions and learning in players. However, the constraints-led approach and related theories provide a framework for coaches that goes beyond their intuitive processes when designing learning environments (for reviews, see Chow et al., 2015; Otte et al., 2021; O Sullivan et al., 2021).

### Games-based approaches

A few games-based approaches (GBAs) to skill acquisition in sport exist, particularly those from the physical education field (e.g., Teaching Games for Understanding (TGFU); Games Sense; and Play Practice; for a review, see Kinnerk et al., 2018), but also more recently from outside of that field (e.g., Video-game Design; for a review, see

## 150 Paul R. Ford and A. Mark Williams

*Table 9.3* Some examples of manipulations to the rules of small-sided games (e.g., 4 vs. 4) so that players practice specific perceptual-motor skills more frequently than normal

| Motor skill | Game manipulations |
| --- | --- |
| Dribbling | Remove goals and have players score by dribbling across their opposition's goal touch lines. |
| Passing | All small-sided games contain a lot of passing, although to encourage one and two-touch passing, the coach can limit touches (e.g., "2-touch"). |
| Long passing | Make the pitch very long but not too wide. Alternatively, have two very small goals with no goalkeepers and a "no go" penalty area. |
| Forward passing | Remove goals and replace with two relatively large American Football style "end zones". Players score by passing the ball into the path of a teammate who runs into the opposition's end zone. Use the touchline that marks the start of the "end zone" as an "offside line". |
| Switch-play passing | Make the pitch wide but short. Plus, remove goals and replace with two smaller goals at each goal line, which are placed on the goal lines extending in from both corners. Players must score by dribbling the ball through one of the two small goals. |
| Turning | Allow both teams to score at either end of the pitch. |
| Shooting | Place large goal nets at either end of the pitch. |
| Crossing | Place corridors along the touchlines from which players who play for whichever team is in possession can cross the ball without opposition. Perhaps limit the number of players allowed in the "penalty area". |

Price et al., 2018). There is a large volume of literature outlining and assessing GBA. Kinnerk et al. (2018) conducted one of several systematic reviews of GBA studies in which researchers have evaluated outcomes in competitive team sport settings. They located 23 studies that included 21 studies assessing invasion game sports, from which eight studies were soccer-based. There were 13 studies with youth participants and 14 studies contained interventions of which six were longer-term. There were six studies utilising systematic observation tools to assess post-intervention improvements in participant game performance. Altogether, five out of those six studies reported significant improvements in various aspects of decision-making and tactical ability. There were two out of six studies that found significant improvements in technical ability in soccer, specifically passing (four out of six studies found no improvement here). Transfer to match-play was assessed in two out of six studies. Those two studies (Pizarro et al., 2017; Práxedes et al., 2016) contained the longest interventions (12 weeks), with most studies having shorter interventions (4–5 weeks) and no test of transfer to match-play. Moreover, the two studies (Pizarro et al., 2017; Práxedes et al., 2016) contained the same age players (U11/12) and skill level (intermediate). Both studies found significant post-intervention match-play performance improvement in decision-making and technical ability. The use of questioning coaching behaviours varied between the six studies, there was an overall lack of detail on the actual game activities, and there was a lack of control groups, confounding findings. Overall, we consider there to be medium-strength evidence for the use of GBA, particularly with younger players. Intervention studies contain limitations and mainly assess the TGFU approach, as opposed to other GBA. It is likely the application of GBA and the activities in Figure 9.2 are context-specific in that it will depend on several current contextual factors surrounding the bout of activity/ies, such as the current age stage of the players or their current strengths and weaknesses, etc. Coaches who work with specialists in skill acquisition may be best placed to optimally design practice activities for player improvement within a specific context (Williams & Ford, 2009).

## Future directions and conclusions

There are two immediate priorities for researchers in this area that have been outlined in detail by Williams et al. (2020). First, there are several theoretical ideas on optimal potential activities for players, many of which have been outlined in this chapter. Researchers need to provide a rigorous quasi-experimental assessment of these ideas, using robust study designs and methods more common to medicine, such as randomised control trials (for an example in soccer, see Roberts et al., 2020; see also Miller et al., 2016). Second, a standardised method to measure player performance in matches and small-sided games is required to assess the causal effects of potential optimal activities and interventions in these research studies. Researchers need to validate this reliable standard method to measure player performance in matches and small-sided games. Performance analysis may provide the best tools to achieve this goal and some research has already been published on this topic (e.g., van Maarseveen et al., 2017).

The practice and other activities in which players engage influence their development and attainment. In this chapter, we reviewed theory and research on this topic and outlined implications for coaches and other interested persons involved in the design of practice activities and environments for players. We recommend aspiring soccer players to progress from mostly soccer-specific play-type activities in childhood to mostly deliberate practice activities in adolescence and adulthood. We advocate that specialists in skill acquisition are employed by clubs and national associations to provide support with the design of practice environments. Regardless, the publication of research and theory in this area will continue and we recommended it focuses on robustly testing theoretical ideas using accepted experimental designs and creating a standard method to measure player performance in matches that can be used to measure the effects of these ideas.

## References

Andersson, H., Ekblom, B., & Krustrup, P. (2008). Elite football on artificial turf versus natural grass: movement patterns technical standards, and player impressions. *Journal of Sports Sciences, 26,* 113–122.

Baker, J, Cobley, S., & Fraser-Thomas, J. (2009). What do we know about early sport specialization? Not much! *High Ability Studies*, 20, 77–89.

Button, C., Seifert, L., Chow, J. Y., Araújo, D., & Davids, K. (2020). *Dynamics of Skill Acquisition: An Ecological Dynamics rationale* (2nd Ed.). Champaignl: Human Kinetics.

Chow, J. Y., Davids, K., Button, C., & Renshaw, I. (2015). *Nonlinear Pedagogy in Skill Acquisition: An Introduction.* London: Routledge.

Clemente, F. M. & Sarmento, H. (2020). The effects of small-sided soccer games on technical actions and skills: A systematic review. *Human Movement, 21,* 100–119.

Davids, K., Button, C., & Bennett, S. (2008). *Dynamics of Skill Acquisition: A Constraints-led Approach.* Champaign, IL: Human Kinetics.

Eccles, D. W., Leone, E. J., & Williams, A. M. (2020). Deliberate practice: What is it and how can I use it? *Journal of Sport Psychology in Action, 13, 16–26*

Ericsson, K. A. (Ed.) (1996). The acquisition of expert performance: an introduction to some of the issues. In K. A. Ericsson (Ed.), *The Road to Excellence: The Acquisition of Expert Performance in the Arts and Sciences, Sports and Games* (pp. 1–50). Hillsdale, NJ: Lawrence Erlbaum.

Ericsson, K. A. (1998). The scientific study of expert levels of performance: General implications for optimal learning and creativity. *High Ability Studies, 9*, 75–100.

Ericsson, K. A. (2003). Development of elite performance and deliberate practice: an update from the perspective of the expert performance approach. In J. L. Starkes & K. A. Ericsson (Eds.), *Expert Performance in Sports: Advances in Research on Sport Expertise* (pp. 49–84). Champaign: IL, Human Kinetics.

Ericsson, K. A. (2006). The influence of experience and deliberate practice on the development of superior expert performance. In K. A. Ericsson, N. Charness, P. Feltovich, & R. R. Hoffman (Eds.), *Cambridge Handbook of Expertise and Expert Performance* (pp. 683–703). Cambridge, UK: Cambridge University Press.

Ericsson, K. A. (2007). Deliberate practice and the modifiability of body and mind: toward a science of the structure and acquisition of expert and elite performance. *International Journal of Sport Psychology, 38*, 4–34.

Ericsson, K. A. (2013). Training history, deliberate practice and elite sports performance: an analysis in response to Tucker and Collins review – what makes champions? *British Journal of Sports Medicine, 47*, 533–535.

Ericsson, K. A. (2016). Summing up hours of any type of practice versus identifying optimal practice activities: Commentary on Macnamara, Moreau, & Hambrick (2016). *Perspectives on Psychological Science, 11*, 351–354.

Ericsson, K. A. (2017). Summing up hours of any type of practice versus identifying optimal practice activities: commentary on Macnamara, Moreau, & Hambrick (2016). *Perspectives on Psychological Science, 11*, 351–354.

Ericsson, K. A. (2020). Towards a science of the acquisition of expert performance in sports: Clarifying the differences between deliberate practice and other types of practice. *Journal of Sports Sciences, 38*, 159–176.

Ericsson, K. A., Krampe, R. T., & Tesch-Römer, C. (1993). The role of deliberate practice in the acquisition of expert performance. *Psychological Review, 100*, 363–406.

Ericsson, K. A. & Towne, T. J. (2010). Expertise. *Wiley Interdisciplinary Reviews Cognitive Science, 1*, 404–416.

Ericsson, K. A. & Pool, R. (2016). *Peak: Secrets From the New Science of Success*. Boston, USA: Houghton Mifflin Harcourt.

Fenoglio, R. (2003). The Manchester United 4 v 4 pilot scheme for U9s. *Insight: The FA Coaches Association Journal, 6 (3)*, 18–19.

Ford, P. R., Carling, C., Garces, M., Marques, M., Miguel, C., Farrant, A., Stenling, A., Moreno, J., Le Gall, F., Holmström, S., Salmela, J. H., & Williams, A. M. (2012). The developmental activities of elite soccer players aged under-16 years from Brazil, England, France, Ghana, Mexico, Portugal and Sweden. *Journal of Sports Sciences, 30*, 1653–1663.

Ford, P. R. & Coughlan, E. (2019). Operationalizing deliberate practice for performance improvement in sport. In A. M. Williams & N. J. Hodges (Eds.), *Skill Acquisition in Sport: Research, Theory and Practice*. 3rd Edn. London: Routledge.

Ford, P. R., Coughlan, E. K., Hodges, N. J., & Williams, A. M. (2015). Deliberate practice in sport. In J. Baker & D. Farrow (Eds.), *The Handbook of Sport Expertise* (pp. 347–362). London: Routledge.

Ford, P. R., Hodges, N. J., & Williams, A. M. (2013). Creating champions: the development of expertise in sports. In S. B. Kaufman (Ed.), *Beyond Talent: The Complexity of Greatness* (pp. 391–414). Oxford: Oxford University Press.

Ford, P. R., Hodges, N. J., Broadbent, D., O'Connor, D., Scott, D., Datson, N., Andersson, H. A., & Williams, A. M. (2020). The developmental and professional activities of female international soccer players from five high-performing nations. *Journal of Sports Sciences, 38*, 1432–1440.

Ford, P. R., Ward, P., Hodges, N. J., & Williams, A. M. (2009). The role of deliberate practice and play in career progression in sport: the early engagement hypothesis. *High Ability Studies, 20*, 65–75.

Ford, P. R. & Whelan, J. (2016). Practice activities during coaching sessions in elite youth football and their effect on skill acquisition. In W. Allison, A. Abraham, & A. Cale (Eds.), *Advances in Coach Education and Development: From Research to Practice* (pp. 112–123). London: Routledge.

Ford P. R., & Williams A. M. (2017). Sport activity in childhood: early specialisation and diversification. In J. Baker, S. Cobley, J. Schorer, & N. Wattie (Eds.), *Handbook of Talent Identification and Development* (pp. 117–132). London: Routledge.

Ford, P. R., Yates, I. & Williams, A. M. (2010). An analysis of practice activities and instructional behaviours used by youth soccer coaches during practice: exploring the link between science and application. *Journal of Sports Sciences, 28*, 483–495.

Guadagnoli, M. A, & Lee, T. D. (2004). Challenge point: a framework for conceptualizing the effects of various practice conditions in motor learning. *Journal of Motor Behavior, 36*, 212–224.

Güllich, A. (2019). "Macro-structure" of developmental participation histories and "microstructure" of practice of German female world-class and national-class football players. *Journal of Sports Sciences, 37*, 1347–1355.

Haywood, K., & Getchell, N. (2001). *Life Span Motor Development.* Champaign, IL: Human Kinetics.

Hendry, D., Williams, A. M., Ford, P. R., & Hodges, N. J. (2019). Developmental activities and perceptions of challenge for national and varsity women soccer players in Canada. *Psychology of Sport and Exercise, 43*, 210–218.

Hodges, N. J. & Lohse, K. R. (2022). An extended challenge-based framework for practice design in sports coaching. *Journal of Sports Sciences.* Advance online publication. DOI: 10.1080/02640414.2021.2015917

Horn, R., & Williams, A. M. (2004). Rate limiters in the development of football skills. *Insight: The FA Coaches Association Journal, 7 (1)*, 59–62.

Hornig, M., Aust, F. & Güllich, A. (2016). Practice and play in the development of German top-level professional football players. *European Journal of Sport Science, 16*, 96–105.

Kinnerk, P., Harvey, S., MacDonncha, C., & Lyons, M. (2018). A review of the game-based approaches to coaching literature in competitive team sport settings. *Quest, 70*, 401–418.

Macnamara, B. N., Moreau, D., & Hambrick, D. Z. (2016a). The relationship between deliberate practice and performance in sports: a meta-analysis. *Perspectives on Psychological Science, 11*, 333–350.

Macnamara, B. N., Hambrick, D. Z., & Moreau, D. (2016b). How important is deliberate practice? Reply to Ericsson (2016b). *Perspectives on Psychological Science, 11*, 355–358.

Miller, A., Harvey, S., Morley, D., Nemes, R., Janes, M., & Eather, N. (2016). Exposing athletes to playing form activity: outcomes of a randomised control trial among community netball teams using a game-centred approach. *Journal of Sports Sciences, 35*, 1846–1857.

Newell, A., & Rosenbloom, P. S. (1981). Mechanisms of skill acquisition and the law of practice. In J. R. Anderson (Ed.), *Cognitive Skills and Their Acquisition* (pp. 1–55). Hillsdale, NJ: Erlbaum.

Newell, K. M. (1986). Coordination, control, and skill. In D. Goodman, R. B. Wilberg, & I. M. Franks (Eds.), *Differing Perspectives in Motor Learning, Memory and Control* (pp. 295–317). Amsterdam: Elsevier.

O' Connor, D., Larkin, P., & Williams, A. (2018). Observations of youth football training: how do coaches structure training sessions for player development? *Journal of Sports Sciences, 36*, 39–47

O' Sullivan, M. O., Woods, C. T., Vaughan, J., & Davids, K. (2021). Towards a contemporary player learning in development framework for sports practitioners. *International Journal of Sports Science & Coaching, 16*, 1214–1222.

Otte, F. W., Davids, K., Millar, S. K., & Klatt, S. (2021). Understanding how athletes learn: integrating skill training concepts, theory, and practice from an ecological perspective. *Applied Coaching Research Journal, 7.* Retrieved January 12, 2022 from https://www.ukcoaching.org/getattachment/Resources/Topics/Research/Applied-Coaching-Research-Journal-April-2021/Research-Journal-Vol-7-Understanding-How-Athletes-Learn.pdf?lang=en-GB

Partington, M., & Cushion, C. (2011). An investigation of the practice activities and coaching behaviors of professional top-level youth soccer coaches. *Scandinavian Journal of Medicine and Science in Sports, 23,* 374, 382.

Patterson, J. T., & Lee, T. (2008). Organizing practice: the interaction of repetition and cognitive effort for skilled performance. In D. Farrow, J. Baker, & C. McMahon (Eds.), *Developing Sports Expertise: Researchers and Coaches put Theory into Practice* (pp. 119–134). London: Routledge.

Pizarro, A. P., Domínguez, A. M., Serrano, J. S., García-González, L., & Del Villar Álvarez, F. (2017). The effects of a comprehensive teaching program on dribbling and passing decision-making and execution skills of young footballers. *Kinesiology, 49,* 74–83.

Práxedes, A., Moreno, A., Sevil, J., García-González, L., & Del Villar, F. (2016). A preliminary study of the effects of a comprehensive teaching program, based on questioning, to improve tactical actions in young footballers. *Perceptual & Motor Skills, 122,* 742–756.

Price, A., Collins, D., Stoszkowski, J., & Pill, S. (2018). Learning to play soccer: lessons on meta-cognition from video game design. *Quest, 70,* 321–333.

Rees, T., Hardy, L., Güllich, A., Abernethy, B., Côté, J., Woodman, T., … Warr, C. (2016). The Great British Medalists Project: a review of current knowledge on the development of the world's best sporting talent. *Sports Medicine, 46,* 1041–1058.

Renshaw, I., Araujo, D., Button, C., Chow, J., Davids, K., & Moy, B. (2016). Why the constraints-led approach is not teaching games for understanding: a clarification. *Physical Education and Sport Pedagogy, 21,* 459–480.

Renshaw, I. & Chow, J. (2019). A constraint-led approach to sport and physical education pedagogy. *Physical Education and Sport Pedagogy, 24,* 103–116.

Renshaw, I., Chow, J., Davids, K., & Hammond, J. (2010). A constraints-led perspective to understanding skill acquisition and game play: a basis for integration of motor learning theory and physical education praxis? *Physical Education and Sport Pedagogy, 15,* 117–137.

Renshaw, I., Davids, K., Newcombe, D., & Roberts, W. (2019). *The Constraints- Led Approach: Principles for Sports Coaching and Practice Design* London: Routledge.

Roberts, S. J., Rudd, J. R., & Reeves, M. J. (2020). Efficacy of using non-linear pedagogy to support attacking players' individual learning objectives in elite-youth football: a randomised cross-over trial. *Journal of Sports Sciences, 38,* 1454–1464.

Roca, A. & Ford, P. R. (2020). Decision-making practice during coaching sessions in elite youth football across European countries. *Science and Medicine in Football, 4,* 263–268.

van Maarseveen, M. J., Oudejans, R. R., & Savelsbergh, G. J. (2017). System for notational analysis in small-sided soccer games. *International Journal of Sports Science & Coaching, 12,* 194–206.

Williams, A. M. & Ford, P. R. (2009). Promoting a skills-based agenda in Olympic sports: the role of skill-acquisition specialists. *Journal of Sports Sciences, 27,* 1381–1392.

Williams, A. M., Drust, B., & Ford, P. R. (2020). Talent identification and development in soccer since the millennium. *Journal of Sports Sciences, 38,* 1199–1210.

# 10 Sociological influences on the identification and development of players

*Matthew J. Reeves and Simon J. Roberts*

## Introduction

Soccer is the world's most popular sport and subsequently an important sociocultural driver. One of the key factors in the sport's worldwide dominance has been the creation of professional leagues and the emergence of teams as powerful commercial brands and, for some (i.e., investors/owners), a substantive financial opportunity. The current context is a far cry from the local, amateur activity that emerged from the middle of the 19th century (cf. Elliott, 2017). At the highest levels of soccer, the frenzied environment is more akin to the entertainment business; whilst at the lowest levels of soccer competition, the game is concerned with continued delivery of a quality product that offers hope, aspiration, and expectation. Regardless of whether competing for the highest international honours available (e.g., the World Cup and the European Champions League), or to remain competitive within a national league structure, there is the requirement for clubs to field a team that can perform.

Due to the ever-increasing costs associated with purchasing players from another club, it is unsurprising that clubs prefer to look at their own talent identification and development (TID) processes and practices (Reeves & Roberts, 2020). Alongside club-driven methodologies for talent identification and development, national and international federations have brought about rule changes. For over a decade, efforts have been made with the broad intention of increasing the quality and quantity of players developed by clubs to support their, and in some instances the national federation's, aspirations. Some examples of these changes include the Deutscher Fußball-Bund (DFB) mandating that all German clubs in the top three tiers must operate an academy; the Fédération Française de Football (FFF) and Ligue de Football Professionnel (LPF) implementing the 'Charte du Football Professionnel'; and the Premier Leagues 'Elite Player Performance Plan' (EPPP). There have, however, also been other, somewhat, controversial, and wide-ranging rule changes, such as UEFAs 'Level Playing Field' initiative, more often referred to as Financial Fair Play (FFP), which has polarised clubs and fans and, seemingly, done little that it set out to achieve.

While there have been numerous influences on clubs and their talent identification and development processes and practices, researchers continue to question the productivity of academies in developing players who can transition to the first team (Morris, Todd & Oliver, 2015). The purpose and different structures of academies across Europe have been well-documented (see Relvas et al., 2010). The range of specialist practitioners within these structures, that help guide player development, has been expanded, though their individual and combined influence remains to be fully

DOI: 10.4324/9781003148418-12

## 156  *Matthew J. Reeves and Simon J. Roberts*

understood. As the breadth of influence (i.e., specialist practitioners) on an individual, from a club or academy environment increases, so too does the need to better understand that influence. It is important to note that the impact of sociological factors on talent identification and development in soccer has received less attention than other disciplines/areas of investigation (Reeves et al., 2018b). However, seven sociological factors have been proposed as potential predictors of future, adult, high performance in soccer (cf. Williams & Reilly, 2000; Williams, Ford & Drust, 2020). In this chapter, we consider several of those factors and attempt to explain how practitioners and researchers can, with an enhanced understanding of the issues explored, more effectively manage processes and practices that ultimately lead to better outcomes in terms of player identification, development, productivity, and club success.

### The role of family

The role of the family unit, but particularly parents, has been of interest to researchers from both participation and performance perspectives (Hoyle & Leff, 1997; for a historical review, see Dorsch et al., 2021). Understandably, parents make a significant contribution to their child's (non)involvement in any sport or activity and there is a body of work that has sought to understand this issue across various sports. Scientists have examined several broad issues including parents' experiences in youth soccer (Clarke & Harwood, 2014; Clarke, Harwood & Cushion, 2016; Newport, Knight & Love, 2020), children's preferences for parental involvement and enjoyment (Furusa et al., 2020), and the role of siblings during talent development (Taylor, Carson & Collins, 2018), though the importance and role of the family do not just concern young players. For example, findings from other studies have highlighted the role of family support in dealing with issues of mental ill-health amongst professional players (Wood, Harrison & Kucharska, 2017), and the impact of job relocation on families (Molnar & Maguire, 2008; Roderick, 2012, 2013).

Scientists that have investigated parents' experiences in youth soccer have reported several common features, including increased sense of parental responsibility and an embodied sense of closeness. An increased sense of parental responsibility has been shown to occur due to enhanced parental identity, linked to their child's role as an academy player (Clarke & Harwood, 2014; Clarke, Harwood & Cushion, 2016). Parents feel that their child being identified and labelled as a junior-elite soccer player reflects their parenting ability and, thus, their identity as a parent. The proximity to parental identity and their child's transition through different stages of development programmes and environments has also been noted to affect parents' identity (Clarke & Harwood, 2014; Clarke, Harwood & Cushion, 2016). In addition to changes in identity, parents must carefully navigate their position within the academy environment (Reeves et al., 2018b), seeking to understand the landscape and manage their exchanges with a range of other actors within the environment. Furthermore, interactions between parents have been suggested to require mediation of expectations regarding their child's transition to becoming an elite athlete. The high attrition rate of junior-elite soccer players means that parents, like their child(ren), require careful management of self within the development environment.

Managing identity, expectations, and self within a talent development environment has been closely linked to notions of socialisation and conforming to norms, practices, and expectations within the established culture. These norms, it is suggested, are heightened through parents' interactions with coaches and other parents; meaning that the quality of a parent's relationship with their child's coach, or other parents, might affect the comments they make, the questions they pose, and the role they take in coaching their own child (Clarke & Harwood, 2014). Clarke and Harwood's (2014) study found that parents had to adjust to the shift in power to, and increased involvement from, their child's coach(es) while negotiating the expectations placed on them, and how this all personally affected their identity. Parents suggested that they experienced difficulties controlling their behaviours while watching competitive games from the side-line and ensuring that they adhered to the sociocultural norms of 'not interfering' despite competition being an emotionally loaded aspect of a parent's role (Dorsch, Smith & McDonough, 2015) and one that can influence both the parent's and child's experience (Knight et al., 2016).

In their study of parents' experiences of the youth soccer journey, Newport, Knight, and Love (2020) sought to understand parental experiences at different transitions of youngsters through an academy environment. Parents detailed an ever-changing journey through the academy environment that included a dual relationship that ranged from enjoyment and opportunity to sacrifice and consequences. Those dualistic experiences coincided with an evolving experience of the implications of the environment, which ranged from initial excitement and amazement to focusing on the future (see Figure 10.1).

In addition, Newport and colleagues proposed several recommendations for academies that included creating a parent-supportive culture, facilitating an environment that is welcoming for parents, respecting, and appreciating parents' commitment, valuing input and feedback from parents, and delivering a programme of support for parents. All these suggestions have resonance with the broader talent development literature (Furusa, Knight, & Hill, 2020), such as the need to support and educate parents on multiple factors relating to their child's involvement and development in the academy environment. Parents blindly trust the academy to do what is best as 'they're

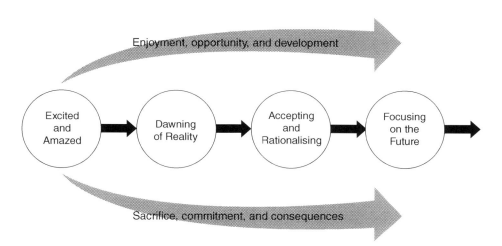

*Figure 10.1* Parents' experiences of the youth soccer academy parenting journey.
Source: Adapted from Newport et al. (2020)

the experts', but acknowledge that they would like to know more to be able to engage with their child in an understanding manner (Reeves et al., 2018c).

While efforts to be more inclusive for parents are certainly warranted, we should not assume that the role of family is only impacted by and through the academy systems and environments. Families themselves have been shown to exercise influence in the decision of whether a young player engages within a talent development programme or not. In their study of young soccer players in Ghana, van der Meij and Darby (2017) found that players believed that being recruited to an academy[1] was necessary to help them to migrate as a professional soccer player to one of the more lucrative leagues, often in Europe. Their ability to take-up the offer of a place at an academy, however, was fraught with delicate negotiations with their families. These negotiations often revolved around the perceived value of soccer and its role in facilitating international mobility as it related to a broader, longer-term livelihood strategy for the whole family. Such studies offer a sort of balance to the standard thinking around engagement in academies and professional soccer, particularly within developing nations.

The role of the family, as a focus of investigation in talent identification and development in soccer, is of great importance. As key stakeholders in the lives of young and established players, their potential influence on myriad factors that have direct or knock-on effects to other domains (i.e., psychological) and ultimately performance cannot be underestimated.

### Coach-athlete relationship

There is a large body of work that underpins our knowledge of the coach-athlete relationship, though its importance was, for a long time, ignored (Yang & Jowett, 2016). Coaches spend a significant amount of time with their players, involved in on- and off-field learning and development activities; this is coupled with the input of other specialist coaches and support staff (e.g., strength and conditioning coaches, performance analysts, and nutritionists). There are also other instances where coaches and players spend long periods of time together, such as travelling to games, where relationships can be affected. The coach-athlete relationship includes all situations where a coach's and athlete's feelings, thoughts, and/or behaviours are inter-related (Jowett, 2007). The relationship between a player and their coach is of great importance and can affect multiple facets of a player's life, including their happiness (Lafrenière et al., 2011), ability to cope (Nicholls et al., 2016), and performance (Jowett & Cockerill, 2003; Murray et al., 2020). However, much of the research in this area has been conducted with elite players or athletes, and so our understanding of the coach-athlete relationship within talent development programmes is sparse.

In recent years, there have been efforts to better understand the coach-athlete relationship within junior-elite soccer. Nicholls and colleagues (2017) sought to explore whether the coach-athlete relationships were able to longitudinally predict the attainment of mastery achievement goals. The study surveyed 104 male academy players aged between 9 and 20 years old and using two measures, the Coach-Athlete Relationship Questionnaire (CART-Q; Jowett & Ntoumanis, 2004) and the Attainment of Sport Achievement Goal Scale (A-SAGS; Amiot, Gaudreau & Blanchard, 2004). The coach-athlete relationship did not change over a 6-month period and the quality of the relationship remained relatively stable. Players who perceived a stronger relationship with their coach were more likely to note higher perceived levels of mastery goal

*Sociological influences* 159

achievement – goals that are aimed at attaining a level of competence defined by skill development or self-improvement – 6 months later. Nicholls et al. (2017) concluded that the coach-athlete relationship might be an important predictor of mastery goal achievement and that academies might maximise its benefit by incorporating coach-athlete relationship training within coach development programmes.

A similar study examined the link between the transformational behaviours of parents and coaches, and the impact of age (Murray et al., 2020). Transformational behaviours of parents and coaches were assessed using the Transformational Parenting Questionnaire (TPQ; Morton et al., 2011) and the Differentiated Transformational Leadership Inventory (DTLI; Hardy et al., 2010), respectively; and players' mental toughness was measured using the Mental Toughness Index (MTI; Gucciardi et al., 2015), and their physical performance through seven field-based fitness tests commonly used to assess physical performance in adolescent soccer players (Paul & Nassis, 2015). A total of 334 male players, aged 10–17 years participated. Multi-level modelling examined the interaction between age and transformational leadership behaviours of parents and coaches on players' mental toughness and physical performance. The father's transformational leadership was positively associated with the mental toughness of younger players, while the coach's transformational leadership behaviours were positively associated with the physical performance of older players. The influence shifts from parent to coach at an older age, and so implications for the coach-athlete relationship and how those dynamics change and, thus, require different behaviours. There remains a need to understand the causal pathways for these shifts in influence and to understand their potential impact on engagement and performance, particularly as young players transition between different phases of player development (i.e., training to train/deliberate play through to training to compete/deliberate practice; Côté, 1999). The results of this study touch on the influence of family and how it might further influence relationships and decision-making between the three groups.

Such influence might also affect how relationships evolve and manifest. As such, there has been an increased interest in the notion of 'care', as a lens by which we can understand relationships between players and coaches. Noddings' (1988) seminal work in education drew on feminist theory to suggest that care should be the central tenet of the teacher-student relationship; an idea that has now been extended to coach-athlete relationships (see Annerstedt & Lindgren, 2014; Jones, 2009). Care has been shown to be an essential component of pedagogy (Cronin, Knowles & Enright, 2019) and thus, the development and maintenance of relationships. However, soccer environments are typically characterised as harsh and uncaring, with myriad micropolitical factors for individuals to contend with (Potrac et al., 2012).

In their case study of an EPL soccer player's relationship with a strength and conditioning coach during a period of long-term injury, Cronin and colleagues (2019) propose three important findings. First, that the coach *'cared for'* the player through a rules-based approach that adopted elements of Noddings' (1988) *pedagogical caring relation* but was largely driven by utilisation of scientific measures and logical rules in a 'care-full' manner. Second, both coach and player appeared to be engaged in a caring relationship that was positioned in a broader milieu shaped by external and internal pressures that included others' employment status, financial pressures associated with league position, and an aggressive blame culture. Thus, how the player was cared for and how that care was received by the player was a complex interplay of factors that reinforce the notion of care as an integrated, not isolated, activity. Finally, while care

160  *Matthew J. Reeves and Simon J. Roberts*

is suggested as being central to pedagogical endeavours, the care given can be defined, limited, or enabled by other actors within their social context (e.g., other coaches, players, agents, etc.). Consequently, this study highlights that for coaches to care, there needs to be a shared understanding with players.

Communication is suggested as a critical component of care with all involved needing to embrace authentic dialogue that involves a genuine effort to listen to individuals (Noddings, 2005). In complex environments, like professional soccer clubs, it is suggested that there is a need to genuinely listen and involve players in order that they receive and accept an appropriate form of care (Cronin, Knowles, & Enright, 2019). Moreover, the involvement of medical staff, soccer-specific coaches, strength and conditioning coaches, sports psychologists, nutritionists, data scientists, and others – all of whom have a role in assessing, monitoring, supporting, and caring for players – it might be better to care through an integrated approach, creating a climate, or web, of care that surrounds players with staff and teammates (Gano-Overway, 2014; Cronin, Knowles, & Enright, 2019).

### Cultural background

The process of globalisation in professional soccer has been driven by increased television and media rights, sponsorship, and merchandise sales which has, in turn, manifested in the global migration of players (Magee & Sudgen, 2002; Poli, 2010; Relvas et al., 2010). In recent years, there have been initiatives by some federations to increase the numbers of indigenous players in club squads. UEFA introduced the *home-grown* rule in 2006, with quota rules to be met by clubs for the start of the 2008–2009 season. Evidence from the six major European leagues (England, France, Germany, Holland, Italy, and Spain) showed that opportunities for *home-grown players* (i.e., minutes played and appearances) between 1999 and 2015 were mixed. Only Germany saw significant increases in playing opportunities for indigenous players when comparing before and after the introduction of the rule; England and Italy saw significant decreases, and all other countries saw decreased, though not statistically significant, opportunities (Bullough et al., 2016). During the 2015–2016 season, approximately 50% of players from the top five European leagues (as above but excluding Holland) were foreign (Gerhards & Mutz, 2017) compared to 20% in 1995–1996, and 39% in 2005–2006.

Cultural diversity in soccer teams around the world has increased over the last few decades (Poli, 2010), though research efforts to understand the impact have only relatively recently begun to appear and the implications are broad. What can be recognised already is that players from different countries, with different cultural backgrounds, languages, social and behavioural norms, are frequently integrated into, and expected to perform effectively, as a team. It has been suggested that the differences noted above increase the likelihood of misunderstandings and conflicts (Lazear, 1999), which might stem from an individual's own or, indeed, his/her cultural prejudices that inhibit willingness to cooperate with others.

When examining the 'big five' leagues, Maderer, Holtbrügge, and Schuster (2014), found that culturally homogenous teams achieved higher average performances. They concluded that managers of more culturally and ethnically diverse teams should consider the potential costs associated with achieving integration and instead should strive to embed young players from the club's own academy. The effect of cultural heterogeneity, as observed in the Bundesliga, has been shown to negatively (Haas & Nüesch,

2012) and positively (Andresen & Altmann, 2006) affect team performance. Looking beyond the macro-level make-up of a team's cultural diversity, Brandes and colleagues (2009) have suggested a more complex interaction of cultural influence on team performance. When accounting for playing positions, more homogenous defensive formations performed better, whereas the opposite was true for striker formations. However, when the performance of teams from the big five leagues in the European Champions League games was examined, diverse and valuable teams tended to outperform less diverse and less valuable ones (Ingersoll et al., 2017), suggesting that the cost of players acted as a mediator to performance outcome alongside cultural diversity.

As the results and findings surrounding cultural and ethnic diversity are inconclusive and evidence is, at best, mixed, it is safe to say that we need to know more about this issue. While it appears that a non-linear relationship exists between cultural and ethnic diversity and team performance, with some teams benefitting from diversity in their teams' makeup, it is not clear where the tipping point between benefits and disadvantages lie or what or how much other factors might be of influence (e.g., team value). While the impact of diversity on team performance has been examined across the top 12 European leagues (Gerhards & Mutz, 2017), a team's market value might be a stronger predictor of success, particularly in leagues with greater financial inequalities amongst clubs. While market value and relative team salary have been shown to have a positive effect on performance and squad size a negative effect, cultural diversity has no significant correlation. These studies have been largely confined to elite teams rather than development environments. While the latter has been examined in relation to the impact of geographic location on talent identification and talent development practices, there has been no attempt to understand the influence of cultural background at this critical time-point in young soccer players' development. There are no studies that have sought to understand the implications of cultural background on teams or individuals within academic environments. Such studies would be welcomed and would undoubtedly have value as soccer's globalised state continues to grow and interest, participation, and investment increases from countries that have, previously, had little influence in soccer, such as China and the Arab States of the Persian Gulf.

### Socioeconomic background

The influence of socioeconomic background has been largely overlooked within soccer talent identification and development research. While there is strong evidence relating to engagement in, and drop out from, grassroots sport based on social class (Pabayo et al., 2014; Pabayo, Molnar et al., 2014; Lammle, Worth, & Bos, 2012; Vandendriessche et al., 2012), there is little examination of this issue from a talent development or elite performance perspective. In other sports, scientists have reported that sociodemographic markers, such as race and relative access to wealth, favour white, privately educated athletes (Lawrence, 2017; Winn et al., 2017). However, this change within soccer has been slow to occur; since inception, soccer has been the quintessential working-class sport. Less than two decades ago, it was suggested that in Ireland, young soccer players tended to be targeted from working-class families (Bourke, 2003), perhaps, due to soccer's historical roots as one of the few sporting opportunities available to those from lower socioeconomic backgrounds (Hodkinson & Sparkes, 1997), though current evidence challenges that notion.

In the United States, there have been material, geographic, and cultural changes in soccer since the 1970s that have included the expansion of private leagues, pushing competitive leagues into the suburbs and away from larger cities with obvious implications for the demographic of players participating (Andrews, 1999; Andrews et al., 1997; Reck & Bruce, 2015). A recent study of the socioeconomic, racial, and geographic composition of professional female soccer players in the United States (Allison & Barranco, 2021) found support for these claims. The study examined longitudinal data including National Women's Super League (NWSL) rosters and combined these with US Census data and concluded that those at the highest levels of women's soccer in the United States come from 'places ("hometowns") that are whiter, less black or Latino, more suburban, and less socioeconomically disadvantaged than the national average, with higher per capita, median household, and median family incomes' (p. 464–465). Also, studies of academies within the United Kingdom indicate that youngsters entering soccer talent development programmes are perceived by scouts and recruitment staff as being increasingly from middle-class backgrounds (Reeves et al., 2018a).

There is only one study, of which we are aware, that has specifically focussed on issues of socioeconomic status of academy soccer players from Europe (Kelly et al., in review). This study explored socioeconomic status and psychological characteristics in academy players in England. Players' home postcodes were used to determine socioeconomic status and the Psychological Characteristics for Developing Excellence Questionnaire (PCDEQ) to explore psychological constructs of coach-rated 'high' and 'low' potential players. Players rated as having a higher potential were from families with a significantly lower socioeconomic status ($P < 0.05$) and scored higher on factor three of the PCDEQ (i.e., coping with performance and developmental pressures ($P < 0.05$), compared to players considered to have lower potential. These results suggest a possible causal link between socioeconomic status, psychological characteristics, and perceived potential to become a professional player. Similar findings have recently been reported in Brazil, where it was suggested that the poverty of young soccer players might help shape their level of skill and expertise (Uehara et al., 2021). The authors suggested that poverty created an ecosystem in which young players increased the likelihood of participation in soccer-specific activities and, thus, their engagement in deliberate practice and play (e.g., Ford, Ward, Hodges, & Williams 2009; Hornig, Aust, & Güllich, 2016), which have both been shown to facilitate the development of expertise. Such situational factors might facilitate some psychological characteristics, such as overcoming adversity, motivation, mental toughness, and resilience.

There are obvious differences between the socioeconomic status of players and their families around the world, but it is imperative that those involved in academies and development programmes recognise the influence that socioeconomic status might have when designing, implementing, and evaluating talent development pathways (Rees et al., 2016).

## Future directions and conclusions

In this chapter, we explored how sociological influences on talent identification and talent development in soccer can have widespread implications. The range, breadth, and interconnectedness of these factors can be a confounding factor and researchers have only recently begun to explore some of these issues. Social factors do not occur in isolation, and so neither can our efforts to examine these issues. We suggest that the

*Sociological influences* 163

impact on the development and performance of individuals and teams can be greatly influenced by sociological factors.

One of the largest contributory factors is the role of family in talent identification and development. Family have been shown to be crucial in providing a range of resources and support to youngsters. But they have also been identified as key in determining (non)engagement in academy/development programme environments and, as such, should be viewed as one of the most crucial stakeholders in their child's talent development pathway. Where players and their families do engage in academies, evidence has indicated that there needs to be a better appreciation of how families are welcomed, appreciated, and valued. Another critical relationship exists between player and coach. This relationship has been shown to be significant in terms of the time spent together, both on and off the pitch – and in soccer, involving multiple coaches and support staff. The coach-athlete relationship has been linked to player happiness, ability to cope, and performance. Recently, the ability of coaches to show care to players has been highlighted as an important factor in how the relationship can manifest but for care to manifest, there must first be a shared understanding of what care is and what it means between the coach and player. The effect of cultural factors in coach-athlete relationships is yet to be explored; and due to the inconclusive and mixed nature of findings from studies examining cultural diversity in soccer, we have a long way to go before we can fully understand and appreciate the complexity of cultural heritage and its impact on talent identification and talent development. Similarly, we have a limited understanding of the role socioeconomic status plays in identification and development. The limited, yet growing data, paints a picture of an increased number of middle-class participants, from less diverse backgrounds entering academies and development programmes in developed countries. However, it is noted that poverty in developing nations, like Brazil, is suggested to be at least in part responsible for the development of more skilful players, through promotion of an ecosystem that promotes deliberate play and practice. That said, the causal relationship between poverty and skill development in soccer has not been established, despite calls for such examinations in the literature.

We must recognise that not all academies and development programmes are created equal and that the social determinants have a significant role to play in the identification and development of soccer players. In order that we, as researchers and practitioners, do not miss or prevent any individual from succeeding in soccer, we must continue to enhance our understanding of the complexity and interconnectedness of social factors with psychological, technical, tactical, and physical determinants of talent in soccer.

## Note

1 It is important to distinguish between the European-style academies, typically owned and operated by professional clubs with no associated costs to players and their families, from the African- (and other-) style academies, which are fee-paying private academies. This highlights a clear distinction in the sport development models operated around the world but is not for further discussion here.

## References

Allison, R., & Barranco, R. (2021). 'A rich white kid sport?' Hometown socioeconomic, racial, and geographic composition among U.S. women's professional soccer players. *Soccer & Society*, *22*(5), 457–469. https://doi.org/10.1080/14660970.2020.1827231

Amiot, C. E., Gaudreau, P., & Blanchard, C. M. (2004). Self-Determination, coping, and goal attainment in sport. *Journal of Sport and Exercise Psychology, 26*(3), 396–411. https://doi.org/10.1123/jsep.26.3.396

Andresen, M., & Altmann, T. (2006). Diversity and success in professional football. *Leadership Organization Magazine, 75*(6), 325–332.

Andrews, D. L. (1999). Contextualizing suburban soccer: consumer culture, lifestyle differentiation and suburban America. *Cultural Sport Society, 2*(3), 31–53. https://doi.org/10.1080/14610989908721846

Andrews, D. L., Pitter, R., Zwick, D., & Ambrose, D. (1997). Soccer's racial frontier: sport and the suburbanization of contemporary America. In G. Armstrong & R. Giulianotti (Eds.), *Entering the Field: New Perspectives on World Football* (pp. 261–282). New York, NY: Berg.

Annerstedt, C., & Lindgren, E.-C. (2014). Caring as an important foundation in coaching for social sustainability: a case study of a successful Swedish coach in high-performance sport. *Reflective Practice, 15*(1), 27–39. https://doi.org/10.1080/14623943.2013.869204

Bourke, A. (2003). The dream of being a professional soccer player. *Journal of Sport and Social Issues, 27*(4), 399–419. https://doi.org/10.1177/0193732503255478

Brandes, L., Franck, E. P., & Theiler, P. (2009). The effect from national diversity on team production – empirical evidence from the sports industry. *Schmalenbach Business Review, 61*(225–246).

Bullough, S., Moore, R., Goldsmith, S., & Edmondson, L. (2016). Player migration and opportunity: examining the efficacy of the UEFA home-grown rule in six European football leagues. *International Journal of Sports Science & Coaching, 11*(5), 662–672. https://doi.org/10.1177/1747954116667104

Clarke, N. J., & Harwood, C. G. (2014). Parenting experiences in elite youth football: a phenomenological study. *Psychology of Sport and Exercise, 15*(5), 528–537. https://doi.org/10.1016/j.psychsport.2014.05.004

Clarke, N. J., Harwood, C. G., & Cushion, C. J. (2016). A phenomenological interpretation of the parent-child relationship in elite youth football. *Sport, Exercise, and Performance Psychology, 5*(2), 125–143. https://doi.org/10.1037/spy0000052

Côté, J. (1999). The Influence of the Family in the Development of Talent in Sport. *The Sport Psychologist, 13*(4), 395–417. https://doi.org/10.1123/tsp.13.4.395

Cronin, C., Knowles, Z. R., & Enright, K. (2019). The challenge to care in a premier league football club. *Sports Coaching Review, 9*(2), 123–146. https://doi.org/10.1080/21640629.2019.1578593

Dorsch, T. E., Smith, A. L., & McDonough, M. H. (2015). Early socialization of parents through organized youth sport. *Sport, Exercise and Performance Psychology, 4*(1), 3–18. https://doi.org/10.1037/spy0000021

Dorsch, T. E., Wright, E., Eckardt, V. C., Elliott, S., Thrower, S. N., & Knight, C. J. (2021). A history of parent involvement in organized youth sport: a scoping review. *Sport, Exercise and Performance Psychology, 10*(4), 536–557. https://doi.org/10.1037/spy0000266

Elliott, R. (Ed.). (2017). *The English Premier League: A socio-cultural analysis.* Routledge: Oxon.

Ford, P. R., Ward, P., Hodges, N. J., & Williams, A. M. (2009). The role of deliberate practice and play in career progression in sport: The early engagement hypothesis. *High Ability Studies, 20(1)*, 65–75. https://doi.org/10.1080/13598130902860721

Gano-Overway, L. A. (2014). The caring climate: how sport environments can develop empathy in young people. In K. Pavlovich & K. Krahnke (Eds.), *Organising Through Empathy* (pp. 166–183). New York, NY: Routledge.

Gerhards, J., & Mutz, M. (2017). Who wins the championship? Market value and team composition as predictors of success in the top European football leagues. *European Societies, 19*(3), 223–242. https://doi.org/10.1080/14616696.2016.1268704

Gucciardi, D. F., Hanton, S., Gordon, S., Mallett, C. J., & Temby, P. (2015). The concept of mental toughness: tests of dimensionality, nomological network, and traitness. *Journal of Personality, 83*(1), 26–44. https://doi.org/10.1111/jopy.12079

Haas, H., & Nüesch, S. (2012). Are multinational teams more successful? *The International Journal of Human Resource Management*, *23*(15), 3105–3113. https://doi.org/10.1080/09585192.2011.610948

Hardy, L., Arthur, C. A., Jones, G., Shariff, A., Munnoch, K., Isaacs, I., & Allsopp, A. J. (2010). The relationship between transformational leadership behaviors, psychological, and training outcomes in elite military recruits. *The Leadership Quarterly*, *21*(1), 20–32. https://doi.org/10.1016/j.leaqua.2009.10.002

Hodkinson, P., & Sparkes, A. C. (1997). Careership: a sociological theory of career decision making. *British Journal of Sociology of Education*, *18*(1), 29–44. https://doi.org/10.1080/0142569970180102

Hornig, M., Aust, F., & Güllich, A. (2016). Practice and play in the development of German top-level professional football players. *European Journal of Sport Science*, 16(1), 96 -105. https://doi.org/10.1080/17461391.2014.982204

Hoyle, R. H., & Leff, S. S. (1997). The role of parental involvement in youth sport participation and performance. *Adolescence*, *32*(125), 233–243.

Ingersoll, K., Malesky, E., & Saiegh, S. M. (2017). Heterogeneity and team performance: evaluating the effect of cultural diversity in the world's top soccer league. *Journal of Sports Analytics*, *3*(2), 67–92. https://doi.org/10.3233/JSA-170052

Jones, R. L. (2009). Coaching as caring (the smiling gallery): accessing hidden knowledge. *Physical Education & Sport Pedagogy*, *14*(4), 377–390. https://doi.org/10.1080/17408980801976551

Jowett, S. (2007). Interdependence analysis and the 3+1Cs in the coach-athlete relationship. In S. J. and D. Lavallee (Ed.), *Social Psychology in Sport* (pp. 15–27). Champaign, IL: Human Kinetics.

Jowett, S., & Cockerill, I. M. (2003). Olympic medallists' perspective of the athlete–coach relationship. *Psychology of Sport and Exercise*, *4*(4), 313–331. https://doi.org/10.1016/S1469-0292(02)00011-0

Jowett, S., & Ntoumanis, N. (2004). The coach-athlete relationship questionnaire (CART-Q): development and initial validation. *Scandinavian Journal of Medicine and Science in Sports*, *14*(4), 245–257. https://doi.org/10.1111/j.1600-0838.2003.00338.x

Kelly, A., Williams, C. A., Jackson, D. T., Turnnidge, J., Reeves, M. J., Dugdale, J., & Wilson, M. R. (in press). Exploring the role of socioeconomic status and psychological characteristics in talent development in an English soccer academy. *Science & Medicine in Football*.

Knight, C. J., Dorsch, T. E., Osai, K. V., Haderlie, K. L., & Sellars, P. A. (2016). Influences on parental involvement in youth sport. *Sport, Exercise, and Performance Psychology*, *5*(2), 161–178. https://doi.org/10.1037/spy0000053

Lafrenière, M.-A. K., Jowett, S., Vallerand, R. J., & Carbonneau, N. (2011). Passion for coaching and the quality of the coach–athlete relationship: the mediating role of coaching behaviors. *Psychology of Sport and Exercise*, *12*(2), 144–152. https://doi.org/10.1016/j.psychsport.2010.08.002

Lammle, L., Worth, A., & Bos, K. (2012). Socio-demographic correlates of physical activity and physical fitness in German children and adolescents. *The European Journal of Public Health*, *22*(6), 880–884. https://doi.org/10.1093/eurpub/ckr191

Lawrence, D. W. (2017). Sociodemographic profile of an Olympic team. *Public Health*, *148*, 149–158. https://doi.org/10.1016/j.puhe.2017.03.011

Lazear, E. P. (1999). Globalisation and the market for team-mates. *The Economic Journal*, *109*(-454), 15–40. https://doi.org/10.1111/1468-0297.00414

Maderer, D., Holtbrügge, D., & Schuster, T. (2014). Professional football squads as multicultural teams. *International Journal of Cross Cultural Management*, *14*(2), 215–238. https://doi.org/10.1177/1470595813510710

Magee, J., & Sugden, J. (2002). The world at their feet. *Journal of Sport and Social Issues*, *26*(4), 421–437. https://doi.org/10.1177/0193732502238257

Molnar, G., & Maguire, J. (2008). Hungarian footballers on the move: Issues of and observations on the first migratory phase. *Sport in Society, 11*(1), 74–89. https://doi.org/10.1080/17430430701717798

Morris, R., Tod, D., & Oliver, E. (2015). An analysis of organizational structure and transition outcomes in the youth-to-senior professional soccer transition. *Journal of Applied Sport Psychology, 27*(2), 216–234. https://doi.org/10.1080/10413200.2014.980015

Morton, K. L., Barling, J., Rhodes, R. E., Mâsse, L. C., Zumbo, B. D., & Beauchamp, M. R. (2011). The application of transformational leadership theory to parenting: questionnaire development and implications for adolescent self-regulatory efficacy and life satisfaction. *Journal of Sport and Exercise Psychology, 33*(5), 688–709. https://doi.org/10.1123/jsep.33.5.688

Murray, R. M., Dugdale, J. H., Habeeb, C. M., & Arthur, C. A. (2020). Transformational parenting and coaching on mental toughness and physical performance in adolescent soccer players: the moderating effect of athlete age. *European Journal of Sport Science, 21*(4), 580–589. https://doi.org/10.1080/17461391.2020.1765027

Newport, R. A., Knight, C. J., & Love, T. D. (2021). The youth football journey: Parents' experiences and recommendations for support. *Qualitative Research in Sport, Exercise and Health, 13(6)*, 1006-1026. https://doi.org/10.1080/2159676X.2020.1833966

Nicholls, A. R., Levy, A. R., Jones, L., Meir, R., Radcliffe, J. N., & Perry, J. L. (2016). Committed relationships and enhanced threat levels: perceptions of coach behavior, the coach–athlete relationship, stress appraisals, and coping among athletes. *International Journal of Sports Science & Coaching, 11*(1), 16–26. https://doi.org/10.1177/1747954115624825

Nicholls, A. R., Earle, K., Earle, F., & Madigan, D. J. (2017). Perceptions of the Coach -Athlete Relationship Predict the Attainment of Mastery Achievement Goals Six Months Later: A Two-Wave Longitudinal Study among F. A. Premier League Academy Soccer Players. *Frontiers in Psychology, 8*, 684. https://doi.org/10.3389/fpsyg.2017.00684

Noddings, N. (2005). *The Challenge to Care in Schools: An Alternative Approach to Education* (2nd ed.). New Jersey, NY: Teachers College Press.

Noddings, N. (1988). An ethic of caring and its implications for instructional arrangements. *American Journal of Education, 96*(2), 215–230. https://doi.org/10.1086/443894

Pabayo, R., Janosz, M., Bisset, S., & Kawachi, I. (2014). School social fragmentation, economic deprivation and social cohesion and adolescent physical inactivity: a longitudinal study. *PLoS ONE, 9*(6), e99154. https://doi.org/10.1371/journal.pone.0099154

Pabayo, R., Molnar, B. E., Cradock, A., & Kawachi, I. (2014). The relationship between neighborhood socioeconomic characteristics and physical inactivity among adolescents living in Boston, Massachusetts. *American Journal of Public Health, 104*(11), e142–e149. https://doi.org/10.2105/AJPH.2014.302109

Paul, D. J., & Nassis, G. P. (2015). Physical fitness testing in youth soccer: issues and considerations regarding reliability, validity, and sensitivity. *Pediatric Exercise Science, 27*(3), 301–313. https://doi.org/10.1123/pes.2014-0085

Poli, R. (2010). Understanding globalization through football: the new international division of labour, migratory channels and transnational trade circuits. *International Review for the Sociology of Sport, 45*(4), 491–506. https://doi.org/10.1177/1012690210370640

Potrac, P., Jones, R. L., Gilbourne, D., & Nelson, L. (2012). 'Handshakes, BBQs, and bullets': self-interest, shame and regret in football coaching. *Sports Coaching Review, 1*(2), 79–92. https://doi.org/10.1080/21640629.2013.768418

Reck, G. G., & Bruce, A. (2015). *American Soccer: History, Culture, Class.* Jefferson, NC: McFarland & Company, Inc.

Rees, T., Hardy, L., Güllich, A., Abernethy, B., Côté, J., Woodman, T., ... Warr, C. (2016). The great British medalists project: a review of current knowledge on the development of the world's best sporting talent. *Sports Medicine, 46*(8), 1041–1058. https://doi.org/10.1007/s40279-016-0476-2

Reeves, M. J., Enright, K. J., Dowling, J., & Roberts, S. J. (2018a). Stakeholders' understanding and perceptions of bio-banding in junior-elite football training. *Soccer & Society*, *19*(8), 1–17. https://doi.org/10.1080/14660970.2018.1432384

Reeves, M. J., Littlewood, M. A., McRobert, A. P., & Roberts, S. J. (2018b). The nature and function of talent identification in junior-elite football in English category one academies. *Soccer & Society*, *19*(8), 1122–1134. https://doi.org/10.1080/14660970.2018.1432385

Reeves, M. J., McRobert, A. P., Littlewood, M. A., & Roberts, S. J. (2018c). A scoping review of the potential sociological predictors of talent in junior-elite football: 2000–2016. *Soccer & Society*, *19*(8), 1–21. https://doi.org/10.1080/14660970.2018.1432386

Reeves, M. J., & Roberts, S. J. (2020). A bioecological perspective on talent identification in junior-elite soccer: a Pan-European perspective. *Journal of Sports Sciences*, *38*(11–12), 1259–1268. https://doi.org/10.1080/02640414.2019.1702282

Relvas, H., Littlewood, M., Nesti, M., Gilbourne, D., & Richardson, D. (2010). Organizational structures and working practices in elite European professional football clubs: understanding the relationship between youth and professional domains. *European Sport Management Quarterly*, *10*(2), 165–187. https://doi.org/10.1080/16184740903559891

Roderick, M. (2013). Domestic moves: an exploration of intra-national labour mobility in the working lives of professional footballers. *International Review for the Sociology of Sport*, *48*(-4), 387–404. https://doi.org/10.1177/1012690212442497

Roderick, M. J. (2012). An unpaid labor of love. *Journal of Sport and Social Issues*, *36*(3), 317–338. https://doi.org/10.1177/0193723512445283

Taylor, R. D., Carson, H. J., & Collins, D. (2018). The impact of siblings during talent development: a longitudinal examination in sport. *Journal of Applied Sport Psychology*, *30*(3), 272–287. https://doi.org/10.1080/10413200.2017.1384938

van der Meij, N., & Darby, P. (2017). Getting in the game and getting on the move: Family, the intergenerational contract and internal migration into football academies in Ghana. *Sport in Society*, *20*(11), 1580–1595. https://doi.org/10.1080/17430437.2017.1284807

Vandendriessche, J. B., Vandorpe, B. F. R., Vaeyens, R., Malina, R. M., Lefevre, J., Lenoir, M., & Philippaerts, R. M. (2012). Variation in sport participation, fitness and motor coordination with socioeconomic status among Flemish children. *Pediatric Exercise Science*, *24*(1), 113–128. https://doi.org/10.1123/pes.24.1.113

Williams, A. M., Ford, P. R., & Drust, B. (2020). Talent identification and development in soccer since the millennium. *Journal of Sports Sciences*, *38*(11–12), 1199–1210. https://doi.org/10.1080/02640414.2020.1766647

Williams, A. M., & Reilly, T. (2000). Talent identification and development in soccer. *Journal of Sports Sciences*, *18*(9), 657–667. https://doi.org/10.1080/02640410050120041

Winn, C. O. N., Ford, P. R., McNarry, M. A., Lewis, J., & Stratton, G. (2017). The effect of deprivation on the developmental activities of adolescent rugby union players in Wales. *Journal of Sports Sciences*, *35*(24), 2390–2396. https://doi.org/10.1080/02640414.2016.1271136

Wood, S., Harrison, L. K., & Kucharska, J. (2017). Male professional footballers' experiences of mental health difficulties and help-seeking. *The Physician and Sports Medicine*, *45*(2), 120–128. https://doi.org/10.1080/00913847.2017.1283209

Yang, S. X., & Jowett, S. (2016). Understanding and enhancing coach–athlete relationships through the 3 + 1Cs model. In R. Thelwell, C. Harwood, & I. Greenlees (Eds.), *The Psychology of Sports Coaching* (pp. 54–67). Abingdon, OX: Routledge.

# 11 Player wellbeing and career transitions

*Carolina Lundqvist and David P. Schary*

## Introduction

In this chapter, we focus on wellbeing and wellbeing promotion among soccer players from youth to the professional level. Organized sport, such as soccer, is a social phenomenon, which when properly structured, can promote wellbeing, quality of life, and develop protective psychosocial resources (e.g., self-esteem, life skills, and social relationships) for mental health among young athletes (Cronin & Allen, 2018; Eime et al., 2013; Swann et al., 2018; Wold et al., 2013). When the level of competition increases and the player becomes more committed to soccer, the psychosocial demands become more complex, posing increased challenges for players to sustain their wellbeing over time (McKay et al., 2022; Reverberi et al., 2020). Scientists have shown that professional soccer players self-report symptoms of psychological distress, anxiety, depression, and insomnia (Gouttebarge et al., 2015; Junge & Feddermann-Demont, 2016; Junge & Prinz, 2019; Kilic et al., 2022). Moreover, deselection and early career termination are associated with an increased risk of identity loss and distress among elite adolescent soccer players (Blakelock et al., 2016; Brown & Potrac, 2009; Wilkinson, 2021).

Sport-related risk factors and situations that decrease wellbeing and are related to elevated symptoms of, for example, psychological stress or depression, often occur during challenging life or sport events (e.g., sports injuries, transition phases, deselections, and performance barriers). These challenging events require life or sports adjustment beyond the usual changes normally expected (Appaneal et al., 2009; Blakelock et al., 2016; Roiger et al., 2015). Certain factors can protect a player's wellbeing during these challenges, like fulfilled basic needs and career satisfaction, resilience, social support, positive relationships, and mental health literacy (MHL) (Kilic et al., 2021; Kuettel et al., 2021; Lundqvist & Sandin, 2014; Madsen et al., 2021). In addition, the dynamic interplay and relationships between various participants in the environment (e.g., players, coaches, staff, family members, and school) pose an impact on player wellbeing (Larsen et al., 2013). Thus, wellbeing variations and outcomes found among athletes may not only be linked to individual factors but also to structural and social elements in the players' sport and/or general life.

Regardless of age or skill level, players' health and performance will benefit when given opportunities to improve or sustain their wellbeing. Mental health promotion involves support to increase players' psychosocial resources and competencies to cope with the demands, obstacles, and challenges naturally occurring in sports and life (Barry, 2001). Efforts are already underway to raise awareness of mental health in soccer at the global level. For example, supported by the World Health Organization (WHO), FIFA, and FIFPRO launched the campaigns "#ReachOut" (FIFA, 2021) and

DOI: 10.4324/9781003148418-13

"Are you ready to talk" (FIFPRO, 2021a). Given this level of international attention, in this chapter, we aim to help researchers and practitioners understand mental health and wellbeing, focusing on strategies and interventions to promote wellbeing, particularly during times of transition. We begin by defining wellbeing, then provide a brief overview of the literature on wellbeing promotion and transitions in soccer. We finish with some suggestions for future research and applied implications.

## Wellbeing – the positive side of mental health

Wellbeing has been associated with a variety of positive outcomes like improved health, recovery, and longevity (Diener et al., 2017; Iasiello et al., 2019; Keyes, 2017; Schotanus-Dijkstra et al., 2019). Moreover, improvements in wellbeing are linked to a reduced risk of developing mental illness in non-clinical populations (Keyes et al., 2010; Wood & Joseph, 2010). Within the general psychology literature, wellbeing is conceptualized as independent from, but related to, mental illness. As a result, psychological interventions can act to change levels of wellbeing, illbeing, or both (Iasiello et al., 2019; van Agteren et al., 2021). The study of wellbeing is nevertheless complex. Several biopsychosocial factors interact, like genetic vulnerability, stress reactivity, attitudes, cognitions, moods/affects, health behaviors, coping skills, family background, social support, and environments (Diener et al., 2017; Lundqvist, 2021).

Progress on the topic of wellbeing was initially hampered because of inconsistent and ambiguous definitions, combined with atheoretical approaches and varied assessments (Lundqvist, 2011). Although definitions and assessments still vary, current research is becoming more intentional in the operationalization and assessment of wellbeing as a defined construct in sports (Giles et al., 2020; Kuettel et al., 2021). Within sport psychology, wellbeing is generally seen as a subdimension of mental health, reflecting a positive and desirable state where the player is functional in life and sports, copes successfully with daily challenges, and subsequently experiences happiness and life satisfaction on a regular basis (Keyes, 2007; Lundqvist & Andersson, 2021). Any deviations from this functional state of wellbeing could be regarded as the negative subdimension of mental health, varying from non-clinical mental health concerns to diagnosed mental disorders (for various theoretical perspectives on mental health, see Lundqvist & Andersson, 2021) (Figure 11.1).

### Hedonic and eudaimonic wellbeing

Two different philosophical perspectives on wellbeing dominate the literature, the hedonic and eudaimonic orientation views. The hedonic view adopts the label subjective or emotional wellbeing and considers it synonymously with pleasure and comfort (Diener, 2009; Huta & Ryan, 2010). The central components of subjective wellbeing are life satisfaction and happiness (Diener, 2009; Diener et al., 2009; Huta & Ryan, 2010). Life satisfaction refers to the cognitive evaluation or judgment of the perceived discrepancies between one's actual and desired life. Happiness refers to the presence of positive affect in the relative absence of negative affect (Diener et al., 2009; Huta & Ryan, 2010). Thus, hedonic wellbeing is generally treated as an emotional outcome and measured by how a player subjectively feels. Scholars have nevertheless cautioned that momentary responses assessed in relation to specific activities (i.e., episodic happiness) may not endure long-term, or even be representative of what a person perceives as a meaningful life (Raibley, 2012). Moreover, it is known that a multitude of variables

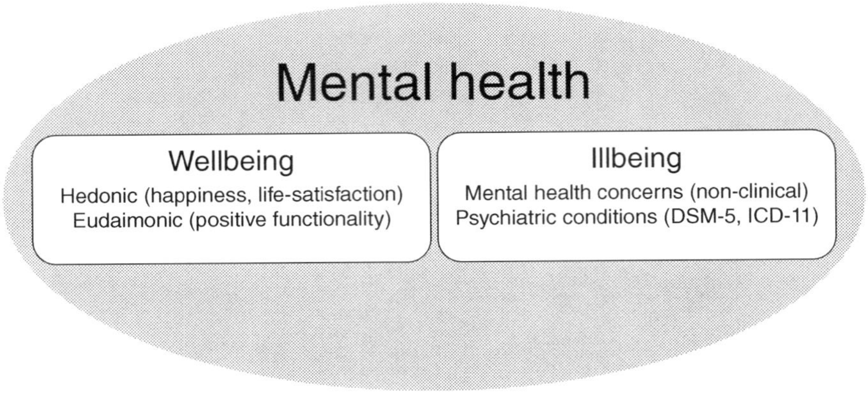

## Mental health

**Wellbeing**
Hedonic (happiness, life-satisfaction)
Eudaimonic (positive functionality)

**Illbeing**
Mental health concerns (non-clinical)
Psychiatric conditions (DSM-5, ICD-11)

*Figure 11.1* An overview of mental health as an umbrella term for both wellbeing and illbeing.

(e.g., context, physiology, and health behaviors) mediate the association between subjective wellbeing and health outcomes (Diener et al., 2017).

The eudaimonic perspective focuses on positive functionality and self-realization of individual talents. Since life inherently involves adversity, the eudaimonic perspective considers how people create meaning during times of difficulty (Keyes & Annas, 2009; Ryff et al., 2004; Ryff, 2014). Personal growth and development are essential components of wellbeing, regardless of their association with positive or negative affect (Huta & Waterman, 2014). Psychological and social wellbeing are common conceptualizations of the eudaimonic orientation. Psychological wellbeing refers to Ryff's (2014) six dimensions of a person's positive functioning: autonomy; environmental mastery; personal growth; positive relations with others; purpose in life; and self-acceptance. Social wellbeing refers to functionality and flourishing in social life, conceptualized by Keyes (1998) as social acceptance, social actualization, social contribution, social coherence, and social integration.

Although distinct, hedonic, and eudaimonic wellbeing are overlapping constructs (Keyes et al., 2002). Eudaimonia is often regarded as a predictor (i.e., how the person lives or behaves) and hedonia as an outcome (i.e., happiness and life-satisfaction) associated with living a well-functioning life (Ryan et al., 2008). Moreover, hedonic wellbeing might provide more immediate benefits to an individual, whereas eudaimonic wellbeing might develop more long-term benefits, suggesting their combination has the greatest effect on an individual's overall wellbeing (Huta & Ryan, 2010). In sport, Lundqvist and Andersson (2021) suggest that hedonic and eudaimonic perspectives together could be regarded as "the athlete's psychosocial functionality and ability to nurture individual talents in the lived elite sports environment, subsequently also increasing the probability of the elite athlete regularly experiencing positive affect and life-satisfaction" (p. 3). We briefly summarize subdimensions of hedonic and eudaimonic wellbeing in Table 11.1.

### Strengthening wellbeing: mental health promotion and prevention

Organized sports, and particularly team sports, is an avenue where wellbeing among youths can be strengthened by use of mental health interventions (Swann et al., 2018). Until recently, sport-specific approaches that attempted to build wellbeing and increase protective factors among sports populations received little attention (Breslin

*Table 11.1* A summary of various subdimensions of hedonic and eudaimonic perspectives on wellbeing (based on Diener, 2009; Keyes, 1998; Ryff, 2014)

| *Hedonic wellbeing (emotional outcome)* | | *Eudaimonic Wellbeing (positive functionality)* | | | |
|---|---|---|---|---|---|
| *Subjective (emotional) wellbeing* | | *Psychological wellbeing* | | *Social wellbeing* | |
| Happiness | Perceives that positive affect outweighs negative affect | Autonomy | Is self-determined and independent with self-referenced standards for behavioral regulation and self-evaluation. Can withstand social pressure. | Social acceptance | Has a positive view of human kindness. Feels comfortable with and trusts other people. |
| Life satisfaction | A cognitive overall evaluation of the lived life and the perceived discrepancy between the desired and the existent life | Environmental mastery | Manages the environment effectively and can use or create opportunities in the external environment to satisfy and realize personal needs and goals. | Social actualization | Is hopeful about future social evolution and think it has potential. Perceives citizens as assets for the societal progress. |
| | | Personal growth | Perceives development and growth as a person. Is open to new experiences and perceives continued improvements in self-knowledge and effectiveness. | Social contribution | Has a perception of being valuable to the society with important contributions to the world. |
| | | Positive relations with others | Cares about others' welfare. Has trusting, empathetic, and sincere relationships with others. | Social coherence | Has an ambition to understand and make sense of what is happening in the world although it may not always be perfect. Sees the world as organized and possible to understand. |
| | | Purpose in life | Perceives that life has a meaning and purpose with directedness and goals. | Social integration | Perceives being part of a social reality, with quality in relationships with society and community and things in common with others. |
| | | Self-acceptance | Accepts and has a positive view of own qualities and various aspects of the self. Has a positive view of past life. | | |

et al., 2017; Kuettel & Larsen, 2020; Rice et al., 2016). As seen in Figure 11.2, interventions targeting wellbeing and mental health can focus on mental health promotion by strengthening competencies and resources that act to increase positive mental health and flourishing (e.g., necessary support, life skills, social and emotional learning, and resources to overcome adversity and fulfill their potential in sports and life (Barry, 2001; Barry et al., 2013). Interventions can also focus on the prevention and reduction of a risk factor for mental health concerns, for example, decreasing the risk for depression, anxiety, substance abuse, and behavioral problems (Barry, 2001; Jacobsson & Timpka, 2015). Prevention is further classified as: (a) primary prevention before pathology is established; (b) secondary prevention focused on reducing the duration of diagnosed pathology; and (c) tertiary prevention used to reduce long-term impairment of clinical disorders (Barry, 2001; Jacobsson & Timpka, 2015). Moreover, universal prevention is recommended for everyone. Selective prevention targets certain subgroups of athletes who at group level are identified by various risk indicators (e.g., age, sex, socio-demographic variables, and sport type), and indicated prevention is delivered to those individuals which have a higher-than-average risk to develop clinical issues (Jacobsson & Timpka, 2015).

Evidence-based recommendations for supporting wellbeing are limited for athletes in general, and soccer players specifically, because there are few rigorous interventions (i.e., randomized controlled trials) evaluating the efficacy and feasibility of these wellbeing strategies and therapies (Breslin et al., 2017). Yet, despite these limitations, we provide a brief, non-comprehensive overview of the current wellbeing strategies for soccer players in the next section.

### *Self-care and health behaviors*

The World Health Organization (WHO, 2022) suggests self-care strategies as critical for enhancing mental health across all populations and sleep, diet, and exercise are described as the big three health behaviors for mental health (Wickham et al., 2020). Unfortunately, professional soccer players may engage in adverse health behaviors that diminish their wellbeing over time like alcohol misuse, smoking, and poor nutrition

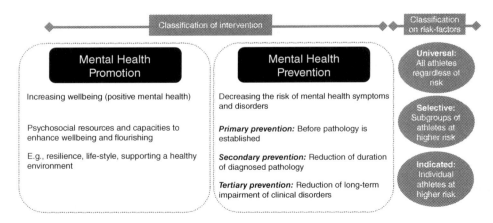

*Figure 11.2* Classifications of interventions based on their overall target and risk factors (based on Barry, 2001; Jacobsson & Timpka, 2015).

(Gouttebarge et al., 2015). Prioritizing healthy habits and behaviors is essential in building and sustaining wellbeing. Good sleep (i.e., both sleep duration and quality) has, for example, been associated with wellbeing and performance optimization (Walsh et al., 2021). Proper sleep habits and regular sleep routines among elite soccer players may nevertheless be challenged by several sport-specific factors (e.g., travels, inconsistency in match schedules, hyper-arousal after matches, early and late training sessions, and high training load), as well as common cultural factors such as smartphones and social media (Fullagar et al., 2016; Nédélec et al., 2015; Walsh et al., 2021).

Scientists have indicated that sleep dysfunction and subsequently insufficient recovery and symptoms of negative mental health are prevalent among both male and female professional and collegiate soccer players (Abbott et al., 2022; Benjamin et al., 2020; Kilic et al., 2021). For clinical and non-clinical populations suffering from sleep problems, cognitive behavioral therapy (CBT) sleep interventions have strong evidence and are commonly recommended (Friedrich & Schlarb, 2018; Rios et al., 2019). Sport-specific sleep interventions for athletes are nascent, but so far include strategies like improving sleep hygiene, sleep education, sleep screening, and managing jetlag (see review Walsh et al., 2021).

### Mental health literacy

MHL evolved as an extension of health literacy primarily used within health care, referring to an individual's ability to understand and effectively use medical information and adhere to medication treatments (Kutcher et al., 2016). Early MHL definitions focused on pathological mental health conditions; for example, Jorm et al. (1997) described it as the "knowledge and beliefs about mental disorders which aid their recognition, management or prevention" (p. 182). However, a one-sided approach focused on relieving symptoms of illbeing or mental disorders is inadequate and does not consider people who do not struggle with illbeing but still experience suboptimal mental health (van Agteren et al., 2021). MHL includes mental health promotion and emphasizes: (a) how positive mental health can be derived and maintained; (b) reduction of stigma of mental health; and (c) knowledge of help-seeking (e.g., when and where), self-management skills, and other competences needed to sustain or improve mental health (Kutcher et al., 2016).

Researchers have evaluated MHL programs and intervention among adolescent soccer players. Liddle et al. (2021) found support for a brief 45-min MHL intervention ("Help Out a Mate") delivered to community male soccer players in Australia. In comparison to the control group, participants significantly improved their knowledge of mental illness, increased intentions, or attitudes towards help-provision to friends with mental health problems, and their help-seeking and problem recognition. Similarly, Vella et al. (2021a) found support for the effectiveness of a multicomponent MHL sports program called "The Ahead of the Game", which included a coach and a parent education program. The program was developed to promote early intervention, resilience, and help-seeking among adolescent males from various sports, including soccer, and the results showed improved outcomes in depression and anxiety literacy, help-seeking intentions from formal but not informal sources, and confidence in seeking mental health information, resilience, and wellbeing.

### Miscellaneous wellbeing interventions

Wellbeing interventions vary greatly in content, goals, and theoretical underpinnings. Interventions found in the literature may include, for example, exercises or wellbeing

## 174  *Carolina Lundqvist and David P. Schary*

therapies which originate in positive psychology (e.g., character strengths, gratitude, and optimism), clinical or general psychology (e.g., self-compassion, acceptance-commitment-therapy, mindfulness-based interventions, CBT, and relaxation), or sports psychology (e.g., psychological skills training; see reviews by Galante et al., 2021; van Agteren et al., 2021). CBT-based approaches and mindfulness-based interventions may support young and professional players by giving them psychological skills to cope with stress and improve wellbeing (Miçooğullari & Ekmekci, 2017; Olmedilla et al., 2019; Shannon et al., 2019). Other researchers have argued for the benefits of re-silience interventions and stress-exposure training or pressure-training interventions for both performance and wellbeing purposes (Low et al., 2021; Madsen et al., 2021).

## Career transitions and wellbeing

Within sport psychology, the field of career transitions is a well-researched area (for a more thorough review of the literature, see Stambulova et al., 2021). Over the years, researchers have found that athletes face two general types of transitions – normative and non-normative (Petitpas et al., 2013; Stambulova, 2010; Wylleman & Lavallee, 2004). Normative transitions are more predictable and expected, occurring within sport (e.g., moving from junior to senior level) and outside of sport (e.g., moving from college/university to the workplace). In contrast, non-normative transitions are less predictable and usually unexpected, but occur within (e.g., deselection from a team) and outside of sport (e.g., moving to a new country).

Both types of career transitions can affect performance and wellbeing, regardless of whether they are inside or outside of sport. Much of the research focuses on the nega-tive effects of transitions and challenges. It is well-documented that during career tran-sitions, athletes can struggle with a variety of challenges like identity loss, adjustment difficulties, social/relationship issues, and financial hardship (Stambulova et al., 2021). To protect wellbeing, athletes need the right resources and support to effectively cope with a major transition (Lundqvist et al., 2022; Samuel & Tenenbaum, 2011; Schloss-berg, 1981). Individual athletes vary, however, in how they experience and react to the same career transitions, producing intraindividual variation of coping skills, needed resources, and outcomes for mental health (Wilkinson, 2021).

### *Common career transitions in soccer*

Most of the career transition research in soccer focuses on career termination, primar-ily at the elite or professional level (Barth et al., 2021). Due to the highly competitive nature of the sport, and the diminishing opportunities for players at each subsequent level, career termination is inevitable for even the most talented players. Since career transitions like termination can pose a serious threat to wellbeing, soccer players need to prepare early for this critical transition especially because most players will not become a professional. Almost all players in the United Kingdom who receive a schol-arship to play at a soccer academy believe they will become a professional (Platts & Smith, 2010), but 85% of them will not receive a contract, and of those that do, only a fraction will play for a top professional team (Brown & Potrac, 2009). In addition, FIFPRO (2021b) found that out of 89 former soccer players from around the world, close to half retired unexpectedly from professional soccer. Given the competitive and unexpected nature of soccer, players of all ages need to prepare and cultivate a life outside of soccer.

## Psychological consequences of forced retirement

Having an identity and life outside of soccer is important because many players will end their careers through deselection or injury. These forced retirements can be a traumatic experience because most players are unprepared and/or receive little support from their clubs (Fortunato & Marchant, 1999). Although players who had the opportunity to voluntarily retire after long and successful careers have a less traumatic experience (Gervis et al., 2019), over 80% have no post-career plan (Barth et al., 2021). Similarly, FIFPRO (2021b) found that 50% of current professional players had not started to prepare for the transition out of soccer. The respondents' primary reasons for not preparing for a post-playing career were the wish to focus on their current playing career and the perception that their transition to a different career is too far away (FIFPRO, 2021b).

This type of thinking is dangerous because whether forced or voluntary, experiencing career termination without a plan or support can lead to higher levels of psychological distress and lower levels of wellbeing. Blakelock et al. (2016) found that 55% of elite adolescent soccer players (ages 15–18) experienced clinical levels of psychological distress 21 days after being released, with many requiring psychosocial treatments from a mental health professional. The most common mental health issues were loss of confidence, social dysfunction, anxiety, and depression.

Similarly, Brown and Potrac (2009) found that four players that joined their soccer club between the ages of 10 and 13 struggled with the loss of identity following their deselection after years of participation. Their identity had become one-dimensional, centered on their athletic skills and team performances. Suddenly removing this sole identity during their formative adolescent years, without developing the psychosocial skills to overcome the challenges, likely led to the players experiencing feelings of loss, uncertainty, and failure.

Soccer clubs are now putting systems in place to prevent and treat mental health issues. This includes making an independent mental health professional available to meet with players in a confidential space. Unfortunately, the mental health resources are for those still associated with the club or team, there is still little support for deselected players (Wilkinson, 2021). For elite players, most received support from a player's association (FIFPRO, 2021b), but that option may not be available for younger players. In addition, the resources are reactionary, trying to improve negative mental health outcomes, instead of proactive like wellbeing promotion. Calvin (2017) stated that since players and their families sacrifice a significant part of their lives and resources pursuing their soccer careers, clubs and academies have a duty of care for all their players, particularly supporting them before and after career transitions like deselection and injury. Historically, clubs have been unwilling to provide clarification to parents after releasing a player, let alone provide professional support or wellbeing promotion (e.g., Wilkinson, 2021).

## Psychological benefits of dual-career programs

Dual-career programs, where athletes combine their sports career with another domain specific to the athletes' life phase (e.g., education, employment, and family), can protect players from negative outcomes by providing them opportunities to build a more robust identity, broader repertoire of life skills, balanced lifestyle, and greater social networks. As a result, these programs can, if properly structured, help to improve wellbeing by providing players with psychosocial resources and safety to handle career termination and positively adapt to life after sports (Breslin et al., 2019; Storm et al., 2021). Many soccer players are involved in another career (academic or employment). FIFPRO (2021b) reported that 46% of active player respondents were engaged in a dual career (27% in education and 19% in employment). As a result, clubs and academies need a culture that supports this reality and concentrates on developing wellbeing. Larsen et al. (2013) found that young soccer players in Denmark thrived in a holistic environment that went beyond winning to prioritize things like healthy coach-athlete relationships, overall development, and academic responsibilities. Building a supportive culture is important, but these Danish programs established an intervention program to intentionally assist their younger players with the challenges of career transitions by strengthening the ties between elite and youth players, as well as facilitating a workshop series to introduce and train psychosocial skills (Larsen et al., 2014). This program helped younger players understand the demands and expectations involved in transitioning to the more elite levels.

Although programs that emphasize realistic expectations prepare young players for the harsh realities of elite-level soccer, it does not help them develop or balance another career. These types of programs should also help players manage dual careers, teaching skills like time management, study skills, and financial literacy. Mentorship, advising, and presentations from retired players with successful non-athletic careers can also help players of all ages understand the challenges and rewards that await them after their soccer careers. Finally, coaches and club officials can promote and encourage non-athletic activities like academics and/or outside employment.

## Future directions and conclusions

Wellbeing promotion and preventative strategies for mental health issues are increasingly getting attention both in applied sports psychology services to athletes and in sports research. Undoubtedly, protecting soccer players' mental health and stimulating wellbeing should be prioritized in sports. Psychosocial factors, exemplified in Figure 11.3, have the potential to protect and increase soccer players' wellbeing regardless of age, skill, or competitive level but are still relatively unexplored in the research literature. Similarly, evidence-based interventions developed for athletes, and soccer players specifically, are presently sparse. Researchers are, therefore, encouraged to focus on increasing the empirical knowledge of essential psychosocial factors for athletes' wellbeing and to increase the availability of tailored and evidence-based wellbeing interventions that can be implemented in soccer from the grass-root level to the professional level.

In addition, mental health is a complex construct. Cultural and social factors in sports and society, which change over time, influence what gets characterized as mental health (Bolton & Bhugra, 2021; Lundqvist & Andersson, 2021). There is also a lack of consensus among governing organizations on the definition and theoretical perspectives of mental health and wellbeing in sports (Vella et al., 2021b), making it difficult for practitioners to provide correct interventions or recommendations. Bringing clarity to this area will help soccer professionals (e.g., coaches, managers, and support personnel) and organizations (e.g., clubs, unions, and schools) know the best strategies for helping their players improve wellbeing and prevent psychological distress.

In the future, researchers need to explore more diverse populations. Currently, most of the research on mental health focuses on European and North American males playing at the professional or elite levels. It would be helpful for the knowledge development within this research field to include more youth, amateur, recreational,

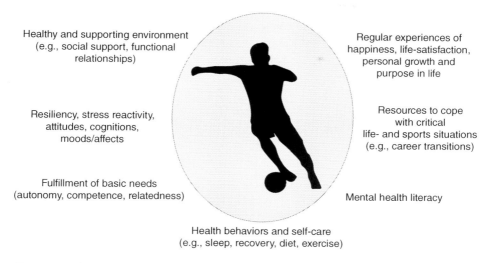

*Figure 11.3* Overview of essential factors for players' wellbeing.

women, and non-European/North American populations (e.g., African, Asian, and South American) in studies and investigate wellbeing related to sociocultural factors. In addition, more researcher-practitioner collaboration could improve the applicability and effectiveness of wellbeing interventions across all competitive levels.

In conclusion, wellbeing reflects an athlete's positive psychosocial functionality and life satisfaction within the lived life circumstances. While soccer players face many challenges across their careers, times of transition are especially demanding on their mental health, particularly forced or unexpected retirement. These players are at higher risk for developing psychological distress and lower wellbeing, especially if they have no plan or access to mental health resources. While more research and consensus are still needed, there are several interventions and resources that can provide athletes with the tools necessary to overcome and thrive amidst the challenges inherent in soccer. For soccer players' wellbeing to become a priority for all ages and abilities, commitment and action from all stakeholders are required.

## References

Abbott, W., Brett, A., Watson, A. W., Brooker, H., & Clifford, T. (2022). Sleep restriction in elite soccer players: Effects on explosive power, wellbeing, and cognitive function. Research Quarterly for Exercise and Sport, 93(2), 325–332. https://doi.org/10.1080/02701367.2020.1834071

Appaneal, R. N., Levine, B. R., Perna, F. M., & Roh, J. L. (2009). Measuring postinjury depression among male and female competitive athletes. *Journal of Sport and Exercise Psychology*, 31(1), 60–76. https://doi.org/10.1123/jsep.31.1.60

Barry, Margaret M. (2001). Promoting positive mental health: theoretical frameworks for practice. International Journal of Mental Health Promotion, 3(1), 25–34.

Barry, M. M., Clarke, A. M., Jenkins, R., & Patel, V. (2013). A systematic review of the effectiveness of mental health promotion interventions for young people in low and middle income countries. *BMC Public Health*, 13(1), 835. https://doi.org/10.1186/1471-2458-13-835

Barth, M., Güllich, A., Forstinger, C. A., Schlesinger, T., Schröder, F., & Emrich, E. (2021). Retirement of professional soccer players: a systematic review from social sciences perspectives. *Journal of Sports Sciences*, 39(8), 903–914. https://doi.org/10.1080/02640414.2020.1851449

Benjamin, C. L., Curtis, R. M., Huggins, R. A., Sekiguchi, Y., Jain, R. K., McFadden, B. A., & Casa, D. J. (2020). Sleep dysfunction and mood in collegiate soccer athletes. *Sports Health*, *12*(3), 234–240. https://doi.org/10.1177/1941738120916735

Blakelock, D. J., Chen, M. A., & Prescott, T. (2016). Psychological distress in elite adolescent soccer players following deselection. *Journal of Clinical Sport Psychology*, *10*(1), 59–77. https://doi.org/10.1123/jcsp.2015-0010

Bolton, D., & Bhugra, D. (2021). Changes in society and young people's mental health. *International Review of Psychiatry*, *33*(1–2), 154–161. https://doi.org/10.1080/09540261.2020.1753968

Breslin, G., Shannon, S., Haughey, T., Donnelly, P., & Leavey, G. (2017). A systematic review of interventions to increase awareness of mental health and well-being in athletes, coaches and officials. *Systematic Reviews*, *6*(1), 177. https://doi.org/10.1186/s13643-017-0568-6

Breslin, G., Smith, A., Donohue, B., Donnelly, P., Shannon, S., Haughey, T. J., Vella, S. A., Swann, C., Cotterill, S., Macintyre, T., Rogers, T., & Leavey, G. (2019). International consensus statement on the psychosocial and policy-related approaches to mental health awareness programmes in sport. *BMJ Open Sport & Exercise Medicine*, *5*(1), e000585. https://doi.org/10.1136/bmjsem-2019-000585

Brown, G., & Potrac, P. (2009). 'You've not made the grade, son': de-selection and identity disruption in elite level youth football. *Soccer & Society*, *10*(2), 143–159. https://doi.org/10.1080/14660970802601613

Calvin, M. (2017). No hunger in paradise. The players. The journey. The dream. London: Arrow Books.

Cronin, L. D., & Allen, J. (2018). Examining the relationships among the coaching climate, life skills development and well-being in sport. *International Journal of Sports Science & Coaching*, *13*(6), 815–827. https://doi.org/10.1177/1747954118787949

Diener, E. (2009). Introduction – The science of well-being: Reviews and theoretical articles by Ed Diener. In: Diener, E. (Ed.). The Science of Well-Being. Social Indicators Research Series, vol 37. Springer, Dordrecht. https://doi.org/10.1007/978-90-481-2350-6_1

Diener, E., Oishi, S., & Lucas, R. E. (2009). Subjective well-being: the science of happiness and life satisfaction. In *Oxford Handbook of Positive Psychology* (2nd ed.) (pp. 187–194). Oxford University Press.

Diener, E., Pressman, S. D., Hunter, J., & Delgadillo-Chase, D. (2017). If, why, and when subjective well-being influences health, and future needed research. *Applied Psychology: Health and Well-Being*, *9*(2), 133–167. https://doi.org/10.1111/aphw.12090

Eime, R. M., Young, J. A., Harvey, J. T., Charity, M. J., & Payne, W. R. (2013). A systematic review of the psychological and social benefits of participation in sport for children and adolescents: Informing development of a conceptual model of health through sport. *International Journal of Behavioral Nutrition and Physical Activity*, *10*(1), 98. https://doi.org/10.1186/1479-5868-10-98

FIFA. (August, 2, 2021). FIFA launches #ReachOut campaign for better mental health. https://www.fifa.com/about-fifa/medical/news/fifa-launches-reach-out-campaign-for-better-mental-health

FIFPRO. (June 1, 2021). FIFPRO video about mental health: Are you ready to talk? https://fifpro.org/en/supporting-players/health-and-performance/mental-health/fifpro-video-about-mental-health-are-you-ready-to-talk/

FIFPRO (2021b). Mind the gap. https://fifpro.org/en/supporting-players/development-beyond-football/project-mind-the-gap/mind-the-gap-67-percent-of-footballers-unsure-of-second-career-path-fifpro-survey-finds/

Fortunato, V., & Marchant, D. (1999). Forced retirement from elite football in Australia. *Journal of Personal and Interpersonal Loss*, *4*(3), 269–280. https://doi.org/10.1080/10811449908409735

Friedrich, A., & Schlarb, A. A. (2018). Let's talk about sleep: a systematic review of psychological interventions to improve sleep in college students. *Journal of Sleep Research*, *27*(1), 4–22. https://doi.org/10.1111/jsr.12568

Fullagar, H. H. K., Skorski, S., Duffield, R., Julian, R., Bartlett, J., & Meyer, T. (2016). Impaired sleep and recovery after night matches in elite football players. *Journal of Sports Sciences*, *34*(14), 1333–1339. https://doi.org/10.1080/02640414.2015.1135249

Galante, J., Friedrich, C., Dawson, A. F., Modrego-Alarcón, M., Gebbing, P., Delgado-Suárez, I., Gupta, R., Dean, L., Dalgleish, T., White, I. R., & Jones, P. B. (2021). Mindfulness-based programmes for mental health promotion in adults in nonclinical settings: A systematic review and meta-analysis of randomised controlled trials. PLoS Medicine, 18(1), e1003481. https://doi.org/10.1371/journal.pmed.1003481

Gervis, M., Pickford, H. C., & Hau, T. (2019). Professional footballer: association counselor perceptions of the role long-term injury plays in mental health issues presented by current and former players. Journal of Clinical Sport Psychology, 13(3), 451–468. https://doi.org/10.1123/jcsp.2018-0049.

Giles, S., Fletcher, D., Arnold, R., Ashfield, A., & Harrison, J. (2020). Measuring well-being in sport performers: where are we now and how do we progress? Sports Medicine, 50(7), 1255–1270. https://doi.org/10.1007/s40279-020-01274-z

Gouttebarge, V., Backx, F. J. G., Aoki, H., & Kerkhoffs, G. M. M. J. (2015). Symptoms of common mental disorders in professional football (Soccer) across five European countries. Journal of Sports Science & Medicine, 14(4), 811–818.

Huta, V., & Ryan, R. M. (2010). Pursuing pleasure or virtue: the differential and overlapping well-being benefits of hedonic and eudaimonic motives. Journal of Happiness Studies, 11(6), 735–762. https://doi.org/10.1007/s10902-009-9171-4

Huta, V., & Waterman, A. S. (2014). Eudaimonia and its distinction from hedonia: developing a classification and terminology for understanding conceptual and operational definitions. Journal of Happiness Studies, 15(6), 1425–1456. https://doi.org/10.1007/s10902-013-9485-0

Iasiello, M., Agteren, J. van, Keyes, C. L. M., & Cochrane, E. M. (2019). Positive mental health as a predictor of recovery from mental illness. Journal of Affective Disorders, 251, 227–230. https://doi.org/10.1016/j.jad.2019.03.065

Jacobsson, J., & Timpka, T. (2015). Classification of prevention in sports medicine and epidemiology. Sports Medicine, 45(11), 1483–1487. https://doi.org/10.1007/s40279-015-0368-x

Jorm, A. F., Korten, A. E., Jacomb, P. A., Christensen, H., Rodgers, B., & Pollitt, P. (1997). "Mental health literacy": a survey of the public's ability to recognise mental disorders and their beliefs about the effectiveness of treatment. The Medical Journal of Australia, 166(4), 182–186. https://doi.org/10.5694/j.1326-5377.1997.tb140071.x

Junge, A., & Feddermann-Demont, N. (2016). Prevalence of depression and anxiety in top-level male and female football players. BMJ Open Sport & Exercise Medicine, 2(1), e000087. https://doi.org/10.1136/bmjsem-2015-000087

Junge, A., & Prinz, B. (2019). Depression and anxiety symptoms in 17 teams of female football players including 10 German first league teams. British Journal of Sports Medicine, 53(8), 471. https://doi.org/10.1136/bjsports-2017-098033

Keyes, C. L. M. (1998). Social well-being. Social Psychology Quarterly, 61(2), 121–140. https://doi.org/10.2307/2787065

Keyes, C. L. M. (2007). Promoting and protecting mental health as flourishing: a complementary strategy for improving national mental health. American Psychologist, 62(2), 95–108. https://doi.org/10.1037/0003-066X.62.2.95

Keyes, C. L. M., & Annas, J. (2009). Feeling good and functioning well: distinctive concepts in ancient philosophy and contemporary science. The Journal of Positive Psychology, 4(3), 197–201. https://doi.org/10.1080/17439760902844228

Keyes, C. L. M., Dhingra, S. S., & Simoes, E. J. (2010). Change in level of positive mental health as a predictor of future risk of mental illness. American Journal of Public Health, 100(12), 2366–2371. https://doi.org/10.2105/AJPH.2010.192245

Keyes, C. L. M., Shmotkin, D., & Ryff, C. D. (2002). Optimizing well-being: the empirical encounter of two traditions. Journal of Personality and Social Psychology, 82(6), 1007–1022. https://doi.org/10.1037/0022-3514.82.6.1007

Kilic, Ö., Carmody, S., Upmeijer, J., Kerkhoffs, G. M. M. J., Purcell, R., Rice, S., & Gouttebarge, V. (2021). Prevalence of mental health symptoms among male and female Australian

180  *Carolina Lundqvist and David P. Schary*

professional footballers. *BMJ Open Sport & Exercise Medicine*, 7(3), e001043. https://doi.org/10.1136/bmjsem-2021-001043

Kuettel, A., & Larsen, C. H. (2020). Risk and protective factors for mental health in elite athletes: A scoping review. *International Review of Sport and Exercise Psychology*, 13(1), 231–265. https://doi.org/10.1080/1750984X.2019.1689574

Kuettel, A., Pedersen, A. K., & Larsen, C. H. (2021). To flourish or languish, that is the question: exploring the mental health profiles of Danish elite athletes. *Psychology of Sport and Exercise*, 52, 101837. https://doi.org/10.1016/j.psychsport.2020.101837

Kutcher, S., Wei, Y., & Coniglio, C. (2016). Mental health literacy: past, present, and future. *The Canadian Journal of Psychiatry*, 61(3), 154–158. https://doi.org/10.1177/0706743715616609

Larsen, C. H., Alfermann, D., Henriksen, K., & Christensen, M. K. (2013). Successful talent development in soccer: the characteristics of the environment. *Sport, Exercise, and Performance Psychology*, 2(3), 190–206. https://doi.org/10.1037/a0031958

Larsen, C. H., Alfermann, D., Henriksen, K., & Christensen, M. K. (2014). Preparing footballers for the next step: an intervention program from an ecological perspective. *The Sport Psychologist*, 28(1), 91–102. https://doi.org/10.1123/tsp.2013-0015

Liddle, S.K., Deane, F.P., Batterham, M. & Vella S.A. (2021). A brief sports-based mental health literacy program for male adolescents: A cluster-randomized controlled trial. Journal of Applied Sport Psychology, 33(1), 20–44. https://doi.org/10.1080/10413200.2019.1653404

Low, W. R., Sandercock, G. R. H., Freeman, P., Winter, M. E., Butt, J., & Maynard, I. (2021). Pressure training for performance domains: A meta-analysis. Sport, Exercise, and Performance Psychology, 10(1), 149–163. https://doi.org/10.1037/spy0000202

Lundqvist, C. (2011). Well-being in competitive sports—The feel-good factor? A review of conceptual considerations of well-being. International Review of Sport and Exercise Psychology, 4(2), 109–127. https://doi.org/10.1080/1750984X.2011.584067

Lundqvist, C. (2021). Well-being and quality of life. In R. Arnold & D. Fletcher (Eds.), *Stress, Well-being and Performance in Sport* (pp. 131–147). New York: Routledge.

Lundqvist, C., & Andersson, G. (2021). Let's talk about mental health and mental disorders in elite sports: a narrative review of theoretical perspectives. *Frontiers in Psychology*, 12, 700829. https://doi.org/10.3389/fpsyg.2021.700829

Lundqvist, C., Sandin, F., (2014), Well-being in elite sport: Dimensions of hedonic and eudaimonic well-being among elite orienteers at a global and sport specific level, The Sport psychologist, 28(3), 245–254. https://doi.org/10.1123/tsp.2013-0024

Madsen, E. E., Krustrup, P., Larsen, C. H., Elbe, A. M., Wikman, J. M., Ivarsson, A., & Lautenbach, F. (2021). Resilience as a protective factor for well-being and emotional stability in elite-level football players during the first wave of the COVID-19 pandemic. Science & Medicine in Football, 5 (supl), 62–69. https://doi.org/10.1080/24733938.2021.1959047

McKay, A., Cropley, B., Mullen, R., Shearer D., & Hanton, S. (2022) Psychosocial demands and situational properties of the club-to-international transition in male youth football, Journal of Applied Sport Psychology, 34 (6), 1272-1294. https://doi.org/10.1080/10413200.2021.1972495

Miçooğullari, B. O., & Ekmekci, R. (2017). Evaluation of a psychological skill training program on mental toughness and psychological wellbeing for professional soccer players. *Universal Journal of Educational Research*, 5, 2312–2319.

Nédélec, M., Halson, S., Abaidia, A.-E., Ahmaidi, S., & Dupont, G. (2015). Stress, sleep and recovery in elite soccer: a critical review of the literature. *Sports Medicine*, 45(10), 1387–1400. https://doi.org/10.1007/s40279-015-0358-z

Lundqvist, C., Sandin, F., (2014), Well-being in elite sport: Dimensions of hedonic and eudaimonic well-being among elite orienteers at a global and sport specific level, The Sport psychologist, 28(3), 245–254. https://doi.org/10.1123/tsp.2013-0024

Olmedilla, A., Moreno-Fernández, I. M., Gómez-Espejo, V., Robles-Palazón, F. J., Verdú, I., & Ortega, E. (2019). Psychological intervention program to control stress in youth soccer players. *Frontiers in Psychology*, 10, 2260. https://doi.org/10.3389/fpsyg.2019.02260

Petitpas, A., Van Raalte, J. L., & Brewer, B. W. (2013). Athletes' careers in the United States: Developmental programming for athletes in transition. In N. B. Stambulova & T. V. Ryba (Eds.), *Athletes' careers across cultures* (pp. 222–234). New York: Routledge/Taylor & Francis Group.

Platts, C., & Smith, A. (2010). 'Money, money, money?' The development of financial inequalities in English professional football. *Soccer & Society*, *11*(5), 643–658. https://doi.org/10.1080/14660970.2010.497365

Raibley, J. R. (2012). Happiness is not well-being. *Journal of Happiness Studies: An Interdisciplinary Forum on Subjective Well-Being*, *13*(6), 1105–1129. https://doi.org/10.1007/s10902-011-9309-z

Reverberi, E., D'Angelo, C., Littlewood, M. A., & Gozzoli, C. F. (2020). Youth football players' psychological well-being: the key role of relationships. *Frontiers in Psychology*, *11*, 567776. https://doi.org/10.3389/fpsyg.2020.567776

Rice, S. M., Purcell, R., De Silva, S., Mawren, D., McGorry, P. D., & Parker, A. G. (2016). The mental health of elite athletes: a narrative systematic review. *Sports Medicine*, *46*(9), 1333–1353. https://doi.org/10.1007/s40279-016-0492-2

Rios, P., Cardoso, R., Morra, D., Nincic, V., Goodarzi, Z., Farah, B., Harricharan, S., Morin, C. M., Leech, J., Straus, S. E., & Tricco, A. C. (2019). Comparative effectiveness and safety of pharmacological and non-pharmacological interventions for insomnia: an overview of reviews. *Systematic Reviews*, *8*(1), 281. https://doi.org/10.1186/s13643-019-1163-9

Roiger, T., Weidauer, L., & Kern, B. (2015). A longitudinal pilot study of depressive symptoms in concussed and injured/nonconcussed national collegiate athletic association division i student-athletes. *Journal of Athletic Training*, *50*(3), 256–261. https://doi.org/10.4085/1062-6050-49.3.83

Ryan, R. M., Huta, V., & Deci, E. L. (2008). Living well: a self-determination theory perspective on eudaimonia. *Journal of Happiness Studies*, *9*(1), 139–170. https://doi.org/10.1007/s10902-006-9023-4

Ryff, C. D. (2014). Psychological well-being revisited: advances in the science and practice of Eudaimonia. *Psychotherapy and Psychosomatics*, *83*(1), 10–28. https://doi.org/10.1159/000353263

Ryff, C. D., Singer, B. H., & Dienberg Love, G. (2004). Positive health: connecting well-being with biology. *Philosophical Transactions of the Royal Society of London. Series B: Biological Sciences*, *359*(1449), 1383–1394. https://doi.org/10.1098/rstb.2004.1521

Samuel, R. D., & Tenenbaum, G. (2011). The role of change in athletes' careers: a scheme of change for sport psychology practice. *The Sport Psychologist*, *25*(2), 233–252. https://doi.org/10.1123/tsp.25.2.233

Schotanus-Dijkstra, M., Keyes, C. L. M., de Graaf, R., & Ten Have, M. (2019). Recovery from mood and anxiety disorders: The influence of positive mental health. Journal of Affective Disorders, 252, 107–113. https://doi.org/10.1016/j.jad.2019.04.051

Shannon, S., Hanna, D., Haughey, T., Leavey, G., McGeown, C., & Breslin, G. (2019). Effects of a mental health intervention in athletes: applying self-determination theory. *Frontiers in Psychology*, *10*, 1875. https://doi.org/10.3389/fpsyg.2019.01875

Stambulova, N. (2010). Professional culture of career assistance to athletes: a look through contrasting lenses of career metaphors. In Tatiana V. Ryba, Robert J. Schinke, Gershon Tenenbaum (Eds.), *The Cultural Turn in Sport Psychology* (pp. 285–312). Morgantown, WV: Fitness Information Technology. http://urn.kb.se/resolve?urn=urn:nbn:se:hh:diva-4882

Stambulova, N. B., Ryba, T. V., & Henriksen, K. (2021). Career development and transitions of athletes: the international society of sport psychology position stand revisited. *International Journal of Sport and Exercise Psychology*, *19*(4), 524–550. https://doi.org/10.1080/1612197X.2020.1737836

Storm, L. K., Henriksen, K., Stambulova, N. B., Cartigny, E., Ryba, T. V., De Brandt, K., Ramis, Y., & Cecić Erpič, S. (2021). Ten essential features of European dual career development environments: a multiple case study. *Psychology of Sport and Exercise*, *54*, 101918. https://doi.org/10.1016/j.psychsport.2021.101918

Swann, C., Telenta, J., Draper, G., Liddle, S., Fogarty, A., Hurley, D., & Vella, S. (2018). Youth sport as a context for supporting mental health: adolescent male perspectives. *Psychology of Sport and Exercise, 35*, 55–64. https://doi.org/10.1016/j.psychsport.2017.11.008

van Agteren, J., Iasiello, M., Lo, L., Bartholomaeus, J., Kopsaftis, Z., Carey, M., & Kyrios, M. (2021). A systematic review and meta-analysis of psychological interventions to improve mental wellbeing. *Nature Human Behaviour, 5*(5), 631–652. https://doi.org/10.1038/s41562-021-01093-w

Vella, S. A., Swann, C., Batterham, M., Boydell, K. M., Eckermann, S., Ferguson, H., Fogarty, A., Hurley, D., Liddle, S. K., Lonsdale, C., Miller, A., Noetel, M., Okely, A. D., Sanders, T., Schweickle, M. J., Telenta, J., & Deane, F. P. (2021a). An intervention for mental health literacy and resilience in organized sports. Medicine and Science in Sports and Exercise, 53(1), 139–149. https://doi.org/10.1249/MSS.0000000000002433

Vella, S.A., Schweickle, M.J., Sutcliffe, J.T., Swann, C. (2021b). A systematic review and meta-synthesis of mental health position statements in sport: Scope, quality and future directions. Psychology of Sport Exercise,55:101946. https://doi.org/10.1016/j.psychsport.2021.101946

Walsh, N. P., Halson, S. L., Sargent, C., Roach, G. D., Nédélec, M., Gupta, L., Leeder, J., Fullagar, H. H., Coutts, A. J., Edwards, B. J., Pullinger, S. A., Robertson, C. M., Burniston, J. G., Lastella, M., Le Meur, Y., Hausswirth, C., Bender, A. M., Grandner, M. A., & Samuels, C. H. (2021). Sleep and the athlete: narrative review and 2021 expert consensus recommendations. *British Journal of Sports Medicine, 55*(7), 356–368. https://doi.org/10.1136/bjsports-2020-102025

Wickham, S.-R., Amarasekara, N. A., Bartonicek, A., & Conner, T. S. (2020). The big three health behaviors and mental health and well-being among young adults: a cross-sectional investigation of sleep, exercise, and diet. *Frontiers in Psychology, 11*, 579205. https://doi.org/10.3389/fpsyg.2020.579205

Wilkinson, R. J. (2021). A literature review exploring the mental health issues in academy football players following career termination due to deselection or injury and how counselling could support future players. *Counselling and Psychotherapy Research, 21*, 859-868. https://doi.org/10.1002/capr.12417

Wold, B., Duda, J. L., Balaguer, I., Smith, O. R. F., Ommundsen, Y., Hall, H. K., Samdal, O., Heuzé, J.-P., Haug, E., Bracey, S., Castillo, I., Ramis, Y., Quested, E., & Krommidas, C. (2013). Comparing self-reported leisure-time physical activity, subjective health, and life satisfaction among youth soccer players and adolescents in a reference sample. *International Journal of Sport and Exercise Psychology, 11*(4), 328–340. https://doi.org/10.1080/1612197X.2013.830433

Wood, A. M., & Joseph, S. (2010). The absence of positive psychological (eudemonic) well-being as a risk factor for depression: a ten year cohort study. *Journal of Affective Disorders, 122*(3), 213–217. https://doi.org/10.1016/j.jad.2009.06.032

World Health Organization (2022). WHO guideline on self-care interventions for health and well-being, 2022 revision. Geneva: World Health Organization.

Wylleman, P., & Lavallee, D. (2004). A developmental perspective on transitions faced by athletes. In *Developmental Sport and Exercise Psychology: A Lifespan Perspective.* (pp. 503–523). Morgantown, WV: Fitness Information Technology.

# 12  Developing (adaptive) coaching expertise

*Christopher J. Cushion and Anna Stodter*

## Introduction

The study of coach development pathways is of interest to those seeking understand how expert coaches develop their skills and knowledge. Knowing and understanding what the journey to coaching expertise looks like enables coach educators to help coaches transition from novice to expert status, thus raising the quality of coaching practice across all areas of the game (grassroots, academy, and professional) and in different coaching domains (participation, development, and performance). That said, recent years have seen developments in coach education, with its evaluation and effectiveness supported by rapid growth in research on coach learning, creating a 'hotbed' of scholarly activity (Lyle & Cushion, 2017). This growth has occurred alongside a gradual paradigm shift whereby coach education based on 'knowledge transfer' from experienced, 'expert' coaches to novices, has moved towards attempts to provide facilitation of more participatory 'learner-centred' approaches to coach development. In this chapter, we explore coach learning alongside a contemporary understanding of expertise as it applies to coaching in soccer. We consider how findings about current coach development may, or may not, contribute to the development of coaching expertise. We then present evidence-informed guidance for coach development focusing on developing adaptive coaching expertise.

## Expertise in coaching

Governing bodies in soccer, through hierarchical accreditation systems, appear to view expertise in part as a function of experience and coaching competencies. Coaching expertise can be conceptualised in this outcome-focused way, or as Berry (2020) suggests, as a process, reflecting definitional challenges in the expertise literature (Farrington-Darby & Wilson, 2006). An outcome conceptualisation is consistent with the definition of expertise as 'reproducible superior performance' (Ericsson & Charness, 1994, p. 726). This concept of routine expertise is referred to as the ability to master domain-specific skills without error (Carbonell et al., 2016). In this regard, routine expertise can be considered analogous to the level- or stage-based competency frameworks embedded within soccer's formal accreditation systems. This approach has largely been adopted in coaching research where it is well established that 'reproducible superior performance' in coaching is not innate, but instead is developed through learning from idiosyncratic combinations of experiences over time (Schempp & McCullick, 2010). In other words, for those striving to advance in coaching and transition from novice to

DOI: 10.4324/9781003148418-14

expert status, the past twenty or so years of scholarly activity have suggested that coaches can become 'more expert' through learning effectively from their experiences.

Deliberate practice has been found to be a mediating factor in the development of expertise in sport. It is a specific form of practice designed to improve performance through a cyclical process involving the repetition of skills at the edge of one's ability, refined by feedback (Berry, 2020). Critiques of formal coach education provide a persuasive argument that the factors necessary for deliberate practice are currently absent. Not least, the amount of time spent engaged in coach education renders it 'low impact', and within coach education itself the time spent practising coaching and receiving appropriate feedback is limited (Stodter & Cushion, 2017, 2019a). Moreover, as Cushion et al. (2021) argue, coaches' experiences show that courses exhibit a number of common features: a single style or formula for coaching; 'sacred texts' prescribing what and how to coach; 'rites of passage' from one level to the next; 'instrumental design' driven by passing of assessments; and on course 'time-crunch' limiting space for spontaneous discussion, challenge, or meaningful feedback to facilitate improvement (Downham & Cushion, 2020; Piggott, 2012; Williams & Bush, 2019; Dempsey et al., 2020; *inter-alia*). Townsend et al. (2021) contend that while research on coach education has significantly increased over the last decade, much of this work reiterates that coach education remains a low-impact endeavour perceived to lack relevance for coaches. As a result, coaching knowledge and practices are still being derived overwhelmingly from experiential, informal, and non-formal sources, with this effect magnified in marginalised coaching spaces such as disability (Townsend et al., 2021). It is unclear if the current conceptions of coach education can legitimately claim to constitute deliberate practice, and the applicability of the deliberate practice model to develop expertise in coaching may currently be questioned.

Coaching in soccer is an impactful and complex activity requiring the flexible balance of numerous changeable tasks, interactions, and relationships (Jones, Bailey, & Thompson, 2013), and applying knowledge appropriate to the context often under competitive pressure. The 'art' of coaching appears instinctive, yet researchers have suggested the use of tacit knowledge to reliably plan, predict outcomes, solve problems, communicate, self-monitor, and make intuitive decisions (Lyle & Cushion, 2017; Nash & Collins, 2006). Superior knowledge, a key characteristic of expert coaching, developed through learning from years of experience, seems to underpin these qualities in consistently bringing about positive outcomes for players.

Given this understanding of the nature of coaching, and useful for coaching an interactive team game like soccer, is a shift in thinking about expertise towards a more process-oriented view (Berry, 2020; Turner, Nelson & Potrac, 2012). In this view, expertise is less a personal characteristic than the product of an interaction between the person and the environment (Turner et al., 2012). From this perspective, experts have been shown to distinguish themselves in their ability to perceive meaningful patterns in their coaching environments that novices cannot (Cushion et al., 2010; Farrington-Darby & Wilson, 2006; Schempp & McCullick, 2010). In essence, a different definition of expertise has different implications for its relevance and application within coaching and coach education. A process view is supportive of the ability of coaches to develop adaptive expertise, the ability to master novel tasks and transfer skills to different and unknown contexts (Barnett & Koslowski, 2002; Sonnentage et al., 2006). As Mees, Sinfield, Collins, and Collins (2020) explain, adaptive expertise builds on, yet contrasts, with routine expertise (Hatano & Inagaki, 1986; Hatano & Oura, 2003).

Both notions of expertise demand the capacity to perform standard tasks and routine functions without error (Mees et al., 2020). Adaptive expertise is less about repeating standardised tasks to a high standard, and more concerned with developing more nuanced planning, situational awareness, reflection, metacognition, and problem-solving skills characterised by efficiency and innovation in applying knowledge to new situations and challenges (Berry, 2020, Bransford et al., 2005; Hutton et al., 2017; Mees et al., 2020). This approach seems relevant to soccer coaching, where coaching is increasingly seen as the orchestration of dynamic problems to be solved rather than simply imparting skills.

Fundamental to an adaptive expertise framework is the need to analyse and develop practitioner decision-making; that of the player and the coach, understanding 'why they do what they do' (Bachkirova & Smith, 2015, p. 135). Adaptive expertise is built on routine expertise, yet individuals with adaptive expertise do not rely solely on rule-based decision-making and know when not to rely on automatic processes like intuition (Berry, 2020; Carbonell et al., 2016). This notion is consistent with Bachkirova and Smith's (2015) argument that competency models oversimplify the demands placed on a coach and fail to account for the complexity of thinking. Complexity within the coaching context underpins the need to focus on process (i.e., reasoning) rather than outcome (Owen & Lindley, 2010). Expertise then becomes about developing cognitive skills, managing complexity, and adapting to new contexts (cf. Cruickshank et al., 2018; Martindale & Collins, 2013; Turner et al., 2012).

## Exploring coach development pathways

Like the broader expertise literature, most researchers have centred on the general characteristics of expertise and knowledge, with less focus on the detail or processes of their acquisition, development, and/or construction over time. What needs to be developed is identified, but not *how* or whether it is an endpoint that can be achieved, meaning it is often difficult to extrapolate informative guidance for coach learning. In considering how coach development pathways develop expertise, coaching as an academic area of study has been characterised by a concern for the description and classification of experiences into the situations or contexts in which coaches' learning, and the development of expertise, supposedly occurs. Scholars have typically echoed Trudel and Gilbert's (2006) use of Sfard's (1998) dichotomous learning framework, exploring the acquisition of knowledge through formal (institutionalised) and non-formal education programmes (occurring outside of broader initiatives), or focusing on learning through participation in informal daily experiences and interacting with the environment and others.

## Informal learning/apprenticeship

Coaches frequently report that informal learning grounded in everyday experiences has much more influence on their development in comparison to the impact of formalised coach education (e.g., Blackett et al., 2019; Mallett, Trudel, Lyle & Rynne, 2009; Stodter & Cushion, 2014; *inter-alia*). Informal learning encapsulates the aggregated effect of the conscious and subconscious knowledge acquired through experiences (Blackett et al., 2019; Cushion et al., 2010; Trudel, Culver & Werthner, 2013). Researchers repeatedly illustrate that much of the knowledge acquired by coaches is picked up through 'apprenticeships of observation' as players, and subsequent experiential learning and mentoring as coaches (Cushion, 2019). Findings over time reinforce the view that coaches mainly learn on the job. Embedded within context and responsive to the everyday realities of practice, coaches spend much more time accumulating these experiences than engaging in formal coach education.

This accumulated coaching knowledge has been considered to be incidental, unguided, unstructured, and uncritical (Cushion et al., 2003; Blackett et al., 2019; Lemyre, Trudel & Durand-Bush, 2007; Mallett et al., 2009; *inter-alia*), occurring within particular socio-cultural contexts. Blackett et al. (2019) argue that coach learning and therefore the development of expertise is bound to the informal socio-cultural norms of the sport's (or club's) sub-culture (Townsend & Cushion, 2017; Barker-Ruchti et al., 2016; Lemyre et al., 2007). The implications are that learning through observation and experience can promote and reinforce certain ideological interpretations of knowledge and practice, resulting in behaviour guided by uncritical inertia, with potentially outdated knowledge and behaviours passed on and reproduced. In addition, the importance placed on informal or 'embodied learning' (Blackett et al., 2019) can create 'one-dimensional' (Brown & Potrac, 2009, p. 155) coach identities. This latter notion has implications for coach development, where coaches may not fully engage in purposeful reflection or critical thinking – both of which are significant aspects of adaptive expertise and its development (Mees, et al., 2020). At the same time, such experience does substantially contribute to the development of sport-specific coaching content knowledge (Blackett et al., 2019; Cushion et al., 2003; Mallett, et al., 2009). This factor then acts in developing tacit knowledge of the sport and coaching practices (Nash & Collins, 2006).

Often, these learning processes connect to a 'default' coaching role, and the behaviours and knowledge that coaches engage with are linked to the issues surrounding 'traditional' coaching, the espoused club culture and socialisation experiences (Cushion, 2019). This issue is problematic for soccer coaching, resulting in an extraordinary sameness in coaching practice with findings of contemporary research tending to mirror work conducted over the last 35 years (e.g., Potrac, Jones & Cushion, 2007; Ford et al., 2010; Lacy & Darst, 1985; O'Connor et al., 2017, 2018). It appears that 'traditional' coaching in soccer is unchangeable, 'what is expected' within the coaching role by coaches, players, parents, and clubs (Cushion, 2013, 2019; Potrac et al., 2007). Potrac et al. (2007, p. 40) claim "the consequence of such action is that athletes are increasingly socialised into expecting instructional behaviours from coaches, and thus resist other coaching methods". As a result, coaching becomes a historical and traditional thread where experiences are powerful, long-lasting, and have a continual influence over pedagogical perspectives, practices, beliefs, and behaviours (Cushion, 2019, 2013; Cushion et al., 2003; Potrac et al., 2007). Therefore, coach socialisation needs to be examined before drawing conclusions about what might constitute good coaching knowledge and practice (Cushion, 2010, 2019).

## Formal learning

Although they are often treated as conceptually distinct, regulated formal coach certification and education programmes occur in combination with informal learning (Werthner & Trudel, 2009) and against a similarly influential cultural backdrop (Stodter & Cushion, 2014). Typically, programmes entail certain prerequisites, are built around compartmentalised, standardised curricula over short blocks of time and result in certification, but in soccer, there is huge variation in their extent and duration.

Researchers have tended to report coaches' perceptions of formal learning opportunities, with much criticism directed at the use of prescriptive teaching strategies aligned to a simplistic 'instruction' paradigm, decontextualised delivery, and limited relevancy or influence on the 'real-world' dynamic demands of coaching. Chapman et al. (2020) described soccer coach education courses as decontextualised (i.e., divorced from the coaches' own coaching context), inadequate (i.e., failing to meet learners' needs) and bureaucratic (Mallett et al., 2009; Sawiuk, Taylor, & Groom, 2016). In other words, not providing the conditions to develop adaptive expertise or its cognitive facets such as flexible planning, nuanced situational awareness, in-action reflection, and metacognition allow for deep self-awareness (Mees et al., 2020). Coaches may merely abide by strict rules on courses to gain certification (cf. Chesterfield, Potrac, & Jones, 2010), missing out on 'deliberate practice'. In contrast, a recent review found that coaches report positive perceptions of more participatory, interactive, and reflective teaching strategies and contextualised assessment processes in line with a 'learning' paradigm (Ciampolini et al., 2019). Such approaches would appear to align with what Mees et al. (2020) outline as valued by adaptive experts, namely, learning and applying knowledge that is motivated to solving novel situation-specific problems (Bransford et al., 2005).

In recent years, there has been a trend towards more 'learner-centred' perspectives (Dempsey et al., 2020) tending to promote a more constructivist-informed epistemology. Knowledge is assumed to be socially constructed in interaction and must be experienced rather than acquired, with the coach positioned more as a non-directive facilitator and, within certain constraints, the player (learner) largely controls their own development. This emphasises the coach's facilitative behaviours, not *instructing* per se but *constructing* experiences for players. In this case, coaches would provide limited amounts of instructional feedback but engage in helping the learner solve problems and construct knowledge experientially through, for example, questioning, summarising, reflecting, and listening – methods more aligned with developing adaptive expertise. Paquette and Trudel (2018) described coach education approaches informed by constructivist epistemology as those that involve facilitation, group work, localised problem-solving, and the sharing of ideas (Dempsey et al., 2020), and these learning principles have become more established in the recent history of coach education (Ciampolini et al., 2019). Moreover, in England, the Football Association has continued a clear move towards coach education being informed by social constructivism (Chapman et al., 2020; Dempsey et al., 2020).

However, as Dempsey et al. (2020) and Cushion (2013) demonstrate, understanding of learning strategy(s) and the theory that informs it varies. Constructivist approaches are not prescriptions for methods or strategies of teaching and a focus on methods rather than underlying philosophical positions can result in a naïve constructivism, placing an inordinate faith in the ability of the learner to structure their own learning (Cushion, 2013, 2019). This notion equates learning exclusively with activity and involvement alone as a sufficient and necessary condition for learning (Kirschner, Sweller & Clark, 2006). Coach development and the education of coach developers themselves rely on assumed learning through such 'active learning opportunities', in line with preferences for experiential learning involving interaction with other coaches (Stodter & Cushion, 2019b).

Meaningful learning occurs when the learner is able to connect to, and make sense of, what is to be learned, identify relevant knowledge and information, organise it into a coherent structure, and integrating it with existing knowledge (Mayer, 2004). Experts progress through levels of knowledge acquisition, but for information to become knowledge, the learner must share some context and meaning with those imparting the knowledge (Cushion et al., 2010; Swap et al., 2001). Therefore, providing meaningful learning experiences is crucial in developing expertise. Learning requires skilful and progressive instruction that assists metacognition and self-monitoring, helping each learner to reflect on answers, and giving feedback that focuses learners on the task. However, a 'one-size-fits-all' approach to learning regardless of individual differences, with very little variation in practice, remains prevalent in soccer (Stodter & Cushion, 2019b). Not all learners are the same, nor are circumstances and contexts, and advocating a singular approach seems to contradict learner-centeredness, conflict with the characteristics of adaptive expertise, and deny or minimise difference (Cushion, 2010, 2013). Engagement with 'naïve constructivism as method' may inadvertently impose arbitrary ideology and values through practice, rather than providing that which will best meet the learner's needs. Importantly, despite the popularity of, and prescriptions *for,* outwardly 'learner-centred' approaches, the evidence of increased impact on learning, knowledge, practice, or the development of expertise is not clear (Paquette & Trudel, 2018).

Cope, Cushion, Harvey, and Partingon (2021) argue that only a handful of studies spread over 20 years have attempted to show how formal coach education has changed knowledge and practice. Stodter and Cushion (2019a) looked at a level three soccer course and reported changes in the use of knowledge around tactics, and engaging with individual players, reflected in an altered proportion of technical to tactically related questions, and more behaviours directed at individual players. Course participants also had changed knowledge of practice structures, challenges and questioning, learning principles and reflection, although corresponding behaviours and practice activities generally remained consistent. The minimal impact of learning on observed coaching behaviour, alongside interview data, revealed some disconnect between knowledge and situated action, suggesting a lack of deep learning. Coaches were able to adopt and reinforce knowledge without challenging deeply held assumptions, reflecting common criticisms of coach education in generating meaningful change. This process is not supportive of developing adaptive expertise which fosters a willingness to challenge and replace prior assumptions and recognise gaps in knowledge, drawing on the individual's reflective and metacognitive capacities (Mees et al., 2020; Bransford et al., 2005). 'Deep-seated' practices can be resistant to change, and changing behaviour is particularly challenging using short, formal coach education courses. While some impact was evidenced, the findings pose questions to the duration, design, and follow-up of educational episodes.

Behavioural research reports a continued disconnect between coaches' intentions and their practice suggesting low self-awareness, and illustrates soccer coaches as directive, instructional, or prescriptive, with the coach deciding when and how players should perform specified skills or movements (cf. O'Connor et al., 2017, 2018). Furthermore, analysis by Cope et al. (2016) showed that coaches engage in limited dialogic behaviour and ask few questions, typically between 2% and 5% of overall reported coaching behaviours. Studies also demonstrate that coaches predominantly ask convergent rather than divergent questions (e.g., Harvey et al., 2011; Partington & Cushion,

*Developing (adaptive) coaching expertise* 189

2013) with the latter seen as pivotal in learning to develop higher-order thinking and the application of adaptive expertise.

## Developing coaching practice and adaptive expertise

Clearly, how coaches are educated in soccer has a direct influence on the nature of their practice of adaptive expertise (Mees et al., 2020). Developing adaptive coaching expertise requires building, then moving beyond, proceduralised practice and competency toward in-context practices that are more flexible, decision-based, and reflective. This change includes developing a range of practices that avoid promoting one approach to coaching as superior to another, as different approaches will be appropriate in different situations. A balance is required between impacting the development of decision-making, problem-solving, and creative skills (Potrac & Cassidy, 2006) with acquiring levels of knowledge and understanding that are immature, incorrect, and may lead to the neglect of key skills (Cushion, 2019; Cushion et al., 2012a; Potrac & Cassidy, 2006).

Potrac and Cassidy (2006) argue that to develop self-regulating and autonomous learners requires "more than either the one-directional transmission of knowledge … or the total ownership by learners of their own development" (p. 40). Thus, being highly adaptive and context-specific, means there is no single all-encompassing approach. Coaches need to be free to interact and behave in a variety of ways and in attempting to adhere to a particular way of coaching, may lose sight of the fact that they need to act to create optimal conditions for learning. In other words, there is a need to be responsive to individual differences where the most valuable coaching practices correspond with developmental needs and individual particularities, requiring a diverse range of approaches (Cushion, 2010, 2019). Adaptive expert, learner-centred coaches should be continuously engaged with evidence-informed approaches and reflection as to how their players learn effectively, being primarily concerned about whether their coaching impairs or facilitates learning (Cushion, 2019; Cushion et al., 2012a).

At the very least, a starting point to a discussion around recommendations/ guidelines for developing coach expertise is a need to emphasise that coaches should be aware of their actual behaviour and the assumptions about learning underpinning their practice (Cushion, 2019). Crucial in raising coach self-awareness, this aspect is a feature of adaptive experts who demonstrate the capacity to self-assess their expertise, knowledge, learning, and problem-solving ability (Mees et al., 2020). While evidence suggests this quality is lacking in soccer, it seems essential if coaches are to grasp the implications of their coaching (good or bad). Coaches can develop a better conceptual understanding by reflecting on why they coach as they do and related underlying assumptions. Alongside critical reflection on their socialisation experiences and the culturally accepted coaching behaviours of soccer, this puts coaches in a strong position to transcend 'traditional' behaviour and develop their own informed approach to expertise. All of which require high cognitive flexibility, deep thinking skills, and metacognitive ability (Mees et al., 2020).

However, established practices in coaching are difficult to change because many coaches "find it difficult to reflect upon, and possibly critique, taken for granted practices that have become integral to their sense of self" (Cassidy, 2010, p. 143). The process of relying solely on one's self-perception of what works closes conversations, blunts knowledge and stifles creativity, which, if left unchallenged, produces stagnation and a climate of self-referential, self-justifying knowledge structures (Cushion, 2019; Abraham et al., 2006). There is a need to use more objective methods that allow coaches to reflect on their practice; robust changes to coaching practice rely on reflection. Systematic observation is a means of analysing what behaviours coaches employ and these data can be used to support reflection through discussions about practice. Partington et al. (2015) tracked five elite soccer coaches over three seasons (approximately 30 months) using the Coach Analysis Intervention System (Cushion et al., 2012b) and video feedback. The study reported significant differences over time in four behaviours: instruction; feedback; silence; and questioning. Objective data and video feedback provided a structure for reflective conversations, improved self-awareness, and triggered behaviour change. There are further examples of coaches developing and changing their coaching behaviour and practice structures when accessing behavioural data combined with reflective practice (e.g., Harvey et al., 2010, 2011). However, changes in practice and behaviour were not totally adopted, with customary practices resisting change. Cope et al. (2021) worked with coaches to develop a learning programme, where the participants perceived changes in their way of thinking about developing as coaches and reported changes in their coaching practice, substantiated by observational data. These studies show that by providing coaches with an opportunity to discuss issues specific to their practice and supporting them to think more critically about their coaching (e.g. through reflective conversations), changes can and do occur (Cope et al., 2021).

Reflective practice is important in developing expertise as well as being a feature of adaptive expertise. There are many types of reflection (e.g., descriptive and creative), but the key type in coach development is critical reflection (Cushion et al., 2012a). Critical reflection necessitates that coaches question and challenge current practices, habits, routines, values, and beliefs. Ghaye (2001, p. 10) calls this "asking the 'why-type' question: 'why do I/we coach in this way?'" Critical reflection enables coaches to integrate various sources of knowledge they encounter into their repertoire, a process necessary to transform behaviours. For coaches with well-developed beliefs, information acquired may contradict their current practice, presenting the dilemma of revising their thinking through 'conceptual change' (Cushion et al., 2012a; Schraw, Crippen, & Hartley, 2006). The ability to engage in critical reflection (i.e., questioning and challenging current practices, habits, routines, values, and beliefs) is therefore a fundamental process for a coach.

Coaches, therefore, require the 'tools' (i.e., reflection, self-regulation, and aligned epistemological beliefs) to deal with the many different and evolving situations that they come across, with coaches appearing to develop and refine strategies through cycles of experimentation and evaluation (Gilbert & Trudel, 2001; Stodter & Cushion, 2017). Expert coaches learn more from events because they critically reflect rather than simply accumulating experience. Such reflection enables a comparison of problem-solving processes with those who are deemed 'more expert' and provides a conceptualisation of adaptive expertise (Hatano & Inagaki, 1986; Nash, Martindale, Collins, & Martindale, 2012) that allows a comparison towards the behaviour of an adaptive expert (Mees et al., 2020). Coaches can become "more expert" by mastering the skill of learning from their experiences through reflective practice (Schempp & McCullick, 2010, p. 230). To develop adaptive expertise, coach education should provide an environment where practice, and the practice of others, can be interrogated and assumptions made explicit, providing the skills and resources to enable reflection and to critically

*Developing (adaptive) coaching expertise* 191

examine the inadequacies of different conceptions of practice (cf. Lyle & Cushion, 2017). However, learning in this way is beyond existing conceptions of soccer coach education which is largely an additive re-tooling (grafting new 'skills'/knowledge onto an existing repertoire) rather than critically transformative (deconstructing taken-for-granted beliefs, assumptions, knowledge and habits, and rebuilding practice; Cushion, 2013, 2019).

## Conclusions and future directions

Ericsson and Charness (1994) argue that expertise is developed by learning through doing and is characterised by pattern recognition based on experience. Coaches can develop expert skills, behaviours, and practices based on highly interconnected knowledge structures, through conscious investment in, and refinement of, experiences. However, these suppositions remain largely untested in the coaching literature (Cushion, 2019). Taking a more process-oriented view, adaptive experts possess extensive, integrated knowledge differentiating them from routine experts (Hatano & Inagaki, 1986). Adaptive experts appear to focus on acquiring new domain knowledge and skills to apply across changing contexts as opposed to learning procedures; suggesting their training and development require a non-routine approach (Mees et al., 2020). Currently, in soccer, coach socialisation is the dominant means of sharing experiences and creating tacit knowledge, largely through informal processes. In recognition of this fact, linear, functionalist, and unproblematic coaching pathway models do not accurately reflect coaching reality, which is 'messy', 'fragmented', and situation-specific (Jones, Armour & Potrac, 2004, p. 1; Blackett et al., 2019). Currently, then, within coach education structures, it is unclear how coaches can engage in targeted 'deliberate' coaching practice to develop specific, context-relevant knowledge and skills and progress towards adaptive expertise.

Research into coach learning has suggested that rather than try to classify the best learning situation or source of coaching knowledge, it is more important to understand the complementarity of different learning situations in contributing to the development of expertise (Trudel et al., 2010). This blending rather than separation is key (Cushion et al., 2010). Contested processes of coach socialisation currently contour coach development by significantly influencing which information is initially acquired and then contextualised into useable knowledge (Blackett et al., 2019). These circumstances greatly influence the nature and likelihood of expertise being developed. Importantly for coaches, time constrains the amount and intensity of formal development that could enable the transfer of knowledge, yet acquiring experience is equally important. There remains, therefore, a requirement to disaggregate experience as a coach from coach education to help understand how coaches may develop requisite levels of expertise.

A need for more thorough, integrated, practical, and conceptually informed approaches to investigating how coaches develop and use their knowledge and skills in context is also apparent. What is clear is that the critical skills of adaptive expertise, including deep knowledge of the content domain, metacognitive skills and problem-solving across differing environments, require formal learning approaches that more accurately resemble continuous deliberate practice, employing explicit and unambiguous means of communication and feedback for coaches. More evidence is needed to say much with certainty about the most appropriate feedback to support coaches' developing adaptive expertise, but reflective conversations – repeated cycles of problem

192 *Christopher J. Cushion and Anna Stodter*

(re)appreciation, strategy generation, experimentation, and evaluation – based on specific practice issues and grounded in everyday experiences, appear to offer the potential for structuring feedback and learning in coaching. Reflective conversations can be embedded into coach development opportunities, notably supported by skilled coach developers to help coaches connect to and make sense of what is to be learned in their own changing environments, thereby facilitating more individually meaningful learning opportunities (Stodter, Cope & Townsend, 2021).

Video recordings of practice and systematic observation of coaching behaviour can also be built into the above process as a powerful catalyst to enhance coaches' self-awareness and metacognitive skills, ultimately working towards changing behaviour and practice in line with adaptive expertise. The significance of helping coaches to understand their own practice, their view of learning, and deliberately 'learning to learn' as part of learner-centred coach education has been noted (e.g., Paquette & Trudel, 2018) and this could be a fruitful but as yet under-evidenced area to develop adaptive expertise in coaching. Overall, rather than a rigid level- and competency-based formal coach education system reflecting the concept of expertise as an outcome, a shift in focus towards the processes of adaptive expertise and varied situations that facilitate learning of these in combination suggests a need for more aligned pedagogic agility in coach development (Mees et al., 2020).

## References

Abraham, A., Collins, D., & Martindale, R. (2006). The coaching schematic: validation through expert coach consensus. *Journal of Sports Sciences, 24*, 549–564.

Bachkirova, T., & Smith, C. (2015). From competencies to capabilities in the assessment and accreditation of coaches. *International Journal of Evidence Based Coaching and Mentoring, 13*(2), 123–140. https://radar.brookes.ac.uk/radar/items/a7515cd5-e58f-4aa6-b504-a1f9c6b92268/1/

Barker-Ruchti, N., Barker, D., Rynne, S. B., & Lee, J. (2016). Learning cultures and cultural learning in high-performance sport: opportunities for sport pedagogues. *Physical Education and Sport Pedagogy, 21*, 1–9.

Barnett, S., & Koslowski, B. (2002). Adaptive expertise: effects of type of experience and the level of theoretical understanding it generates. *Thinking & Reasoning, 8*(4), 237–267. https://doi.org/10.1080/13546780244000088

Berry, P. (2020). An alternative conceptualisation of coach expertise. *Coaching: An International Journal of Theory, Research and Practice, 14*(2), 202-213. DOI: 10.1080/17521882.2020.1853189

Blackett, A. D., Evans, A. B., & Piggott, D. (2019). "They have to toe the line": a Foucauldian analysis of the socialisation of former elite athletes into academy coaching roles. *Sports Coaching Review, 8*(1), 83–102, DOI: 10.1080/21640629.2018.1436502

Bransford, J., Derry, S., Berliner, D., Hammerness, K., & Beckett. K. L. (2005). Theories of learning and their roles in teaching. In L. Darling-Hammond & J. Bransford (Eds.). *Preparing Teachers for a Changing World: What Teachers Should Learn and Be Able to Do* (pp. 40–87). San Francisco: Jossey-Bass.

Brown, G., & Potrac, P. (2009). "You've not made the grade, son": de-selection and identity disruption in elite level youth football. *Soccer & Society, 10*, 143–159.

Carbonell, K., Könings, K., Segers, M., & van Merriënboer, J. (2016). Measuring adaptive expertise: development and validation of an instrument. *European Journal of Work and Organizational Psychology, 25*(2), 167–180. https://doi.org/10.1080/1359432X.2015.1036858

Cassidy, T. (2010). Understanding athlete learning and caching practice: utilising 'practice theories' and 'theories of practice'. In J. Lyle & C. Cushion (Eds.), *Sports Coaching Professionalization and Practice* (pp. 177–192). London: Churchill Livingstone Elsevier.

Chapman, R., Richardson, D., Cope, E., & Cronin, C. (2020). Learning from the past; a Frierean analysis of FA coach education since 1967. *Sport, Education and Society, 25* (6),618–697.

Chesterfield, G., Potrac, P., & Jones, R. L. (2010). 'Studentship' and 'impression management': coaches' experiences of an advanced soccer coach education award. *Sport, Education and Society, 15*, 299–314.

Ciampolini, V., Milistetd, M., Rynne, S. B., Brasil, V. Z., & do Nascimento, J. V. (2019). Research review on coaches' perceptions regarding the teaching strategies experienced in coach education programs. *International Journal of Sports, Science and Coaching, 14*(2), 216–228. https://doi.org/10.1177/1747954119833597

Cope, E., Cushion, C. J., Harvey, S., & Partington, M. (2021). Investigating the impact of a Freirean informed coach education programme. *Physical Education and Sport Pedagogy, 26*(1), 65–78. DOI: 10.1080/17408989.2020.1800619

Cope, E., Partington, M., Cushion, C. J., & Harvey, S. (2016). An investigation of professional top-level youth football coaches' questioning practice. *Qualitative Research in Sport, Exercise and Health, 8(4)*, 380–393. DOI: 10.1080/2159676X.2016.1157829

Cruickshank, A., Martindale, A., & Collins, D. (2018). Raising our game: the necessity and progression of expertise-based training in applied sport psychology. *Journal of Applied Sport Psychology, 32(3)*, 237–255. https://doi.org/10.1080/10413200.2018.1492471

Cushion. C. J. (2019). Observing coach behaviours: developing coaching practice and coach education? In Thelwell R., & Dicks M., (Eds). *Professional Advances in Sports Coaching: Research and Practice* (pp. 358–376). London: Routledge.

Cushion, C. J. (2013). Applying game centered approaches to coaching: a critical analysis of the 'dilemmas' of practice impacting change. *Sports Coaching Review, 2*(1), 61–76

Cushion, C. J., (2010). Coach behaviour. In. J. Lyle, & C. J. Cushion (Eds.), *Sports Coaching Professionalization and Practice* (pp. 43–62). London: Elsevier.

Cushion, C. J., Armour, K. M., & Jones, R. L. (2003). Coach education and continuing professional development: experience and learning to coach. *Quest, 55*(3), 215–230.

Cushion, C. J., Ford, P. R., & Williams, A. M. (2012a). Coach behaviours and practice structures in youth soccer: implications for talent development. *Journal of Sports Sciences, 30*(15), 1631–164.

Cushion, C. J., Harvey, S., Muir, B., & Nelson, L. (2012b). Developing the coach analysis and intervention system (CAIS): establishing validity and reliability of a computerised systematic observation instrument. *Journal of Sports Sciences, 30*(2), 203–218.

Cushion, C. J., Nelson, L., Armour, K., Lyle, J., Jones R. L., Sandford, R., & O'Callaghan, C. (2010). *Coach Learning and Development: A Review of Literature.* Leeds: Sports Coach.

Cushion, C. J., Stodter, A. & Clarke, N. J. (2021). 'It's an experiential thing': the discursive construction of learning in high-performance coach education. *Sport Education and Society, 27(7)*, 844–861. DOI: 10.1080/13573322.2021.1924143

Dempsey, N. M., Richardson, D. J., Cope, E., & Cronin, C. J. (2020). Creating and disseminating coach education policy: a case of formal coach education in grassroots football. *Sport, Education and Society, 26(8)*, 917–930. DOI:10.1080/13573322.2020.1802711

Downham, L., & Cushion, C. J., (2020). Reflection in a high-performance sport coach education programme: a Foucauldian analysis of coach developers. *International Sport Coaching Journal, 7(3)*, 347–359. https://doi.org/10.1123/iscj.2018-0093

Ericsson, K., & Charness, N. (1994). Expert performance: its structure and acquisition. *American Psychologist, 49*(8), 725–747. https://doi.org/10.1037/0003-066X.49.8.725

Farrington-Darby, T., & Wilson, J. (2006). The nature of expertise: a review. *Applied Ergonomics, 37*(1), 17–32. https://doi.org/10.1016/j.apergo.2005.09.001

Ford, P. R., Yates, I., & Williams, A. M. (2010). An analysis of practice activities and instructional behaviours used by youth soccer coaches during practice: exploring the link between science and application. *Journal of Sports Sciences, 28*, 483–495.

Ghaye, T. (2001). Reflective practice. *Faster, Higher, Stronger, 10*, 9–12.

Gilbert, W. D. & Trudel, P. (2001). Learning to coach through experience: reflection in model youth sport coaches. *Journal of Teaching in Physical Education, 21*, 16–34.

Harvey, S., Cushion, C. J., Wegis, H. M., & Massa-Gonzalez, A. N. (2010). Teaching games for understanding in American high-school soccer: a quantitative data analysis using the game performance assessment instrument. *Physical Education and Sport Pedagogy, 15*, 29–54.

Harvey, S., Cushion, C. J., & Massa-Gonzalez, A. N. (2011). Learning a new method: teaching games for understanding in the coaches' eyes. *Physical Education and Sport Pedagogy, 15*, 361–382.

Hatano, G., & Inagaki, K. (1986). Two courses of expertise. In H. Stevenson, H. Azuma, & K. Hakuta (Eds.), *Child Development and Education in Japan* (pp. 262–272). New York: Freeman. doi:10.1002/ccd.10470.

Hatano, G., & Oura, Y. (2003). Commentary: reconceptualizing school learning. *Educational Researcher, 32*(8), 26–29. doi:10.3102/0013189X032008026.

Hutton, R., Ward, P., Gore, J., Turner, P., Hoffman, R., & Conway, G. (2017). Developing adaptive expertise: a synthesis of literature and implications for training. In *13th International Conference on Naturalistic Decision Making* (pp. 81–86). Bath, UK.

Jones, R. L., Armour, K. M., & Potrac, P. (2004). Constructing expert knowledge: a case study of a top-level professional soccer coach. *Sport, Education and Society, 8*, 213–229.

Jones, R. L., Bailey, J., & Thompson, A. (2013). Ambiguity, noticing and orchestration: further thoughts on managing the complex coaching context. In P. Potrac, W. Gilbert & J. Denison (Eds.), *Routledge Handbook of Sports Coaching* (pp. 271–283). Abingdon, UK: Routledge.

Kirschner, P. A., Sweller J., & Clark, R. E. (2006). Why minimal guidance during instruction does not work: an analysis of the failure of constructivist, problem based, experiential and inquiry-based teaching. *Educational Psychologist, 41*(2), 75–86.

Lacy, A. C., & Darst, P. W. (1985). Systematic observation of behaviours of winning high school head football coaches. *Journal of Teaching in Physical Education, 4*, 256–270.

Lemyre, F., Trudel, P., & Durand-Bush, N. (2007). How youth-sport coaches learn to coach. *The Sport Psychologist, 21*, 191–209.

Lyle, J., & Cushion, C. J. (2017). *Sports Coaching Concepts: A Framework for Coaching Practice* (2nd ed). London: Routledge.

Mallett, C., Trudel, P., Lyle, J., & Rynne, S. (2009). Formal vs. informal coach education. *International Journal of Sports Science & Coaching, 4*(3), 325–364. doi:10.1260/174795409789623883

Martindale, A., & Collins, D. (2013). The development of professional judgment and decision-making expertise in applied sport psychology. *The Sport Psychologist, 27*(4), 390–399. https://doi.org/10.1123/tsp.27.4.390

Mayer, R. E. (2004). Should there be a three strikes rule against pure discovery learning? *American Psychologist, 59*(1), 14–19.

Mees, A., Sinfield, D., Collins, D., & Collins, L., (2020). Adaptive expertise: a characteristic of expertise in outdoor instructors? *Physical Education and Sport Pedagogy, 25*(4), 423–438.

Nash, C., & Collins, D. (2006). Tacit knowledge in expert coaching: science or art? *Quest, 58*, 465–477.

Nash, C., Martindale, R., Collins, D., & Martindale. A. (2012). Parameterising expertise in coaching: past, present and future. *Journal of Sports Sciences, 30*(10), 985–994. doi:10.1080/02640414.2012.682079.

O'Connor, D., Larkin, P., & Williams, M. (2017). Observations of youth football training. How do coaches structure training sessions for player development? *Journal of Sport Sciences, 36*(1), 39–47.

O'Connor, D., Larkin, P., & Williams, M. (2018). What earning environments help improve decision-making? *Physical Education and Sport Pedagogy, 22*(6), 647–660.

Owen, J., & Lindley, L. (2010). Therapists' cognitive complexity: review of theoretical models and development of an integrated approach for training. *Training and Education in Professional Psychology, 4*(2), 128–137. https://doi.org/10.1037/a0017697

Paquette, K., & Trudel, P. (2018). Learner-centered coach education: practical recommendations for coach development administrators. *International Sport Coaching Journal*, 5(1), 169–175.

Partington, M., & Cushion, C. (2013). An investigation of the practice activities and coaching behaviors of professional top-level youth soccer coaches. *Scandinavian Journal of Medicine & Science in Sports, 13*, 1–9.

Partington, M., Cushion, C. J., Cope, E., & Harvey, S. (2015). The impact of video feedback on professional youth football coaches' reflection and practice behaviour: a longitudinal investigation of behaviour change. *Reflective Practice: International and Multidisciplinary Perspectives, 16(5),* 700–716. DOI: 10.1080/14623943.2015.1071707.

Piggott, D. (2012). Coaches' experiences of formal coach education: a critical sociological investigation. *Sport, Education and Society, 17*(4), 535–554.

Potrac P., & Cassidy, T. (2006). The coach as 'more capable other'. In R. L. Jones (ed.), *The Sports Coach as Educator Re-conceptualising Sports Coaching* (pp 39–50). London: Routledge.

Potrac, P., Jones, R. L., & Cushion, C. J., (2007). Understanding power and the coach's role in professional English soccer: a preliminary investigation of coach behaviour. *Soccer and Society, 8*, 33–49.

Sawiuk, R., Taylor, W., & Groom, R. (2016). Exploring formalized elite coach mentoring programmes in the UK. *Sport, Education and Society, 23*(6), 619–631. doi:10.108 0/13573322.2016.1248386

Schempp, P. G., & McCullick, B. (2010). Coaches' expertise. In J. Lyle & C. Cushion (Eds.), *Sports Coaching: Professionalisation and Practice* (pp. 221–231). China: Elsevier.

Schraw, G. S., Crippen, K. J., & Hartley, K. (2006). Promoting self-regulation in science education: metacognition as part of a broader perspective on learning. *Research in Science Education, 36,* 111–139.

Sfard, A. (1998). On two metaphors for learning and the dangers of choosing just one. *Educational Researcher, 27*, 4–13.

Sonnentage, S., Niessen, C., & Volmer, J. (2006). Expertise in software design. In A. Ericsson, N. Charness, P. Feltovich, & R. Hoffman (Eds.), *The Cambridge Handbook of Expertise and Expert Performance* (pp. 373–389). Cambridge University Press, Cambridge, UK.

Stodter, A., & Cushion, C. J. (2014). Coaches' learning and education: a case study of cultures in conflict. *Sports Coaching Review, 3*(1), 63–79.

Stodter, A., & Cushion, C. J. (2017). What works in coach learning, how, and for whom? A grounded process of soccer coaches' professional learning. *Qualitative Research in Sport, Exercise and Health, 9*(3), 321–338.

Stodter, A., & Cushion, C. J. (2019a). Evidencing the impact of coaches' learning: changes in coaching knowledge and practice over time. *Journal of Sports Sciences, 37*(18), 2086–2093.

Stodter, A., & Cushion. C. J. (2019b). Layers of learning in coach developers' practice theories, preparation and delivery. *International Sport Coaching Journal, 6*(3), 307–316.

Anna Stodter, Ed Cope & Robert C. Townsend (2021) Reflective conversations as a basis for sport coaches' learning: a theory-informed pedagogic design for educating reflective practitioners, Professional Development in Education, DOI: 10.1080/19415257.2021.1902836

Swap, D., Leonard, D., Shields, M., & Abrams, A. (2001) Using mentoring and storytelling to transfer knowledge in the workplace. *Journal of Management Information Systems, 18*(1), 95–114.

Townsend, R. C., & Cushion, C. (2017). Elite cricket coach education: a Bourdieusian analysis. *Sport, Education and Society, 4*, 528–546.

Townsend, R. C., Huntley, T. D., Cushion, C. J., & Culver, D. (2021). Infusing disability into coach education and development: a critical review and agenda for change. *Physical Education and Sport Pedagogy, 27(3),* 247–260. DOI: 10.1080/17408989.2021.1873932

Trudel, P., Culver, D., & Werthner, P. (2013). Looking at coach development from the coach-learner's perspective: considerations for coach development administrators. In P. Potrac, W.

Gilbert & J. Denison (Eds.), *Routledge Handbook of Sports Coaching* (pp. 375–387). London: Routledge.

Trudel, P., & Gilbert, W. (2006). Coaching and coach education. In D. Kirk, D. Macdonald & M. O'Sullivan (Eds.), *The Handbook of Physical Education*. London: Sage.

Trudel, P., Gilbert, W., & Werthner, P. (2010). Coach education effectiveness. In J. Lyle & C. Cushion (Eds.) *Sports Coaching: Professionalisation and Practice* (pp. 135–152). China: Elsevier.

Turner, D., Nelson, L., & Potrac, P. (2012). The journey *is* the destination: reconsidering the expert sports coach. *Quest, 64*, 313–325.

Werthner, P., & Trudel, P. (2009). Investigating the idiosyncratic learning paths of elite Canadian coaches. *International Journal of Sports Science & Coaching, 4*, 433–449.

Williams, S., & Bush, A. J. (2019). Connecting knowledge(s) to practice: a Bernsteinian theorising of a collaborative coach learning community project. *Sport, Education and Society, 24*(4), 375–389.

# Section C

# Sports Medicine and Biomechanics

# 13 Injury epidemiology, monitoring, and prevention

*Ian Beasley*

## Introduction

Soccer is a contact sport, involving running, jumping, and changing direction suddenly (known as 'cutting'), whereas for goalkeepers it involves diving with unprotected landing. It follows, therefore, that injury is part of playing the sport, and this can be related to any of the above activities or by way of contact with other players, or on-pitch/off-pitch hardware, such as goalposts or advertising hoardings. Professional players train for up to 3 h daily and play competitive matches (at least) twice a week, placing upon them what might be considered unreasonable physiological and psychological stress.

Most practitioners working in professional soccer can identify players that seem to be more susceptible to injury than others, and some who seem to take longer than others to recover from injury. Suffice to say that like the general population, players are a 'mixed bag' and idiosyncratically respond to the demands of the sport, both in performance and susceptibility to, and recuperation from, injury. The mechanism of injury may be of use when trying to assess severity, and in the modern game, there are video recordings of incidents that can be evaluated 'live' by staff on the team bench and help guide management of injuries via radio link with the practitioners attending the injury. Concussion is often best observed from the stand, and 'spotters' are now deployed with video replay facilities, as well as a better vantage point to view the field of play, enabling them to deliver real-time information to those delivering emergency aid to the injured player on the field, for instance, regarding whether the player concerned lost consciousness.

## Epidemiology of injury

The largest body of work in this field is the UEFA Champions League (UCL) studies (Ekstrand et al., 2020), which have been running since 2001. These studies include data from professional clubs in European Leagues that are involved in the pan-European competitions run by UEFA. The findings have highlighted the most common injury patterns in soccer (Ekstrand et al., 2016), as well as injury trends (Ekstrand et al., 2016), and average time loss from injury. From a practitioner's point of view, this information is valuable when predicting re-availability/return to play (RTP) (Ekstrand et al., 2020, Lubberts et al., 2019). Availability of players within a squad has been shown to contribute to success of a team (Ekstrand, 2013).

There are now many epidemiological studies from different leagues and competitions across the globe revealing underlying injury patterns (Ekstrand et al., 2020;

DOI: 10.4324/9781003148418-16

200 *Ian Beasley*

Mosler et al., 2018; Tabben et al., 2021). It is useful also, within a league, to understand what the 'normal' (in a Gaussian distribution sense) injury rates are. Any research into injury patterns within a league should be shared between clubs/teams, so that any glaring differences can be examined, and acted upon so that players are protected from injury.

Within clubs, epidemiological studies are useful in understanding which injuries are more common, when injury risk is highest (e.g., with higher match frequency), and which player positions are most susceptible to injury. Planning and preparation within a medical and sports science multi-disciplinary team (MDT) on where the 'pinch points' are in a season, and which injuries are more common, helps in advising coaching staff when players might be at greater risk.

## Screening/profiling and injury mitigation

There have been endless discussions about screening/periodic health evaluation and whether it prevents injury (Bahr, 2016; Boles et al., 2015), and whether we profile or screen. Wilson and Jungner (1968) described the criteria in Public Health circles for mass screening programmes (e.g., cervical cancer screening) and some of their principles apply when screening in this context, and this is where profiling, rather than screening comes into the picture. For instance, one of Wilson and Jungners' criteria states, *'The natural history of the disease or condition should be adequately understood, the disease or condition well defined, and there should be a detectable pre-clinical phase'*. This is clearly often not the case in musculoskeletal injury. This has ramifications, in explaining why a condition was not picked up in a pre-signing medical, or a pre-season screening session, despite investigating things to the full. The use of the term profiling/screening is probably more appropriate, with the emphasis on the stroke. There may be some things that are detectable, but certainly not all. We can measure quite well but are unable to always predict. It is fair to say that screening can identify some susceptibilities (e.g., hypermobility, Paccy et al., 2010); cardiac risk (Malhotra et al., 2017), but soccer is an unpredictable sport, and injuries and other issues will occur, hence the use of 'injury and illness mitigation' rather than injury prevention.

Most professional clubs will carry out profiling/screening activity, which may consist only of statutory cardiac screening, or may consist of cardiac, medical, musculoskeletal, nutritional, and psycho-social components. Screening/profiling resources and is usually carried out during the pre-season conditioning period. This process can coincide with times when coaches require players to be available for training, hence planning the screening/profiling with coaching staff is important so that it can take place without the pressure of players having to be available for other activities. A proper and honest assessment of the time needed for adequate profiling/screening should be agreed upon within the medical and science MDT, and presented to team management, and a timetable agreed.

The epidemiological literature will outline what the most common injuries are (Ekstrand et al., 2016; Tabben et al., 2021) whereas other research findings will indicate what susceptibilities might be implicated. As more publications appear, possible causations as well as treatments change or are refined, so a constant surveillance of current knowledge is important. The published evidence will guide screening practice, so that any prevention/mitigation of injury can be achieved by acting on findings during the screening session.

At the end of the session, all the information gathered should be collated and reviewed. For instance, a certain player may be weak or lack flexibility in an area where they have (perhaps) sustained an injury in the past. The issue(s) can be explained to the player, and an agreed programme to address weaknesses can be made. A set period is given before a reassessment of the issue to review progress, and further action/maintenance plan.

## Muscle injury

Muscle injuries are common in soccer (Ekstrand et al., 2012), and mostly non-contact in origin, with the hamstring being the most frequently injured (see Figure 13.1; Ekstrand et al., 2012)

Muscle injury occurs when the muscle is stretched beyond its capacity to resist the excessive stretching force applied to it, causing tearing and disruption of the muscle fibres, the connective tissue, and the tendons associated with the muscle. Some tendons are intramuscular, that is, within the muscle itself (e.g., in the soleus muscle). When a muscle injury occurs, the player will often describe hearing or feeling something 'go'. This should not be taken as necessarily indicating a more severe injury, but is an important issue for the player, as they perceive it as such. The extent of muscle injury, as one might expect, has a bearing on when a player might RTP. The amount of damage is graded so that prognostication is more accessible. The first question asked by players, coaches, and fans alike is – how long will it be before RTP!

There have been many grading systems described and Grassi et al. (2016) gives a comprehensive overview of the evolution of the grading systems, and how imaging modalities and research findings (e.g., of tendon involvement influencing the time of RTP) have necessitated modifications and additions to each system, leading to the creation of new categories and gradings. As mentioned, with grading, a more accurate prediction of RTP (Ardern et al., 2016) can be made, and this is of psychological benefit to the

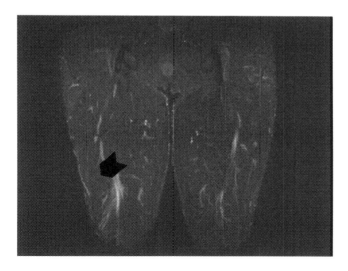

*Figure 13.1* Hamstring injury.

202 *Ian Beasley*

athlete and of practical worth to the coaching staff, who may need to plan to recruit a replacement.

Imaging is undoubtedly useful in the management of muscle injuries. Armed with the extent of muscle damage, cross-referencing this with which grade the injury can be assigned to help not only to prognosticate RTP but also to guide practitioners in the rehabilitation process. When treating muscle injuries, the aim is to return the player to full activity while avoiding a recurrence of the injury. Recurrence is a well-known hazard of muscle injury, often taking longer to recover than the initial injury (Donmez et al., 2020). As radiological imaging techniques have improved, it is now possible to grade the extent of a muscle injury using MRI or ultrasonography (Pollock et al., 2014; Hamilton et al., 2015; Lee & Healy, 2004). Muscle damage, as with any healing tissue, results in some scarring. Scar tissue is non-contractile and is at risk of being torn during normal muscle action during the RTP process or when the player has returned to play. While this is not usually a significant problem, repeated injury at or near the site of an original injury is worrisome and can interrupt successful RTP.

Myositis ossificans is a well-known complication of muscle injury, often resulting from direct trauma to the muscle in a tackle, or with collision with pitch-side apparatus. The trauma prompts the formation of ectopic bone in the muscle. It takes 2–3 weeks to establish itself and can take up to a year to resolve spontaneously (https://orthobullets.com/pathology/8042/myositis ossificans). The calcification can be seen on plain radiographs, but often the manual examination findings are more impressive than the x-ray appearance. Ultrasound examination is a much more sensitive way to view this injury and following progress of resolution can be better monitored using this modality, as well as avoiding repeated radiation exposure (Lacout et al., 2012).

## Treatment

Treatment of muscle injuries is well-established. The acronyms POLICE (Bleakley et al., 2012) or PRICE (Brooks et al., 1981) give a guide to initial/first aid treatment regimens (see Table 13.1).

*Table 13.1* The POLICE/PRICE guidelines to initial/first-aid treatment

| |
| --- |
| P= ***Protection*** *from further injury, which usually means withdrawing the player from performing is standard in all first-aid advice.* |
| OL/R = ***Optimal Loading,*** *or* ***Rest****. This amounts to the same thing. A player can weight bear if they are not going to injure the part more.* |
| I = ***Ice****, to reduce inflammation and pain.* |
| C = ***Compression*** *to reduce bleeding at the site of injury.* |
| E = ***Elevation,*** *to help drain any accumulating inflammatory oedema causing congestion around the injury that potentially inhibits early local biochemical activity that leads to efficient healing.* |
| P = ***Protection*** *from further injury, which usually means withdrawing the player from performing is standard in all first-aid advice.* |
| OL/R = ***Optimal Loading,*** *or* ***Rest****. This amounts to the same thing. A player can weight bear if they are not going to injure the part more.* |
| I = ***Ice****, to reduce inflammation and pain.* |
| C = ***Compression*** *to reduce bleeding at the site of injury.* |
| E = ***Elevation,*** *to help drain any accumulating inflammatory oedema causing congestion around the injury that potentially inhibits early local biochemical activity that leads to efficient healing.* |

*Injury epidemiology, monitoring, and prevention* 203

After being withdrawn from the field of play, and first aid treatment administered, and the diagnosis confirmed by investigation, the next steps in management of the injury are made by the medical and sports science MDT, and a plan formulated with a prediction of RTP. Early predictions, as in any branch of medicine, are not definitive. Communication to team management staff of the possible deviations from a prospective timeline should be explained so that there are no surprises when things, as is often the case, do not progress in the desired linear fashion.

The next phase in managing an injured player is where the MDT planning becomes most important. Physiotherapy treatment in the early stages forms the basis of physical treatment. To make sure that healing and adapting tissues have the right environment to optimally recover, performance nutrition is an important tool to use. Early deployment is essential so that the different phases of inflammation, through to the healing of an injury are supported by appropriate supplementation of the normal diet.

Psychological support is warranted, as the player will inevitably have concerns about recovery, any threat an injury might have to their career, and whether an injury may impact income. Following mood and sleep patterns and addressing any 'bumps in the road' is important in helping the player cope with the evolution of an injury towards RTP. As implied above, recovery from injury does not follow straight lines, and there will be times when the rate of progress is slower than the athlete wishes. For long-term injuries, such as anterior cruciate ligament (ACL) reconstruction or severe fracture, there is evidence that psychological support is important, despite not all clubs having resources to offer this support (Gervis et al., 2020). A more thorough understanding of players' fears and anxieties is valuable in the holistic/MDT approach to care. This is oft best obtained using a psychologist, who may have better-interviewing skills and more time to use them. Sharing knowledge obtained can be invaluable when planning the varying care pathway. Once the player is 'off the couch' the sports science and fitness coach teams become more heavily involved, the pathway to RTP is usually clearer, but, of course, beware the ups and downs of rehabilitation.

## Joint injury

In soccer, ankle and knee joints are the commonest injury (Lopez-Valenciano et al., 2020) with shoulder, elbow, and hand/wrist more common in goalkeepers (Ekstrand et al., 2013). Joint injuries can result in damage that causes problems in later life with knee and hip osteoarthritis being more common in ex-players as is the need for arthroplasty for these two joints in retired professional population (Fernandes et al., 2018; Van den Noort et al., 2021). Each joint is different, but there are some commonalities. Joints are enclosed in a joint capsule, and mostly with a synovial membrane within the capsule producing synovial fluid, which helps nourish the joint. Joint surfaces are covered in hyaline (articular) cartilage, which is a glass-like substance consisting of type II collagen and chondromucoprotein (www.medcell.med.yale.edu/histology/connective_tissue_lab/hyaline_cartilage.php) which when under compression 'evens out' the effects of pressure by moving water within the substance of the hyaline cartilage away from the point of pressure. After the pressure is removed during the completion of a movement, the water returns to the area, which helps prevent wearing at those areas of the joint surface experiencing most use.

The bones forming the joint are held together by ligaments which attach to the bones on each side. These stabilising ligaments are usually called collateral ligaments.

In general, the bigger the joint, the more complex the ligaments. The bones forming the knee joint, for instance, the biggest joint in the body, must weight bear and the ligaments must manage multi-directional forces. It has collateral ligaments and cruciate ligaments, as well as some accessory ligaments to ensure that during ambulation, and sometimes at speed, the knee retains its integrity.

Joint injuries cause inflammation, which is usually associated with joint swelling due to fluid collection within the joint caused when the synovial membrane over-produces fluid – this inflammation is its normal response to injury. Bleeding into the joint (called a haemarthrosis) caused by tearing of tissues within the joint also causes swelling. Taking an accurate history from the player about the injury is important. Immediate (or within an hour or so) swelling indicates a haemarthrosis and indicates significant damage to the joint. Quite apart from the injury that has caused bleeding into the joint, blood in the joint is damaging to the joint surfaces. For this reason, it may be reasonable to attempt to aspirate the joint to minimise the irritation.

Examination of joints should be approached with a routine in mind that is reproducible. The examiner should have an idea of what normal function is, and if possible, the contralateral joint should be assessed as a 'normal' control. It is helpful to first make sure that you, as the examiner, are not going to cause so much discomfort to the player that they are unable to comply with the examination and are guarding so much that no useful information can be obtained – despite the accurate history that you will have already obtained.

## Knee injury

### *Meniscus injuries*

There are two menisci (medial and lateral) in the knee. They are made of fibrocartilage. The lateral is smaller than the medial. They sit on top of the tibia, and act as a cushion, as well as making the relatively flat top of the tibia a better fit with the more rounded condyles of the femur. They are susceptible to injury when the femur rotates on a fixed tibia, for instance, when the foot is planted on the turf (and stuck because of boot studs) and cannot rotate. Characteristically, the knee swells within 12 h, often the player wakes with swelling the next day, describing it as 'it looked like a grapefruit'.

There are many types of meniscal injuries, or tears (see Figures 13.2 and 13.3; Nguyen et al., 2014), and the ongoing management of this injury can depend on the type of tear. The meniscus has a blood supply, richer in the periphery, which declines with age. It follows that it may be possible to repair/suture together a meniscal tear if it is in a zone where there is a blood supply; named, for obvious reasons, the 'red zone'. Resection of significant amounts of a meniscus, or total meniscectomy results in the knee becoming more susceptible to degenerative change, and earlier onset of osteoarthritis (see Figure 13.4; Ardern, 2013).

## Cruciate ligament injuries

There are two cruciate ligaments, anterior and posterior. The 'anterior' and 'posterior' refer to where the respective ligaments are attached to the tibial spine; this the prominence/line on the tibial plateau which bisects the medial and lateral parts (or condyles) of the tibial plateau. The ACL is injured more often than the posterior

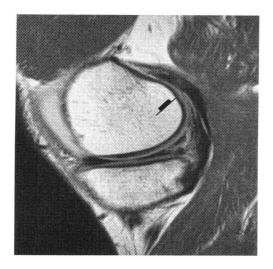

*Figure 13.2* Meniscal tear.

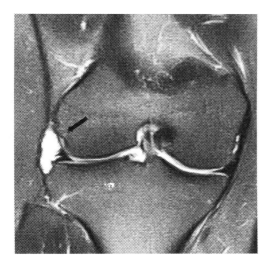

*Figure 13.3* Meniscal cyst.

cruciate ligament (PCL), and results in a haemarthrosis (see Figure 13.5). The incidence of ACL-related knee injuries has been quoted to be as high as 50% (Joseph et al., 2013). The mechanism of injury is by an external tibial rotational force with knee valgus strain, usually non-contact, and often when 'cutting'. The player often hears a 'pop' in the knee at the time of injury. An ACL rupture is almost invariably managed with surgery. There is some research evidence that shows that players can RTP without surgery (Ardern, 2013), but rehabilitation without surgical intervention

206 *Ian Beasley*

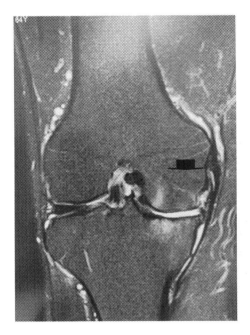

*Figure 13.4* Degenerative change after meniscectomy.

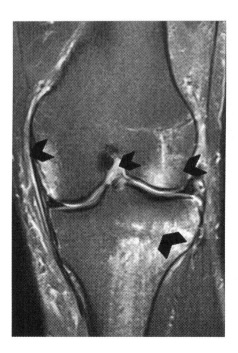

*Figure 13.5* ACL rupture, with bone bruising, and medial collateral ligament injury

from this injury can take 3 months or more, and if rehabilitation fails and surgery is required, the RTP time is much longer. The longer time span from the advent of the injury to RTP is undesirable in the professional game, but may be more acceptable in the recreational player.

ACL injury is often combined with other damage to intra-articular structures. O'Donoghue (1950) described an 'unhappy triad' of ACL rupture, medial collateral ligament (MCL) tear, and medial meniscus disruption (see Figure 13.6). It is essential that any management considers the condition of the whole joint when planning treatment. At professional level, 83% return to the same level as prior to injury (Lai et al., 2018). Median time to RTP in professional sport is 6–13 months (Lai et al., 2018), but it should be borne in mind that players in this situation have physiotherapy and rehabilitation daily, something that may not be available to all at the recreational level.

PCL injuries are uncommon, with an incidence of 0.65–3% of all sports-related knee injuries (Longo et al., 2021) usually caused by a direct blow to the front of the tibia, and around the tibial tuberosity, on a flexed knee forcing the tibia backwards, and tearing the PCL (described as a 'dashboard injury' from the days before seat belts). Isolated PCL injuries are often managed without surgery, but this injury can be associated with damage to other stabilising structures at the postero-lateral corner (PLC) of the joint. Proper assessment of the joint needs to be carried out to ascertain if this is the case. Surgery may be needed with complex injuries of this type, or at least bracing, depending on the severity. It can be confusing to hear that a player has a PCL/PLC injury!

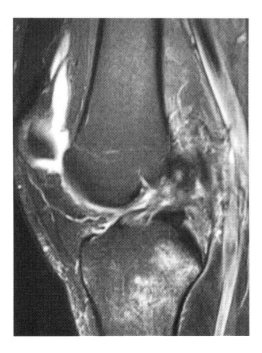

*Figure 13.6* ACL rupture sagittal.

## Medial collateral ligament (MCL)

The MCL is a large ligament that originates at the superior part of the medial femoral condyle and extends to a hand's width below the joint line of the knee to an attachment on the tibia. It journeys slightly forwards to its attachment, resisting lateral tibial rotation as well as the valgus strain of the knee. Injury to this ligament is usually because of a forced valgus strain, with external rotation of the tibia often involved. This causes the ligament to tear and become laxer, and the extent of the laxity directs the grading of the tear. The injury is graded I–III, with treatment driven by the grading, although recently a novel grading has been reported with five grades of tear, with the aim of refining treatment regimens (Makhmalbaf et al., 2018). Treatment includes bracing to prevent extension of the injury and on occasion surgery, but physiotherapy with rehabilitation is the mainstay of treatment.

## Ankle

The ankle is held together by a complex array of ligaments. The tibia and fibula are bound together near the joint by strong ligaments at the front and back (the anterior and posterior inferior tibiofibular ligaments – AITFL and PITFL) with the interosseus membrane in between the two bones, as its name suggests. These three elements are known as ankle syndesmosis. The MCL of the ankle joint is a strong band of tissue consisting of two layers. The superficial layer consists of the tibionavicular, tibiospring, tibiocalcaneal, and superficial posterior tibiotalar ligaments. The deep layer consists of the anterior tibiotalar ligament and the deep posterior tibiotalar ligament. The lateral ligament complex comprises three parts; the anterior talofibular ligament (ATFL), the calcaneofibular ligament (CFL), and the posterior talofibular ligament (PTFL). The lateral ligament complex, particularly the ATFL, is the most injured, and the usual mechanism is a forced inversion of the ankle, often when landing after jumping (see Figure 13.7).

Complete rupture of the ATFL can lead to anteroposterior instability of the ankle, and place extra strain on the other structures around the ankle, causing recurrent swelling and pain – the 'chronic ankle'. Rehabilitation is the key to mitigating the effect of the ATFL deficiency and continued topping up of the rehabilitation process is necessary – even when the player has returned to playing and training fully.

The three elements of rehabilitation are stretch, strength, and proprioception. Proprioception is an ability of the tissues around the joint to avoid damage by acting on a spinal reflex initiated by stretch receptors that are present in all tissues. If it appears that the joint is in a position where it may be injured, the stretch receptors prompt a change in body posture to avoid damage. Think of the situation where, on occasion, you may have tripped and almost injured on your ankle whilst walking along on an uneven surface, but somehow, and without conscious effort, you manage to re-gain balance before falling and injuring yourself. This is a system that is damaged when the joint itself is damaged, but it is something that can be trained back so that further harm to the joint is prevented. Any player who has twisted their ankle will be seen on various pieces of apparatus in the rehabilitation gym trying to maintain balance on the injured ankle (see Figure 13.8). This encourages the neural pathways to re-engage with the aim of keeping the patient upright, as well as preventing further damage to the ankle. Occasionally, if an ATFL-deficient ankle persists in swelling and with dysfunction, surgical intervention may be necessary to try and stabilise the joint.

*Injury epidemiology, monitoring, and prevention* 209

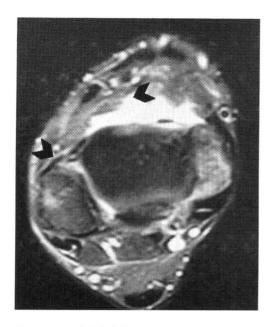

*Figure 13.7* Ankle injury.

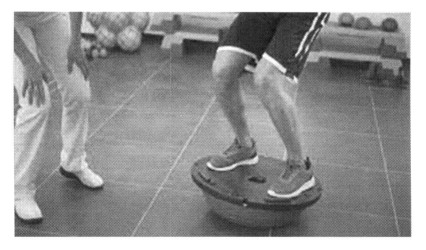

*Figure 13.8* Wobble (balance) board to improve proprioception

210  *Ian Beasley*

'High ankle sprains' is a term used to describe injury to the AITFL, PITFL, and the interosseus membrane-the ankle syndesmosis. The mechanism for this injury is often a forced external rotation of the joint, often combined with dorsiflexion. The three parts of the ligament complex tend to get damaged in sequence, AITFL, then interosseus membrane, and then PITFL. The MCL complex is usually damaged to some extent at the same time. These injuries are best assessed, after taking a history and examining the joint, by imaging with MRI scanning. The full extent of the damage can be difficult to assess clinically, certainly in the acute phase, and usually, management is driven by MRI appearances. In general, if all three of the syndesmosis elements are markedly injured, surgery may be opted for; a loose syndesmosis leads to joint instability. Stabilising and immobilising the joint while the ligaments have healed is the aim of surgery.

## Tendon injury

Tendons are made of type 1 collagen (65–80%) and elastin (1–2%) embedded in a proteoglycan-water matrix (Kannus, 2000). The tendon has a microstructure of cross-linkage and bundling to form the whole tendon, which is surrounded by a sheath called the paratenon. Tendons are structures that attach a muscle to a bone. When a muscle contracts, it pulls on the bone via the tendon and the limb/part concerned moves. Tendon injuries are not uncommon in soccer with varying degrees of damage from strains to tears, to complete rupture, and often in conjunction with muscle injury, for instance, the intramuscular tendon of the rectus femoris. Some tendons, such as the Achilles and patellar tendons are prone to overuse causing degenerative change within the tendon substance.

The issue with tendon disruption of any kind is that blood supply is low and so healing is slow. Even though not commonplace, tendon ruptures, such as those of the Achilles (Tarantino et al., 2020), require surgical intervention, at least in professional and academy players. Achilles tendon rupture in the recreational player is often treated conservatively with the ankle in equinus (toes pointing down-full plantar flexion) initially, and gradually reducing back to a normal position (Holm et al., 2015). This is achieved using a heel wedge (or wedges) in a boot plastic boot. The size or number of wedges is gradually reduced until the neutral position is reached.

Tendinopathy is an overuse condition of a tendon, where, in response to overload, the tendon tries to adapt, and produces more tenocytes and supportive matrix to cope with the excess load (Sharma & Maffulli, 2006). This results in a tendon less able to withstand this extra burden, which leads to pain and dysfunction. In soccer, Achilles and patellar tendon (see Figure 13.9) involvement are the most common, but goalkeepers may suffer the same issues with rotator cuff tendons of the shoulder, and wrist extensor or flexor tendons at the elbow.

Although MRI imaging will help exclude other diagnoses in the region of pain (e.g., co-existing fat pad syndrome or bursitis in the case of patellar tendinopathy), ultrasound is the investigation of choice for tendons, and the feature in tendinopathy that is best seen with ultrasound is neovascularisation. This is visualised with the use of Doppler software and can show dramatic changes within the tendon. The neovascular changes represent the endeavours of the tendon to heal, with the new vessels growing in to aid the process (see Figure 13.10).

Ultrasound tissue characterisation (UTC) scanning is another technique using ultrasound, but shows the damaged/degenerative areas of the tendon involved in more

Injury epidemiology, monitoring, and prevention 211

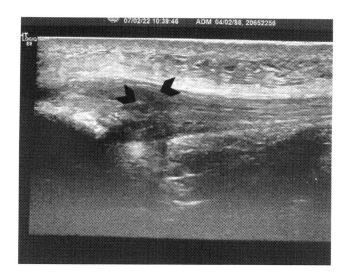

*Figure 13.9* Patellar tendinopathy.

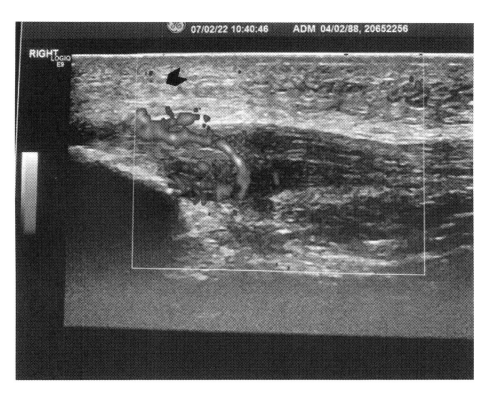

*Figure 13.10* Patellar tendinopathy with Doppler© 2022 Christoph Spang, Lorenzo Masci and Håkan Alfredson. https://www.mdpi.com/1648-9144/58/5/601/htm

detail than the standard 'grey-scale' ultrasound used regularly in clinical practice (Winter Bee et al., 2017). Following progress using UTC gives a better idea of the restoration of normalised anatomy, helping to guide the rehabilitation process towards normal function.

Treatment revolves around physiotherapy. When seeing patients in the clinic, they will often give a long history with periods of enforced rest due to pain, thinking that rest will help heal the issue. This is one of the situations where (graded) exercise is curative, but rest is not. Disused tendons show similar histological changes as overuse tendinopathic ones (Cook & Purdam, 2018). The physiotherapist will initiate the graded exercise programme, often starting with isometric 'holds', where the player resists a weight, but holds (in the case of Achilles tendinopathy) the ankle joint in neutral, with the muscle not lengthening or shortening. Weight and time of holding are incremental and done so whilst monitoring symptoms and reaction to each session. The exercise that most will know is then brought in, which is 'eccentric exercises'. This produces load for the tendon, which hopefully will promote healing (Rees et al., 2008; Grigg et al., 2009). Eccentric exercise is a muscle contraction while the muscle/tendon unit lengthens – think of putting something heavy down on the ground after lifting. Lengthening your muscles to do this equates to an eccentric contraction. Other treatments involve extra-corporeal shockwave therapy (Abdelkader et al., 2021), and injection therapy using differing chemical (e.g., corticosteroid and hyaluronic acid) and biochemical (e.g., platelet-rich plasma and other orthobiologics) agents (Madhi et al., 2020; Jiang et al., 2020; Nuhmani, 2020; Lopez-Royo et al., 2020; Saif Azmy et al., 2021).

## Bone injury

Bone injury falls into two categories, acute and overuse. Professional teams can expect one to two fractures per season (Larsson et al., 2016). Most are traumatic in nature due to contact with another player or an object on the field (e.g., goal post) or near the field (e.g., advertising hoardings), but can be due to falling or landing awkwardly when jumping. The commonest bones injured are lower limb in outfield players and upper limb in goalkeepers (study of Qatar Super League players: personal communication). Bones bleed when fractured, and localised swelling is an early indication that the injury may be a fracture. The investigation of choice if a fracture is suspected is plain x-ray, although often an MRI is ordered as the diagnosis is not clear from either mechanism or history and examination. If a fracture is reported then appropriate further imaging may be required, which may be plain x-ray or CT scan. As with any other type of injury, once a definitive diagnosis and grading/extent of the fracture (e.g., displacement/comminuted or not) is made, further management can be planned.

The reported time loss for this type of injury depends, as one might expect, on the bone injured, and the type of fracture, open or closed (an open fracture is one where the skin is breached), comminuted or not (a comminuted fracture is one where the bone is in many pieces), or displaced or not. All these factors are considered when planning further management and whether the player may need surgery. Decisions should be made in a shared and multi-disciplinary environment. These injuries can be career-threatening, and all those concerned in player care, which includes coaching staff, should be involved in the process and be aware of the issues. In general, although the absence after fracture is quoted as 32 days (median), the range is much greater, between 1 and 278 days (Larsson et al., 2016).

*Injury epidemiology, monitoring, and prevention* 213

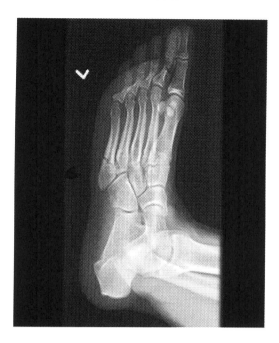

*Figure 13.11* Jones fracture.

Overuse bony injuries are stress fractures and occur at approximately one-tenth the incidence of traumatic fractures, although appear to take longer before the player returns to action (Larsson et al., 2016). The initial investigation of choice once again will be x-ray but will often not yield a diagnosis. MRI will demonstrate the subtle signs of a stress injury or stress fracture to bone and is quoted as the 'gold standard' in diagnosis (Saunier & Chapurlat, 2018). Stress injuries and fractures to bone have a grading system which helps to prognosticate when managing this type of injury (Fredericson et al., 1995; Kijowski et al., 2012).

Conservative treatment is the cornerstone of fracture management of any kind, with immobilisation in a cast or other device mandatory while the bones heal. However, there are instances where surgical intervention is required, and fixation of the bones in a position where healing can take place. Surgical intervention can be necessary in either traumatic fractures (e.g., tibia and fibula fracture) or overuse fractures (e.g., navicular stress fracture). For most stress injuries, however, a period of relative rest is often enough to allow the bone to heal without intervention. This can entail a period of non-weight bearing (e.g., pelvic stress fracture) or immobilisation (e.g., metatarsal stress fracture).

One well-known type of stress fracture is that of the fifth metatarsal, the eponymous 'Jones fracture'. After some high-profile players sustained this injury, it gained some renown (figure 13.11).

At the time, there were some changes in boot design that seemed to pre-dispose to sustaining this injury (Kijowski et al., 2012). Biomechanics, boot design, and nutrition status must all be considered when planning a prevention, or mitigation strategy.

214 *Ian Beasley*

Professional players have highly lucrative contracts with boot companies, and it is sometimes necessary to liaise with these companies to make sure there the player will not fall foul of a new boot design which may not suit their biomechanical makeup.

## Women's soccer

The injuries are the same, but female soccer warrants a separate section because of a slightly different pattern of injury (Larruskain. et al., 2018), and an explanation regarding some of the reasons why, and the prevention strategies that might be employed. It is well-documented now that differing levels of oestrogen during the menstrual cycle influence injury incidence (Chidi-Ogbolu et al., 2019; Martin et al., 2021). It is well-established that ACL rupture is more common in women (Larruskain. et al., 2018), and in part this is due to the ACL becoming laxer, with anteroposterior translation increasing incrementally until the pre-ovulatory phase (Belanger et al., 2013; Shultz et al., 2005), making the ligament more prone to stretch and rupture. Another factor in the increased incidence of ACL rupture in women is that an increase in hip varus and knee valgus when cutting and landing exposes the ligament to increased stress. Preventative measures with re-training of core neuromechanics have reduced the incidence (Mandelbaum et al., 2005; Steffen et al 2013).

Oestrogen inhibits an enzyme called lysyl oxidase, which facilitates collagen cross-linkages which normally help stiffen a ligament. Inhibition of this enzyme, especially in the pre-ovulatory phase of the menstrual cycle, when oestrogen levels approach their zenith, reduces the stiffness and resilience of tendons and ligaments (Cassandra et al., 2015). There has been some research showing that women using the oral contraceptive were less likely to undergo ACL surgery (Rahr-Wagner et al., 2014), which may mean conferring protection, although the research was undertaken surveying a group of women who underwent surgery, so it is not prospective in nature.

In a study carried out in track and field athletics, men were found to have twice the risk of muscle injuries (Edouard et al., 2016). This may be due to tendon compliance being higher (i.e., less stiff) due to the limitations of cross-linkage as described above. Achilles rupture is less common in pre-menopausal women, compared with men and their post-menopausal counterparts. Post-menopausal women and men share similar incidences. Muscle and tendon injuries occur twice as often in the days before ovulation (Martin et al., 2021).

Although treatments for injuries have no gender differences, the risk of injury seems to differ with the phase of the menstrual cycle. There are some individual and genetic differences in the way tissues respond to their hormonal milieu but having knowledge of the stage each player is at may be able to help plan training sessions, and guide more closely rehabilitation sessions (e.g., the first twist and turn session with the ball for, say, an ankle sprain may be best carried out post-ovulation). Although it may seem intrusive, there may be some merit in tracking individual risk profiles to avoid injury.

## Age-specific soccer

The advent of soccer as a route to general fitness and better health outcomes for women (Krustrup et al., 2018) and men (Bangsbo et al., 2015), with reviews hailing recreational soccer at any age to be 'medicine against non-communicable disease' (Sarmento

*Injury epidemiology, monitoring, and prevention*   215

et al., 2020), has meant greater involvement in soccer in advancing years, with walking soccer now well-established.

The physical sequelae from playing soccer are poorly understood in the recreational arena, but are becoming more appreciated in the ex-professional. In males, ex-players experience twice as much knee pain and degenerative changes on x-ray as the general population. They also experience knee symptoms 10–15 years before those in the general population and require three times as many knee replacements (Fernandes et al., 2018). Hip arthritis is of a similar incidence range as in the general population (0.3–8% general population vs. 2–8.3% in ex-players), but it has been noted that quality of life is affected more in ex-players with hip degenerative disease (Van den Noort et al., 2021).

Runacres et al. (2021) reviewed over 38,000 articles on longevity and concluded that mixed-event athletes such as soccer players lived longer, by virtue of a reduction in cardiovascular disease and cancer. Mental health has been a focus in ex-soccer players, and Van Ramele (2017) noted that the incidence of common mental health disorders was high when compared with the general population. Overall, it appears that soccer is an appropriate source of exercise throughout life and fulfils WHO recommendations (http://www.who.int/dietphysicalactivity/factsheet).

## Concussion

A concussion is an injury to the brain, which can occur because of a blow to the head, or trauma to any part of the body that might cause a perturbing force to be transmitted to the brain within the skull. Most sports-related concussions resolve within 7–10 days, but recovery can take longer. On occasion, the trauma is severe enough to cause bleeding around the brain or its coverings (called the meninges), causing an increase in pressure within the skull. This constitutes a medical emergency and may require surgical intervention to remove any collection of blood.

The brain sits inside the skull, and when injured, cannot be directly examined in the same way joints and soft tissue can. The clinician assesses neurological (i.e., brain) function, and this gives them an indirect view of how the brain is doing. An International Conference on Concussion in Sport has been held since 2001, the first being in Vienna, with multi-sport collaboration producing guidelines on sports-related concussion management from injury to RTP (Aubry et al., 2002). Since then, similar conferences have been held with the latest being in Berlin in 2016 (McCrory et al., 2017). The consensus of concussion recognition and management from these conferences has become the cornerstone of concussion guidelines issued by federations and international bodies.

Pitch-side management of concussion is based around the mantra 'if in doubt, sit them out'. Clinicians entering the field of play for a suspected concussion will assess the various brain/neurological functions that will demonstrate whether there has been a concussion and should remove the player if there is any doubt about their ability to continue to take part in the match/session. The player will not be allowed to take part in any activity from that point, until cleared to do so by a clinician.

Knowing the player and understanding the player's usual demeanour are important in this situation. The effects of concussion can cause mood changes, and these can be difficult to pick up unless the clinician knows what a player is usually like. An understanding of the mechanism of the injury will be helpful and may be available from a

216  *Ian Beasley*

*Table 13.2* Summary of information on CRT-5 form

---

Step 1-Red flags: These are indications that the injury is a serious one, and the player needs urgent transfer to hospital
Step 2-Observable signs (e.g., Gait disturbance, slow to get up)
Step 3-Symptoms (e.g., What is the player feeling? Dazed? Headache?)
Step 4-Memory assessment (e.g., Maddocks questions; Maddocks et al., 1995)
Step 1-Red flags: These are indications that the injury is a serious one, and the player needs urgent transfer to hospital
Step 2-Observable signs: e.g. Gait disturbance, slow to get up
Step 3-Symptoms: e.g., What is the player feeling? Dazed? Headache?
Step 4-Memory assessment: e.g., Maddocks questions (Maddocks et al., 1995)

---

player or the referee (e.g., 'he was knocked out' and 'he got a real bang on his head'). A reliable history, even though second-hand, will help the clinician come to a decision. A systematic approach to the examination is always advisable, and aide memoires are helpful here. The Concussion Recognition Tool 5 (CRT-5) (BJSM, 2017) (Table 13.2) should be in every 'run-on' bag to aid assessment.

Once the player has been removed from the field of play, they should be taken to a quiet location to undergo a more thorough examination which in the acute stage is done by using the SCAT5 (Sports Concussion Assessment Tool 5) which covers similar areas to the CRT-5, but in more detail. Players should undergo a SCAT5 examination at the beginning of the season as a baseline, so comparisons can be made.

If a concussion is diagnosed, the player must enter a graduated RTP process. This begins with a period of rest, followed by a graduated exercise programme until back in full training and eligible for selection. The English Football Association (http://uptonjfc.org/wp-content/uploads/2021/05/the-fa-concussion-guidelines-2019-changes-highlighed.pdf) has published guidelines which include an RTP protocol, which differs for junior and senior players, as junior players are more susceptible to the effects of concussion, as are women (Gomez et al., 2013). The player must be signed off as fit to RTP by the team physician, or a physician experienced in the management of sports concussion. Although RTP decisions can be made purely using serial SCAT 5 examinations until there is a return to baseline, there are audio-visual tools that allow assessment of players' neurocognitive functions that are used in professional soccer (Schatz et al., 2006). These can be helpful if there are language barriers or observer bias.

If a player suffers more than one concussion in a season, they should be reviewed in a specialist multi-disciplinary clinic, with a comprehensive examination to include vestibular function as well as imaging and neurological assessment. The player with multiple concussions should be counselled as to the possible long-term effects of (repeated) brain injury. There are many cases of ex-soccer players suffering from dementia that have been reported in the national press. Ling et al. (2017) described the post-mortem appearances of ex-professional soccer players who had been suffering from dementia. They found a greater incidence of chronic traumatic encephalopathy in two-thirds, where the normal amount would have been one-eighth approximately. Their conclusion was that this difference was due to heading the ball. This study comprised of low numbers, however. A large study in Scotland found that there was a three-fold increase in death from neurodegenerative diseases in ex-soccer players, compared with normal, matched, and controls.

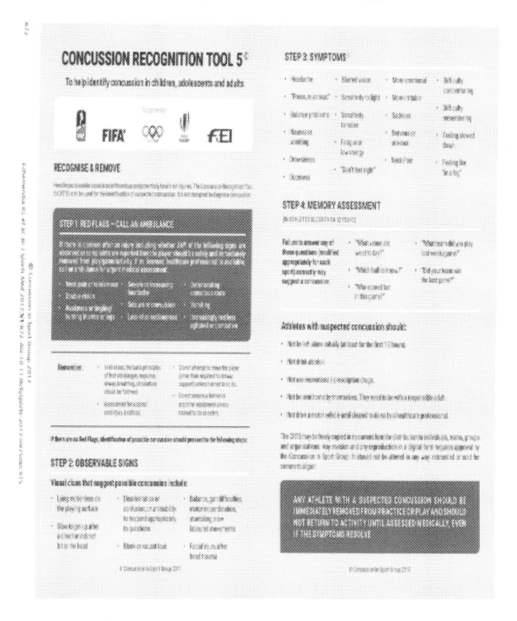

*Figure 13.12* Pocket Concussion recognition tool-5.

The debate rages on whether heading the ball in soccer is too much of a risk, with the accumulative effects of sub-concussive events leading to damage to the brain, resulting eventually in an increased incidence of neurological disease. Lipton et al. (2013) counted headers in a group of amateur soccer players and followed them with MRI scanning and memory testing. They demonstrated that there was white matter damage and neurocognitive effects for those having headed the ball more than 1,800 times in a

218   *Ian Beasley*

year. There is, however, no doubt that not every soccer player suffers in this way, and there seems to be a genetic susceptibility to concussion (Antrobus et al., 2021). Until there is a clearer understanding of the risks, and who might be more prone to the long-lasting effects of a career in soccer, it would seem prudent to give advice based on our current level of knowledge.

## Future directions and conclusions

The increase in sports science input into soccer is remarkable, and the advent of GPS has meant that it is now possible to monitor physical load much more accurately and predict when a player might be reaching a point where they are liable to get injured. It seems apparent that undertrained players are more likely to get injured, they reach a breaking point in matches much easier. It is also apparent that overtrained players get injured more often. This group is 'nearer the edge'. It follows that there is a 'sweet spot', which is individual of course. This is the classic 'J-shaped curve of risk' (Gabbett, 2016). GPS helps science and medical staff understand where each player is on this continuum, and its refined use will aid injury prevention in the future, enabling coaches to train players more efficiently and safely.

At present, soccer players are not counselled regarding the possible effects of a career playing the game professionally. Degenerative joint disease (Fernandes et al., 2018; Van den Noort et al., 2021) is more common, with symptoms earlier in life than normal, and there is the spectre of repeated brain trauma leading to dementia or other neurodegenerative diseases. While the players performing in the top teams in their respective countries may enjoy a good standard of living, most players are not in this category and have less choice when it comes to weighing the pros and cons of giving up their livelihood without the certain knowledge that playing soccer might be detrimental to their health later in life. However, we are not at a point where we can easily predict and advise prospective players. Gouttebarge et al. (2019) have begun a prospective study looking at all these aspects so that we can advise players, as well as governing bodies and national and international federations on how we might support players in retirement. We have a duty of care to players who have entertained us all (Carmody et al., 2019).

## References

Abdelkader NA, Helmy MNK, Fayaz NA, Saweeres ESB. Short- and intermediate-term results of extracorporeal shockwave therapy for noninsertional achilles tendinopathy. *Foot Ankle Int.* 2021;42(6):788–797.

Antrobus MR, Brazier J, Stebbings GK, Day SH, Heffernan SM, Kilduff LP, Erskine RM, Williams AG. Genetic factors that could affect concussion risk in elite rugby. *Sports (Basel).* 2021 Jan 22;9(2):19.

Ardern C. Reconstruction surgery is not always necessary for active young people who rupture their anterior cruciate ligament. *J Physiother.* 2013 Sep;59(3):209.

Ardern CL, Glasgow P, Schneiders A, et al. Consensus statement on return to sport from the first world congress in sports physical therapy, Bern. *Br J Sports Med.* 2016;50:853–864.

Aubry M, Cantu R, Dvorak J, et al. Summary and agreement statement of the first international conference on concussion in Sport, Vienna 2001. *Br J Sports Med.* 2002;36:6–7.

Bahr R. Why screening tests to predict injury do not work—and probably never will ...: a critical review. *Br J Sports Med.* 2016;50:776–780.

Bangsbo J, Hansen PR, Dvorak J, et al. Recreational football for disease prevention and treatment in untrained men: a narrative review examining cardiovascular health, lipid profile, body composition, muscle strength and functional capacity. *Br J Sports Med.* 2015;49:568–576.

Belanger L, Burt D, Callaghan J, Clifton S, Gleberzon BJ. Anterior cruciate ligament laxity related to the menstrual cycle: an updated systematic review of the literature. *J Can Chiropr Assoc.* 2013;57(1):76.

Bentley JA, Ramanathan AK, Arnold GP, Wang W, Abboud RJ. Harmful cleats of football boots: a biomechanical evaluation. *Foot Ankle Surg.* 2011 Sep;17(3):140–144.

Bleakley CM, Glasgow P, MacAuley DC. PRICE needs updating, should we call the POLICE? *Br J Sports Med.* 2012;46:220–221.

Boles, Andrew & Potts, Alex & Hodgson, Lisa. The functional movement screening tool does not predict injury in football. *Progr Orthop Sci.* 2015;1:1.

Brooks SC, Potter BT, Rainey JB. Treatment for partial tears of the lateral ligament of the ankle: a prospective trial. *Br Med J (Clin Res Ed).* 1981;21282(6264):606.

Carmody S, Jones C, Malhotra A, et al. Put out to pasture: what is our duty of care to the retiring professional footballer? Promoting the concept of the 'exit health examination' (EHE). *Br J Sports Med.* 2019;53:788–789.

Cassandra A. Lee, Ann Lee-Barthel, Louise Marquino, Natalie Sandoval, George R. Marcotte, Keith Baar. Estrogen inhibits lysyl oxidase and decreases mechanical function in engineered ligaments. *J Appl Physiol.* 2015 March;118:1250–1257.

Chidi-Ogbolu Nkechinyere, Baar Keith. Effect of estrogen on musculoskeletal performance and injury. *Risk Front Physiol.* 2019; 9:1834.

Cook JL, Purdam CR. Is tendon pathology a continuum? A pathology model to explain the clinical presentation of load-induced tendinopathy. *Br J Sports Med.* 2018;43:409–416.

Dönmez G, Kudaş S, Yörübulut M, Yıldırım M, Babayeva N, Torgutalp SS. Evaluation of muscle injuries in professional football players: does coach replacement affect the injury rate? *Clin J Sport Med.* 2020 Sep;30(5):478–483.

Edouard P, Branco P, Alonso J. Muscle injury is the principal injury type and hamstring muscle injury is the first injury diagnosis during top-level international athletics championships between 2007 and 2015. *Br J Sports Med.* 2016;50:619–630.

Ekstrand J. Keeping your top players on the pitch: the key to football medicine at a professional level. *Br J Sports Med.* 2013;47:723–724.

Ekstrand J, Hägglund M, Törnqvist H, et al. Upper extremity injuries in male elite football players. *Knee Surg Sports Traumatol Arthrosc.* 2013;21:1626–1632.

Ekstrand J, Hägglund M, Waldén M. Epidemiology of muscle injuries in professional football (soccer). *Am J Sports Med.* 2012;39(6):1226–1232

Ekstrand J, Krutsch W, Spreco A, et al. Time before return to play for the most common injuries in professional football: a 16-year follow-up of the UEFA elite club injury study. *Br J Sports Med.* 2020;54:421–426.

Ekstrand J, Waldén M, Hägglund M. Hamstring injuries have increased by 4% annually in men's professional football, since 2001: a 13-year longitudinal analysis of the UEFA elite club injury study. *Br J Sports Med.* 2016;50:731-737.

Fernandes GS, et al. Prevalence of knee pain, radiographic osteoarthritis and arthroplasty in retired professional footballers compared with men in the general population: a cross-sectional study. *Br J Sports Med.* 2018;52:678–683.

Fredericson M, Bergman AG, Hoffman KL, Dillingham MS. Tibial stress reaction in runners. Correlation of clinical symptoms and scintigraphy with a new magnetic resonance imaging grading system. *Am J Sports Med.* 1995;23(4):472–81.

Gabbett TJ. The training—injury prevention paradox: should athletes be training smarter and harder? *Br J Sports Med.* 2016;50:273–280.

Gervis M, Helen Pickford, Thomas Hau, Meghan Fruth. A review of the psychological support mechanisms available for long-term injured footballers in the UK throughout their rehabilitation. *Sci Med Footb.* 2020;4(1):22–29.

Gómez JE, Hergenroeder AC, et al. New guidelines for management of concussion in sport: special concern for youth. *J Adol Health*. 2013;53(3):311–313.

Gouttebarge V, et al Monitoring the health of transitioning professional footballers: protocol of an observational prospective cohort study BMJ Open Sport & Exercise Medicine 2019;5:e000680. doi: 10.1136/bmjsem-2019-000680

Grassi A, Quaglia A, Canata GL, Zaffagnini S. An update on the grading of muscle injuries: a narrative review from clinical to comprehensive systems. *Joints*. 2016;4(1):39–46.

Grigg NL, Wearing SC, Smeathers JE. Eccentric calf muscle exercise produces a greater acute reduction in Achilles tendon thickness than concentric exercise. *Br J Sports Med*. 2009;43:280–283.

Hamilton B, Valle X, Rodas G, et al. Classification and grading of muscle injuries: a narrative review. *Br J Sports Med*. 2015;49:306.

Holm C, Kjaer M, Eliasson P. Treatment of achilles tendon ruptures. *Scand J Med Sci Sports*. 2015;25:e1–e10. https://www.orthobullets.com/pathology/8042/myositis-ossificans

Jiang G, Wu Y, Meng J, et al. Comparison of leukocyte-rich platelet-rich plasma and leukocyte-poor platelet-rich plasma on achilles tendinopathy at an early stage in a rabbit model. *Am J Sports Med*. 2020;48(5):1189–1199.

Joseph AM, Collins CL, Henke NM, Yard EE, Fields SK, Comstock RD. A multisport epidemiologic comparison of anterior cruciate ligament injuries in high school athletics. *J Athl Train*. 2013;48(6):810–817. doi:10.4085/1062–6050-48.6.03

Kannus, P. Structure of tendon and connective tissue. *Scan J Med Sci Sports*. 2000 Dec;10(6):312–320.

Kijowski R, Choi J, Shinki K, Del Rio AM, De Smet A. Validation of MRI classification system for tibial stress injuries. *AJR Am J Roentgenol*. 2012;198(4):878–884.

Krustrup P, Helge EW, Hansen PR, et al. Effects of recreational football on women's fitness and health: adaptations and mechanisms. *Eur J Appl Physiol*. 2018;118:11–32.

Lacout Alexis, et al. Myositis ossificans imaging: keys to successful diagnosis. *Ind J Radiol Imag*. 2012;22(1):35–39.

Lai CCH, Ardern CL, Feller JA, et al. Eighty-three per cent of elite athletes return to preinjury sport after anterior cruciate ligament reconstruction: a systematic review with meta-analysis of return to sport rates, graft rupture rates and performance outcomes. *Br J Sports Med*. 2018;52:128–138.

Larruskian J, Lekue JA, Diaz N, Odriozola A, Gil SM. A comparison of injuries in elite male and female football players: a five-season prospective study. *Scand J Med Sci Sports*. 2018;28:237–245.

Larsson D, Ekstrand J, Karlsson MK. Fracture epidemiology in male elite football players from 2001 to 2013: how long will this fracture keep me out?. *Br J Sports Med*. 2016;50:759–763.

Lee JC, Healy J. Sonography of lower limb muscle injury. *Am J Roentgenol*. 2004;182(2):341–351.

Ling H, et al. Mixed pathologies including chronic traumatic encephalopathy account for dementia in retired association football (soccer) players. *Acta Neuropathol*. 2017;133:337–352.

Lipton ML, Kim N, Zimmerman ME, Kim M, Stewart WF, Branch CA, Lipton RB. Soccer heading is associated with white matter microstructural and cognitive abnormalities. Radiology. 2013 Sep;268(3):850-7.

Longo UG, Viganò M, Candela V, de Girolamo L, Cella E, Thiebat G, Salvatore G, Ciccozzi M, Denaro V. Epidemiology of posterior cruciate ligament reconstructions in Italy: a 15-year study. *J Clin Med*. 2021;10(3):499.

López-Royo MP, Ortiz-Lucas M, Gómez-Trullén EM, Herrero P. The Effectiveness of Minimally Invasive Techniques in the Treatment of Patellar Tendinopathy: A Systematic Review and Meta-Analysis of Randomized Controlled Trials. Evid Based Complement Alternat Med. 2020 Sep 5;2020

López-Valenciano A, Ruiz-Pérez I, Garcia-Gómez A, et al. Epidemiology of injuries in professional football: a systematic review and meta-analysis. *Br J Sports Med*. 2020;54:711–771.

*Injury epidemiology, monitoring, and prevention* 221

Lubberts B, D'Hooghe P, Bengtsson H, et al. Epidemiology and return to play following isolated syndesmotic injuries of the ankle: a prospective cohort study of 3677 male professional footballers in the UEFA elite club injury study. *Br J Sports Med.* 2019;53:959–964.

Maddocks DL, Dicker GD, Saling MM. The assessment of orientation following concussion in athletes. *Clin J Sport Med.* 1995;5(1):32–35.

Madhi I, et al. The use of PRP in treatment of achilles tendinopathy: a systematic review of literature. Study design: systematic review of literature. *Ann Med Surg.* 2020;55:320–326.

Makhmalbaf H, Shahpari O, et al. medial collateral ligament injury; a new classification based on MRI and clinical findings: a guide for patient selection and early surgical intervention. *Arch Bone Jt Surg.* 2018;6(1):3–7.

Malhotra A, Sharma S, et al. Hypertrophic cardiomyopathy in athletes. *Eur Cardiol.* 2017;12(2):80–82.

Mandelbaum BR, Silvers HJ, Watanabe DS, et al. Effectiveness of a neuromuscular and proprioceptive training program in preventing anterior cruciate ligament injuries in female athletes: 2-year follow-up. *Am J Sports Med.* 2005;33(7):1003–1010.

Martin Dan, Timmins Kate, Cowie Charlotte, Alty Jon, Mehta Ritan, Tang Alicia, Varley Ian. Injury incidence across the menstrual cycle in international footballers. *Front Sports Act Liv.* 2021;3:17.

McCrory P, Meeuwisse WH, Dvořák J, et al. 5th International conference on concussion in sport (Berlin). *Br J Sports Med.* 2017;51:837.

Mosler AB, Weir A, Eirale C, et al. Epidemiology of time loss groin injuries in a men's professional football league: a 2-year prospective study of 17 clubs and 606 players. *Br J Sports Med.* 2018;52:292–297.

Nguyen JC, Arthur A De Smet, Ben K Graf, Humberto G Rosas. MR imaging–based diagnosis and classification of meniscal tears. *Radio Graph.* 2014;34(4):981–999.

Nuhmani S. Injection therapies for patellar tendinopathy. *Phys Sportsmed.* 2020;48(2):125–130.

O'Donoghue D. Surgical treatment of fresh injuries to the major ligaments of the knee. *J Bone Joint Surg Am.* 1950;32(A4):721–738.

Paccy V, Nicholson LL, Adams RD, Munn J, Munns CF. Generalized joint hypermobility and risk of lower limb joint injury during sport: a systematic review with meta-analysis. *Am J Sports Med.* 2010;38(7):1487–1497.

Pollock N, James SLJ, Lee JC, et al. British athletics muscle injury classification: a new grading system. *Br J Sports Med.* 2014;48:1347–1351.

Rahr-Wagner L, Thillemann TM, Mehnert F, Pedersen AB, Lind M. Is the use of oral contraceptives associated with operatively treated anterior cruciate ligament injury?: a case-control study from the Danish knee ligament reconstruction registry. *Am J Sports Med.* 2014;42(12):2897–2905.

Rees JD, Lichtwark GA, Wolman RL, Wilson AM. The mechanism for efficacy of eccentric loading in achilles tendon injury; an *in vivo* study in humans. *Rheumatology.* 2008 Oct;47(10):1493–1497.

Runacres A, Mackintosh KA, McNarry MA. Health consequences of an elite sporting career: long-term detriment or long-term gain? a meta-analysis of 165,000 former athletes. *Sports Med.* 2021 Feb;51(2):289–301.

Saif Azmy M, Ibtesam K Ali, Ahmed R Radwan, Mohammed Ali Ismail. Efficacy of hyaluronic acid injections versus steroid injections on painful tendinopathies. *Egyptian J Hosp Med.* 2021 Autumn;85(2):3551–3556.

Sarmento H, Manuel Clemente F, Marques A, Milanovic Z, David Harper L, Figueiredo A. Recreational football is medicine against non-communicable diseases: a systematic review. *Scand J Med Sci Sports.* 2020;30:618–637.

Saunier J, Roland Chapurlat R. Stress fracture in athletes. *Joint Bone Spine.* 2018;85(3):307–310.

Schatz P, et al. Sensitivity and specificity of the impact test battery for concussion in athletes. *Arch Clin Neuropsychol.* 2006 Jan;21(1):91–99.

222 *Ian Beasley*

Sharma P, Nicola Maffulli. Understanding and managing achilles tendinopathy. *Br J Hosp Med*. 2006;67(2):64–67.

Shultz SJ, Sander TC, Kirk SE, Perrin DH. Sex differences in knee joint laxity change across the female menstrual cycle. *J Sports Med Phys Fitness*. 2005 Dec;45(4):594–603.

Steffen K, Emery CA, Romiti M, et al. High adherence to a neuromuscular injury prevention programme (FIFA 11+) improves functional balance and reduces injury risk in Canadian youth female football players: a cluster randomised trial. *Br J Sports Med*. 2013;47:794–802.

Tabben M, Eirale C, Singh G, et al. Injury and illness epidemiology in professional Asian football: lower general incidence and burden but higher ACL and hamstring injury burden compared with Europe. *Br J Sports Med*. 2021 Jan; Published Online First.

Tarantino D, Palermi S, Sirico F, Corrado B. Achilles tendon rupture: mechanisms of injury, principles of rehabilitation and return to play. *J Funct Morphol Kinesiol*. 2020;5(4):95.

Van den Noort D, et al. Clinical hip osteoarthritis in current and former professional footballers and its effect on hip function and quality of life. *J Sports Science Med*. 2021;20:284–290.

Van Ramele S, et al. Mental health in retired professional football players: 12-month incidence, adverse life events and support. *Psychol Sport Exer*. 2017 Jan;28:85–90.

Wilson JMG, Jungner G. *Principles and practice of screening for disease*. Geneva: WHO; 1968.

Winter Bee W, Ubhi J, Kumar B. Subcategories of tendinopathy using ultrasound tissue characterization (utc): dorsal mid-portion achilles tendinopathy is more severe than ventral achilles tendinopathy. *Br J Sports Med*. 2017 May;Published Online First.

# 14 Infectious diseases

*Monica Duarte Muñoz and Tim Meyer*

## Introduction

At first sight, players may be considered at high risk of acquiring and spreading infectious diseases considering the typical circumstances of their training and competition. The most relevant aspects seem to be the proximity to teammates and opponents, travel requirements, and possibly some detrimental effects on the immune system from intense sport. However, there is little research available on this topic, which might be due to the predominant presence of traumatology-oriented members of the medical staff around teams. The importance of infections can be underestimated due to their lower incidence compared to that of injuries (Bjørneboe et al., 2016). Nevertheless, infectious diseases have the potential to interfere with training and match performance and produce time loss. While a mild cold may seem trivial for a white-collar worker, this will hardly be the case for elite athletes, where even mild symptoms can impair performance. Infections may even have potentially life-threatening complications without adequate treatment. Finally, infections may lead to an increased number of injuries in the following weeks. Therefore, timely identification and proper management of infectious diseases are of high relevance in soccer.

## Epidemiology and clinical presentation of infections in players

As with the rest of the general population – and other athletes – the most common infections among soccer players are those of the upper respiratory tract (URTI), ranging from 40% to 74% of all illnesses in professional players (Orhant et al., 2010; Bjørneboe et al., 2016; Dvorak et al., 2011). The same is true in other codes of football, such as American football, rugby, and Australian Rules football (Chesson et al., 2020). It is noteworthy that epidemiological data about infections in soccer are scarce, and the available information from the UEFA Champions League and FIFA World Cups (Bjørneboe et al., 2016; Dvorak et al., 2011) reflects the highest level of play only (and, thus, a high level of medical care).

URTI symptoms include runny nose, nasal congestion, cough, sore throat, malaise, and fever. In most cases, these are caused by viral agents. In professional players, the average incidence of URTI episodes has been found to be 1.5 per 1,000 player days, leading to an average training absence of 3 days per episode (Bjørneboe et al., 2016). As a result, such infections are not considered a major cause of time loss. However, a single URTI may mean the loss of an important match and performance impairment after infectious episodes remain uninvestigated. On the other hand, a player might not

224 *Monica Duarte Muñoz and Tim Meyer*

report mild symptoms or may go undiagnosed. The absence of diagnosis should be avoided given that training or playing during an acute infection has the potential to cause severe consequences.

The second most common infection in soccer players – as well as in the rest of the population – is gastrointestinal illness (GI) (Orhant et al., 2010; Bjørneboe et al., 2016; Dvorak et al., 2011). It is often caused by bacteria like *Escherichia coli* types, but sometimes by viruses (e.g., norovirus) and other agents. Symptoms of GI include diarrhea, stomachache, and malaise. GI account for approximately 13–28% of all infectious episodes in professional soccer (Orhant et al., 2010; Bjørneboe et al., 2016; Dvorak et al., 2011). Less than one episode per 1,000 player days is reported with an absence of 1 day per 1,000 player-days (Bjørneboe et al., 2016). Malaise is more frequent in GI than in URTI, and it is generally easier for players to accept the need for adequate rest. Fluids lost due to fever, vomiting, or diarrhea, need to be replaced before safely returning to play. Therefore, weight control is among the important measures of GI management. Players must be weighed as soon as possible after the onset of symptoms and before returning to play to ensure that fluid loss has been sufficiently replaced. Adequate hand hygiene is critical in preventing the occurrence and spread of GI.

Skin infections are much less common, but they are the main source of "outbreaks" in sport settings (Fontanilla et al., 2010; Turbeville et al., 2006). Their relevance for soccer players is mainly dependent on their location and severity (i.e., acuteness and degree of inflammation). Skin lesions, such as infected blisters, at the players' feet can represent a very serious problem because of their interference with wearing proper shoes and possibly because of the resulting pain during training and match play. Skin infections are often caused by *Streptococcus pyogenes* (e.g., erysipela) *and Staphylococcus aureus*, including methicillin-resistant *S. aureus* (MRSA) (Romano et al., 2006; Shaban et al., 2020). *S. aureus* is often harbored in asymptomatic athletes in the nares, oropharynx, axilla, and groin. This so-called "asymptomatic colonization" is more common in contact sports athletes than in non-contact sports athletes (Jimenez-Truque et al., 2017). Other skin infections such as onychomycosis, tinea pedis, and pityriasis versicolor are more common in professional soccer players than in the general population (Buder et al., 2018).

## Less common infections (vector-borne, blood-borne)

Less common infectious diseases that occur in soccer players include dental, eye, and sexually transmitted infections, among others. These rarely cause severe complications, at least not immediately, but they do interfere with overall wellbeing and, therefore, with performance. Thus, as is the case with the above-mentioned diseases, they require medical evaluation and treatment which may exceed the protocols typically employed for such infections.

There are no specific considerations for *vector-borne infectious diseases* like malaria or yellow fever besides the ones in place for all persons traveling to countries where they are endemic (see Table 14.1). Some infections can be prevented via vaccination. Possibly a bit more surprisingly, infections that can be transmitted via body fluids (usually excluding sweat) and, therefore, also by blood, do not warrant specific precautions in addition to the ones usually taken by medical staff. The reason is the very low transmission rate under soccer-specific conditions. This is not only true for HIV but also for the much more contagious hepatitis B.

*Infectious diseases* 225

*Table 14.1* Prevention of vector-borne infectious diseases (*Tickborne Encephalitis*, 2022; *Yellow Fever*, 2022)

| | |
|---|---|
| Prevent mosquito bites | Use insect repellent (DEET, picaridin/icaridin, etc.) |
| | Minimize skin exposure (long-sleeve shirts, long pants, closed shoes, tucking clothes in, etc.) |
| | Use bed nets |
| | Treat clothes with permethrin |
| Control mosquitoes | Use screens on windows and doors |
| | Stop mosquitoes from laying eggs (empty and clean items that can hold water) |
| | Use air conditioning |
| | Insecticides and spatial repellents |
| Check for ticks | Inspect body and clothing after visiting a tick-infested area |

## Prevention of infectious diseases

The most "definite" approach for prevention of infectious diseases is vaccination. Little is sport-specific about vaccinations, but statements can be made about performance-oriented athletes. The "disadvantage" of vaccinations is that they only prevent one specific infectious disease and do not provide a broader protection (although this is sometimes purported). Therefore, they must be supplemented by other – less-specific – measures.

## Vaccination

Guidelines available in most countries provide a vaccination scheme to be followed by the general population, including elite athletes. However, some cases require specific recommendations according to exposure circumstances, such as travel or living conditions. A few specific considerations apply to elite athletes as a group (Gärtner & Meyer, 2014). Planning vaccinations early enough before travel is critical in soccer players, as there are diseases that are endemic in certain areas and countries may require vaccinations to be applied prior to travel (see Table 14.2).

With each vaccine, there are risks of side effects. However, certain circumstances in soccer players require special attention. For example, pain in the site of inoculation, which is one of the most common side effects of vaccines, may interfere with training or playing. Therefore, whenever possible, a vaccine should be applied in a region that does not hinder training or playing; for example, the deltoid might be preferred over the intra-gluteal route (except for goalkeepers), plus, the vaccine should be applied on the non-dominant extremity. An adequate application technique is also fundamental to minimize pain afterwards. These considerations also apply in lower levels of play.

Severe side effects can occur, albeit infrequently. For example, vaccine-specific symptoms may appear with live vaccines. Anaphylactic reactions or syncopes can have serious consequences and require advanced medical attention, although athletes are not at higher risk of presenting with these side effects than the rest of the population. However, as with infectious illnesses, the consequences of such side effects may appear more disabling in athletes. An ideal time for vaccination is during or shortly prior to the winter and summer breaks (Gärtner & Meyer, 2014). This timing ensures that, should a complication or side-effects arise, it will not interfere with the players' schedules. When this is not feasible, no specific interruptions or adjustments of the

226 *Monica Duarte Muñoz and Tim Meyer*

*Table 14.2* Preventive measures

| | |
|---|---|
| Adequate hand hygiene | Isolation of sick players |
| Avoid sharing personal objects | Use of antibacterial gel |
| Adequate coughing and sneezing etiquette | Bottled water when water quality is unknown |
| Load monitoring | Ensure food is not contaminated |

training schedule are required. Training sessions or matches do not relevantly affect induction of the immune response to vaccination in elite athletes or modify the occurrence of side effects (Stenger et al., 2020). The optimal time point for a vaccination during ongoing training seems to be the day after a match.

## Other preventive measures

Other measures can and should be taken to prevent the occurrence and spread of infectious diseases (Table 14.2). Ensuring adequate hand hygiene might be the most obvious measure, yet it is not always respected. Players should also be reminded not to share their personal objects, such as towels, water bottles, and cutlery. One of the main ways in which certain pathogens spread is through respiratory droplets and aerosols, therefore, athletes should follow an adequate coughing and sneezing etiquette. It will also be important to monitor load, as there may be periods of high match and training load (e.g., during pre-season), which may make players prone to infections (Schwellnus et al., 2016; Piggot et al., 2009; Jones et al., 2017). Finally, sick players should usually be isolated. Many of these measures are common sense although their efficacy has not been scientifically proven. Evidence only comes from a few papers in other sports (Schwellnus et al., 2016; Hanstad et al., 2011).

The above-mentioned measures can be applied under any circumstances. There are certain additional actions that can be taken during traveling. The use of antibacterial and hand disinfectants has been widely promoted (Kratzel et al., 2020; Tamimi et al., 2015; Henriey et al., 2014) given that it is a simple and effective measure. In countries with warm climates and inadequate hygiene, where tournaments and training camps frequently take place, it is recommended to drink only bottled water and be cautious with food preparation.

Certain improper – yet common – practices in soccer may contribute to spreading infections and other pathogens. Some examples are sharing personal objects (e.g., drinking bottles and towels) and use of a single towel for several players (by medical personnel and physiotherapists) (Shaban et al., 2020). Correctly managing open wounds (which may occur frequently) is also crucial, and in such cases, players must refrain from using communal baths. In addition to this, following the recommendations from the Centers for Disease Control and Prevention (CDC) is strongly suggested (Table 14.3).

## Drugs to prevent infectious diseases

Most approaches to reduce the number of infectious diseases by intake of drugs claim to boost or improve the immune response. Candidates for such pharmaceutical actions include echinacea (Wang et al., 2006; Karsch-Völk et al., 2015), umckaloabo (Timmer et al., 2013; Roth et al., 2019; Jekabsone et al., 2019), and several other plant

*Table 14.3* CDC recommendations for athletes for prevention of spread of MRSA (*MRSA*, 2019)

| **Wash hands often with soap and water or use alcohol-based sanitizer** | **Cover skin cuts and wounds** |
|---|---|
| • Before and after playing sports<br>• After using shared weight-training equipment<br>• After caring for wounds<br>• After using the toilet<br>**Shower immediately after exercise**<br>• Avoid sharing bar soap or towels<br>**Wash your uniform and clothing after each use**<br>• Dry clothes completely (in a dryer) | • With clean, dry bandages or other dressings recommended by healthcare provider until healed.<br>• Follow healthcare provider's instructions on change of bandages and dressings.<br>**Wear protective clothing or gear designed to prevent skin abrasions or cuts**.<br>**Do not share items that come into contact with your skin**<br>• Personal items<br>• Ointments applied by placing your hand in the container<br>• Use a barrier (e.g., a towel) between your skin and shared equipment (e.g., sauna, weight-training) |

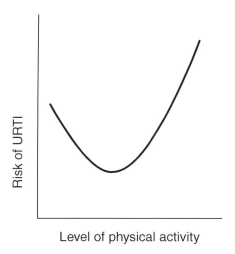

*Figure 14.1* The risk of URTI is lower with moderate levels of physical activity when compared to more sedentary people. The risk of URTI increases progressively with higher levels of physical activity Adapted from Nieman, 1994.

compounds as well as probiotics (Pyne et al., 2015) and zinc (Hojyo & Fukada, 2016; Wessels et al., 2017). Little evidence is available, and many researchers do not utilize appropriate control conditions or prefer target parameters from the blood to the "real currency", that is the incidence of infectious diseases. Moreover, most of these studies are sponsored by companies, which creates the potential for publication bias.

## Soccer-specific influences on the likelihood of infectious diseases

Certain factors may make players more prone to infectious diseases than the general population. These include high training loads, close interaction with teammates and opponents, and frequent travel. However, these negative factors must be weighed against the fact that most players are healthy and young, which gives them a potentially robust immune system. First, we address the high training and match loads to which players are subjected and the impact they may have on the immune response. There are indications that an acquisition of infections is more likely in the immediate aftermath of intense exercise (like matches and hard training sessions). This factor is summarized in the "open window theory". The theory states that there is a decreased immune response in athletes during the first hours after exercise (Pedersen & Ullum, 1994) and refers to the concentrations of some lymphocyte subpopulations – like natural killer cells (Kakanis et al., 2010; Shek et al., 1995) – as well as salivary immunoglobin A (sIgA) (Fahlman & Engels, 2005) (a mucosal defense mechanism) which fall below pre-exercise baseline values. It follows from such considerations that players who frequently undergo strenuous exercise have multiple "windows" through which infectious agents might enter their bodies.

There is an accompanying theory about the long-term ("chronic") consequences of repeated exercise bouts. The J-shaped curve (Nieman, 1994) states that moderate exercisers are at a lower risk of URTI when compared to athletes who exercise at high intensities (Pedersen & Bruunsgaard, 1995). It would seem, therefore, that elite players are prone to infectious illness both acutely and chronically. sIgA, which is part of the initial (or acute) immune response to pathogens entering the body via the mucosae, decreases progressively in soccer players when matches are scheduled too close to each other (Morgans et al., 2014). This factor might suggest a chronically increased susceptibility to infectious diseases. However, there is currently no consensus about the significance of both theories for soccer. It is of relevance whether training and competition stimuli as they typically occur in professional soccer are of sufficient intensity, duration, and frequency to compromise the immune response. At least at the semi-professional and recreational level, it is unlikely that proneness to infections exceeds that of the general population.

A second inherent risk is the close interaction that occurs between teammates and opponents – particularly when combined with periods of impaired immunity like during an "open window". Players come into close contact with their opponents during matches. Tackling, yelling, heavy breathing, and touching one's face may contribute to increasing the risk of pathogen transmission through airborne particles. However, during a match, players were found within 1.5 m or less of both, teammates, and opponents, for an average total time of 1 min and a half (87.8 s) (Knudsen et al., in press), with most interactions lasting less than 3 s (Egger, in press). This exposure may not be sufficient time to spread pathogens through close contact, at least not the less contagious ones. Another publication from the Netherlands documented those other interactions on the pitch such as goal celebrations and corner kicks contributed the most to the risk (Knudsen, et al., 2022).

Third, traveling may increase the risk of infections in professional players. Naturally, some areas of the world pose risks (Table 14.4). Therefore, it is essential to be informed before travel to prepare accordingly. For example, vaccination can be required in certain areas with endemic diseases. This applies to competition as well as to training camps, which often take place in developing/warm countries. In such countries, there may be a higher risk of GI due to lower hygiene standards. Thus, adequate hand hygiene and ensuring food and water safety are of considerable importance. Another risk in such countries is vector-transmitted diseases, such as malaria, for which mosquito repellents (among other measures) can be useful (see Table 14.1). However, there is an additional inherent risk in traveling itself. Long-haul air travel for tournaments and competition poses an increased risk, although responsible mechanisms remain speculative at this moment. Among the

*Infectious diseases* 229

*Table 14.4* Infectious diseases to consider in traveling athletes

| Disease | Cause | Where? |
|---|---|---|
| Tick-borne encephalitis (TBE) (*Tickborne Encephalitis*, 2022) | Tick bite (*Ixodes ricinus, I. persulcatus*) TBEV (*Flaviviridae*) | Eastern, Central, and Northern Europe Europe, Northern China, Mongolia, and the Russian Federation |
| Hepatitis A (*Hepatitis A*, 2022) | Ingesting contaminated food or water, direct contact. HAV | Low- and middle-income countries with poor sanitary conditions and hygiene practices |
| Yellow fever (*Yellow Fever*, 2022) | Mosquito bite (*Aedes* or *Haemagogus*) *Flavivirus* | Africa and some tropical parts of South America |
| Typhoid fever (*Typhoid Fever*, 2022) | Poor hygiene *Salmonella typhi* | Asian regions of Russia and neighboring countries, parts of South and South-East Asia, Africa, and South America |
| Dengue (*Dengue*, 2023) | Dengue virus, mosquito bite (*Aedes aegypti* or *Aedes albopictus*) | Caribbean, Mexico, Central and South America, Southeast Asia, and Pacific Islands |
| Zika (*Zika*, 2019, 2022) | Zika virus, mosquito bite (*Aedes aegypti* or *Aedes albopictus*) | North, Central and South America, France, Africa, and Asia |
| Helminthes (*Helminth infections*, 2023) | Soil-transmitted parasites (*Ascaris lumbricoides, Trichuris trichiura, Necator americanus*, etc.) | Tropical and subtropical areas, sub-Saharan Africa, the Americas, China, and East Asia |
| Chagas (*Chagas*, n.d.) | Bite, urine, or feces of triatomines (*Trypanosoma cruzi*) | Mexico, Central and South America (currently widespread) |

candidate factors are proximity to fellow passengers in an enclosed environment (cabin of the plane), stress, and possibly lack of sleep. Moreover, crossing a high number of time zones seems to contribute to the risk of infections (Schwellnus et al., 2012) with a direction away from home being another aggravating factor. Finally, differing spectrums of infectious agents between countries may challenge an immune system further.

Finally, inadequate nutrition and difficult intra- and inter-personal or family situations can likewise contribute to a decreased function of the immune system and increase the risk of infections. Therefore, it is important that medical and other staff keep track of the general wellbeing of players.

## Diagnosis of infectious diseases

Usually, diagnosis is initiated and guided by symptoms of infection. It does not make sense to screen for infectious diseases without any suspicious complaints (possibly except for pandemic situations like COVID-19). It is well possible that a diagnosis can be made based on history and physical findings alone. At least in professional players, it is advisable to consider taking a venous blood sample to determine blood count and C-reactive protein (CRP; possibly additionally liver enzymes and other organ-targeted parameters). This procedure may help assess the severity of the condition and be valuable for later decisions about the return-to-play when the question arises whether the course of the disease has reached its climax (Scharhag & Meyer, 2014).

230 *Monica Duarte Muñoz and Tim Meyer*

A major focus of initial diagnosis is always to determine if the infection is local or generalized. Also, an assessment must be made about contagiousness (to allow for proper management in a team setting). This is usually only possible by a summarizing view on all available findings and has to be carried out by a trained physician. The presence of generalized symptoms (fever, malaise, and swollen lymph nodes) speaks in favor of non-eligibility for any kind of physical activity. When contagiousness must be assumed, an isolation of the affected player is usually wise or at least strict advice on how tosss behave towards teammates.

## Consequences of infectious diseases

Infectious symptoms have the potential to interfere with training, competition, and in general with the performance of players. In contrast to a white-collar worker, a player will likely notice even minor symptoms and perceive them as inconvenient. This is not only true for upper respiratory symptoms but also for symptoms in other organs. It follows that players should be thoroughly examined and questioned to safely determine whether they are eligible again for training and match play. Also, symptomatic treatment is still important even when medical constraints for return-to-play have disappeared.

After URTI or any other infection has been diagnosed, proper treatment and recovery are fundamental. A recovery and resting period of a few days will be required in many cases (Scharhag & Meyer, 2014). This process can have important consequences for the affected player as well as for his/her teammates. Even during short recovery periods, this may mean the absence of a player for an important match. Furthermore, when a longer resting period is required, the outcome for the affected player can be a decrease in physical condition and skill. The extent of this temporary loss in performance will naturally be different depending on the time of the season. Notwithstanding, return to play and training should take place gradually and only after the player is symptom-free (Börjesson et al., 2018). Sufficient recovery is of utmost importance given the possible and severe consequences that can come from training and competing during a viral infection (i.e., the affection of other organs).

One of the most feared complications is myocarditis – an inflammation of the heart muscle. Infectious agents – such as viruses (influenza, coxsackie, adeno, and herpes), bacteria (meningococcus and streptococcus), and fungus (aspergillosis) among others – are the most common causes of myocarditis (Basso et al., 2007). Physical activity during viral replication may cause myocardial necrosis and death. Although this has only been experimentally shown in mice (Gatmaitan et al., 1970), we should assume the same effect in humans.

Some illnesses require a prolonged recovery period. One such case is infectious mononucleosis, which has a higher incidence in athletes from 15 to 25 years of age (Becker & Smith, 2014). Athletes who have suffered from this disease may have an enlarged spleen for weeks after the initial infection, with an increased risk of splenic rupture, which can happen with minor trauma or even spontaneously. Other diseases, such as glandular fever (Epstein–Barr virus), Lyme disease (*Borrelia burgdorferi*), or Q fever (*Coxiella burnetii*), have been linked to chronic post-infective fatigue states (Hickie et al., 2006). A player should have full resolution of fatigue and other associated symptoms (Becker & Smith, 2014) before returning to full training load and competition. It is recommended that physical activity progresses gradually to prevent complications. Close follow-up of players who have presented an infectious illness is therefore imperative.

## Treatment of infectious diseases

There is a plethora of drugs utilized for the treatment of infectious diseases. Most of them do not interfere with training or match activity. It is the severity of each infectious disease that must be assessed to conclude about medical eligibility (Scharhag & Meyer, 2014). This is true for antibiotic treatment as well. The application of antibiotics alone does not preclude participation in training or competition. However, the severity of an illness is usually high when antibiotic treatment is considered. Although these drugs are only effective against bacteria, they are sometimes used to prevent bacterial superinfections or because uncertainty exists about the infectious agent.

Another medication class that is often used to alleviate infection symptoms is nonsteroidal anti-inflammatory drugs (NSAIDs). They are available as over-the-counter drugs in most countries and, therefore, much less controlled by medical staff. It needs to be considered that frequent intake of NSAIDs may lead to gastroduodenal ulcers and renal damage, which means that players and staff members with medical conditions at these organs should employ particular care. Another consideration is that NSAIDs can cover infectious symptoms and lead to a falsely positive reception of one's clinical status.

## Return-to-training and return-to-play after infectious diseases

Naturally, the question arises of how to determine whether a player can continue to train and compete. There exists a thumb rule that may be of use: the so-called "neck check" (Eichner, 1993; Primos, 1996). This rule simply states that if a player has symptoms "above the neck" (i.e., sore throat and runny nose) they can be, in general, allowed to train and compete; whereas when "below the neck" symptoms are present (i.e., fever and muscle ache) it is advisable to restrict the player (Primos, 1996). This is, as stated before, only a rule of thumb. It is merely to be used as an initial reference and by no means should substitute an adequate medical examination (Scharhag & Meyer, 2014).

Like with injuries, there is a trade-off between a quick return to training and competition and medical safety. A few recommendations have been published (Scharhag & Meyer, 2014) and many considerations are sport – rather than soccer-specific. A return too early imposes the risk of underperformance as well as complicated and lengthy courses of the infection. In the worst case, organ affections like hepatitis or even myocarditis can arise. The most reliable indicators of sufficient recovery are cessation of symptoms and normalization of laboratory values, the latter being the more objective ones, of course. These may be of importance particularly in professional soccer because there is some financial attractiveness in participating in the next match which may lead to dissimulation. CRP can be considered the most reliable indicator (Scharhag & Meyer, 2014), particularly when it has been determined repeatedly.

## Specific considerations for COVID-19

Professional leagues have been able to restart their competitions with costly hygiene protocols, including repeated PCR testing and elaborate measures to allow for distancing and to avoid virus transmission within a team and its staff (Meyer et al., 2021; Schumacher et al., 2021). However, for all leagues which are unable to afford such protocols, a major question arose around the likelihood of SARS-CoV-2 transmission under "normal" conditions on a pitch. Early studies investigated the distance between players during a match and found that player-player contacts at less than 2 m mostly have a duration below 1 min, some of them even lower (Knudsen et al., in press; Van Duivenbode & Goes, 2020). This finding was later complemented by more detailed analyses of the players' behavior including mucosae contacts and direction of the face during contacts (Egger, in press). SARS-CoV-2 transmissions during football play are unlikely, whereas simulations or commentaries partly concluded the opposite. Corner kicks and goal celebrations were the activities with the longest close contact.

Of course, the experimental approach – letting infected persons play soccer and assess the degree of transmission directly – is unethical. Therefore, the only way of addressing real transmissions is to analyze retrospectively cases where contagious players have participated in matches unintentionally (e.g., in error about testing results or due to failure of the information chain). Such a study was carried out by Egger (in press). Their thorough follow-up revealed not a single transmission case on the pitch, confirming the match analysis data. The study has been mirrored in English rugby players (Jones et al., in press). The fact that they did not find transmissions in a discipline with very close body contact makes a strong point in favor of soccer being a low-risk sport for acquiring respiratory infections on the pitch.

## Conditions that may appear to be of infectious origin

While it is important not to miss a diagnosis of a URTI, it is equally important to not to "over-diagnose" upper respiratory symptoms (URS) as URTI in players. An increase in minute ventilation during exercise can produce significant stress on the respiratory tract (Hull et al., 2017). This factor can cause certain typically URTI-associated symptoms, such as cough. Extreme conditions, such as cold air and high-intensity exercise, may promote airway hyper-responsiveness (Hull et al., 2017).

Increased airflow also increases exposure to allergens present in the air, which can trigger an allergic response. It has also been suggested that a reactivation of the Epstein–Barr virus (EBV) may cause transient symptoms. We do not agree with the assumption that such reactivations which may be seen in immunocompromised patients occur in healthy soccer players. However, allergic conditions may mimic infectious diseases and may partly account for a relatively short duration of symptoms (Gleeson & Pyne, 2016).

## Future directions and conclusions

Some research has been done pertaining to infectious diseases and soccer. However, much of the information that is currently available about the topic of infectious diseases and sport comes from disciplines other than soccer (e.g., cycling, running, and skiing). Therefore, there is a need for more studies conducted specifically in soccer, and more importantly, in female and male players at different levels of play, as well as different age groups. Moreover, the SARS-CoV-2 pandemic, although it has already fueled much research in the immunology of exercise, will demand even further investigations as the situation progresses and when it finally comes to an end.

In conclusion, the most common infections in soccer players are URTI, followed by GI. Other endemic diseases (such as vector-borne diseases) should be thought of before traveling to competitions or training camps. Preventive measures include vaccinations, hand hygiene, and ensuring food and water quality. Certain factors increase the risk of infectious diseases, for example, proximity to teammates and opponents. However, it seems that match play does not pose an increased risk for URTI. Laboratory parameters (such as leukocytes and CRP), as well as signs and symptoms, aid in the diagnosis of infectious diseases. Players with generalized symptoms should refrain from physical activity. An infectious episode might lead to a loss of the sick player for important trainings or matches. However, the consequences of an inadequate period of rest and recovery are potentially far worse. Common drugs used as part of a treatment include antibiotics and NSAIDs. Most of the drugs used do not impede training or playing per se. After an infectious episode, return-to-play and return-to-training should take place when the player is symptom-free and should be gradual depending on the circumstances of each individual case. There seems to be very little risk of SARS-CoV-2 spread during a match. Avoiding under-diagnosing is as important as avoiding over-diagnosing. Some URS may occur after strenuous exercise, it is important that these are not mistaken for URTI.

## References

Basso, C., Carturan, E., Corrado, D., & Thiene, G. (2007). Myocarditis and dilated cardiomyopathy in athletes: diagnosis, management, and recommendations for sport activity. *Cardiol Clin*, 25(3), 423–429, vi. https://doi.org/10.1016/j.ccl.2007.08.008

Becker, J. A., & Smith, J. A. (2014). Return to play after infectious mononucleosis. *Sports Health*, 6(3), 232–238. https://doi.org/10.1177/1941738114521984

Bjørneboe, J., Kristenson, K., Waldén, M., Bengtsson, H., Ekstrand, J., Hägglund, M., Rønsen, O., & Andersen, T. E. (2016). Role of illness in male professional football: not a major contributor to time loss. *Br J Sports Med*, 50(11), 699–702. https://doi.org/10.1136/bjsports-2015-095921

Börjesson M., Arvidsson D., Rensburg C.J.V., Schwellnus M. (2018). Return to Play After Infectious Disease. In: Musahl V., Karlsson J., Krutsch W., Mandelbaum B., Espregueira-Mendes J., d'Hooghe P. (Eds), *Return to Play in Football: An Evidence-Based Approach* (755–769). Springer, Berlin, Heidelberg. https://doi.org/10.1007/978-3-662-55713-6_56

Buder, V., Augustin, M., Schäfer, I., Welsch, G., Catala-Lehnen, P., & Herberger, K. (2018). [Prevalence of dermatomycoses in professional football players: A study based on data of German Bundesliga fitness check-ups (2013–2015) compared to data of the general population]. *Hautarzt*, 69(5), 401–407. https://doi.org/10.1007/s00105-017-4120-3

Bury, T., Marechal, R., Mahieu, P., & Pirnay, F. (1998). Immunological status of competitive football players during the training season. *Int J Sports Med*, 19(5), 364–368. https://doi.org/10.1055/s-2007-971931

Centers for Disease Control and Prevention. (2019, May 20). *About Zika*. Centers for Disease Control and Prevention. Retrieved February 27, 2023, from https://www.cdc.gov/zika/about/index.html

Centers for Disease Control and Prevention. (2023, February 9). *Dengue*. Centers for Disease Control and Prevention. Retrieved February 27, 2023, from https://www.cdc.gov/dengue/index.html#print

Centers for Disease Control and Prevention. (2019, January 31). *Methicillin-resistant Staphylococcus aureus (MRSA)*. For Athletes. Centers for Disease Control and Prevention. Retrieved February 27, 2023, from https://www.cdc.gov/mrsa/community/team-hc-providers/advice-for-athletes.html#

Centers for Disease Control and Prevention. (2022, November 14). *Prevention of yellow fever*. Centers for Disease Control and Prevention. Retrieved February 27, 2023, from https://www.cdc.gov/yellowfever/prevention/index.html

Centers for Disease Control and Prevention. (2020, July 1). *Ticks. Preventing tick bites*. Centers for Disease Control and Prevention. Retrieved February 28, 2023, from https://www.cdc.gov/ticks/avoid/on_people.html

Centers for Disease Control and Prevention. (2022, September 16). *Traveler's Health. Hepatitis A*. Centers for Disease Control and Prevention. Retrieved February 27, 2023, from https://wwwnc.cdc.gov/travel/diseases/hepatitis-a

Centers for Disease Control and Prevention. (2022, May 6). *Traveler's Health. Tick-borne encephalitis*. Centers for Disease Control and Prevention. Retrieved February 27, 2023, from https://wwwnc.cdc.gov/travel/diseases/tickborne-encephalitis

Centers for Disease Control and Prevention. (2022, September 16). *Traveler's Health. Typhoid fever*. Centers for Disease Control and Prevention. Retrieved February 27, 2023, from https://wwwnc.cdc.gov/travel/diseases/typhoid

Centers for Disease Control and Prevention. (2022, September 22). *Traveler's Health. Yellow Fever*. Centers for Disease Control and Prevention. Retrieved February 27, 2023, from https://wwwnc.cdc.gov/travel/diseases/yellow-fever

Chesson, L., Whitehead, S., Flanagan, K., Deighton, K., Matu, J., Backhouse, S. H., & Jones, B. (2021). Illness and infection in elite full-contact football-code sports: A systematic review. *Journal of science and medicine in sport, 24*(5), 435–440. https://doi.org/10.1016/j.jsams.2020.11.001

Dvorak, J., Junge, A., Derman, W., & Schwellnus, M. (2011). Injuries and illnesses of football players during the 2010 FIFA World Cup. *Br J Sports Med, 45*(8), 626–630. https://doi.org/10.1136/bjsm.2010.079905

Egger, F., Faude, O., Schreiber, S., Gärtner, B. C., & Meyer, T. (2021). Does playing football (soccer) lead to SARS-CoV-2 transmission? - A case study of 3 matches with 18 infected football players. *Science & medicine in football, 5*(supl), 2–7. https://doi.org/10.1080/24733938.2021.1895442

Eichner, E. R. (1993). Infection, Immunity, and Exercise. *Phys Sportsmed, 21*(1), 125–135. https://doi.org/10.1080/00913847.1993.11710319

Fahlman, M. M., & Engels, H. J. (2005). Mucosal IgA and URTI in American college football players: a year longitudinal study. *Med Sci Sports Exerc, 37*(3), 374–380. https://doi.org/10.1249/01.mss.0000155432.67020.88

Figueiredo, P., Nassis, G. P., & Brito, J. (2019). Within-Subject Correlation Between Salivary IgA and Measures of Training Load in Elite Football Players. International journal of sports physiology and performance, 14(6), 847–849. https://doi.org/10.1123/ijspp.2018-0455

Fontanilla, J. M., Kirkland, K. B., Talbot, E. A., Powell, K. E., Schwartzman, J. D., Goering, R. V., & Parsonnet, J. (2010). Outbreak of skin infections in college football team members due to an unusual strain of community-acquired methicillin-susceptible Staphylococcus aureus. *J Clin Microbiol, 48*(2), 609-611. https://doi.org/10.1128/JCM.02297-09

Gatmaitan, B. G., Chason, J. L., & Lerner, A. M. (1970). Augmentation of the virulence of murine coxsackie-virus B-3 myocardiopathy by exercise. *J Exp Med, 131*(6), 1121–1136. https://doi.org/10.1084/jem.131.6.1121

Gleeson, M., & Pyne, D. B. (2016). Respiratory inflammation and infections in high-performance athletes. *Immunol Cell Biol, 94*(2), 124–131. https://doi.org/10.1038/icb.2015.100

Gärtner, B. C., & Meyer, T. (2014). Vaccination in elite athletes. *Sports Med, 44*(10), 1361–1376. https://doi.org/10.1007/s40279-014-0217-3

Hanstad, D. V., Rønsen, O., Andersen, S. S., Steffen, K., & Engebretsen, L. (2011). Fit for the fight? Illnesses in the Norwegian team in the Vancouver Olympic Games. *Br J Sports Med, 45*(7), 571–575. https://doi.org/10.1136/bjsm.2010.081364

Henriey, D., Delmont, J., & Gautret, P. (2014). Does the use of alcohol-based hand gel sanitizer reduce travelers' diarrhea and gastrointestinal upset?: A preliminary survey. *Travel Med Infect Dis, 12*(5), 494–498. https://doi.org/10.1016/j.tmaid.2014.07.002

Hickie, I., Davenport, T., Wakefield, D., Vollmer-Conna, U., Cameron, B., Vernon, S. D., Reeves, W. C., Lloyd, A., & Group, D. I. O. S. (2006). Post-infective and chronic fatigue syndromes precipitated by viral and non-viral pathogens: prospective cohort study. *BMJ, 333*(7568), 575. https://doi.org/10.1136/bmj.38933.585764.AE

Hojyo, S., & Fukada, T. (2016). Roles of Zinc Signaling in the Immune System. *J Immunol Res, 2016*, 6762343. https://doi.org/10.1155/2016/6762343

Hull, J. H., Dickinson, J. W., & Jackson, A. R. (2017). Cough in exercise and athletes. *Pulm Pharmacol Ther, 47*, 49–55. https://doi.org/10.1016/j.pupt.2017.04.005

Jekabsone, A., Sile, I., Cochis, A., Makrecka-Kuka, M., Laucaityte, G., Makarova, E., Rimondini, L., Bernotiene, R., Raudone, L., Vedlugaite, E., Baniene, R., Smalinskiene, A., Savickiene, N., & Dambrova, M. (2019). Investigation of Antibacterial and Antiinflammatory Activities of Proanthocyanidins from *Pelargonium sidoides* DC Root Extract. *Nutrients, 11*(11), 2829. https://doi.org/10.3390/nu11112829

Jiménez-Truque, N., Saye, E. J., Soper, N., Saville, B. R., Thomsen, I., Edwards, K. M., & Creech, C. B. (2017). Association Between Contact Sports and Colonization with Staphylococcus aureus in a Prospective Cohort of Collegiate Athletes. *Sports Med, 47*(5), 1011–1019. https://doi.org/10.1007/s40279-016-0618-6

Jones, C. M., Griffiths, P. C., & Mellalieu, S. D. (2017). Training Load and Fatigue Marker Associations with Injury and Illness: A Systematic Review of Longitudinal Studies. *Sports Med, 47*(5), 943-974. https://doi.org/10.1007/s40279-016-0619-5

Jones, B., Phillips, G., Kemp, S., Payne, B., Hart, B., Cross, M., & Stokes, K. A. (2021). SARS-CoV-2 transmission during rugby league matches: do players become infected after participating with SARS-CoV-2 positive players?. *British journal of sports medicine, 55*(14), 807–813. https://doi.org/10.1136/bjsports-2020-103714

Kakanis, M. W., Peake, J., Brenu, E. W., Simmonds, M., Gray, B., Hooper, S. L., & Marshall-Gradisnik, S. M. (2010). The open window of susceptibility to infection after acute exercise in healthy young male elite athletes. *Exerc Immunol Rev, 16*, 119–137.

Karsch-Völk, M., Barrett, B., & Linde, K. (2015). Echinacea for preventing and treating the common cold. *JAMA, 313*(6), 618-619. https://doi.org/10.1001/jama.2014.17145

Knudsen, N. S., Thomasen, M. M. D., & Andersen, T. B. (2022). Modelling the potential spread of virus during soccer matches. *BMJ open sport & exercise medicine, 8*(2), e001268. https://doi.org/10.1136/bmjsem-2021-001268

Kratzel, A., Todt, D., V'kovski, P., Steiner, S., Gultom, M., Thao, T. T. N., Ebert, N., Holwerda, M., Steinmann, J., Niemeyer, D., Dijkman, R., Kampf, G., Drosten, C., Steinmann, E., Thiel, V., & Pfaender, S. (2020). Inactivation of Severe Acute Respiratory Syndrome Coronavirus 2 by WHO-Recommended Hand Rub Formulations and Alcohols. *Emerg Infect Dis, 26*(7), 1592–1595. https://doi.org/10.3201/eid2607.200915

Maya, J., Marquez, P., Peñailillo, L., Contreras-Ferrat, A., Deldicque, L., & Zbinden-Foncea, H. (2016). Salivary Biomarker Responses to Two Final Matches in Women's Professional Football. Journal of sports science & medicine, 15(2), 365–371.

Meyer, T., Mack, D., Donde, K., Harzer, O., Krutsch, W., Rössler, A., Kimpel, J., von Laer, D., & Gärtner, B. C. (2021). Successful return to professional men's football (soccer) competition after the COVID-19 shutdown: a cohort study in the German Bundesliga. *Br J Sports Med, 55(1)*, 62-66. https://doi.org/10.1136/bjsports-2020-103150

Moreira, A., Bradley, P., Carling, C., Arruda, A. F., Spigolon, L. M., Franciscon, C., & Aoki, M. S. (2016). Effect of a congested match schedule on immune-endocrine responses, technical performance and session-RPE in elite youth soccer players. Journal of sports sciences, 34(24), 2255–2261. https://doi.org/10.1080/02640414.2016.1205753

Morgans, R., Orme, P., Anderson, L., Drust, B., & Morton, J. P. (2014). An intensive Winter fixture schedule induces a transient fall in salivary IgA in English premier league soccer players. *Research in sports medicine (Print), 22*(4), 346–354. https://doi.org/10.1080/15438627.2014.944641

Mutebi, J. P., & Gimnig, J. E. (2020). Mosquitoes, Ticks & Other Arthropods. In Brunette, G. W. and Nemhauser, J. B. (Eds.), CDC *Yellow Book 2020: Health Information for International Travel.* New York: Oxford University Press; 2017. https://wwwnc.cdc.gov/travel/yellowbook/2020/noninfectious-health-risks/mosquitoes-ticks-and-other-arthropods

Nieman, D. C. (1994). Exercise, infection, and immunity. *Int J Sports Med, 15 Suppl 3*, S131–141. https://doi.org/10.1055/s-2007-1021128

Orhant, E., Carling, C., & Cox, A. (2010). A three-year prospective study of illness in professional soccer players. *Res Sports Med, 18*(3), 199–204. https://doi.org/10.1080/15438627.2010.490462

Pedersen, B. K., & Bruunsgaard, H. (1995). How physical exercise influences the establishment of infections. *Sports Med, 19*(6), 393–400. https://doi.org/10.2165/00007256-199519060-00003

Pedersen, B. K., & Ullum, H. (1994). NK cell response to physical activity: possible mechanisms of action. *Med Sci Sports Exerc, 26*(2), 140–146. https://doi.org/10.1249/00005768-199402000-00003

Piggott, B., Newton, M., McGuigan, M. (2009). The relationship between training load and incidence of injury and illness over a pre-season at an Australian Football League Club. *JASC, 17*(3), 4–17.

Primos, W. A. (1996). Sports and Exercise During Acute Illness. *Phys Sportsmed, 24*(1), 44–54. https://doi.org/10.1080/00913847.1996.11947895

Pyne, D. B., West, N. P., Cox, A. J., & Cripps, A. W. (2015). Probiotics supplementation for athletes - clinical and physiological effects. *Eur J Sport Sci, 15*(1), 63–72. https://doi.org/10.1080/17461391.2014.971879

Romano, R., Lu, D., & Holtom, P. (2006). Outbreak of community-acquired methicillin-resistant Staphylococcus aureus skin infections among a collegiate football team. *J Athl Train, 41*(2), 141–145.

Roth, M., Fang, L., Stolz, D., & Tamm, M. (2019). Pelargonium sidoides radix extract EPs 7630 reduces rhinovirus infection through modulation of viral binding proteins on human bronchial epithelial cells. *PLoS One, 14*(2), e0210702. https://doi.org/10.1371/journal.pone.0210702

Scharhag, J., & Meyer, T. (2014). Return to play after acute infectious disease in football players. J Sports Sci, 32(13), 1237–1242. https://doi.org/10.1080/02640414.2014.898861

Schlagheck, M. L., Walzik, D., Joisten, N., Koliamitra, C., Hardt, L., Metcalfe, A. J., Wahl, P., Bloch, W., Schenk, A., & Zimmer, P. (2020). Cellular immune response to acute exercise: Comparison of endurance and resistance exercise. European journal of haematology, 105(1), 75–84. https://doi.org/10.1111/ejh.13412

Schumacher, Y. O., Tabben, M., Hassoun, K., Al Marwani, A., Al Hussein, I., Coyle, P., Abbassi, A. K., Ballan, H. T., Al-Kuwari, A., Chamari, K., & Bahr, R. (2021). Resuming professional football (soccer) during the COVID-19 pandemic in a country with high infection rates: a prospective cohort study. *British journal of sports medicine, 55*(19), 1092–1098. https://doi.org/10.1136/bjsports-2020-103724

Schwellnus, M., Soligard, T., Alonso, J. M., Bahr, R., Clarsen, B., Dijkstra, H. P., Gabbett, T. J., Gleeson, M., Hägglund, M., Hutchinson, M. R., Janse Van Rensburg, C., Meeusen, R., Orchard, J. W., Pluim, B. M., Raftery, M., Budgett, R., & Engebretsen, L. (2016). How much is too much? (Part 2) International Olympic Committee consensus statement on load in sport and risk of illness. *Br J Sports Med, 50*(17), 1043–1052. https://doi.org/10.1136/bjsports-2016-096572

Schwellnus, M. P., Derman, W. E., Jordaan, E., Page, T., Lambert, M. I., Readhead, C., Roberts, C., Kohler, R., Collins, R., Kara, S., Morris, M. I., Strauss, O., & Webb, S. (2012). Elite athletes travelling to international destinations >5 time zone differences from their home country have a 2-3-fold increased risk of illness. *Br J Sports Med, 46*(11), 816–821. https://doi.org/10.1136/bjsports-2012-091395

Shaban, R. Z., Li, C., O'Sullivan, M. V. N., Kok, J., Dempsey, K., Ramsperger, M., Brown, M., Nahidi, S., & Sotomayor-Castillo, C. (2021). Outbreak of community-acquired Staphylococcus aureus skin infections in an Australian professional football team. *Journal of science and medicine in sport, 24*(6), 520–525. https://doi.org/10.1016/j.jsams.2020.11.006

Shek, P. N., Sabiston, B. H., Buguet, A., & Radomski, M. W. (1995). Strenuous exercise and immunological changes: a multiple-time-point analysis of leukocyte subsets, CD4/CD8 ratio, immunoglobulin production and NK cell response. *Int J Sports Med, 16*(7), 466–474. https://doi.org/10.1055/s-2007-973039

Springham, M., Williams, S., Waldron, M., Strudwick, A. J., Mclellan, C., & Newton, R. U. (2021). Salivary Immunoendocrine and Self-report Monitoring Profiles across an Elite-Level Professional Football Season. Medicine and science in sports and exercise, 53(5), 918–927. https://doi.org/10.1249/MSS.0000000000002553

Stenger, T., Ledo, A., Ziller, C., Schub, D., Schmidt, T., Enders, M., GÄrtner, B. C., Sester, M., & Meyer, T. (2020). Timing of Vaccination after Training: Immune Response and Side Effects in Athletes. *Med Sci Sports Exerc, 52*(7), 1603–1609. https://doi.org/10.1249/MSS.0000000000002278

Tamimi, A. H., Maxwell, S., Edmonds, S. L., & Gerba, C. P. (2015). Impact of the use of an alcohol-based hand sanitizer in the home on reduction in probability of infection by respiratory and enteric viruses. *Epidemiol Infect, 143*(15), 3335–3341. https://doi.org/10.1017/S0950268815000035

Timmer, A., Günther, J., Motschall, E., Rücker, G., Antes, G., & Kern, W. V. (2013). Pelargonium sidoides extract for treating acute respiratory tract infections. *The Cochrane database of systematic reviews 2013*, Issue 10. Art. No.: CD006323. https://doi.org/10.1002/14651858.CD006323.pub3

Turbeville, S. D., Cowan, L. D., & Greenfield, R. A. (2006). Infectious disease outbreaks in competitive sports: a review of the literature. *Am J Sports Med, 34*(11), 1860–1865. https://doi.org/10.1177/0363546505285385

Van Duivenbode, V; Goes, F. (2020). "Social Distancing" in Football (Powerpoint slides). Koninklijke Nederlandse Voetbal Bond: https://www.mayouthsoccer.org/assets/61/6/knvb_research_social_distancing.pdf

Wang, C. Y., Chiao, M. T., Yen, P. J., Huang, W. C., Hou, C. C., Chien, S. C., Yeh, K. C., Yang, W. C., Shyur, L. F., & Yang, N. S. (2006). Modulatory effects of Echinacea purpurea extracts on human dendritic cells: a cell- and gene-based study. *Genomics, 88*(6), 801-808. https://doi.org/10.1016/j.ygeno.2006.08.011

Wentz, L. M., Nieman, D. C., McBride, J. E., Gillitt, N. D., Williams, L. L., & Warin, R. F. (2018). Carbohydrate Intake Does Not Counter the Post-Exercise Decrease in Natural Killer Cell Cytotoxicity. Nutrients, 10(11), 1658. https://doi.org/10.3390/nu10111658

Wessels, I., Maywald, M., & Rink, L. (2017). Zinc as a Gatekeeper of Immune Function. *Nutrients, 9*(12), 1286. https://doi.org/10.3390/nu9121286

World Health Organization. (n.d.). *Chagas disease (American trypanosomiasis)*. World Health Organization. Retrieved February 27, 2023, from https://www.who.int/health-topics/chagas-disease

World Health Organization. (2023, January 18). *Soil-transmitted helminth infections*. World Health Organization. Retrieved February 27, 2023, from https://www.who.int/news-room/fact-sheets/detail/soil-transmitted-helminth-infections

World Health Organization. (2022, December 8). *Zika virus*. World Health Organization. Retrieved February 27, 2023, from https://www.who.int/news-room/fact-sheets/detail/zika-virus

# 15 Biomechanical assessments

*Mark A. Robinson, Katherine A.J. Daniels and Jos Vanrenterghem*

## Introduction

Biomechanics is the study of the effect of forces on the body. In soccer, a player experiences or generates many types of forces. The external forces come from outside of the body and include reaction forces from contact with the ground, ball, or opponents. The internal forces are generated inside the body through muscular contractions which cause movement and prepare the body to cope with external forces. Soccer match play is highly dynamic with activities such as jumping, landing, sprinting, and turning requiring players to generate and dissipate high forces. Biomechanics has two broad applications for soccer. First, to maximise performance during these tasks. Second, to reduce injury/re-injury risk. Several comprehensive reviews exist that have covered these applications in depth both holistically (Lees & Nolan, 1998; Nunome et al., 2017), and specifically, for example, related to kicking (Kellis & Katis, 2007; Lees et al., 2010), heading (Caccese & Kaminski, 2016), surfaces, and equipment (Lees & Lake, 2003). In this chapter, we focus on practical tests and measurements that are used in soccer and are interpreted in a biomechanical context. A suite of measurement tools and techniques exists to provide detailed, objective, and quantitative data to understand and evaluate the physical status and biomechanical effectiveness of players. Specifically, we consider four areas based on assessments that could be performed by a sports scientist with equipment that would typically be available in a professional and academy club setting. Where low-cost alternatives exist, these will be considered.

## Evaluating jump performance

The evaluation of jump performance has traditionally been part of pre-season screening. While typically this is done as part of the assessment of players' physical fitness, the truth is that for many teams the recorded jump heights are perhaps not much more than a stimulus for players to compete for the team record. Nonetheless, the trainer, coach, and possibly physiotherapist, often have their own ideas on why screening for jump performance may be relevant. They may, for example, have an interest in age-dependent performance changes in the context of talent identification, seasonal variations in performance, or obtaining a baseline performance against which to compare future evaluations (e.g., during rehabilitation). What is certain is that in all cases, practitioners who have worked out why they wish to evaluate jump performance will have asked the following questions: which type of jump should I test? Which technology should I use? How will I use the test outcomes to change my training/rehabilitation

DOI: 10.4324/9781003148418-18

*Biomechanical assessments* 239

approach? In this section, we provide a brief overview of some supportive evidence to help answer those questions.

## Considerations for data collection

Decisions about which type of jump to test are typically interlinked with the available time and technology. An overview of common jump test approaches is provided in Table 15.1. While the Sargent 'jump and reach test' is the cheapest, the flight time method has arguably been the most popularly used test in soccer. In the 1980s, Carmelo Bosco described a simple procedure with the calculation of flight height ($H_{flight}$) from measured flight time ($t_{flight}$), derived from the motion equations related to parabolic flight (Bosco et al., 1983).

$$H_{flight} = \frac{1}{2}\left(\frac{t_{flight}}{2}\right)^2$$

*Table 15.1* A schematic overview of commonly used jump evaluation approaches

| Method | Equipment | Outcome | Main pro | Main con |
|---|---|---|---|---|
| Sargent vertical jump (reach distance method) | Chalk on wall with measuring tape; vertec$^{TM}$ with horizontally rotating vanes | Distance between reach height marked at peak of flight relative to standing reach height | Cheapest vertical jump test | Need to have a good arm coordination during jumping |
| Vertical jump height based on flight time recording (flight time method) | Jump mat (e.g., just jump); opto jump$^{TM}$; my jump$^{TM}$ phone app | Flight height; Stretch-shortening cycle index; repetitive jump performance (avg contact time and flight height) | Quick setup and accurate if recorded at a high enough frame rate (>100 Hz) | Need to land the jump in a controlled fashion |
| Jump height based on ground reaction force recording (impulse method) | Any floor-mounted force platform, some portable force platforms | Same as flight time methods; push-off mechanics (e.g., rate of force development, counter movement depth); broad jump horizontal take-off velocity | In-depth data on mechanical quality of the push-off | Expensive equipment and need for tightly standardised procedures to have valid results |
| Standing broad jump (flight distance method) | Tape-measure on non-slip surface | Jump distance based on foot contact | Relevance for sprint-related performance indicators | Landing coordination can interfere with push-off performance |

Practically, the flight time method is most applied using a 'jump mat' which measures flight time from contact switches. The main constraint with this method is that body configuration at the instant of landing needs to be the same as at the instant of take-off. Practitioners may sometimes confuse a 'jump mat' with a force platform (which measures forces). While a force platform could be used to measure flight time directly, the main advantage is that it allows take-off velocity ($V_{\text{takeoff}}$) to be calculated. To achieve this aim, force signals are integrated over time to calculate the impulse, which is proportional to the change in velocity of the body centre of mass (hence referred to as the impulse method). Using the same motion equations related to parabolic flight, flight height can be calculated independent of whether the athlete returns onto the force platform.

$$H_{\text{flight}} = \left( \frac{V_{\text{takeoff}}}{2g} \right)^2 \qquad \text{with } g = 9.81 \, ms^{-2}$$

The impulse method allows for many other variables related to the push-off to be calculated. Rate of force development metrics are likely to be the most relevant performance determinants; peak power has been suggested to be highly relevant, but this is a misconception stemming from commonly used terminology ('explosive power') (Ruddock & Winter, 2016). However, the impulse method does come with some concerns, requiring stricter data collection procedures and more advanced data processing routines to counter undesirable measurement artefacts (Vanrenterghem et al., 2001).

In terms of the type of jump, endless variations exist concerning starting configuration (from standing, from deep squat, following pre-hop, and after box-drop), use of the arms (with arm swing, holding arms in front of chest or akimbo, holding a bar across the shoulders, and holding added handheld weights), direction of the jump (vertical, broad, and lateral), single versus double legged push-off, or jump repetitions (reactive strength, reactive strength endurance, and agility ladder jumps). The target population often determines one's choices. For example, evaluating the differences in jump performance with and without the use of the arms may be relevant in goalkeepers more so than in field players. Also, in soccer players unilateral jumps in horizontal directions may be more relevant than the commonly used two-legged vertical jump to assess explosive muscular capacity (Murtagh et al., 2018).

## Considerations for data interpretation

Whether or not a test outcome should trigger a change in training plan depends on two interlinked questions. First, how confident can I be that my test result is valid (against a gold standard test), reliable (variation within a session), and repeatable (variation between sessions)? This provides me with an overall noise estimate on my measure (standard deviation), allowing me to estimate the sensitivity of the test outcome for detecting a meaningful change, that is, the Minimal Detectable Change. Second, I must decide which criterion value (e.g., normative data and a player's own reference data) to use to detect the change against. Whilst it is impossible to accurately summarise the existing evidence related to these questions (and its scientific quality), some practical advice may be in place.

- An application with more outcome measures does not make it better, rather, it often promotes cherry-picking to confirm pre-existing beliefs rather than truly supporting the practitioner.

- A player's own historical test results are more valuable than the comparison against peers or a normative dataset (except perhaps when evaluating the relationship between physical growth and functional development as part of health screening in young players).
- Routinely incorporating an easy but trusted jump evaluation in the training process has greater chances of generating relevant information about player fitness and/or fatigue than running a fully comprehensive jump evaluation with dozens of test outcome measures once in the season.
- The added value of jump tests as part of regular screening may not only lie in assessing a player's fitness, but in the biopsychosocial facets of player management (Bahr, 2016), none the least that it can promote good-natured banter between players and staff.

## Muscle activity assessment with electromyography

Electromyography (EMG) is used to measure and evaluate the electrical activity of a muscle. It provides a way of understanding the behaviour of a muscle during a given task. Observing muscle contraction and relaxation provides an insight into the dynamic function of the muscle. Muscular contraction is the product of action potentials moving along muscle fibres. The change in electrical activity of a muscle fibre can be detected by electrodes. The EMG signal, therefore, describes the recruitment and firing pattern detected within a muscle (Konrad, 2006). Different types of electrodes can be used to detect muscular activity. Finewire electrodes are invasively placed into the muscle (inserted with a needle) and require specialist training to use but are sometimes needed for the detailed clinical assessment of individual muscles, particularly if these muscles are not near the skin surface. High-density electrodes are an array of electrodes placed on the skin, covering a large surface of the muscle, and can provide a detailed insight into motor unit firing and progression of the action potentials through the muscle. The most-used electrodes are surface electrodes. These electrodes by comparison are non-invasive and simply require two electrodes to be placed on the skin above the muscle belly.

Within soccer, surface EMG has been applied in injury prevention and rehabilitation contexts, for example, to investigate muscular fatigue, neuromuscular characterisation, and training, or hamstring injury risk. While electromyography is primarily a research tool, EMG is becoming increasingly more accessible to soccer clubs. Wireless signal transmission directly from the muscle belly has become the norm, and even electrodes embedded in clothing allow for more applied applications (Finni et al., 2007). Nonetheless, the implementation of EMG in an applied context remains complex because of the large number of considerations for data collection and treatment.

## Considerations for data collection

We can draw many different questions and conclusions from EMG analysis. Practical questions can allow comparisons within and between individuals, as well as within and between muscles (Vigotsky et al., 2018). All of which need careful consideration of the data collection and interpretation.

The primary constraint of surface EMG is that it is not suitable for all muscles. Careful palpation of the central portion of the muscle belly located closest to the surface of

242    *Mark A. Robinson et al.*

the skin is needed to avoid 'cross-talk' from other muscles nearby. Skin preparation is required to reduce the electrical resistance of the skin and maximise the quality of the EMG signal. Typically, this process will involve shaving areas on the muscle belly that have excess hair and wiping with an alcohol swab. A good skin preparation will have a resistance of <5 Ohms between the electrodes.

The most evident application in the practical setting is to provide real-time feedback on whether and how a muscle is functioning during activities, typically in a rehabilitation context. If the intention is to compare the magnitude of activation between muscles (e.g., medial and lateral hamstring muscles) or between sessions (before and after a therapeutic intervention) it is necessary to first 'calibrate' the raw EMG signals. A common calibration method is to express the magnitude of the EMG signal against the muscle's maximal activation level, for which a maximum voluntary contraction (MVC) is recorded. Obtaining a reliable MVC can be challenging, as it depends on the ability of the individual to do a maximal effort muscle contraction which they are not used to. It is advised to collect multiple attempts to verify the data are representative. Also, the calibration process typically needs to be done in post-processing, so calibrated data are not available real-time.

Another application is the identification of muscles that are being activated too late or too early in a movement, for example, around the time of impact with the ground. To identify the timings of activation with respect to key movement phases, it will be necessary to synchronise the EMG equipment with other devices such as motion capture systems, force platforms, or wearable inertial measurement systems. Prior to purchasing an EMG system, check that your intended system is compatible with the relevant devices.

**Considerations for data interpretation**

The raw (unprocessed) EMG signal is generally not used for any quantitative data analysis as the higher-frequency components of the signal are not reproducible. It is common to focus on the general shape of the EMG signal with high-frequency signals removed. This type of analysis focuses on the time domain of the signal and is used to address questions relating to the magnitude and timing of the signal. The second type of analysis focuses on the frequency domain of the signal, basically identifying how fast spikes follow one another. This measure is used to address questions relating the signal 'drive' to the muscle, for example, revealing the impact of fatigue on the ability to fully recruit one's muscles.

### How do I process the EMG signal?

For time domain analysis, you will typically need to use three processes: bandpass filter your signal (10–500 Hz) to remove high-frequency (for example, coming from electronic devices) and low-frequency (for example, movement artefacts) signals that are not related to muscle activation; full-wave rectification to convert negatives to positives; then create a linear envelope (a smooth outline of the signal). The root mean square is a common choice to create this linear envelope, with a time window of 20 ms for very rapid movements such as jumping, landing, or running, or up to 100 ms for slower movements such as walking (Figure 15.1). For a frequency domain analysis, the unfiltered signal should be used.

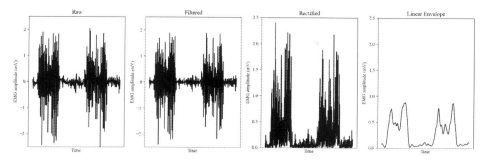

*Figure 15.1* The processing stages of a raw EMG signal.

## *How should I calibrate the EMG signal?*

By expressing the processed EMG as a percentage of the above-mentioned MVC value for a time domain analysis is a common fourth step. This is not always easily obtained in a practical setting, and expressing the signal relative to the activation level of a standard activity such as walking or a maximal vertical jump may be preferred, depending somewhat on the goal of the analysis (Burden, 2010). It is not uncommon for dynamic contractions to exceed the 100% value of an MVC recording.

## *What metrics can I use?*

Typical metrics for a time-domain analysis are the mean or maximal signal, the time-to-peak activation, time between onset and offset, or the area under the curve (integrated EMG). For the frequency domain, the median frequency is often used to represent changes in EMG due to fatigue. It is worthwhile identifying which of these can be readily extracted from the software that comes with commercially available EMG systems, potentially saving a lot of time and headaches. It may also be possible to extract the raw data for your own processing in Microsoft Excel, for example, using the Biomechanics Toolbar, a freely available post-processing add-in (www.biomechanicstoolbar.org).

An excellent general guide for all aspects of EMG is 'The ABC of EMG' (Konrad, 2006).

The SENIAM project http://www.seniam.org/ has sensor location recommendations for 30 individual muscles.

The International Society of Electrophysiology and Kinesiology (ISEK) is a multi-disciplinary organisation interested in EMG https://isek.org/. Their reports are a must-read for reporting EMG data in scientific publications: https://isek.org/-wp-content/uploads/2015/05/Standards-for-Reporting-EMGData.pdf

## Muscle strength assessment

Muscular strength is a key component of physical performance and injury prevention. An isokinetic dynamometer (IKD) is a sophisticated tool used to assess muscle strength under controlled circumstances, most commonly at a constant (isokinetic) velocity of joint angular rotation (Figure 15.2). Within soccer, it would be used by a

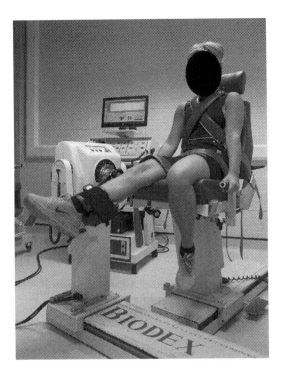

*Figure 15.2* An isokinetic dynamometer set-up for right knee testing.

sports scientist, physiotherapist, or strength and conditioning coach either for general health screening purposes, evaluation of training progress, or as part of return to sport decision-making (e.g., establishing interlimb asymmetry). The most assessed muscle groups are the quadriceps and hamstrings. Other devices are also popular for strength assessment, but these are generally limited to a (quasi) isometric evaluation (e.g., handheld dynamometer), assessment of one muscle group only (e.g., NordBord), or closed-chain actions (e.g., portable force platform in combination with a Smith machine). The IKD by comparison is large and heavy, but nonetheless often available in professional environments. We highlight some practical considerations for data collection, treatment, and interpretation, which aim to complement other more detailed resources (e.g., Baltzopoulos, 2008).

## Considerations for data collection

For simplicity, we focus on the assessment of knee flexion-extension as depicted in Figure 15.2, though many other actions in the lower and upper limbs can be evaluated.

### *Preparation*

The collection of accurate IKD data is reliant on the correct set-up of the player prior to testing. The three key requirements are: (1) the fixed body segments (i.e., thigh and

Biomechanical assessments 245

upper body) must be firmly fixated to avoid unwanted movements of the knee-joint axis or confounding actions of biarticular muscles crossing both hip and knee (i.e., rectus femoris and hamstrings); (2) the rotating axle of the crank arm must be aligned with the knee-joint axis; and (3) the end of the lower leg must be strapped firmly to the crank to maximise the forces transferred to the torque sensor in the IKD. Allowing the player multiple attempts at sub-maximal intensity after preparation would be good practice.

### Protocol selection and settings

An IKD will typically allow the practitioner to select the isokinetic contraction mode, angular range, and angular velocity to be tested. The most common contraction modes used for player assessment are concentric (muscle fibres shortening), eccentric (muscle fibres lengthening), and isometric (zero joint rotation speed and hence no change in the length of the muscle-tendon unit). Angular range for isokinetic modes is typically set to encompass the full-joint active range of motion, while isometric testing can be done at several different joint angles to test different regions of the muscle force-length relationship. The chosen angular velocity of the crank will influence the maximum forces the player can generate based on the force-velocity relationship of muscle. Typical angular velocities reported in the literature include 60, 180, and 300 deg s$^{-1}$. For the higher angular velocities, it should be verified that the player generates the required angular velocity within the permitted range of motion. Alternative options can be available, such as protocols in which the crank arm produces a pre-determined resistance rather than speed (isotonic), but these are more commonly used for exercising than for assessment.

## Considerations for data interpretation

As the player's effort is measured through a torque sensor in the crank arm axle, the main measured variable is the joint moment reported in Newton-metres (Nm) – not muscle force. The key outcome measure of an isokinetic assessment tends to be the peak joint moment. A visual verification that the peak moment occurred when the angular velocity was at the pre-determined speed is important for concentric mode testing, particularly for higher angular velocities (Baltzopoulos, 2008). The software should permit the profiles of joint moment, angle of the crank, and angular velocity of the crank to be reported alongside each other (see Figure 15.3 left panel).

Besides peak joint moment, the IKD can provide detailed insight into the moment-angle profile, that is, how the agonists are able to produce force throughout the joint range of motion. For example, one can look at the joint angle at which the peak joint moment is reached, but also at the general rise and fall of the joint moment because of the force-length characteristics of muscle contraction. For this type of analysis, one needs to present the moment data against joint angular displacement (Figure 15.3 right panel) rather than against time (Figure 15.3 left panel). Some device software has this as a reporting option, but the user does not always have full control over what is and is not included in the report. If practitioners wish to gain more control over this, for example, in the context of applied research, then the use of an application such as IKD1D (www.ikd1d.org) may be preferred.

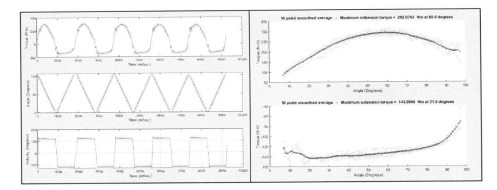

*Figure 15.3* (Left) Visualisation of the joint moment, angle, and angular velocity profiles for a concentric-concentric Quadriceps-Hamstrings protocol with the isokinetic phase highlighted. (Right) Calculation of a 10-point moving average joint moment-angle profile for the multiple trials.

Finally, some practical advice:

- When reporting a joint moment, the moment should be ascribed to the muscle group around the joint (e.g., the quadriceps or triceps surae joint moment, rather than a specific muscle such as the vastus or gastrocnemius moment). Also, while reduced joint moments are typically interpreted as reduced agonist contractile capacity, one should keep in mind that this can sometimes be linked to agonist inhibition (e.g., arthrogenic muscle inhibition immediately in the weeks following ACL reconstruction) or increased antagonist co-contractions as a subconscious protective mechanism following injury to the agonist.
- Joint moments are often expressed as a ratio against the antagonist moment to infer 'balance' about the joint (e.g., the Hamstrings: Quadriceps ratio evaluates the capacity of the hamstring muscle strength against its antagonist the quadriceps). For maximal clarity, it is useful to include the contraction type in the description of such ratio (e.g., $Ham_{con}:Quad_{con}$). For example in soccer, the so-called functional H:Q ratio ($H_{ecc}:Q_{con}$ ratio) is often reported to represent the perceived function of the hamstrings muscle group in stabilising the knee during locomotion. As a safety precaution, the joint angular velocity of the eccentric hamstring evaluation in such $H_{ecc}:Q_{con}$ ratio is typically lower than the concentric quadriceps evaluation (e.g., 30 deg s$^{-1}$ versus 120 deg s$^{-1}$).
- Caution is needed in interpreting maximum joint moments as indicative of dynamic muscle function during athletic tasks. The single-joint action during an IKD assessment eliminates important multi-muscle actions such as the transfer of muscle forces between joints and the capacity to return stored energy very effectively from tendon elastic forces during adequately coordinated multi-joint actions (i.e., stretch-shortening action).

## Injury prevention screening and return to play testing

Systematic physical testing of athletes is increasingly incorporated into training structures within competitive sport, with the aim of minimising overall playing time lost to musculoskeletal injuries. Many of these tests incorporate observations and/or technologies that would typically be used by biomechanists (e.g., timing sensors, force sensors, and video analysis). Testing can be carried out routinely on uninjured athletes to identify individuals presenting with modifiable risk factors for injury (*injury prevention screening*) or can be used to monitor recovery from musculoskeletal injury and inform the timing of an individual athlete's return to competitive play (*return to sport testing*). Athletes identified as 'at risk' through injury prevention screening programmes are often targeted with interventions focused on reducing the likelihood of future injury, while return to sport testing is used to guide decision-making when evaluating the optimum route back to competition after injury or 'clearing' athletes for full participation in sport.

## Considerations for data collection

As it is often desirable to quantify multiple physical qualities, and no single isolated test appears to provide adequate discriminative ability, testing batteries commonly comprise the evaluation of several tasks that can be considered as independent 'pass/fail' components of the assessment or can be used to derive an overall summed score. Some examples of physical tests and testing batteries that have been utilised in soccer for these purposes are listed below (in approximate ascending order of time and equipment demands).

### *Single-limb hop for distance testing*

A series of single-limb hopping tasks commonly used for return to sport testing after lower-limb injury. Routine tests include the single hop (landing on the same foot), the triple hop (three consecutive hops), and the cross-over hop (three consecutive hops with a mediolateral component). For all of these tasks, the aim is to maximise the total distance covered. Timed tests can also be included, for which the athlete is required to hop a given distance in the shortest possible time.

### *The star excursion balance test / Y balance test*

A dynamic balance test in which the participant stands on one leg and attempts to extend the contralateral leg as far as possible in multiple directions. All distances are comprised into a composite reach score which is used to identify athletes that may be at risk of injury, and inter-limb asymmetries can be used to monitor rehabilitation.

### *The functional movement screen (FMS)*

A whole-body testing battery incorporating multiple movement tasks that require stability and controlled movement, such as the straight-leg raise and the deep squat. Each component is rated visually on a four-point scale and the resultant score is used to identify asymmetries and deficits that could indicate an increased risk of future injury.

### *The athletic shoulder (ASH) test*

An upper-limb isometric testing protocol involving the use of a single force platform to measure isometric shoulder strength at multiple orientations. Test results are used

248 *Mark A. Robinson et al.*

to guide return to sport decision-making for overhead and contact sport athletes, such as soccer goalkeepers.

## Considerations for data interpretation

There are two key concepts to understand when interpreting the results of injury prevention screening tests: *sensitivity* and *specificity*. Sensitivity describes the ability of a test to identify a player who will obtain an injury (a 'true positive'), while specificity describes the ability of a test to correctly report a negative result for those who will not obtain an injury ('true negative'). In practice, sensitivity and specificity usually trade-off against each other – high sensitivity is associated with lower specificity, and vice versa. The multifactorial nature of many sports injuries means that physical screening tests tend to have relatively low sensitivity and specificity, limiting their predictive value (Bahr, 2016). Practitioners may, therefore, choose to offer injury prevention programmes to the entire team rather than only to those athletes identified as presenting an elevated individual injury-risk profile.

When physical testing is intended to inform return to sport decision-making after recovery from injury, the injured athlete's test results are commonly compared to 'reference' values to estimate rehabilitation status. The choice of reference data can influence the conclusions drawn and decisions made, so is an important consideration for practitioners. The preferred approach in most circumstances is to compare the athlete's post-injury performance and/or mechanics to their own pre-injury baseline measures. However, this option relies on the existence and availability of appropriate baseline data (hence why clubs may hold team-based pre-season screenings). Alternative approaches are:

(i) to compare the athlete's post-injury data to reference data collected from an uninjured control group; and
(ii) in the case of unilateral injury, to use the athlete's uninjured contralateral limb data as the reference.

Both approaches have limitations. The range of 'normal' values in many strength, biomechanical and performance metrics is large, so it is only possible to compare to a broad 'normal' or 'healthy' control group range. In addition, the choice of control group should be carefully considered as differences in age, training history, and skill level are known to affect many commonly-used assessment metrics. Comparing the injured limb to the athlete's own uninjured limb can circumvent these difficulties, but de-training adaptations experienced by both limbs following injury can lead to overestimation of rehabilitation status. For example, improvements in symmetry metrics can often be partially ascribed to post-injury deterioration of the uninjured limb rather than solely to improvements in the injured limb (Wellsandt et al., 2018).

Finally, some practical advice:

- Performance-based metrics such as task completion time or distance have the advantage of efficiency, as many players can be screened – or testing repeated frequently – without extensive time and staffing requirements but can fail to highlight movement patterns and compensations indicating incomplete rehabilitation or 'high-risk' movement. The increased risk of re-injury from incomplete rehabilitation may justify the cost and time invested in a detailed functional movement assessment (in the same way as MRI is used to obtain a high-resolution structural assessment).

- With the advent of high-resolution high-speed video cameras in smartphones and tablets, there is also a surge of apps to undertake video analysis. Some of these apps claim to measure force-related movement characteristics based on estimations of acceleration. Verifying how these parameters are being calculated/estimated, and what they exactly represent, is paramount to avoiding unfounded (and likely invalid) interpretations.

## Future directions and conclusions

We considered biomechanical assessments that might be undertaken in a professional and academy soccer setting. Many assessments conducted within soccer are underpinned by biomechanics and biomechanical principles. Consideration of these principles alongside the practical considerations within this chapter will allow the sports scientist to be well-informed and critical about how these assessments can help answer soccer-related questions. We, therefore, advise practitioners to be cautious in ensuring: (1) the validity of biomechanical measurements in both the lab and field; (2) that the assessments and measurements undertaken are measuring what you wish to measure and not an unrelated surrogate measure; and (3) that the assessment used is sufficiently reliable to allow changes in performance or rehabilitation to be detected.

Over time, the role of biomechanical assessments within soccer has shifted from primarily technique evaluation to underpinning medical and rehabilitation monitoring. The last decade has seen an increased availability of portable and low-cost biomechanical assessments which will continue. New approaches likely to be applied within soccer include multi-sensor biomechanical assessment and data-fusion for personalised approaches, and novel techniques utilising neural networks for markerless motion capture to measure player movements and estimate forces in field-based settings (Verheul et al., 2020). Recently, a growing interest in biomechanical perspectives on injury prevention and performance enhancement within the general context of player load monitoring has led to increased research efforts to keep up with technological developments (Vanrenterghem et al., 2017). Extensive ongoing efforts between scientists and product developers are expected to continue to make the role of biomechanical assessments in soccer more prominent in the coming decades.

## References

Bahr, R. (2016). Why screening tests to predict injury do not work—and probably never will: a critical review. *Br J Sports Med*, *50*(13), 776–780. https://doi.org/10.1136/bjsports-2016-096256

Baltzopoulos, V. (2008). Biomechanical evaluation of movement in sport and exercise. In C. J. Payton & R. Bartlett (Eds.), *The British Association of Sport and Exercise Sciences Guidelines*. Oxfordshire, UK.

Bosco, C., Luhtanen, P., & Komi, P. V. (1983). A simple method for measurement of mechanical power in jumping. *Eur J Appl Physiol Occup Physiol*, *50*(2), 273–282. https://doi.org/10.1007/BF00422166

Burden, A. (2010). How should we normalize electromyograms obtained from healthy participants? What we have learned from over 25years of research. *J Electromyog Kinesiol*, *20*(6), 1023–1035. https://doi.org/10.1016/j.jelekin.2010.07.004

Caccese, J. B., & Kaminski, T. W. (2016). Minimizing head acceleration in soccer: a review of the literature. *Sports Med, 46*(11), 1591–1604. https://doi.org/10.1007/s40279-016-0544-7

Finni, T., Hu, M., Kettunen, P., Vilavuo, T., & Cheng, S. (2007). Measurement of EMG activity with textile electrodes embedded into clothing. *Physiol Measure, 28*(11), 1405. https://doi.org/10.1088/0967-3334/28/11/007

Kellis, E., & Katis, A. (2007). Biomechanical characteristics and determinants of instep soccer kick. *J Sports Sci Med, 6*(2), 154–165.

Konrad, P. (2006). *The ABC of EMG: A Practical Introduction to Kinesiological Electromyography.* Arizona: Noraxon U.S.A. Inc., Scottsdale, U.S.A.

Lees, A., Asai, T., Andersen, T. B., Nunome, H., & Sterzing, T. (2010). The biomechanics of kicking in soccer: a review. *J Sports Sci, 28*(8), 805–817. https://doi.org/10.1080/02640414.2010.481305

Lees, A., & Lake, M. (2003). The biomechanics of soccer surfaces and equipment. In T. Reilly (Ed.), *Science and Soccer.* Oxfordshire: Routledge.

Lees, A., & Nolan, L. (1998). The biomechanics of soccer: a review. *J Sports Sci, 16*(3), 211–234. https://doi.org/10.1080/026404198366740

Murtagh, C. F., Nulty, C., Vanrenterghem, J., O'Boyle, A., Morgans, R., Drust, B., & Erskine, R. M. (2018). The neuromuscular determinants of unilateral jump performance in soccer players are direction-specific. *Int J Sports Physiol Perform, 13*(5), 604–611. https://doi.org/10.1123/ijspp.2017-0589

Nunome, H., Hennig, E., & Smith, N. (2017). *Football Biomechanics.* Oxfordshire: Routledge.

Ruddock, A. D., & Winter, E. M. (2016). Jumping depends on impulse not power. *J Sports Sci, 34*(6), 584–585. https://doi.org/10.1080/02640414.2015.1064157

Vanrenterghem, J., Clercq, D. D., & Cleven, P. V. (2001). Necessary precautions in measuring correct vertical jumping height by means of force plate measurements. *Ergonomics, 44*(8), 814–818. https://doi.org/10.1080/00140130118100

Vanrenterghem, J., Nedergaard, N. J., Robinson, M. A., & Drust, B. (2017). Training load monitoring in team sports: a novel framework separating physiological and biomechanical load-adaptation pathways. *Sports Med, 47*(11), 2135–2142. https://doi.org/10.1007/s40279-017-0714-2

Verheul, J., Nedergaard, N. J., Vanrenterghem, J., & Robinson, M. A. (2020). Measuring biomechanical loads in team sports – from lab to field. *Sci Med Footb, 4*(3), 246–252. https://doi.org/10.1080/24733938.2019.1709654

Vigotsky, A. D., Halperin, I., Lehman, G. J., Trajano, G. S., & Vieira, T. M. (2018). Interpreting signal amplitudes in surface electromyography studies in sport and rehabilitation sciences. Frontiers in physiology, 8: 985.

Wellsandt, E., Failla, M., & Snyder-Mackler, L. (2018). Limb symmetry indexes can overestimate knee function after ACL injury. *J Orthop Sports Phys Therap, 47*(5), 334–338. https://doi.org/10.2519/jospt.2017.7285.Limb

# Section D

# Analysing and Monitoring Performances

# 16 Analysis of physical performance in match-play

*Christopher Carling and Naomi Datson*

## Introduction

Quantifying physical match performance allows practitioners to use objective information to develop systematic approaches to training prescriptions and create future tactics (Reilly, 2005). Time motion analysis is the predominant method for collecting physical match performance data. Over the last five decades, scientists have progressed from manual video-based coding to sophisticated systems that are commonplace within professional soccer settings (Bradley et al., 2013). These systems include semi-automated multiple-camera systems, radio-based local positioning systems (LPS), and global positioning systems (GPS).

Semi-automated multiple camera systems became popularised in the late 1990s and at the time provided a transformation in approach, with benefits such as multi-player tracking and integration of technical and tactical variables. Pioneers of this technology included AMISCO (Sport Universal Process, Nice, France) and Prozone (Prozone Sports Ltd., Leeds, UK). Subsequently, technological advancements have continued and multi-camera systems such as TRACAB (Chyron Hego, New York, USA) and SportVU (Stats Perform, Chicago, USA) provide real-time analysis. These systems allow practitioners to access in-match objective performance-related data that can help inform decision-making.

Technological innovations have facilitated analysis by enabling players to wear miniaturised sensors during match-play. LPS and GPS allow metabolically taxing activities such as accelerations, decelerations, and changes of direction to be accounted for, thus allowing a more comprehensive understanding of the physiological, metabolic, and mechanical demands of match-play (Bradley et al., 2018). There are practical advantages and disadvantages to LPS and GPS, with LPS such as Inmotio (Inmotio Object Tracking BV, Amsterdam, Netherlands) and Kinexon (Kinexon Precision Technologies, Munich, Germany) offering high sampling rates but requiring a semi-fixed installation, whereas GPS such as Catapult (Catapult Sports, Melbourne, Australia) and STATSports (STATSports Group Limited, Newry, Northern Ireland) do not require any specific installation but may be subject to reduced measurement accuracy inside stadia (Malone et al., 2017).

Due to the inherent practicalities of each system, practitioners often use a combination of systems to gather physical performance data for an individual player. In practice, GPS or LPS sensors are often worn during training, whereas semi-automated multiple-camera systems are routinely used during matches (Buchheit & Simpson, 2017). However, practitioners should be cautious of differences between systems and

DOI: 10.4324/9781003148418-20

254  *Christopher Carling and Naomi Datson*

are recommended to apply calibration equations to enable data integration (Buchheit et al., 2014; Taberner et al., 2020). In 2015, FIFA permitted the use of electronic performance and tracking systems in competitive matches that may support practitioners moving towards a single system for quantifying player physical performance in both training and match-play.

Regardless of the system(s) used, collecting objective physical performance data from training and matches is of benefit when prescribing training and recovery strategies. Such data can assist practitioners as they attempt to maximise player performance and minimise susceptibility to injury or illness. In this chapter, we consider general and position-specific characteristics of match physical performance with examples of published data across multiple forms of soccer. Moreover, we address those factors affecting match physical performance and practical implications of the data.

## General match demands

Total distance covered during a match is perhaps the most-cited metric when considering the physical performance of players. Total distance is indicative of the volume of activity completed by players, providing a global representation of the overall match physical demands. Typically, professional male outfield players cover a total match distance of 11–12 km (Bradley et al., 2013), whereas their elite female counterparts cover 9–11 km (Scott et al., 2020). Total distances covered have been described for other forms of the game including youth, futsal, amputee, and beach soccer. Youth players (U10–U18) cover 5–7 km during 60 min of match-play (Saward et al., 2016), futsal players cover ~4 km during 40 min of match-play (Ribeiro et al., 2020), and amputee players cover ~6 km during 50 min of match-play (Simim et al., 2018). As beach soccer involves unlimited substitutions, players often have a reduced playing time with research showing players cover ~1 km during 12 min of active playing time (Castellano & Casamichana, 2010).

The differences in match duration for various formats of the game make it challenging to draw meaningful conclusions from total distance data. Consequently, the use of relative distance, that is, distance covered relative to match duration, allows more appropriate comparisons between game formats. Approximate relative total distances for each of the above game formats are as follows: elite male (120–130 m min$^{-1}$) (Bradley et al., 2013); elite female (100–120 m min$^{-1}$) (Scott et al., 2020); youth (80–120 m min$^{-1}$) (Saward et al., 2016); futsal (90–100 m min$^{-1}$) (Ribeiro et al., 2020); amputee (110 m min$^{-1}$) (Simim et al., 2018); and beach soccer players (100 m min$^{-1}$) (Castellano & Casamichana, 2010).

Although total distance provides a broad indication of the overall movement demands, it does not provide a comprehensive understanding of physical match performance. To gain a better understanding of exercise intensity, total distance covered is generally sub-divided into activity categories or "zones" that are determined by speed of movement. Common qualitative descriptors for such activity categories include walking, jogging, running, high-speed running, and sprinting. There are generally two approaches for assigning speed thresholds to each activity category: (1) the use of absolute (or arbitrary) thresholds; or (2) the use of individualised (or player-specific) thresholds. While using arbitrary zones may facilitate between-study comparisons if the same thresholds are applied, there remains no consensus within the literature for the definition of movement categories according to running speed. For example, two recent studies involving male players (Curtis et al., 2020; Fereday et al., 2020) classified high-speed running activity as 14.4 km h$^{-1}$ and 19.8 km h$^{-1}$, respectively. In addition, if applying arbitrary zones to youth or female cohorts, then due consideration of potentially adapted speed thresholds is warranted (Malone et al., 2017). Player-specific zones, based on individual fitness attributes have previously been suggested to offer a more specific evaluation of external load in case-study scenarios (Hunter et al., 2015; Lovell & Abt, 2013). However, recent evidence suggests the practice of individualising speed thresholds might not add value in determining the dose response of soccer activity in professional female players (Scott & Lovell, 2018). If player-specific zones are to be used, then numerous challenges exist when considering an individualised approach. For example, the physical performance test(s) that should be used to assist threshold determination and the frequency with which such tests can be administered around the training and competition schedule (Malone et al., 2017). While a definitive consensus remains absent, researchers and practitioners are advised to consider the cohort or individual being assessed when selecting thresholds for activity categories.

Low-speed activity accounts for most of the distance covered in match-play, emphasising the predominantly aerobic nature of the game. English Premier League players and international-level female players have been shown to cover ~75% and ~76%, respectively, of the total distance covered in a match in low-speed activity categories (i.e., walking and jogging) (Bradley et al., 2013; Datson et al., 2017, see Figure 16.1). Values are comparable in youth soccer, with players covering approximately 71% and 76% of total distance in lower-speed categories in male (Saward et al., 2016) and female match-play, respectively (Harkness-Armstrong et al., 2020). Similar values have been demonstrated in both beach soccer (~70%) (Castellano & Casamichana, 2010) and futsal (~79%) (Ribeiro et al., 2020).

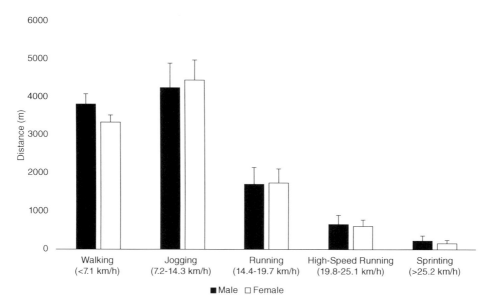

*Figure 16.1* Physical match performance in professional male and female soccer players (adapted from Bradley et al., 2013; Datson et al., 2017).

Although low-speed activities dominate performance profiles in all forms of the game, it is high-speed activities which are often considered critical to the match outcome. These actions frequently precede crucial moments within match-play, such as the movement required to evade the opposition and capitalise on goal-scoring opportunities (Di Salvo et al., 2009). Figure 16.1 shows for professional male and female match-play, approximately 25% of total match performance is spent above 14.4 km h$^{-1}$ (i.e., running, and above) and 9% is spent above 19.8 km h$^{-1}$ (i.e., high-speed running, and above).

Sprints generally occur over short distances with research showing 76% and 95% of all match sprints occur over 5 m and 10 m, respectively, in female players (Datson et al., 2017). Di Salvo and colleagues reported similar findings in male players participating in European Cup competitions with most sprints occurring over short distances (0–10 m) (Di Salvo et al., 2010). Longer-distance sprints (>20 m) do occur, albeit infrequently, as demonstrated by an average sprint distance of 15.1 ± 9.4 m in female players (Vescovi, 2012). Professional male players complete more explosive (characterised by a fast acceleration) than leading (characterised by a gradual acceleration) sprints (Di Salvo et al., 2010), whereas female players perform an even number of both types of sprints (Datson et al., 2017).

Soccer is inherently intermittent in nature as players are required to complete high-speed or sprinting actions with variable recovery periods throughout the match. Scientists have reported that these high-speed actions occur on average every ~70 s in professional male players (Bradley et al., 2010) and every ~40 s in professional female players (Datson et al., 2019). Slight methodological differences exist between these studies which likely account for the differences between sexes, however, both studies emphasise the stochastic nature of match-play. While average data provide valuable information for estimating work-to-rest ratios, practitioners should be mindful of minimum and maximum recovery periods as well as between-position differences (Carling et al., 2012). The ability to produce and recover from high-speed actions in a limited time frame is termed repeated sprint ability (RSA). RSA is broadly defined as multiple high-speed running and/or sprinting bouts within a given time-period. Published reports indicate that, when employing a sprinting threshold, the frequency of RSA is relatively low (one to two bouts per match) (Datson et al., 2019; Schimpchen et al., 2016). However, these data represent the average demands for RSA and may not be reflective of the worst-case scenario that players may encounter. Nevertheless, the low occurrence of RSA bouts suggests this particular fitness component might not be as crucial to success as previously suggested (Carling et al., 2012).

Profiling match performance based on locomotion will underestimate the true workload for a player by neglecting the energy expenditure of sport-specific movements (e.g., accelerations, decelerations, and changes of direction) and actions (e.g., heading, tackling, and running with the ball). For example, a maximum acceleration commencing from a low speed is a high-intensity activity with a high metabolic load (Osgnach et al., 2010). However, this activity would be discounted from traditional definitions that only consider high-intensity movements to be those occurring at high speed. Researchers have shown that accelerations and decelerations occur frequently (~850 per match, at a threshold of >2 m s$^{-2}$) and that players generally perform more high-intensity decelerations compared to accelerations (Harper et al., 2019; Mara et al., 2017b). The energy cost of soccer-specific actions such as running with the ball is not quantifiable when using locomotor-based analyses. However, running with a ball on a pitch at a standard speed of 10 km h$^{-1}$ requires an additional energy cost of

*Table 16.1* Influence of playing position on match physical activity profile in elite female soccer players (data adapted from Datson et al., 2017, 2019)

| | *Central defenders* | *Wide defenders* | *Central midfielders* | *Wide midfielders* | *Attackers* |
|---|---|---|---|---|---|
| Total distance (km) | $9.5 \pm 0.6$ | $10.3 \pm 0.7$ | $11.0 \pm 0.7$ | $10.6 \pm 0.7$ | $10.3 \pm 0.8$ |
| High-speed running (m) | $423 \pm 79$ | $634 \pm 168$ | $683 \pm 170$ | $700 \pm 167$ | $651 \pm 135$ |
| Sprinting (m) | $111 \pm 42$ | $163 \pm 79$ | $170 \pm 69$ | $220 \pm 116$ | $221 \pm 53$ |
| Recovery between high-speed efforts (s) | $54 \pm 9$ | $40 \pm 9$ | $36 \pm 9$ | $35 \pm 8$ | $38 \pm 8$ |

approximately 10% (Piras et al., 2017). Such findings emphasise the importance of an integrated approach to match analysis in soccer (Bradley & Ade, 2018).

## Position-specific match demands

Physical match performance profiles differ distinctly across playing positions in senior male (Aquino et al., 2020b), senior female (Datson et al., 2017), youth male (Abbott et al., 2018), youth female (Harkness-Armstrong et al., 2020), and futsal (Ohmuro et al., 2020) players. Scientists have routinely considered five key outfield playing positions in the 11 *vs.* 11 format: defenders (central and wide); midfielders (central and wide); and attackers. However, further sub-divisions such as central defensive midfielders, central attacking midfielders (Dellal et al., 2011), and "second" strikers (Buchheit et al., 2010) have been included in the literature. In futsal, the different playing positions commonly studied are pivots, wingers, and defenders.

Published reports frequently highlight that central defenders complete less total, high-speed, and sprinting activity per match compared to other playing positions (Abbott et al., 2018; Datson et al., 2017). Central midfielders often produce the highest total distances (Abbott et al., 2018; Harkness-Armstrong et al., 2020) and wide attackers the greatest high-speed running and sprinting distances (Ingebrigtsen et al., 2015; Mara et al., 2017a). The recovery duration between isolated and repeated high-speed actions varies with playing position, with longer recovery durations more common in central defenders and shorter recovery durations more common in central and wide midfield players (Carling et al., 2012; Datson et al., 2019). An overview of the physical match performance for different outfield playing positions is shown in Table 16.1. The physical match profile of goalkeepers is less well studied, but recent reports show that English Premier League goalkeepers cover a total distance of ~5.5 km with ~120 m at high speed (>15 km $h^{-1}$) (White et al., 2020). These positional differences in activity profiles are to be expected due to differing tactical roles. For example, central midfielders link attack and defence and are often required to participate in both phases of play. Meanwhile, wide attackers play in less congested areas of the pitch and have a greater opportunity to achieve high-speeds unopposed (Abbott et al., 2018).

## Fatigue and variations in performance

Total match physical performance is often sub-divided into discrete time periods such as 45-min (i.e., between-half), 15-min, and 5-min intervals. Data are then analysed to examine variability in work rate profiles between each time for individuals and teams.

258  *Christopher Carling and Naomi Datson*

*Table 16.2* Total distance covered (m) by soccer players during first and second halves of competitive match-play

| Reference | Total distance (m) | 1st Half (m) | 2nd Half (m) | Difference (m) | Game format | Statistical conclusion |
|---|---|---|---|---|---|---|
| Aquino et al., 2016 | 6,249 | 3,086 | 3,163 | +77 | U16 Male | No change |
| Atan et al., 2016 | 5,434 | 2,997 | 2,437 | −560 | U14 Male | Reduction |
| Bradley et al., 2014 | 10,753 | 5,486 | 5,267 | −219 | Pro female | Reduction |
| Di Salvo et al., 2007 | 11,393 | 5,709 | 5,684 | −25 | Pro male | No change |
| Russell et al., 2016 | 9,457 | 4,891 | 4,566 | −325 | U21 Elite male | Reduction |
| Simim et al., 2018 | 5,660 | 2,920 | 2,740 | −180 | Amputee male | No change |

### Between-half match performance

The evidence of between-half changes in total distance covered remains unclear with some researchers observing reductions in second-half running performance, whereas others report no change (see Table 16.2). Similarly, contradictory findings exist for between-half differences in high-speed running distance, with some evidence of significant second-half reductions (Di Salvo et al., 2009) and others observing no changes (Russell et al., 2016).

### Performance towards the end of each half

While between-half differences in match physical performance provide a broad appreciation of work rate profiles, consideration of shorter time periods, such as 15-min intervals, afford a more comprehensive understanding. Analysis of international female match-play observed a 35% reduction in high-speed running distance from the first to the last 15 min. Furthermore, players completed less high-speed running during the final 15 min of each half compared with the previous 15 min (Datson et al., 2017). Similarly, in male match-play high-speed running distance as well as the number of sprints, accelerations and decelerations were significantly lower in the last 15 min compared to the first 15 min of match-play (Russell et al., 2016).

### Transient fatigue

Variability in match physical performance across 5-min intervals has been shown in elite male and female players, with players completing 40% less high-speed running distance in the 5-min period which follows the peak 5-min period for high-speed running (Carling & Dupont, 2011; Datson et al., 2017). The following 5-min period has been shown to be 6–8% lower than the average 5-min period in Premier League players (Bradley et al., 2009). These 5-min periods were based on pre-defined intervals within analysis software, such as 0–5 min and 5–10 min. However, researchers have shown that there are even larger decrements when using rolling 5-min periods

*Analysis of physical performance in match-play* 259

(i.e., distance covered from every time point for the next 5-min period) (Varley et al., 2012).

### Reasons for variations in performance

The decreases in physical match performance observed in the latter stages of match-play may be a result of glycogen depletion of individual muscle fibres (Krustrup et al., 2006), whereas transient changes after periods of high intensity may be due to intramuscular acidosis or changes in the concentration of potassium in the muscle interstitium (Mohr et al., 2005). There are suggestions that declines in match running performance may be related to mental fatigue (Paul et al., 2015) or the conscious or subconscious employment of pacing strategies to ensure physical readiness for the most challenging periods of a game (Drust et al., 2007).

While variations in player physical performance at different time points within a match may represent fatigue, caution must be exhibited when analysing physical performance without due consideration of technical and tactical indices. Basing fatigue purely on match running performances is likely too simplistic, particularly due to our limited understanding of physiological responses to match demands (Paul et al., 2015). Such a reductionist approach is likely to impede the development of a comprehensive and holistic understanding of match-play demands (Bradley & Ade, 2018). For example, while a reduced physical performance is observed in the final 15 min of match-play compared to the first 15 min, it should be considered that teams will try to establish tactical superiority at the start of a match which may lead to artificially increased values for high-intensity activities during the first 15 min (Weston et al., 2011). Recently, researchers have reported that approximately 58% of the decline in match running performance in matches in the Bundesliga is caused by an increase in game interruptions and cannot be related to physical fatigue (Linke et al., 2018).

Match performance data are generally "noisy" in nature and demonstrate high levels of natural variability in match as well as from one match to the next. The interpretation of findings from time-motion studies can be hampered by the large variability in performance (typically reported as a % coefficient of variation or % CV) within and between players. Gregson et al. (2010) investigating a large sample of Premier League players demonstrated that high-intensity activities varied by ~15–30% from match to match and that the variability was higher for central defenders and midfielders than for wide midfielders and attackers. In a French Ligue 1 team, high collective CV values were found for high-intensity distances of ~32%, ~26%, ~60%, and 24%, respectively when the team was in and out of ball possession, in individual ball possession, and during the peak 5-min activity period. In the same study, individual values for high-intensity distance ranged from 11% in a full back to 26% in a central defender (Carling et al., 2016).

The variability in physical performance is mediated through the inherent demands of the game that are influenced by a myriad of contextual factors (Bush, Archer, Hogg & Bradley, 2015) (Figure 16.2). A large body of research relating to the effects of situational and environmental factors on match-running currently exists. In addition to playing position, the influence of situational factors such as playing formation and tactics, time spent in ball possession, opposition ranking, standard of play, location (home or away match), effective ball-in-play time, pacing strategy, and score status

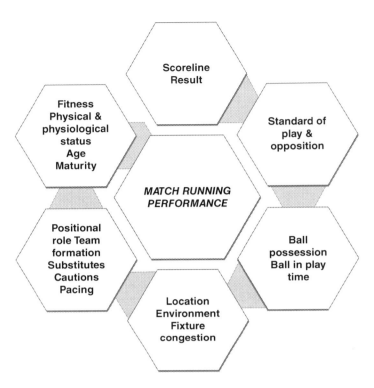

*Figure 16.2* A summary of the numerous factors influencing soccer match-play running performance.

have been comprehensively investigated (see Bush et al., 2015; Trewin et al., 2018). The evidence of a deleterious effect on match-to-match performance when players are exposed to fixture congestion, where multiple matches are played over short and long periods, has not been conclusive (Julian et al., 2020). Environmental factors such as altitude and temperature (both heat and cold) can affect match-running due to physiological limitations and possible subconscious pacing while performing in these environments (Trewin et al., 2018). A recent review synthesises the relationships between match running performance and player anthropometric, maturity, and physical fitness characteristics (Aquino et al., 2020a).

Finally, it is important to mention that studies reporting the influence of situational and environmental factors have generally examined these in an isolated manner. While no single study can comprehensively measure and control all these factors, it is useful to try to verify the relative contribution of the independent variables to the variance in match running performance before making inferences. Recently, researchers have integrated and examined the influence of several contextual factors notably in professional female (Trewin et al., 2018) and youth male players (Aquino et al., 2020b). Moreover, a novel study focusing on the role of substitutes investigated the impact on performance of substitution timing, score line, and match location, helping coaches assess the efficacy of their substitution strategies (Hills et al., 2020b).

## Practical implications of time-motion analyses

### Physical conditioning strategies

As part of the contemporary coaching process, empirical information derived from time–motion analyses of physical performance in competition are essential to provide a platform for making objective decisions relating to fitness training and match preparation. The aim of a soccer physical conditioning programme is to prepare players to cope with the intermittent-endurance demands of match-play and the necessity to perform intense efforts repeatedly and recover from these when called upon, both in and out of ball possession. Time-motion analyses provide information on the overall volume of exercise, represented by the overall distance covered, while the total distances covered at various exercise intensities offer global measures of the physiological strain imposed on players (Strudwick & Iaia, 2018). Information on the ratio of exercise-to-rest periods and high-intensity versus low-intensity outputs (using the time spent and/or distance covered in each) is pertinent. Indices such as high-metabolic load and speed exertion and dynamic stress loads are commonly used.

The creation of a typical match profile can be used as part of the foundation from which daily and weekly training workload is structured and tailored to ensure that players are replicating or over- or under-loading match demands. For example, a practitioner may use a simple 4 *vs.* 4 small-sided game (SSG, pitch size: 25 × 30 m, 3-min duration) to overload mechanical work (accelerations, decelerations, and changes of direction events), whereas a 10 *vs.* 10 SSG (pitch size: 102 × 67 m, 30-min) can overload total and high-intensity distance compared to relative match demands (Lacome et al., 2018b).

Profiling the frequency of repeated high-intensity efforts and time spent in recovery as well as the type of recovery activity (active or passive) between discrete intense bouts of exercise is particularly pertinent when designing high-intensity conditioning drills to simulate match demands. For example, simple isolated repeated high-intensity drills could be designed using work-recovery data derived from match-play analyses. Sets of multiple high-intensity bouts ($>$19.1 km h$^{-1}$) separated by approximately 60-s recovery intervals (Bradley et al., 2009) or incorporating shorter and longer between-bout recovery intervals based on the data reported in Table 16.3. Analysis of the locomotor activity during recovery intervals between consecutive high-intensity efforts can also be used to impact upon high-intensity drill design. Data gathered in France showed that recovery phases were mostly active in nature with 37% of movements performed at velocities ranging from 7.1 to 19.7 km h$^{-1}$ (Carling, Le Gall & Dupont, 2012).

The most intense or peak 5-min blocks of match-play running activity provide critical information for designing field-based conditioning drills. Information collected on these most intense periods of play helps quantify "worst case" match scenarios (Carling et al., 2019). An analysis of the length of recovery and running outputs following peak activity periods can give an indication of player ability to resist transient fatigue, as well as having implications for fitness training regimens. In a group of professional players, following a peak period of activity, high-intensity distance remained reduced by up to 30% in the 5th minute after, in comparison to the match average (Schimpchen, Gopaladesikan & Meyer, 2020). High-intensity conditioning drills can provide the necessary training stimulus to help players respond to such demands. For

## 262 Christopher Carling and Naomi Datson

*Table 16.3* Mean recovery duration between sprints using individualised speed thresholds and frequency of recovery periods according to the time elapsed between consecutive sprints, collectively and in relation to positional role in German Bundesliga players (data adapted from Schimpchen et al., 2016)

| Recovery duration | All players (n = 2514) | Defenders | | Midfielders | | | Centre-forwards (n = 263) |
|---|---|---|---|---|---|---|---|
| | | Central (n = 296) | Fullbacks (n = 559) | Holding (n = 518) | Wide (n = 655) | Attacking (n = 223) | |
| Mean recovery time (s) | 274.3 | 415.8 | 275.1 | 232.8 | 243.7 | 299.2 | 255.7 |
| % <30 s | 12.3 | 7.1 | 11.3 | 20.0 | 9.8 | 10.1 | 12.7 |
| % 30.1–60 s | 6.9 | 4.7 | 6.9 | 5.3 | 6.3 | 6.8 | 8.8 |
| % >60 s | 80.9 | 88.2 | 81.8 | 64.7 | 84.0 | 83.1 | 78.5 |

example, a 4 *vs.* 4 SSG drill ensures players perform the same relative number of accelerations and player load to that observed in a typical 5-min peak match activity period (1.7 *vs.* 1.6 and = 248, *vs.* 227, respectively) (Dalen et al., 2019).

Players must be able to perform at maximum levels consistently throughout matchplay. Running performance is commonly analysed individually or collectively across halves or towards the end of games (e.g., final 15-min interval) to identify whether the team or an individual within the collective unit is susceptible to accumulated fatigue. However, determining to what extent the reduction in running activity across match periods can realistically be considered "meaningful" is problematic (Carling, 2013). Analysis of physical efforts such as in the first 5 min of play of the match and immediately after the half-time pause, might give an idea of physical "readiness" of players and has implications for the intensity and duration of warm-up routines. For example, the quantification of running outputs during warm-up practices in substitutes in English professional soccer led to modification of their pre-pitch-entry routines, subsequently improving physical performance on-pitch-entry (Hills et al. 2020a).

Characterising match demands across age categories can potentially be used to establish age-specific performance profiles. Ramos et al. (2019) reported substantially higher values in match demands in senior versus U/20 and U/17 female Brazilian national team players, suggesting a need to tailor physical preparation for entry into the adult professional game. However, match-running performance develops nonlinearly across age categories with large individual variations (Saward et al. 2016; see Figure 16.3). In addition, match-running activity should not be considered a marker of player potential to "make the grade" (Carling & Collins, 2017) especially as there is generally little association between competitive physical performance and "success" in professional soccer. Nevertheless, it remains pertinent to characterise the demands across different leagues and competitions. The distance covered at high intensities was inferior in the English Premier League when compared with the Championship, while players moving down from the former to compete in the latter demonstrated substantially higher physical outputs (Bradley et al., 2013).

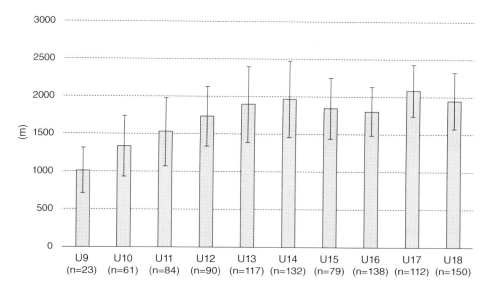

*Figure 16.3* High-intensity match-running performance in elite youth soccer players according to age group (data adapted from Saward et al., 2016).

Finally, time-motion analyses can help tailor physical conditioning programmes to account for the statistically significant differences in athletic demands reported earlier across individual playing positions. Yet, in real-world terms, the "magnitude" of some of these differences is questionable, potentially raising doubts about the practical necessity for position-specific fitness training interventions (Carling, 2013), especially when based solely on simple volume and intensity metrics. An integrated approach assimilating physical, tactical, and technical data is more pertinent for training. Innovative recent work (Bradley et al., 2018, 2019) has translated the movement patterns, technical skills, and tactical actions associated with high-intensity efforts into practical metrics that can be employed to construct position-specific attacking and defending conditioning drills. For example, fullbacks and wide midfielders frequently produce more high-intensity efforts when running to overlap and "run the channel" followed by crosses when compared to other positions.

## *Player monitoring and management*

Sports scientists and fitness practitioners aim to ensure that players perform consistently from one match to the next across the entire season. Current physical fitness levels should always enable them to express themselves tactically and technically, while reducing the risk of injury. Contemporary schedules require participation in one- or two-match weekly micro-cycles. A greater exposure to match-play and subsequent running loads can favour the maintenance and/or improvement of physical capacities relevant to performance (Dalen & Lorås, 2019). This factor has implications for managing preparation of the squad and especially the training requirements of starting and non-starting players, particularly during one-match weeks. High-intensity

264  *Christopher Carling and Naomi Datson*

compensation sessions can be implemented for used or unused substitutes in relation to match-play demands (Buchheit et al., 2020).

Impairments in physical, physiological, and perceptual performance indices can occur for up to 72 h following match-play (Carling et al., 2018). Forty-eight hours after the game is probably the most critical time as muscle soreness tends to be at its highest level although the time course and magnitude of these changes are individual-dependent (Strudwick & Iaia, 2018). Quantifying the physical efforts in any one match can help to ascertain the potential magnitude of ensuing post-match fatigue, hence readiness to train, and management of future exposure and training content. It is noteworthy that for every 100-m run above 19.8 km h$^{-1}$ during soccer match-play, creatine kinase activity measured 24 h post-match can increase by 30% and countermovement jump peak power output can decrease by 0.5% (Hader et el., 2019). Therefore, a larger than usual volume of high-intensity running could incrementally impact on recovery time and subsequently readiness to train.

During congested periods where two matches are played per week, players may be at risk of exposure while not fully recovered, potentially increasing the propensity of underperformance and injury. As such, there is potential for utilising data derived from time-motion analyses to determine the extent to which players are "coping" with such schedules. Yet, collective analyses of match-to-match performance using measures of total distance run and that covered in high-intensity generally report statistically non-significant drops across either short or longer congested schedules, implying that teams are able to maintain running performance (Julian et al., 2020). It has been suggested that these distance-based variables lack sensitivity and alternative measures quantifying the frequency of shorter high-intensity locomotor actions are necessary (Arruda et al., 2015). Strong associations have been reported between the frequency of hard accelerations and changes of direction and the magnitude of post-match fatigue determined by decrements in physical, physiological, and perceptual performance indices (Nedelec et al., 2014).

The large match-to-match variability (% CV) reported generally both across the season, and specifically when successive matches are separated by minimal recovery time (linked in part to the contextual factors discussed earlier in this chapter), potentially masks any "meaningful" drops in collective and individual running profiles across congested periods (Carling et al., 2015). A recent study has attempted to establish the practical significance of individual match-to-match changes in running performance using a Minimum Effects Testing framework to highlight changes beyond "normal" match-to-match variability (Oliva-Lozano et al., 2020). The authors suggested that between-match individual changes of ±~10–15% in measures of total distance, total accelerations and maximum running velocity were of practical significance. A more holistic approach to performance monitoring during fixture congestion is necessary via integration of tactical and technical indices into the match profile.

### Implications for injury prevention

In professional match-play, the mean distance and duration of sprint runs are relatively short with distances rarely exceeding 20 m and 4 s in duration and the occurrence of near-to-maximal speed running bouts is low (Buchheit et al., 2020). However, time-motion analysis has shown a potential link between injury risk and sprinting when the distance and duration of individual sprint runs were substantially greater than the habitual profile of the player. Physical training typically aims to mimic the physical intensity and movement patterns of match-play but can result in under-exposure to high-speed running owing to the use of smaller areas, particularly in small-sided games in training (Buckthorpe et al., 2019). Players may be underprepared to respond on the rare occasions they must perform a longer sprint and, as such, are at increased risk of injury. Accordingly, researchers have shown that exposure to bouts of maximal velocity running (>95% maximum velocity) can produce a protective effect and help reduce hamstring injury risk in team sports players (Malone et al., 2018).

The quantification of peak periods of match locomotor activity is considered important to help prepare players for the most intense periods of match-play. Researchers have demonstrated a harmful association for the volume of sprinting performed prior to injury occurrences in professional soccer match-play (Carling et al., 2010; Gregson et al., 2020). Gregson and colleagues (2020) recommended preparing players to sustain and repeat sprint-type activity during match-play as part of any injury prevention strategy. While exercise bouts requiring multiple sprints repeated over a short time are relatively rare (Schimpchen et al., 2016), players must be able to respond physically and not "break down" when play requires them to perform these "worse case" scenarios.

Finally, time-motion data have potential for use in monitoring running performance on return to competition. Portillo et al. (2020) and Whiteley et al. (2020) reported that following a muscular injury (causing >8 days lay off) match high-intensity outputs (distance covered and/or maximum speed) can be considerably affected.

## Future directions and conclusions

Processes are slowly evolving from the generation of data that provide a rudimentary description of *what has happened* to intelligent systems that attempt to answer *why it happened*, then predict *what might happen* and inform prescription *to make it happen*. Within these processes, current technologies within the contemporary match performance analysis ecocycle are constantly being supplanted by improved or novel tools enabling real-time and simultaneous capture of different sources of information, notably via wearable sensors. These include sensors embedded in smart clothing and footwear or worn as simple patches placed on the skin or even ingested orally. A myriad of information relating to biochemical markers, heart rate patterns, neuromuscular activity, joint speeds, contact forces, and 3D motion is progressively complementing data habitually gathered on running volume and intensity. Irrespective of the technology adopted, it is imperative that strong evidence relating to validity and reliability in addition to safety checks is independently established. In addition, machine or deep learning model approaches to automatise sport movement recognition are showing strong potential to enhance both the efficiency and accuracy of sport performance analysis (Cust et al., 2019). A pertinent and practical example in soccer is work described by Bradley (2020) combining techniques from machine learning and neural network analyses to facilitate the contextualisaton and classification of the tactical purpose of high-intensity activities (e.g., overlapping run for a full back) and collectively for the team (e.g., closing opposition players).

## 266 Christopher Carling and Naomi Datson

Automatised and intelligent systems exist to aid analysis and interpretation of the masses of complex data generated. These notably help to separate the "noise" from the "signal" within datasets to identify meaningful changes in performance outputs, as well as providing insightful key actionable indicators and advanced statistical models. Recently, machine learning techniques have predicted workload responses to aid periodisation of future training sessions (Jaspers et al., 2018, Rossi et al., 2018). Additional work, notably in conjunction with the expert knowledge of elite practitioners, is required to further advance this area. Finally, advanced graphic telestration tools (e.g., Coachpaint by Chyron Hygo) and data visualisation dashboards designed using business intelligence software (e.g., Tableau, Microsoft Power BI) are being increasingly employed by sports scientists and conditioning coaches. These aid translation of data into eye-catching, easy to understand and impactful soccer visuals engaging coach buy-in and supporting decision-making processes (Lacome, Simpson & Buchheit, 2018a).

In this chapter, we provided a brief overview of the different technologies commonly used to collect data on physical performance in contemporary professional soccer match-play. We presented examples of published data from the accumulated scientific knowledge base illustrating general and position-specific demands, the occurrence of fatigue, as well as contextual factors that impact performance in competition. Finally, information on how the data generated from analyses can be used in practice to objectively impact upon decision-making processes by supporting the physical conditioning elements of player development and match preparation was discussed. It is clear that both the knowledge base and expertise relating to physical performance in match-play have grown considerably, particularly over the last decade, playing a key role in aiding sports scientists and practitioners join up the many components underpinning performance in soccer.

## References

Abbott, W., Brickley, G., & Smeeton, N. J. (2018). Physical demands of playing position within English Premier League academy soccer. *Journal of Human Sport and Exercise*, *13*(2), 285–295. https://doi.org/10.14198/jhse.2018.132.04

Aquino, R., Carling, C., Maia, J., Vieira, L. H. P., Wilson, R. S., Smith, N., Almeida, R., Gonçalves, L. G. C., Kalva-Filho, C. A., Garganta, J., & Puggina, E. F. (2020a). Relationships between running demands in soccer match-play, anthropometric, and physical fitness characteristics: a systematic review. *International Journal of Performance Analysis in Sport*, *20*(3), 534–555. https://doi.org/10.1080/24748668.2020.1746555

Aquino, R., Carling, C., Palucci Vieira, L. H., Martins, G., Jabor, G., Machado, J., Santiago, P., Garganta, J., & Puggina, E. (2020b). Influence of situational variables, team formation, and playing position on match running performance and social network analysis in Brazilian professional soccer players. *Journal of Strength and Conditioning Research*, *34*(3), 808–817. https://doi.org/10.1519/jsc.0000000000002725

Aquino, R. L. Q. T., Gonçalves, L. G. C., Vieira, L. H. P., Oliveira, L. P., Alves, G. F., Santiago, P. R. P., & Puggina, E. (2016). Biochemical, physical and tactical analysis of a simulated game in young soccer players. *Journal of Sports Medicine and Physical Fitness*, *56*(12), 1554–1561

Arruda, A. F. S., Carling, C., Zanetti, V., Aoki, M. S., Coutts, A. J., & Moreira, A. (2015). Effects of a very congested match schedule on body-load impacts, accelerations, and running measures in youth soccer players. *International Journal of Sports Physiology and Performance*, *10*(2), 248–252. https://doi.org/10.1123/ijspp.2014-0148

Atan, S. A., Foskett, A., & Ali, A. (2016). Motion analysis of match play in New Zealand U13 to U15 age-group soccer players. *Journal of Strength and Conditioning Research, 30*(9), 2416–2423. https://doi.org/10.1519/JSC.0000000000001336

Bradley, P. S. (2020). *Football Decoded: Using Match Analysis & Context to Interpret the Demands.* Independently published.

Bradley, P. S., & Ade, J. D. (2018). Are current physical match performance metrics in elite soccer fit for purpose or is the adoption of an integrated approach needed? *International Journal of Sports Physiology and Performance, 13*(5), 656–664. https://doi.org/10.1123/ijspp.2017-0433

Bradley, P. S., Carling, C., Gomez Diaz, A., Hood, P., Barnes, C., Ade, J., Boddy, M., Krustrup, P., & Mohr, M. (2013). Match performance and physical capacity of players in the top three competitive standards of English professional soccer. *Human Movement Science, 32*(4), 808–821. https://doi.org/10.1016/j.humov.2013.06.002

Bradley, P. S., Dellal, A., Mohr, M., Castellano, J., & Wilkie, A. (2014). Gender differences in match performance characteristics of soccer players competing in the UEFA Champions League. *Human Movement Science, 33*, 159–171. https://doi.org/10.1016/j.humov.2013.07.024

Bradley, P S, Di Mascio, M., Mohr, M., Fransson, D., Wells, C., Moreira, A., Castellano, J., Gómez, A., & Ade, J. (2018). Can modern football match demands be translated into novel training and testing modes? *Aspetar Sports Medicine Journal, 7*(June), 9–13.

Bradley, P. S., Di Mascio, M., Peart, D., Olsen, P., & Sheldon, B. (2010). High-intensity activity profiles of elite soccer players at different performance levels. *Journal of Strength and Conditioning Research, 24*(9), 2343–235. https://doi.org/10.1519/jsc.0b013e3181aeb1b3

Bradley, P. S., Martin-Garcia, A., Ade, J. D., & Gomez-Diaz, A. (2019). Position specific & positional play training in elite football: context matters. *Football Med & Perform, 29*, 31–35.

Bradley, P. S., Sheldon, W., Wooster, B., Olsen, P., Boanas, P., & Krustrup, P. (2009). High-intensity running in English FA premier league soccer matches. *Journal of Sports Sciences, 27*(2), 159–168. https://doi.org/10.1080/02640410802512775

Buchheit, M., Allen, A., Poon, T. K., Modonutti, M., Gregson, W., & Di Salvo, V. (2014). Integrating different tracking systems in football: multiple camera semi-automatic system, local position measurement and GPS technologies. *Journal of Sports Sciences, 32*(20), 1844–1857. https://doi.org/10.1080/02640414.2014.942687

Buchheit, M., Mendez-Villanueva, A., Simpson, B. M., & Bourdon, P. C. (2010). Repeated-sprint sequences during youth soccer matches. *International Journal of Sports Medicine, 31*(10), 709–716. https://doi.org/10.1055/s-0030-1261897

Buchheit, M., & Simpson, B. M. (2017). Player-tracking technology: half-full or half-empty glass? *International Journal of Sports Physiology and Performance, 12*(s2), S2–S35. https://doi.org/10.1123/ijspp.2016-0499

Buchheit, M., Simpson, B. M., Hader, K., & Lacome, M. (2021). 5(2), 105–110 Occurrences of near-to-maximal speed-running bouts in elite soccer: insights for training prescription and injury mitigation. *Science and Medicine in Football*, 1-6 https://doi.org/10.1080/24733938.2020.1802058

Buckthorpe, M., Wright, S., Bruce-Low, S., Nanni, G., Sturdy, T., Gross, A. S., Bowen, L., Styles, B., Della Villa, S., Davison, M., & Gimpel, M. (2019). Recommendations for hamstring injury prevention in elite football: translating research into practice. *British Journal of Sports Medicine, 53*(7), 449–456. https://doi.org/10.1136/bjsports-2018-099616

Bush, M. D., Archer, D. T., Hogg, R., & Bradley, P. S. (2015). Factors influencing physical and technical variability in the English premier league. *International Journal of Sports Physiology and Performance, 10*(7), 865–872. https://doi.org/10.1123/ijspp.2014-0484

Carling, C. (2013). Interpreting physical performance in professional soccer match-play: should we be more pragmatic in our approach? *Sports Medicine, 43*(8), 655–663. https://doi.org/10.1007/s40279-013-0055-8

Carling, C., Gregson, W., McCall, A., Moreira, A., Wong, delP., & Bradley, P. S. (2015). Match running performance during fixture congestion in elite soccer: research issues and

268  *Christopher Carling and Naomi Datson*

future directions. Sports medicine (Auckland, N.Z.), 45(5), 605–613. https://doi.org/10.1007/s40279-015-0313-z

Carling, C., Bradley, P., McCall, A., & Dupont, G. (2016). Match-to-match variability in high-speed running activity in a professional soccer team. *Journal of Sports Sciences*, 34(24), 2215–2223. https://doi.org/10.1080/02640414.2016.1176228

Carling, C., & Collins, D. (2017). Comment on match analysis of U9 and U10 English premier league academy soccer players using a global positioning system. *Journal of Strength and Conditioning Research*, 31(2), e61–e63. https://doi.org/10.1519/jsc.0000000000000466

Carling, C., & Dupont, G. (2011). Are declines in physical performance associated with a reduction in skill-related performance during professional soccer match-play? *Journal of Sports Sciences*, 29(1), 63–71. https://doi.org/10.1080/02640414.2010.521945

Carling, C., Lacome, M., McCall, A., Dupont, G., Le Gall, F., Simpson, B., & Buchheit, M. (2018). Monitoring of post-match fatigue in professional soccer: welcome to the real world. *Sports Medicine*, 48(12), 2695–2702. https://doi.org/10.1007/s40279-018-0935-z

Carling, C., Le Gall, F., & Dupont, G. (2012). Analysis of repeated high-intensity running performance in professional soccer. *Journal of Sports Sciences*, 30(4), 325–336. https://doi.org/10.1080/02640414.2011.652655

Carling, C., Le Gall, F., & Reilly, T. P. (2010). Effects of physical efforts on injury in elite soccer. *International Journal of Sports Medicine*, 31(03), 180–185. https://doi.org/10.1055/s-0029-1241212

Carling, C., McCall, A., Harper, D., & Bradley, P. S. (2019). The use of microtechnology to quantify the peak match demands of the football codes: a systematic review. *Sports Medicine*, 49(2), 343–345. https://doi.org/10.1007/s40279-018-1032-z

Castellano, J., & Casamichana, D. (2010). Heart rate and motion analysis by GPS in beach soccer. *Journal of Sports Science and Medicine*, 9(1), 98–103. http://www.jssm.org

Curtis, R. M., Huggins, R. A., Benjamin, C. L., Sekiguchi, Y., Adams, W. M., Arent, S. M., Jain, R., Miller, S. J., Walker, A. J., & Casa, D. J. (2020). Contextual factors influencing external and internal training loads in collegiate men's soccer. *Journal of Strength and Conditioning Research*, 34(2), 374–381. https://doi.org/10.1519/jsc.0000000000003361

Cust, E. E., Sweeting, A. J., Ball, K., & Robertson, S. (2019). Machine and deep learning for sport-specific movement recognition: a systematic review of model development and performance. *Journal of Sports Sciences*, 37(5), 568–600. https://doi.org/10.1080/02640414.2018.1521769

Dalen, T., & Lorås, H. (2019). Monitoring training and match physical load in junior soccer players: starters versus substitutes. *Sports*, 7(3), 70. https://doi.org/10.3390/sports7030070

Dalen, T., Sandmæl, S., Stevens, T., Hjelde, G. H., Kjøsnes, T. N., & Wisløff, U. (2021). Differences in acceleration and high-intensity activities between small-sided games and peak periods of official matches in elite soccer players. *Journal of Strength and Conditioning Research*. 35(7), 2018–2024 10.1519/JSC.0000000000003081. Advance online publication.

Datson, N., Drust, B., Weston, M., & Gregson, W. (2019). Repeated high-speed running in elite female soccer players during international competition. *Science and Medicine in Football*, 3(2), 150–156. https://doi.org/10.1080/24733938.2018.1508880

Datson, N., Drust, B., Weston, M., Jarman, I. H., Lisboa, P. J., & Gregson, W. (2017). Match physical performance of elite female soccer players during international competition. *Journal of Strength and Conditioning Research*, 31(9), 2379–2387. https://doi.org/10.1519/JSC.0000000000001575

Dellal, A., Chamari, K., Wong, D. P., Ahmaidi, S., Keller, D., Barros, R., Bisciotti, G. N., & Carling, C. (2011). Comparison of physical and technical performance in European soccer match-play: Fa Premier League and La Liga. *European Journal of Sport Science*, 11(1), 51–59. https://doi.org/10.1080/17461391.2010.481334

Di Salvo, V., Baron, R., Tschan, H., Calderon Montero, F. J., Bachl, N., & Pigozzi, F. (2007). Performance characteristics according to playing position in elite soccer. *International Journal of Sports Medicine*, 28(3), 222–227. https://doi.org/10.1055/s-2006-924294

Di Salvo, V., Gregson, W., Atkinson, G., Tordoff, P., & Drust, B. (2009). Analysis of high intensity activity in premier league soccer. *International Journal of Sports Medicine, 30*(3), 205–212. https://doi.org/10.1055/s-0028-1105950

Di Salvo, V., Baron, R., González-Haro, C., Gormasz, C., Pigozzi, F., & Bachl, N. (2010). Sprinting analysis of elite soccer players during European champions league and UEFA cup matches. *Journal of Sports Sciences, 28*(14), 1489–1494. https://doi.org/10.1080/02640414.2010.521166

Drust, B., Atkinson, G., & Reilly, T. (2007). Future perspectives in the evaluation of the physiological demands of soccer. *Sports Medicine, 37*(9), 783–805. https://doi.org/10.2165/00007256-200737090-00003

Fereday, K., Hills, S. P., Russell, M., Smith, J., Cunningham, D. J., Shearer, D., McNarry, M., & Kilduff, L. P. (2020). A comparison of rolling averages versus discrete time epochs for assessing the worst-case scenario locomotor demands of professional soccer match-play. *Journal of Science and Medicine in Sport, 23*(8), 764–769. https://doi.org/10.1016/j.jsams.2020.01.00

Gregson, W., Drust, B., Atkinson, G., & Salvo, V. (2010). Match-to-match variability of high-speed activities in premier league soccer. *International Journal of Sports Medicine, 31*(04), 237–242. https://doi.org/10.1055/s-0030-1247546

Gregson, W., Di Salvo, V., Varley, M.C., Modonutti, M., Belli, A., Chamari, K., Weston, M., Lolli, L., & Eirale, C. (2020). Harmful association of sprinting with muscle injury occurrence in professional soccer match-play: a two-season, league wide exploratory investigation from the Qatar Stars League. Journal of Science and Medicine in Sport, 23(2), 134–138. https://doi.org/10.1016/j.jsams.2019.08.289

Hader, K., Rumpf, M. C., Hertzog, M., Kilduff, L. P., Girard, O., & Silva, J. R. (2019). Monitoring the athlete match response: can external load variables predict post-match acute and residual fatigue in soccer? a systematic review with meta-analysis. *Sports Medicine – Open, 5*(1), 48.

Harkness-Armstrong, A., Till, K., Datson, N., & Emmonds, S. (2021). Whole and peak physical characteristics of elite youth female soccer match-play. *Journal of Sports Sciences, 39*(12), 1320–1329 https://doi.org/10.1080/02640414.2020.1868669

Harper, D. J., Carling, C., & Kiely, J. (2019). High-intensity acceleration and deceleration demands in elite team sports competitive match play: a systematic review and meta-analysis of observational studies. *Sports Medicine, 49*(12), 1923–1947. https://doi.org/10.1007/s40279-019-01170-1

Hills, S. P., Barrett, S., Hobbs, M., Barwood, M. J., Radcliffe, J. N., Cooke, C. B., & Russell, M. (2020a). Modifying the pre-pitch entry practices of professional soccer substitutes may contribute towards improved movement-related performance indicators on match-day: a case study. *PloS One, 15*(5), e0232611. https://doi.org/10.1371/journal.pone.0232611

Hills, S. P., Barrett, S., Thoseby, B., Kilduff, L. P., Barwood, M. J., Radcliffe, J. N., Cooke, C. B., & Russell, M. (2022). Quantifying the peak physical match-play demands of professional soccer substitutes following pitch-entry: assessing contextual influences. *Research Quarterly for Exercise and Sport, 93*(2), 270-281 https://doi.org/10.1080/02701367.2020.1823308

Hunter, F., Bray, J., Towlson, C., Smith, M., Barrett, S., Madden, J., Abt, G., & Lovell, R. (2015). Individualisation of time-motion analysis: a method comparison and case report series. *International Journal of Sports Medicine, 36*(1), 41–48. https://doi.org/10.1055/s-0034-1384547

Ingebrigtsen, J., Dalen, T., Hjelde, G. H., Drust, B., & Wisløff, U. (2015). Acceleration and sprint profiles of a professional elite football team in match play. *European Journal of Sport Science, 15*(2), 101–110. https://doi.org/10.1080/17461391.2014.933879

Jaspers, A., De Beéck, T. O., Brink, M. S., Frencken, W. G. P., Staes, F., Davis, J. J., & Helsen, W. F. (2018). Relationships between the external and internal training load in professional soccer: what can we learn from machine learning? *International Journal of Sports Physiology and Performance, 13*(5), 625–630. https://doi.org/10.1123/ijspp.2017-0299

Julian, R., Page, R. M., & Harper, L. D. (2021). The effect of fixture congestion on performance during professional male soccer match-play: a systematic critical review with meta-analysis. *Sports Medicine, 51*(2), 255-273 https://doi.org/10.1007/s40279-020-01359-9

Krustrup, P., Mohr, M., Steensberg, A., Bencke, J., Klær, M., & Bangsbo, J. (2006). Muscle and blood metabolites during a soccer game: implications for sprint performance. *Medicine and Science in Sports and Exercise, 38*(6), 1165–1174. https://doi.org/10.1249/01.mss.0000222845.89262.cd

Lacome M., Simpson, B. M., & M. Buchheit. (2018a). Part 2: Monitoring training status with player-tracking technology: still on the road to Rome. *Aspetar Sports Medicine Journal, 7,* 57–66.

Lacome, M., Simpson, B. M., Cholley, Y., Lambert, P., & Buchheit, M. (2018b). Small-sided games in elite soccer: does one size fit all? *International Journal of Sports Physiology and Performance, 13*(5), 568–576. https://doi.org/10.1123/ijspp.2017-0214

Linke, D., Link, D., Weber, H., & Lames, M. (2018). Decline in match running performance in football is affected by an increase in game interruptions. *Journal of Sports Science and Medicine, 17,* 662–667. http://library1.nida.ac.th/termpaper6/sd/2554/19755.pdf

Lovell, R., & Abt, G. (2013). Individualization of time-motion analysis: a case-cohort example. International Journal of Sports Physiology and Performance, 8(4), 456–458. https://doi.org/10.1123/ijspp.8.4.456

Malone, J. J., Lovell, R., Varley, M. C., & Coutts, A. J. (2017). Unpacking the black box: applications and considerations for using GPS devices in sport. *International Journal of Sports Physiology and Performance, 12*(s2), S2–S18. https://doi.org/10.1123/ijspp.2016-0236

Malone, S., Owen, A., Mendes, B., Hughes, B., Collins, K., & Gabbett, T. J. (2018). High-speed running and sprinting as an injury risk factor in soccer: can well-developed physical qualities reduce the risk? *Journal of Science and Medicine in Sport, 21*(3), 257–262. https://doi.org/10.1016/j.jsams.2017.05.016

Mara, J. K., Thompson, K. G., Pumpa, K. L., & Morgan, S. (2017a). Quantifying the high-speed running and sprinting profiles of elite female soccer players during competitive matches using an optical player tracking system. *Journal of Strength and Conditioning Research, 31*(6), 1500–1508. https://doi.org/10.1519/JSC.0000000000001629

Mara, J. K., Thompson, K. G., Pumpa, K. L., & Morgan, S. (2017b). The acceleration and deceleration profiles of elite female soccer players during competitive matches. *Journal of Science and Medicine in Sport, 20*(9), 867–872. https://doi.org/10.1016/j.jsams.2016.12.078

Mohr, M., Krustrup, P., & Bangsbo, J. (2005). Fatigue in soccer: a brief review. *Journal of Sports Sciences, 23*(6), 593–599. https://doi.org/10.1080/02640410400021286

Nedelec, M., McCall, A., Carling, C., Legall, F., Berthoin, S., & Dupont, G. (2014). The influence of soccer playing actions on the recovery kinetics after a soccer match. *Journal of Strength and Conditioning Research, 28*(6), 1517–1523. https://doi.org/10.1519/jsc.0000000000000293

Ohmuro, T., Iso, Y., Tobita, A., Hirose, S., Ishizaki, S., Sakaue, K., & Yasumatsu, M. (2020). Physical match performance of Japanese top-level futsal players in different categories and playing positions. *Biology of Sport, 37*(4), 359–365. https://doi.org/10.5114/BIOLSPORT.2020.96322

Oliva-Lozano, J. M., Muyor, J. M., Fortes, V., & McLaren, S. J. (2021). Decomposing the variability of match physical performance in professional soccer: implications for monitoring individuals. *European Journal of Sport Science,* 21(11), 1588-1596 https://doi.org/10.1080/17461391.2020.1842513

Osgnach, C., Poser, S., Bernardini, R., Rinaldo, R., & Di Prampero, P. E. (2010). Energy cost and metabolic power in elite soccer: a new match analysis approach. *Medicine and Science in Sports and Exercise, 42*(1), 170–178. https://doi.org/10.1249/MSS.0b013e3181ae5cfd

Paul, D. J., Bradley, P. S., & Nassis, G. P. (2015). Factors affecting match running performance of elite soccer players: shedding some light on the complexity. *International Journal of Sports Physiology and Performance, 10*(4), 516–519. https://doi.org/10.1123/IJSPP.2015-0029

Piras, A., Raffi, M., Atmatzidis, C., Merni, F., & Di Michele, R. (2017). The energy cost of running with the ball in soccer. *International Journal of Sports Medicine, 38*(12), 877–882. https://doi.org/10.1055/s-0043-118340

Portillo, J., Abián, P., Calvo, B., Paredes, V., & Abián-Vicén, J. (2020). Effects of muscular injuries on the technical and physical performance of professional soccer players. *The Physician and Sportsmedicine*, *48*(4), 437–441. https://doi.org/10.1080/00913847.2020.1744485

Ramos, G. P., Nakamura, F. Y., Penna, E. M., Wilke, C. F., Pereira, L. A., Loturco, I., Capelli, L., Mahseredjian, F., Silami-Garcia, E., & Coimbra, C. C. (2019). Activity profiles in U17, U20, and senior women's Brazilian national soccer teams during international competitions. *Journal of Strength and Conditioning Research*, *33*(12), 3414–3422. https://doi.org/10.1519/jsc.0000000000002170

Reilly, T. (2005). An ergonomics model of the soccer training process. *Journal of Sports Sciences*, *23*(6), 561–572. https://doi.org/10.1080/02640410400021245

Ribeiro, J. N., Gonçalves, B., Coutinho, D., Brito, J., Sampaio, J., & Travassos, B. (2020). Activity profile and physical performance of match play in elite futsal players. *Frontiers in Psychology*, *11*. https://pubmed.ncbi.nlm.nih.gov/32793058/

Rossi, A., Pappalardo, L., Cintia, P., Iaia, F. M., Fernàndez, J., & Medina, D. (2018). Effective injury forecasting in soccer with GPS training data and machine learning. *PLoS one*, *13*(7), e0201264. https://doi.org/10.1371/journal.pone.0201264

Russell, M., Sparkes, W., Northeast, J., Cook, C. J., Love, T. D., Bracken, R. M., & Kilduff, L. P. (2016). Changes in acceleration and deceleration capacity throughout professional soccer match-play. *Journal of Strength and Conditioning Research*, *30*(10), 2839–2844. https://doi.org/10.1519/JSC.0000000000000805

Saward, C., Morris, J. G., Nevill, M. E., Nevill, A. M., & Sunderland, C. (2016). Longitudinal development of match-running performance in elite male youth soccer players. *Scandinavian Journal of Medicine and Science in Sports*, *26*(8), 933–942. https://doi.org/10.1111/sms.12534

Schimpchen, J., Gopaladesikan, S., & Meyer, T. (2021). The intermittent nature of player physical output in professional football matches: an analysis of sequences of peak intensity and associated fatigue responses. *European Journal of Sport Science*, *21*(6), 793-802 https://doi.org/10.1080/17461391.2020.1776400

Schimpchen, J., Skorski, S., Nopp, S., & Meyer, T. (2016). Are "classical" tests of repeated-sprint ability in football externally valid? A new approach to determine in-game sprinting behaviour in elite football players. *Journal of Sports Sciences*, *34*(6), 519–526. https://doi.org/10.1080/02640414.2015.1112023

Scott, D., Haigh, J., & Lovell, R. (2020). Physical characteristics and match performances in women's international versus domestic-level football players: a 2-year, league-wide study. *Science and Medicine in Football*, *4*(3), 211–215. https://doi.org/10.1080/24733938.2020.1745265

Scott, D., & Lovell, R. (2018). Individualisation of speed thresholds does not enhance the dose-response determination in football training. *Journal of Sports Sciences*, *36*(13), 1523–1532. https://doi.org/10.1080/02640414.2017.1398894

Simim, M. A. M., Da Mota, G. R., Marocolo, M., Da Silva, B. V. C., De Mello, M. T., & Bradley, P. S. (2018). The demands of amputee soccer impair muscular endurance and power indices but not match physical performance. *Adapted Physical Activity Quarterly*, *35*(1), 76–92. https://doi.org/10.1123/apaq.2016-0147

Strudwick, A. J., & Iaia, F. M. (2018). Physical preparation of elite soccer players. In W. Gregson & M. Littlewood (Eds.), *Science in Soccer: Translating Theory into Practice* (pp.63–83). London: Bloomsbury Publishing.

Taberner, M., O'keefe, J., Flower, D., Philips, J., Morgans, R., Cohen, DD., Richter, C., Carling, C. (2020). Interchangeability of position tracking technologies; can we merge the data? *Science & Medicine in Football*, *4*, 76–81. https://doi.org/10.1080/24733938.2019.1634279

Trewin, J., Meylan, C., Varley, M. C., Cronin, J., & Ling, D. (2018). Effect of match factors on the running performance of elite female soccer players. *Journal of Strength and Conditioning Research*, *32*(7), 2002–2009. https://doi.org/10.1519/jsc.0000000000002584

Varley, M. C., Elias, G. P., & Aughey, R. J. (2012). Current match-analysis techniques' underestimation of intense periods of high-velocity running. *International Journal of Sports Physiology and Performance*, 7(2), 183–185. https://doi.org/10.1123/ijspp.7.2.183

Vescovi, J. D. (2012). Sprint profile of professional female soccer players during competitive matches: female athletes in motion (FAiM) study. *Journal of Sports Sciences*, 30(12), 1259–1265. https://doi.org/10.1080/02640414.2012.701760

Weston, M., Batterham, A. M., Castagna, C., Portas, M. D., Barnes, C., Harley, J., & Lovell, R. J. (2011). Reduction in physical match performance at the start of the second half in elite soccer. *International Journal of Sports Physiology and Performance*, 6(2), 174–182. https://doi.org/10.1123/ijspp.6.2.174

White, A., Hills, S. P., Hobbs, M., Cooke, C. B., Kilduff, L. P., Cook, C., Roberts, C., & Russell, M. (2020). The physical demands of professional soccer goalkeepers throughout a week-long competitive microcycle and transiently throughout match-play. *Journal of Sports Sciences*, 38(8), 848–854. https://doi.org/10.1080/02640414.2020.1736244

Whiteley, R., Massey, A., Gabbett, T., Blanch, P., Cameron, M., Conlan, G., Ford, M., & Williams, M. (2021). Match high-speed running distances are often suppressed after return from hamstring strain injury in professional footballers. *Sports Health: A Multidisciplinary Approach*, 194173812096445. 13(3), 290-295 https://doi.org/10.1177/1941738120964456

Lovell, R., & Abt, G. (2013). Individualization of time-motion analysis: a case-cohort example. International Journal of Sports Physiology and Performance, 8(4), 456-458. https://doi: 10.1123/ijspp.8.4.456

Gregson, W., Di Salvo, V., Varley, M.C., Modonutti, M., Belli, A., Chamari, K., Weston, M., Lolli, L., & Eirale, C. (2020). Harmful association of sprinting with muscle injury occurrence in professional soccer match-play: a two-season, league wide exploratory investigation from the Qatar Stars League. Journal of Science and Medicine in Sport, 23(2), 134-138. https://doi.org/10.1016/j.jsams.2019.08.289

# 17 Technical and tactical match analysis

*Allistair P. McRobert, Javier Fernández-Navarro and Laura Seth*

## Introduction

Over the past two decades, match analysis has become an integral part of the coaching process, coupled with an increase in published research on the topic (Sarmento et al., 2018, 2014). The considerable growth of match analysis is due to an increase in performance analysts with specific expertise and developments in software, making it more accessible to coaches, players, clubs, and organisations. The systems have become easier to use through integration of digital video footage and computer technology, so there is no longer a need for analysts with computer science or statistics degrees (James, 2006). Licensed and subscription-based self-coding software such as hudlsportscode (https://hudl.com), nacsport (https://nacsport.com), Dartfish (https://dartfish.com), and LongoMatch (https://longomatch.com) are cost-effective or free platforms that have increased the integration of performance analysis into the coach-athlete-sport science relationship (Drust, 2010; Lago, 2009). In addition, valid and reliable semi-automated computer tracking, local position measurement (LPM), and global position systems (GPS) that log event data and monitor player position, velocity, and movement patterns provide large volumes of technical, tactical, and physical performance data (Bradley, O'Donoghue, Wooster, & Tordoff, 2007; Cummins, Orr, O'Connor, & West, 2013; Frencken, Lemmink, & Delleman, 2010; Olthof, Frencken, & Lemmink, 2018; Valter, Adam, Barry, & Marco, 2006). Companies such as Stats Perform (https://statsperform.com), Second Spectrum (https://secondspectrum.com), and Chyron Hego (https://chyron.com) provide coding and analysis services during and after the match. Whereas LPM and GPS companies like Catapult (https://catapultsports.com), STATSports (https://statsports.com), and Inmotio (https://inmotio.eu) allow sports scientists to monitor players during training and matches.

Prior to these advancements, analysis of technical and tactical performance in team games was completed through game observation. These qualitative game observations were less objective, comprehensive, and systematic. Using the subjective observer impressions slowed the analysis process and relied on the coaches' experiences and expertise. In contrast, quantitative game observations are more objective and comprehensive due to systematic categorisation of behavioural data (Memmert, Lemmink, & Sampaio, 2016). Furthermore, majority of clubs integrate performance analysis data into their workflows so that it informs the decision-making processes of key stakeholders (i.e., coaches and players). Performance analysts often use video and data for pre-match analysis, live feedback, post-match analysis and feedback, opposition analysis, scouting/recruitment analysis, trend data analysis, data visualisation, and video telestration (Jones, Rands, & Butterworth, 2020; Wright, Atkins, Jones, & Todd, 2013).

DOI: 10.4324/9781003148418-21

274 *Allistair P. McRobert et al.*

The earliest published match analysis research was by Reep and Benjamin (1968), and for further background on how Reep influenced soccer notational and performance analysis, see Pollard (2002). Since then, scientific literature has significantly increased and the area now has international societies (e.g., International Society of Performance Analysis of Sport), specialist journals (e.g., International Journal of Performance Analysis in Sport, Journal of Quantitative Analysis in Sports, Science and Medicine in Football), international conferences (e.g., World Congress of Performance Analysis in Sport, World Congress on Science and Soccer), and published books (e.g., Jayal, McRobert, Oatley, & O'Donoghue, 2018; McGarry, O'Donoghue, & Sampaio, 2013). However, there are often disconnects between research and application due to a lack of context (e.g., opposition style of play, home advantage, current score-line, and officiating decisions) and situation-specific information (e.g., the pitch location where actions took place, quality of the pass or ball control, quality of player decision-making and skill) on variables measured (Carling, Wright, Nelson, & Bradley, 2013; Mackenzie & Cushion, 2012; Sarmento et al., 2014). More recently, researchers have access to larger event and positional data sets so that they can use multiple performance indicators to apply analytical approaches such as multivariate statistical approaches, spatiotemporal analysis, machine learning, and social network analysis (for more detail, see Herold, Goes, Nopp, Bauer, Thompson, & Meyer, 2019; Jayal, McRobert, Oatley, & O'Donoghue, 2018; Sarmento et al., 2018).

In this chapter, we describe the role of performance analysis in the coaching process, principles and moments of play, tactics and strategies, key performance indicators, and an overview of match-play research during set plays and open play. Finally, we review some current approaches in soccer performance analysis that use analytical techniques to assess multiple performance indicators.

## Performance analysis in the coaching process

The provision of performance analysis, feedback, and future planning are important considerations in the coaching process. Traditionally, coaching interventions were based on subjective observations, which could potentially be unreliable and inaccurate because they are based on perceptions, biases, and previous experiences. For example, international-level soccer coaches could only recall 30% of key variables that determined match success and were less than 45% correct in a postgame assessment of events (Franks & Miller, 1991). Therefore, a coaching process model was proposed that included performance analysis (Maslovat & Franks, 2008). The primary purpose of video-based performance analysis in the coaching process is to provide objective information and feedback about performance that allow coaches and players to modify technical behaviour and tactical decision-making. After players perform, subjective coach observations and evaluations are combined with objective information captured by the performance analyst. This information is used to identify and enhance strengths or to improve weaknesses. In addition, a database of past events included in the review and interpretation phase can inform the planning and implementation of future practice interventions or competition (see Figure 17.1). Data profiling and benchmarking allow the tracking of performance trends across games and seasons, and the analysis of the opposition so that appropriate strategies and tactics can be prepared.

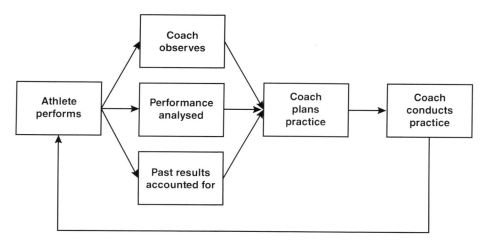

*Figure 17.1* The coaching process.
Source: Adapted from Maslovat & Franks, 2008.

Coaches perceive performance analysis to be beneficial to the coaching process as a support tool that facilities learning and develops mutual understanding between the coach and player (Groom, Cushion, & Nelson, 2011). A survey of elite professional and semi-professional coaches reported that 84% had access to full video or edited clips following most games (16%), or after every game (68%), on the same day (56%), or the following day (16%), and that they shared feedback with the team (86%), individual players (83%), and small groups (73%) (Wright, Atkins, & Jones, 2012). A survey of elite soccer performance analysts reported that they used an external company (70%) and/or a self-coding software (88%) to provide post-match analysis (81%), post-match feedback (71%), pre-match analysis (79%), live analysis (79%), and scouting/opposition analysis (54%) of individuals and team/s (Wright et al., 2013). Finally, coaches, players, and performance analysts suggest that performance analysis impacts team and individual performance, develops game understanding and decision-making and is essential when developing their playing style and tactics (Groom & Cushion, 2005; Reeves & Roberts, 2017; Wright, Atkins, & Jones, 2013).

## Soccer principles and moments of play, tactics, and strategies

Players and team actions are influenced by the cooperation of teammates and the organisation of the opposition, the large degrees of freedom and variability, and the skill of a player to act in specific conditions (Garganta, 2009). Gréhaigne et al. (1997) identified space and time, information, and organisation as the main challenges in soccer. Therefore, tactical match performance depends on the quality of individual players or team actions in space and time during match play to be successful (Memmert, Lemmink, & Sampaio, 2016). Performance analysis, specifically tactical modelling, can be used to identify regular or random game features during attacking and defensive play, providing information on player and team efficacy, and creating benchmarks for training.

To achieve the primary objectives of scoring while not conceding goals, teams maintain ball possession so they can invade space directly in front of the goal (i.e., scoring zone) to score, whereas defending teams reduce available space and attempt to regain possession. Wade (1996) identified attack, defence, and preparation or midfield play as the three main phases of soccer. Teams develop strategies and tactics to plan their own attacking and defensive actions across the phases, while anticipating and responding to their opponents.

Strategy and tactics influence game outcomes and are fundamental to successful performance in soccer (Carling, Williams & Reilly, 2007; Yiannakos & Armatas, 2006). Strategy is defined as the plans, principles of play or action guidelines that inform players and team interactions during the game (Hewitt, Greenham, & Norton, 2016). For example, attacking strategies involve moving players to field positions where they can receive the ball or score, overlap their teammate and defensive player in the direction of the goal to exploit space, or increase the width and depth of team surface area to create space in critical areas and/or a player numerical advantage. In contrast, defensive strategies involve the immediate delaying of opposition attacking play once it regains possession through the restriction of passing options and time to make the pass, and/or the increase of player density, and structure (i.e., defensive shape) in defensive areas.

In addition, strategies are influenced by playing style, defined as the general behaviour of the team to achieve attacking and defensive objectives. Attacking playing styles include direct, possession or elaborate, counterattacking, total soccer, and crossing, whereas defending playing styles include low pressure and high pressure (Bangsbo & Peitersen, 2000; Garganta et al., 1997; Pollard et al., 1988; Wright et al., 2011). Team strategy and specific playing styles inform the subsidiary units (e.g., defending back four) and individual player position roles and responsibilities so that instructions known as tactics can be provided.

Tactics, or tactical decision-making, is defined as specific attacking and defensive actions executed as a solution to anticipated situations influenced by the opposition. In addition, tactical changes occur based on team and player attributes, player injury/substitution, quality of opposition, current match status (i.e., winning, drawing, or losing), and/or match location (i.e., home, or away). Tactics determine how teams manage space and time, and individual (i.e., one-on-one attacking and defending events with or without the ball) and group actions (i.e., the cooperation between subsidiary units to achieve objectives) (Fradua et al., 2013; Garganta, 2009). Tactics are often changed to gain an advantage during competition, influenced by contextual and situational factors, and the interaction between and within the two teams (Rein & Memmert, 2016). Therefore, strategy and tactics inform team, unit, and individual player tactical decision-making prior to and during the game.

In addition, during the game, one team will be in a phase of play that impacts the opposition's phase of play, and vice versa. Dynamical systems theory has been used to describe the interaction between two teams and how perturbations alter the rhythmic flow of attacking and defending (Gréhaigne et al., 1997; McGarry, Anderson, Wallace, Hughes, & Franks, 2002). For example, an attacking phase may influence opposition tactics used in the defensive phase based on the position of players on the field in relation to the ball during a possession transition. However, to describe the playing style and tactics during these phases of play, a framework to segment the game is required. Hewitt et al. (2016) stated that moments of play can be categorised as

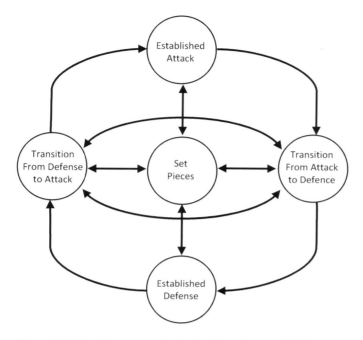

*Figure 17.2* The five moments of play (Hewitt et al., 2016).

one of the following five categories: Established Attack; Transition from Attack to Defence; Established Defence; Transition from Defence to Attack; and Set Plays (see Figure 17.2). For further simplicity, moments of play were grouped into three phases: (1) Established Offense and Defence; (2) Transitional Play; (3) and Set Plays. The terminology used to describe these phases is widely used by coaches, players, analysts, and researchers to describe strategy, playing styles, and tactics.

## Key performance indicators in soccer

Performance indicators are a selection or combination of action variables that describe some or all aspects of performance and should relate to successful or unsuccessful performance of actions or outcome of events (Hughes & Bartlett, 2002). Match analysis is employed to describe and define technical and tactical performance using discrete events (i.e., counts or frequencies) and categorical data (i.e., time and location) to assess how these performance indicators differ between successful and unsuccessful teams, and/or individual players (Nevill, Atkinson, Hughes, & Cooper, 2002). Team analysis provides information on how effectively they applied their playing style, strategies, and tactics, whereas subsidiary unit and individual analysis provide information on their contribution. Tactical and technical performance indicators are analysed, and performance profiles are created so that data can be compared to previous games and opponents. However, caution is required when comparing due to the match-to-match variability found in performance indicators (Gregson, Drust, Atkinson, & Salvo, 2010; Liu, Gomez, Gonçalves, & Sampaio, 2015). Therefore, when presenting a performance profile of a team, subsidiary unit or individual, means of

278    *Allistair P. McRobert et al.*

variables analysed need to have stabilised so that normative profiles can be established (Hughes, Evans & Wells, 2001; O'Donoghue, 2017).

Previously, indicators were classified based on the quality of performance (e.g., passes per possession) and scoring indicators (e.g., goals scored). Researchers attempted to identify key performance indicators associated with successful teams and outcomes in the World Cup (Franks, 2005; Liu, Gomez, Lago-Peñas, & Sampaio, 2015; Ruiz-Ruiz, Fradua, Fernández-Garcĺa, & Zubillaga, 2013), Women's World Cup (Barreira & Da Silva, 2016; Iván-Baragaño, Maneiro, Losada, & Ardá, 2021; Kubayi & Larkin, 2020), Euro Cup (Casal, 2019; Yiannakos & Armatas, 2006), Champions League (Almeida, Ferreira, & Volossovitch, 2014; Lago-Peñas, Lago-Ballesteros, & Rey, 2011), English Premier League (Adams, Morgans, Sacramento, Morgan, & Williams, 2013; Bradley, Lago-Peñas, Rey, & Gomez Diaz, 2013; Bush, Barnes, Archer, Hogg, & Bradley, 2015), Spanish La Liga (Castellano, Alvarez, Figueira, Coutinho, & Sampaio, 2013; Lago-Peñas & Dellal, 2010), and German Bundesliga (Hiller, 2014; Vogelbein, Nopp, & Hökelmann, 2014; Yue, Broich, & Mester, 2014). These studies mostly focused on goals, shots, possession, and passing patterns prior to a goal as an attempt to predict future team outcomes (Franks, 2005; Jones, James, & Mellalieu, 2004; Taylor, Mellalieu, & James, 2005).

## Soccer match-play research

To date, most soccer research has analysed set plays or open play, with the former focusing on corner kicks, penalty kicks, and free kicks, and the latter mainly on attacking play. Implications and effectiveness of defensive strategies and tactics are then inferred based on the opponents attacking play.

### *Analysis of open play*

Since Reep and Benjamin's (1968) seminal work demonstrated that approximately 80% of goals were from passing sequences of three passes or fewer, with a goal scored every 10 shots, there has been a debate on whether longer or shorter passing sequences are more effective strategies, with literature reporting mixed findings. Since then, studies have reported that more goals are scored from shorter passing sequences, which are more frequent than longer passing sequences, however, once the data are normalised, longer passing sequences are more effective (Franks, 2005; Tenga, Holme, Ronglan, & Bahr, 2010a). In addition to passing sequences, longer possession durations are typically associated with successful teams, however, differences in length of passing sequence durations have been reported between international teams and the English Premier League (Carling & Williams, 2008; Jones et al., 2004; Tenga & Sigmundstad, 2011). Furthermore, more goals are scored in the second half of games, and midfielders and forwards score more goals than any other position (Acar et al., 2009; Barreira et al., 2013; Grant et al., 1998; Partridge et al., 1993; Taylor, Mellalieu, & James, 2005; Yiannakos & Armatas, 2006; Yi, Jia, Liu, & Gomez, 2018). Goal scoring and associated scoring variables are measured to determine performance efficiency, however, goal prevalence is low in soccer compared to other invasion games. Therefore, additional behaviour patterns and event data need to be collected and analysed. For example, shots at goal have been measured, specifically shot location, shot outcome (i.e., goal, on-target, off-target, goalkeeper save, and blocked), shot frequency, actions prior to the goal (i.e., pass, cross, free kick, and corner kick), and player/s involved (Lago-Ballesteros & Lago-Peñas, 2010; Bate, 1988; Collet, 2013; Corbellini et al., 2013; Chervenjakov, 1988; Ensum et al., 2005; Franks, 2005; Garganta et al., 1997; Hughes & Churchill, 2005; Hughes & Franks, 2005; Hughes et al., 1988; Lago-Peñas et al., 2011; Mara, Wheeler, & Lyons, 2012; Yi et al., 2018). Shots are more likely to produce a goal if they are taken closer to the goal and in central positions, so attacking third and penalty area entries have been examined. Teams winning games in the World Cup 2006 made more penalty area entries, and that there was a moderate correlation between the number of entries and the likelihood of scoring a goal (Ruiz-Ruiz et al., 2013).

Tenga and colleagues (2010a, 2010b) analysed 1,688 open-play possessions in the Norwegian male professional league. They defined a score box possession as an entry into the score box in front of the goal with a high degree of control (i.e., space and time for the attacking team to perform intended actions). A strong correlation was reported between score box possessions and shooting opportunities, and a 1% scoring probability based on an average of scoring three goals and having 280 possessions per match. In addition, when playing against an imbalanced defence, counterattack possession types were more effective than elaborate possession play (Tenga, Holme, Ronglan, & 2010a; 2010b; Tenga, Ronglan, & Bahr, 2010). However, from the 1,688 open play possessions, only 80 (4.7%) led to scoring opportunities and 167 (9.9%) to score box possessions, whereas other outcomes (i.e., no score box possession, or possession lost in the defensive, middle, or attacking third) occurred for the remaining 1,441 (85.4%) possessions (Tenga, Ronglan, & Bahr, 2010). Therefore, it would be useful to understand what happens during the large proportion of possessions that do not lead to score box possessions or scoring opportunities.

Previously, researchers focusing on ball possession explored the association between successful performance, pitch areas where possession is maintained, and maintenance of possession close to the opponent goal as an indicator of a successful attack (Bell-Walker, McRobert, Ford, & Williams, 2007; Breen, Iga, & Ford, 2006; Franks, 2005; Jones et al., 2004; Lago-Peñas & Dellal, 2010; Tenga & Sigmundstad, 2011). Conversely, having more possessions does not always lead to scoring opportunities and goals (Bate, 1988; Wright et al., 2011). Moreover, like other performance indicators, possession is influenced by contextual factors, such as match location (i.e., home or away), match status (i.e., winning, drawing, or losing), and quality of the opposition (Gomez, Parmar, & Travassos, 2020; Lago-Peñas & Dellal, 2010; Lago-Peñas & Gómez-Lopez, 2014; Lago-Peñas, Gomez, & Pollard, 2017; Paixão, Sampaio, & Almeida, 2015; Taylor, Mellalieu, James, & Shearer, 2008), and once these factors are accounted for, possession becomes a poor predictor of outcome (Collet, 2013).

### *Analysis of set plays*

Researchers have estimated that between 30% and 40% of goals are scored from set plays (Casal, Maneiro, Ardá, Losada, & Rial, 2015). Siegle and Lames (2012) reported an average of 108 interruptions per match, with throw-ins (40), and free kicks (33) the most frequent, whereas goal kicks (17), corner kicks (10), substitutions (4), and kick-offs (3) were less frequent. Set plays such as free kicks, penalty kicks, corners, goal kicks, and throw-ins occur when the ball runs out of the playing area or play is stopped due to a foul. These events have certain advantages because the player of the team executing the restart controls the timing from a stable situation, where the opposition must respect distance rules, therefore, the player has an opportunity to advance the ball into a goal-scoring position or take a shot at goal (Maneiro et al., 2019). Furthermore, successful domestic and international teams were more efficient with a set play-to-goal ratio of 1:7 compared to 1:15 for unsuccessful teams (Carling, Williams, & Reilly, 2005).

Despite the relatively low frequency of corner kicks, they can often be a determining factor in match outcomes. In tournament knockout stages (i.e., UEFA Champions League 2010/2011, World Cup 2010, and Euro 2012), only 26% of corners resulted in an attempt at goal and 2.2% as a goal, however, 76% of matches ended in a draw or win if a goal was scored from a corner (Casal et al., 2015). Similarly, 25% of corners resulted in an attempt at goal and 3.7% as a goal in the 2018 World Cup (Kubayi & Larkin, 2019). In the English Premier League 2011/2012 season, 31% attempts at goal and 13.3% of goals came from corners, whereas 34% attempts at goal and 4.6% of goals came from corners in the FA Women's Super League 2017/2018 season (Beare & Stone, 2019; Pulling, Robins, & Rixon, 2013). In contrast, the top and bottom six teams had only 10% of attempts at goal from corners during the English Premier League 2015/2016 season, with 67% of matches ending in a draw or win if a goal was scored from one (Strafford, Smith, North, & Stone, 2019). Moreover, the likelihood of corner goal attempts increased when attacking strategies involved deliveries to the far post, a dynamic attacking move involving three or four attackers, whereas defensive strategies involving zonal marking slightly reduced goal attempts compared to one-to-one marking (Strafford et al., 2019; Casal et al., 2015; De Baranda & Lopez-Riquelme, 2012; Pulling et al., 2013).

Penalty kicks provide a clear goal-scoring opportunity that can decide the result of a match. The success rates of penalty kicks in professional soccer leagues and tournaments range from 70% to 85% (Almeida, Volossovitch, & Duarte, 2016; Bar-Eli, Azar, Ritov, Keider-Levin & Schein, 2007; Horn, de Waal, & Kraak, 2020; Hughes & Wells, 2002; Lopez-Botella & Palao, 2007). In tournament shoot-outs between 1982–1998 and 2002–2008, penalty kicks had a success rate of 76% and 73%, respectively, whereas success rate during match play between 2002 and 2008 was 68% compared to 85% between 1982 and 1998 (Dalton, Guillon, & Naroo, 2015; McGarry & Franks, 2000). Moreover, the number of penalty kicks awarded and success rate are influenced by strike direction, goalkeeper reaction time, ball speed, foot used, positional role, player age, time period, match status, and venue (Almeida et al., 2016; Fariña, Fábrica, Tambussi & Alonso, 2013; Horn et al., 2020; Jordet, Hartman, Visscher, & Lemmink 2007; Lopez-Botella & Palao, 2007). Jamil et al. (2020) reported variations in individual (i.e., length of run-ups, strike direction, type of shot, and foot used) and situational variables (i.e., time period, match status, and venue) across four European soccer leagues (i.e., English Premier League, Spanish La Liga, German Bundesliga, and Italian Serie A) when analysing penalty kick success.

Free kicks are an important component of performance in soccer, however, there is limited research on this aspect compared to corner and penalty kicks. In tournaments, teams take three indirect free kicks per match aimed at scoring, 21.8% are attempts at goal, 9.3% are on target, and 2.9% were goals (Casal, Maneiro, Ardá, Losada, & Rial, 2014). During the 2007 Women's World Cup, one goal was scored every 4.6 games from free kicks, ball flights times were significantly faster for goals and all goals were scored within 7 m of the goal (Alcock, 2010). In the German Bundesliga, Link et al. (2016) reported 34.9 free kicks per game, 5.8 were less than 35 m from the goal, 22.2%

were attempts at goal, while the remaining resulted in a pass or cross. Moreover, they used geostatistical approaches, specifically variograms of position (2D location of the free kick), density (number of free kicks in each sector), interruption time (time from foul to ball in play), distance to wall, players in the wall, rule violation, laterality, type of play, outcome of shot, and outcome of cross to provide continues spatial profiles of free kicks. In conclusion, free-kick crosses into the penalty area are less likely to result in a goal, and it might be more effective to increase passes from side free kicks and use short passes and dribbles to enter the penalty area.

## Current approaches in soccer performance analysis

Attempting to identify performance indicators to predict performance has generated mixed results, often due to interpretation of definitions, access to appropriate and larger datasets, and the difficulty in including contextual and situational variables (Carling et al., 2013; Mackenzie & Cushion, 2012). Therefore, analysts adopted a reductionist approach in which performance indicators are used to segment the video into critical moments from the game that can provide feedback to the coach and players. More recently, the availability of additional event and positional data has allowed researchers to develop new methods to contextualise performance. Analytical techniques are used to assess multiple performance indicators, such as behaviour indexes, multifactorial statistical approaches, social network analysis, spatiotemporal analysis, and machine learning.

Kempe et al. (2014) developed the Index of Game Control (IGC) and Index of Offensive Behaviour (IOB) to evaluate playing styles and tactics. IGC was calculated using several passing and passing success parameters (i.e., passes per action, passing direction, target player passes, passing success rate, and forward passing success rate), whereas IOB combined IGC, duration and distance of actions, and game speed (i.e., mean passes per attack, game speed, mean time of attack, gain of possession, distance per attack, and relative ball possession). The most successful teams preferred the possession style and had a higher score for ICG. Fernandez-Navarro et al. (2019) developed the Possession Effectiveness Index (PEI) based on expected goals and ball movement points to evaluate playing style effectiveness and the influence of contextual variables (i.e., match status, venue, and quality of opposition). Linear mixed models showed that direct play, counterattack, maintenance, and crossing effectiveness increased when teams were winning by two or more goals. Counterattack increased when winning and reduced when losing by one goal, whereas direct play increased when losing by two or more goals. Playing away negatively affected direct play, maintenance, and high pressure, with all styles reduced when playing stronger opposition.

Factor analysis, specifically principal component analysis can be used to cluster performance indicators into fewer factors that represent playing styles (Fernandez-Navarro, Fradua, Zubillaga, Ford, & McRobert, 2016). They extracted six factors that defined eight attacking (i.e., direct *vs.* possession, crossing *vs.* no crossing, wide *vs.* narrow possession, and fast *vs.* slow progression) and four defending styles (i.e., pressure on wide *vs.* central areas, low *vs.* high pressure) in the English Premier League and Spanish La Liga. Using these factors, playing style profiles can be created (see Figure 17.3), for example, Everton F.C. had an attacking playing style involving direct, no crossing, narrow possession, with fast progression, and a defensive style of low and central areas pressure. In comparison, F.C. Barcelona had an attacking style involving

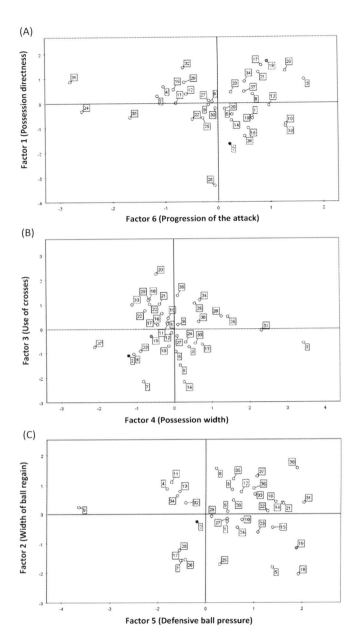

*Figure 17.3* Soccer team's styles of play. Attacking styles of play: (a) factors 1 and 6, (b) factors 3 and 4. Defensive styles of play: (c) factors 2 and 5.

Notes: Numbers assigned to the teams for figure interpretation were: Atletico de Madrid (1), Barcelona (2), Betis (3), Bilbao (4), Celta (5), Deportivo (6), Espanyol (7), Mallorca (8), Osasuna (9), Real Madrid (10), Real Sociedad (11), Sevilla (12), Valencia (13), Zaragoza (14), Arsenal (15), Aston Villa (16), Bolton (17), Chelsea (18), Everton (19), Liverpool (20), Manchester City (21), Manchester United (22), Portsmouth (23), Tottenham (24), West Ham (25), Wigan (26) for season 2006–2007; and Atletico de Madrid (27), Barcelona (28), Bilbao (29), Getafe (30), Levante (31), Osasuna (32), Real Madrid (33), Real Sociedad (34), Valencia (35), Villareal (36), Zaragoza (37) for season 2010–2011.

Barcelona (2006–2007) highlighted in black. Everton (2006–2007) highlighted in grey.

possession, no crossing, narrow possession, fast progression, and a defensive style of high and central pressure. Gomez et al. (2018) included additional performance indicators and examined the effects of venue (i.e., home *vs.* away) and team ranking. They extracted eight factors (i.e., ball possession, ending actions, individual challenges, counterattack, set pieces, transitional play, fouling actions, and free kicks) and reported specific tactical trends based on team rankings and venue.

Social network analysis can provide insights into strategies and tactics by examining passing connectivity between players. Players in this analysis are seen as a network of nodes linked by passing connections to provide team connectivity and cohesiveness metrics, which further understanding of how teams coordinate actions and identify the most connected players (Clemente, Martins, Kalamaras, Wong, & Mendes, 2015; Clemente, Martins, Wong, Kalamaras, & Mendes, 2017; Mclean et al., 2018a). Mclean et al. (2018b) used notational and social network analysis to examine goal-scoring passing networks (GSPN) characteristics in the 2016 Euros as a function of match status and pitch location. GSPN were highly variable, match status influenced the networks, and high team connectivity did not determine the GSPN between successful and unsuccessful teams or the group and knockout stages, however, degree centrality measures can be used to determine prominent pitch zones during matches.

Due to positional tracking data availability, spatiotemporal approaches such as Voronoi diagrams and centroid analysis have been used to analyse tactical behaviours during attacking and defensive phases, transitions, and critical moments such as goals (Fonseca, Milho, Travassos, Araújo, & Lopes, 2013; Frencken, Poel, Visscher, & Lemmink, 2012). Centroid analysis characteristics such as centroid position (average position of the outfield players) provide information on how teams move across the pitch, whereas increases and decreases in team surface area (total space covered by outfield players) provide information on team space control when attacking or defending. Frencken et al. (2012) examined inter-team distance dynamics during critical match events. Match events identified through longitudinal inter-team distance related to defending players moving forwards or backwards after a longitudinal pass, whereas lateral inter-team distance corresponded with defending players moving laterally after a sideways pass. Fonseca et al. (2012) used Voronoi diagrams to understand how opposite teams coordinate player locations to define and adjust their dominate regions during a game. They reported that players from the team in possession were further apart from each other, whereas defending players were closer.

Finally, de Jong et al. (2020) used three different analytical approaches to identify technical determinants of female soccer match outcomes from a larger sample (1,390 team performances) and range of variables (450). First, a data-driven approach used 450 variables for feature selection. Second, a rational approach involved two authors selecting a range of variables (74) relevant to coaches to reduce over-fitting and increase practical application. Third, a literature-driven approach selected 16 variables from previous literature, so comparisons were possible. Match outcome was modelled using generalised linear modelling and decision trees for variables in each analytical approach. They reported that the rational and data-driven approaches outperformed the literature-driven approach when predicting match outcome, with higher prediction accuracies compared to studies on male soccer. Furthermore, the strongest determinants of match outcome were scoring first, intentional assists relative to the opponent, percentage of shots on goal saved by the goalkeeper relative to the opponent, shots on goal relative to the opponent, and the percentage of successful duels.

## Future directions and conclusions

Soccer is a goal-striking invasion game where two opposing teams attempt to score goals while not conceding goals. Therefore, most researchers have analysed performance indicators during set plays and open plays to predict performance. Set plays such as corner, penalty, and free kicks account for 30–40% of goals scored and are often a deciding factor in winning. In addition, due to the dynamic nature of soccer and low prevalence of goals and goal attempts, open play analysis has focused on possession and passing sequences, however, they have produced mixed results when predicting performance. Researchers have included situational and contextual variables such as pitch location, pass quality, skills and decision-making quality, opposition quality and style of play, home advantage, and score line to provide further depth.

More recently, availability of event and positional data, and use of analytical techniques such as behaviour indexes, multifactorial statistical approaches, social network analysis, spatiotemporal analysis, and machine learning provide further insights into playing styles, tactical behaviour, and better contextualise performance. More importantly, spatiotemporal approaches using tracking data provide information on tactical behaviour during defensive and attacking play, whereas previously, defensive effectiveness and tactics have been inferred based on the opponent's attacking play.

In future, researchers should continue to explore the use of these analytical techniques so that we can provide additional information on how teams control space during attacking and defending play. In addition, the recent growth and investment in the women's game means that event and positional data are becoming more available, however, published research is still limited. Recently, in conjunction with FIFA and Adidas, Science and Medicine in Football has announced a women's football special issue.

Performance analysis is an integral part of the coaching process that merges objective data with subjective coach observations so that technical and tactical behaviours can be modified. In addition, databasing information allows tracking of performance trends and analysis of opposition strategy and tactics. Moreover, due to advancements in technology, coaches, players, and analysts access information almost immediately to develop game understanding, decision-making, playing style, and tactics.

## References

Acar, M. F., Yapicioglu, B., Arikan, N., Yalcin, S., Ates, N., & Ergun, M. (2009) Analysis of goals scored in the 2006 World Cup. In T. Reilly & F. Korkusuz (eds.), *Science and Football VI* (pp. 235–242). London: Routledge.

Adams, D., Morgans, R., Sacramento, J., Morgan, S., & Williams, M. D. (2013). Successful short passing frequency of defenders differentiates between top and bottom four English premier league teams. *International Journal of Performance Analysis in Sport, 13*(3), 653–668. http://dx.doi.org/10.1080/24748668.2013.11868678

Alcock, A. (2010). Analysis of direct free kicks in the women's football world cup 2007. *European Journal of Sport Science, 10*(4), 279–284. http://doi.org/10.1080/17461390903515188

Almeida, C. H., Ferreira, A. P., & Volossovitch, A. (2014). Effects of match location, match status and quality of opposition on regaining possession in UEFA champions league. *Journal of Human Kinetics, 41*(1), 1–12. http://doi.org/10.2478/hukin-2014-0048

Almeida, C. H., Volossovitch, A., & Duarte, R. (2016). Penalty kick outcomes in UEFA club competitions (2010-2015): the roles of situational, individual and performance factors. *International Journal of Performance Analysis in Sport, 16*(2), 508–522. http://doi.org/10.1080/24748668.2016.11868905

Bangsbo, J., & Peitersen, B. (2000). *Soccer Systems and Strategies*, Champaign, IL: Human Kinetics.

Bar-Eli, M., Azar, O. H., Ritov, I., Keider-Levin, Y. & Schein, G. (2007). Action bias among elite soccer goalkeepers: the case of penalty kicks. *Journal of Economic Psychology, 28*, 606–621. http://doi.org/10.1016/j.joep.2006.12.001

Barreira, J., & Da Silva, C. E. (2016). National teams in women's soccer world cup from 1991 to 2015: participation, performance and competitiveness. *Journal of Physical Education and Sport, 16*(3), 795-799. http://doi.org/10.7752/jpes.2016.03126

Barreira, D., Garganta, J., Pinto, T., Valente, J., & Anguera, M.T. (2013). Do attacking game patterns differ between first and second halves of soccer matches in the 2010 FIFA world cup? In H. Nunome, B. Drust, & B. Dawson (eds.), *Science and Football VII* (pp. 193–198). London: Routledge.

Bate, R. (1988). Football chance: tactics and strategy. In T. Reilly, A. Lees, K. Davids, & W. J. Murphy (eds.), *Science and Football* (pp. 293–301). London: E & FN Spon.

Beare, H., & Stone, J. A. (2019). Analysis of attacking corner kick strategies in the FA women's super league 2017/2018. *International Journal of Performance Analysis in Sport, 19*(6), 893–903. http://doi.org/10.1080/24748668.2019.1677329

Bell-Walker, J., McRobert, A., Ford, P., & Williams, A. M. (2007). A quantitative analysis of successful teams at the 2006 World Cup finals. *Insight: The FA Coaches Association Journal, Autumn/Winter*, 36–43.

Bradley, P. S., Lago-Peñas, C., Rey, E., & Gomez Diaz, A. (2013). The effect of high and low percentage ball possession on physical and technical profiles in English FA premier league soccer matches. *Journal of Sports Sciences, 31*(12), 1261–1270. http://doi.org/10.1080/02640414.2013.786185

Bradley, P., O'Donoghue, P., Wooster, B., & Tordoff, P. (2007). The reliability of prozone match viewer: a video-based technical performance analysis system. *International Journal of Performance Analysis in Sport, 7*(3), 117–129.

Breen, A., Iga, J., Ford, P., & Williams, A. M. (2006). World cup 2006 – Germany. A quantitative analysis of goals scored. *Insight: The FA Coaches Association Journal, Autumn/Winter*, 44–53.

Bush, M., Barnes, C., Archer, D. T., Hogg, B., & Bradley, P. S. (2015). Evolution of match performance parameters for various playing positions in the English Premier League. *Human Movement Science, 39*, 1–11. https://doi.org/10.1016/j.humov.2014.10.003

Carling, C., & Williams, A. M. (2008). Match analysis and elite soccer performance: integrating science and practice. In T. Reilly (ed.), *Science and Soccer* (pp. 32–47). Maastricht, Netherlands: Shaker Publishing.

Carling, C., Williams, A.M., & Reilly, T. (2005). *Handbook of Soccer Match Analysis: A Systematic Approach to Improving Performance (1st ed.)*. Routledge, London. https://doi.org/10.4324/9780203448625

Carling, C., Wright, C., John Nelson, L., & S Bradley, P. (2013). Comment on performance analysis in football: a critical review and implications for future research. *Journal of Sports Sciences, 32*(1), 2–7. http://doi.org/10.1080/02640414.2013.807352

Casal, C. A. (2019). Offensive Transitions in High-Performance Football: Differences Between UEFA Euro 2008 and UEFA Euro 2016. Fpsyg-10-01230.Tex, 10, 1–10. https://doi.org/10.3389/fpsyg.2019.01230

Casal, A. C., Maneiro, R., Ardá, T., Losada, J. L., & Rial, A. (2014). Effectiveness of indirect free kicks in elite soccer. *International Journal of Performance Analysis in Sport, 14*(3), 744–760. http://doi.org/10.1080/24748668.2014.11868755

Casal, C. A., Maneiro, R., Ardá, T., Losada, J. L. & Rial, A. (2015). Analysis of corner kick success in elite football. *International Journal of Performance in Sport, 15*(2), 430–451. http://doi.org/10.1080/24748668.2015.11868805

Casal, C. A. (2019). Offensive Transitions in High-Performance Football: Differences Between UEFA Euro 2008 and UEFA Euro 2016. *Fpsyg-10-01230.Tex, 10*, 1–10. https://doi.org/10.3389/fpsyg.2019.01230

Castellano, J., Alvarez, D., Figueira, B., Coutinho, D., & Sampaio, J. (2013). Identifying the effects from the quality of opposition in a football team positioning strategy. *International Journal of Performance Analysis in Sport, 13*(3), 822–832.

Chervenjakov, M. (1988). Assessment of the playing effectiveness of soccer players. In T. Reilly, A. Lees, K. Davids, & W. J. Murphy (eds.), *Science and Football* (pp. 288–292). London: E & FN Spon.

Clemente, F. M., Martins, F. M. L., Kalamaras, D., Wong, P. D., & Mendes, R. S. (2015). General network analysis of national soccer teams in FIFA world cup 2014. *International Journal of Performance Analysis in Sport, 15*(1), 80–96. http://doi.org/10.1080/24748668.2015.11868778

Clemente, F. M., Martins, F. M. L., Wong, P. D., Kalamaras, D., & Mendes, R. S. (2017). Midfielder as the prominent participant in the building attack: A network analysis of national teams in FIFA world cup 2014. *International Journal of Performance Analysis in Sport, 15*(2), 704–722. http://doi.org/10.1080/24748668.2015.11868825

Collet, C. (2013). The possession game? A comparative analysis of ball retention and team success in European and international football, 2007–2010. *Journal of Sports Sciences, 31*(2), 123–136. http://doi.org/10.1080/02640414.2012.727455

Corbellini, F., Volossovitch, A., Andrade, C., Fernandes, O., & Ferreira, A. P. (2013). Contextual effects on the free kick performance: a case study with a Portuguese professional soccer team. In H. Nunome, B. Drust, & B. Dawson (eds.), *Science and Football VII* (pp. 217–222). London: Routledge.

Cummins, C., Orr, R., O'Connor, H., & West, C. (2013). Global positioning systems (GPS) and microtechnology sensors in team sports: a systematic review. *Sports Medicine, 43*(10), 1025–1042. http://doi.org/10.1007/s40279-013-0069-2

Dalton, K., Guillon, M., & Naroo, S. A. (2015). An analysis of penalty kicks in elite football post 1997. *International Journal of Sport Coaching, 10*(5), 815–827. http://doi.org/10.1260/1747-9541.10.5.815

De Baranda, P. S., & Lopez-Riquelme, D. (2012). Analysis of corner kicks in relation to match status in the 2006 world cup. *European Journal of Sport Science, 12*(2), 121–129. http://doi.org/10.1080/17461391.2010.551418

de Jong, L. M. S., Gastin, P. B., Angelova, M. B., & Dwyer, D. B. (2020). Technical determinants of success in professional women's soccer: a wider range of variables reveals new insights. *PLoS ONE, 15*(10), e0240992. http://doi.org/10.1371/journal.pone.0240992

Drust, B. (2010). Performance analysis research: meeting the challenge. *Journal of Sports Sciences, 28*(9), 921–922. http://doi.org/10.1080/02640411003740769

Ensum, J., Pollard, R., & Taylor, S. (2005). Applications of logistic regression to shots at goal in association football. In T. Reilly, J. Cabri, & D. Araujo (eds.), *Science and Football V* (pp. 211–218). London: Routledge.

Fariña, A. R., Fábrica, G., Tambussi, P. S., & Alonso, R. (2013). Taking the goalkeeper's side in association football penalty kicks. *International Journal of Performance Analysis in Sport, 13*(1), 96–109. http://doi.org/10.1080/24748668.2013.11868634

Fernandez-Navarro, J., Fradua, L., Zubillaga, A., & McRobert, A. P. (2019). Evaluating the effectiveness of styles of play in elite soccer. *International Journal of Sports Science & Coaching, 14*(4), 514–527. http://doi.org/10.1177/1747954119855361

Fernandez-Navarro, J., Fradua, L., Zubillaga, A., Ford, P. R., & McRobert, A. P. (2016). Attacking and defensive styles of play in soccer: analysis of Spanish and English elite teams. *Journal of Sports Sciences, 34*(24), 2195–2204. http://doi.org/10.1080/02640414.2016.1169309

Fonseca, S., Milho, J., Travassos, B., & Araújo, D. (2012). Spatial dynamics of team sports exposed by Voronoi diagrams. *Human Movement Science, 31*(6), 1652–1659. http://doi.org/10.1016/j.humov.2012.04.006

Fonseca, S., Milho, J., Travassos, B., Araújo, D., & Lopes, A. (2013). Measuring spatial interaction behavior in team sports using superimposed Voronoi diagrams. *International Journal of Performance Analysis in Sport, 13*(1), 179–189.

Fradua, L., Zubillaga, A., Caro, Ó., Iván Fernández-García, Á., Ruiz-Ruiz, C., & Tenga, A. (2013). Designing small-sided games for training tactical aspects in soccer: extrapolating pitch sizes from full-size professional matches. *Journal of Sports Sciences, 31*(6), 573–581. http://doi.org/10.1080/02640414.2012.746722

Franks, I. M. (2005). Analysis of passing sequences, shots and goals in soccer. *Journal of Sports Sciences, 23*(5), 509–514. http://doi.org/10.1080/02640410410001716779

Franks, I. M., & Miller, G. (1991). Training coaches to observe and remember. *Journal of Sports Sciences, 9*(3), 285–297. http://doi.org/10.1080/02640419108729890

Frencken, W. G. P., Lemmink, K. A. P. M., & Delleman, N. J. (2010). Soccer-specific accuracy and validity of the local position measurement (LPM) system. *Journal of Science and Medicine in Sport, 13*(6), 641–645. http://doi.org/10.1016/j.jsams.2010.04.003

Frencken, W., Poel, H. de, Visscher, C., & Lemmink, K. (2012). Variability of inter-team distances associated with match events in elite-standard soccer. *Journal of Sports Sciences, 30*(12), 1207–1213. http://doi.org/10.1080/02640414.2012.703783

Garganta, J. (2009). Trends of tactical performance analysis in team sports: bridging the gap between research, training and competition. *Revista Portuguesa De Ciências Do Desporto, 9*(1), 81–89. http://doi.org/10.5628/rpcd.09.01.81

Garganta, J., Maia, J., & Basto, F. (1997). Analysis of goal-scoring patterns in European top level soccer teams. In J. Bangsbo, T. Reilly & A. M. Williams (eds.), *Science and Football III* (pp. 246–250). London: E & FN Spon.

Gomez, M.-Á., Mitrotasios, M., Armatas, V., & Lago-Peñas, C. (2018). Analysis of playing styles according to team quality and match location in Greek professional soccer. *International Journal of Performance Analysis in Sport, 18*(6), 986–997. http://doi.org/10.1080/24748668.2018.1539382

Gomez, M.-Á., Reus, M., Parmar, N., & Travassos, B. (2020). Exploring elite soccer teams' performances during different match-status periods of close matches' comebacks. *Chaos, Solitons & Fractals, 132*, 109566. http://doi.org/10.1016/j.chaos.2019.109566

Grant, A., Reilly, T., Williams, A. M., & Borrie, A. (1998). Analysis of the goals scored in the 1998 world cup. *Insight: The FA Coaches Association Journal, 2*(1), 18–20.

Gregson, W., Drust, B., Atkinson, G., & Salvo, V. D. (2010). Match-to-match variability of high-speed activities in premier league soccer. *International Journal of Sports Medicine, 31*(4), 237–242. http://doi.org/10.1055/s-0030-1247546

Gréhaigne, J.-F., Bouthier, D., & David, B. (1997). Dynamic-system analysis of opponent relationships in collective actions in soccer. *Journal of Sports Sciences, 15*(2), 137–149. http://doi.org/10.1080/026404197367416

Groom, R., & Cushion, C. (2005). Using of video based coaching with players: a case study. *International Journal of Performance Analysis in Sport, 5*(3), 40–46. http://doi.org/10.1080/24748668.2005.11868336

Groom, R., Cushion, C., & Nelson, L. (2011). The delivery of video-based performance analysis by England youth soccer coaches: towards a grounded theory. *Journal of Applied Sport Psychology, 23*(1), 16–32. http://doi.org/10.1080/10413200.2010.511422

Herold, M., Goes, F., Nopp, S., Bauer, P., Thompson, C., & Meyer, T. (2019). Machine learning in men's professional football: current applications and future directions for improving attacking play. *International Journal of Sports Science & Coaching, 14*(6), 798–817. https://doi.org/10.1177/1747954119879350

Hewitt, A., Greenham, G., & Norton, K. (2016). Game style in soccer: what is it and can we quantify it? *International Journal of Performance Analysis in Sport, 16*(1), 355–372. https://doi.org/10.1080/24748668.2016.11868892

Hiller, T. (2014). The importance of players in teams of the German Bundesliga in the season 2012/2013 – a cooperative game theory approach. *Applied Economics Letters, 22*(4), 324–329. http://doi.org/10.1080/13504851.2014.941527

Horn, M., de Waal, S., & Kraak, W. (2020). In-match penalty kick analysis of the 2009/10 to 2018/19 English premier league competition. *International Journal of Performance Analysis in Sport, 21*(1), 139–155. http://doi.org/10.1080/24748668.2020.1855052

Hughes, M. D., & Bartlett, R. M. (2002). The use of performance indicators in performance analysis. *Journal of Sports Sciences, 20*(10), 739–754. https://doi.org/10.1080/026404102320675602

Hughes, M. D., & Churchill, S. (2005). Attacking profiles of successful and unsuccessful teams in Copa America 2001. In T. Reilly, J. Cabri, & D. Araujo (eds.), *Science and Football V* (pp. 221–224). London: Routledge.

Hughes, M., Evans, S., & Wells, J. (2001). Establishing normative profiles in performance analysis. *International Journal of Performance Analysis in Sport, 1*(1), 1 -26. https://doi.org/10.108 0/24748668.2001.11868245

Hughes, M. D., Robertson, K., & Nicholson, A. (1988). Comparison of patterns of play of successful and unsuccessful teams in the 1986 world cup for soccer. In T. Reilly, A. Lees, K. Davids, & W. J. Murphy (eds.), *Science and Football* (pp. 363–367). London: E & FN Spon.

Hughes, M., & Wells, J. (2002) Analysis of penalties taken in shoot-outs. *International Journal of Performance Analysis in Sport, 2*(1), 55-72. https://doi.org/10.1080/24748668.2002.11868261

Hughes, M., & Franks, I. (2005). Analysis of passing sequences, shots and goals in soccer. *Journal of Sports Sciences, 23*(5), 509–514. https://doi.org/10.1080/02640410410001716779

Iván-Baragaño, I., Maneiro, R., Losada, J. L., & Ardá, A. (2021). Multivariate analysis of the offensive phase in high-performance women's soccer: a mixed methods study. *Sustainability, 13*(11), 6379. http://doi.org/10.3390/su13116379

James, N. (2006). Notational analysis in soccer: past, present and future *International Journal of Performance Analysis in Sport, 6*(2), 67–81.

Jamil, M., Littman, P., & Beato, M. (2020). Investigating inter-league and inter-nation variations of key determinants for penalty success across European football. *International Journal of Performance Analysis in Sport, 20*(5), 892–907. http://doi.org/10.1080/24748668.2020.1794720

Jayal, A., McRobert, A. P., Oatley, G., & O'Donoghue, P. (2018). *Sports Analytics: Analysis, Visualisation and Decision Making in Sports Performance (1st ed.).* Routledge. http://doi.org/10.4324/9781315222783

Jones, D., Rands, S., & Butterworth, A. D. (2020). The use and perceived value of telestration tools in elite football. *International Journal of Performance Analysis in Sport, 20*(3), 373–388. http://doi.org/10.1080/24748668.2020.1753965

Jones, P., James, N., & Mellalieu, S. (2004). Possession as a performance indicator in soccer. *International Journal of Performance Analysis in Sport, 4*(1), 98–102.

Jordet, G., Hartman, E., Visscher, C., & Lemmink, K. A. P. M. (2007). Kicks from the penalty mark in soccer: the roles of stress, skill, and fatigue for kick outcomes. *Journal of Sports Sciences, 25*(2), 121–129. http://doi.org/10.1080/02640410600624020

Kempe, M., Vogelbein, M., Memmert, D., & Nopp, S. (2014). Possession vs. direct play: evaluating tactical behavior in elite soccer. *International Journal of Sports Science, 4*(6a), 35–41. http://doi.org/10.5923/s.sports.201401.05

Kubayi, A., & Larkin, P. (2019). Analysis of teams' corner kicks defensive strategies at the FIFA world cup 2018. *International Journal of Performance Analysis in Sport, 19*(5), 809–819. http://doi.org/10.1080/24748668.2019.1660547

Kubayi, A., & Larkin, P. (2020). Technical performance of soccer teams according to match outcome at the 2019 FIFA women's world cup. *International Journal of Performance Analysis in Sport, 20*(5), 908–916. http://doi.org/10.1080/24748668.2020.1809320

Lago, C. (2009). The influence of match location, quality of opposition, and match status on possession strategies in professional association football. *Journal of Sports Sciences, 27*(13), 1463–1469. http://doi.org/10.1080/02640410903131681

Lago-Ballesteros, J., & Lago-Peñas, C. (2010). Performance in team sports: identifying the keys to success in soccer. *Journal of Human Kinetics, 25*, 85–91.

Lago-Peñas, C., & Dellal, A. (2010). Ball possession strategies in elite soccer according to the evolution of the match-score: the influence of situational variables. *Journal of Human Kinetics*, *25*(1), 293–298. http://doi.org/10.2478/v10078-010-0036-z

Lago-Peñas, C., & Gómez-Lopez, M. (2014). How important is it to score a goal? the influence of the scoreline on match performance in elite soccer. *Perceptual and Motor Skills*, *119*(3), 774–784. http://doi.org/10.2466/23.27.PMS.119c32z1

Lago-Peñas, C., Gomez, M. Á., & Pollard, R. (2017). Home advantage in elite soccer matches. A transient effect? *International Journal of Performance Analysis in Sport*, *17*(1–2), 86–95. http://doi.org/10.1080/24748668.2017.1304024

Lago-Peñas, C., Lago-Ballesteros, J., & Rey, E. (2011). Differences in performance indicators between winning and losing teams in the UEFA champions league. *Journal of Human Kinetics*, *27*, 135–146. http://doi.org/10.2478/v10078-011-0011-3

Link, D., Kolbinger, O., Weber, H., & Stöckl, M. (2016). A topography of free kicks in soccer. *Journal of Sports Sciences*, *34*(24), 2312–2320. http://doi.org/10.1080/02640414.2016.1232487

Liu, H., Gomez, M.-Á., Gonçalves, B., & Sampaio, J. (2015). Technical performance and match-to-match variation in elite football teams. *Journal of Sports Sciences*, *34*(6), 509–518. http://doi.org/10.1080/02640414.2015.1117121

Lopez-Botella, M., & Palao, J. (2007). Relationship between laterality of foot strike and shot zone on penalty efficacy in specialist penalty takers. *International Journal of Performance Analysis in Sport*, *7*(3), 26–36. http://doi.org/10.1080/24748668.2007.11868407

Mackenzie, R., & Cushion, C. (2012). Performance analysis in football: a critical review and implications for future research. *Journal of Sports Sciences*, *31*(6), 639–676. http://doi.org/10.1080/02640414.2012.746720

Maneiro, R., Casal, C. A., Álvarez, I., Moral, J.E., López, S., Ardá, A., & Losada, J. L. (2019). Offensive transitions in high-performance football: differences between UEFA Euro 2008 and UEFA Euro 2016. *Frontiers in Psychology*, *10*, 1230. http://doi.org/10.3389/fpsyg.2019.01230

Mara, J. K., Wheeler, K. W., & Lyons, K. (2012). Attacking strategies that lead to goal scoring opportunities in high level women's football. *International Journal of Sports Science & Coaching*, *7*(3), 565–577. http://doi.org/10.1260/1747-9541.7.3.565

Maslovat, D., & Franks, I. (2008). The need for feedback. In M. Hughes & I. Franks (Eds.), *The Essentials of Performance Analysis: An Introduction* (pp. 1–7). London, UK: Routledge.

McGarry, T., & Franks, I. M. (2000). On winning the penalty shoot-out in soccer. *Journal of Sports Sciences*, *18*(6), 401–409. https://doi.org/10.1080/02640410050074331

McGarry, T., Anderson, D. I., Wallace, S. A., Hughes, M. D., & Franks, I. M. (2002). Sport competition as a dynamical self-organizing system. *Journal of Sports Sciences*, *20*(10), 771–781. http://doi.org/10.1080/026404102320675620

McGarry, T., O'Donoghue, P., & Sampaio, A. J. (2013). *Routledge Handbook of Sports Performance Analysis*. London: Routledge.

Mclean, S., Salmon, P. M., Gorman, A. D., Stevens, N. J., & Solomon, C. (2018b). A social network analysis of the goal scoring passing networks of the 2016 European Football Championships. *Human Movement Science*, *57*, 400–408. http://doi.org/10.1016/j.humov.2017.10.001

Mclean, S., Salmon, P. M., Gorman, A. D., Wickham, J., Berber, E., & Solomon, C. (2018a). The effect of playing formation on the passing network characteristics of a professional football team. *Human Movement*, *19*(5), 14–22. http://doi.org/10.5114/hm.2018.79416

Memmert, D., Lemmink, K. A. P. M., & Sampaio, J. (2016). Current approaches to tactical performance analyses in soccer using position data. *Sports Medicine*, *47*(1), 1–10. http://doi.org/10.1007/s40279-016-0562-5

Nevill, A. M., Atkinson, G., Hughes, M. D., & Cooper, S.-M. (2002). Statistical methods for analysing discrete and categorical data recorded in performance analysis. *Journal of Sports Sciences*, *20*(10), 829–844. http://doi.org/10.1080/026404102320675666

O'Donoghue, P. (2017). Normative profiles of sports performance. *International Journal of Performance Analysis in Sport*, *5*(1), 104–119. http://doi.org/10.1080/24748668.2005.11868319

Olthof, S. B. H., Frencken, W. G. P., & Lemmink, K. A. P. M. (2018). Match-derived relative pitch area changes the physical and team tactical performance of elite soccer players in small-sided soccer games. *Journal of Sports Sciences*, *36*(14), 1557–1563. http://doi.org/10.1080/02640414.2017.1403412

Paixão, P., Sampaio, J., & Almeida, C. H. (2015). How does match status affects the passing sequences of top-level European soccer teams? *International Journal of Performance Analysis in Sport*, *15*(1), 229–240. https://doi.org/10.1080/24748668.2015.11868789

Partridge, D., Mosher, R. E., & Franks, I. (1993). A computer assisted analysis of technical performance – A comparison of the 1990 world cup and intercollegiate soccer. In T. Reilly, J. Clarys, & A. Stibbe (eds.), *Science and Football II* (pp. 221–231). London: E & FN Spon.

Pollard, R. (2002). Charles reep (1904-2002): pioneer of notational and performance analysis in football. *Journal of Sports Sciences*, *20*(10), 853–855. https://doi.org/10.1080/026404102320675684

Pollard, R., Reep, C., & Hartley, S. (1988). The quantitative comparison of playing styles in soccer. In T. Reilly, A. Lees, K. Davids, & W. J. Murphy (eds.), *Science and Football* (pp. 309–315). London: E & FN Spon.

Pulling, C., Robins, M., & Rixon, T. (2013). Defending corner kicks: analysis from the English premier league. *International Journal of Performance Analysis in Sport*, *13*(1), 135–148. https://doi.org/10.1080/24748668.2013.11868637

Reep, C., & Benjamin, B. (1968). Skill and chance in association football. *Journal of the Royal Statistical Society: Series A (General)*, *131*(4), 581–585. https://doi.org/10.2307/2343726

Reeves, M. J., & Roberts, S. J. (2017). Perceptions of performance analysis in elite youth football. *International Journal of Performance Analysis in Sport*, *13*(1), 200–211. http://doi.org/10.1080/24748668.2013.11868642

Rein, R., & Memmert, D. (2016). Big data and tactical analysis in elite soccer: future challenges and opportunities for sports science. *Springer Plus*, *5*(1), 1–13. http://doi.org/10.1186/s40064-016-3108-2

Ruiz-Ruiz, C., Fradua, L., Fernández-García, Á., & Zubillaga, A. (2013). Analysis of entries into the penalty area as a performance indicator in soccer. *European Journal of Sport Science*, *13*(3), 241–248. http://doi.org/10.1080/17461391.2011.606834

Sarmento, H., Clemente, F. M., Araújo, D., Davids, K., McRobert, A. P., & Figueiredo, A. (2018). What performance analysts need to know about research trends in association football (2012–2016): a systematic review. *Sports Medicine*, *48*(4), 799–836. http://doi.org/10.1007/s40279-017-0836-6

Sarmento, H., Marcelino, R., Anguera, M. T., Campanico, J., Matos, N., & Leitão, J. C. (2014). Match analysis in football: a systematic review. *Journal of Sports Sciences*, *32*(20), 1831–1843. http://doi.org/10.1080/02640414.2014.898852

Siegle, M., & Lames, M. (2012). Game interruptions in elite soccer. *Journal of Sports Sciences*, *30*(7), 619–624. http://doi.org/10.1080/02640414.2012.667877

Strafford, B. W., Smith, A., North, J. S., & Stone, J. A. (2019). Comparative analysis of the top six and bottom six teams' corner kick strategies in the 2015/2016 English premier league. *International Journal of Performance Analysis in Sport*, *19*(6), 904–918. http://doi.org/10.1080/24748668.2019.1677379

Taylor, B. J., Mellalieu, D. S., & James, N. (2005). A comparison of individual and unit tactical behaviour and team strategy in professional soccer. *International Journal of Performance Analysis in Sport*, *5*(2), 87–101. http://doi.org/10.1080/24748668.2005.11868329

Taylor, J. B., Mellalieu, S. D., James, N., & Shearer, D. A. (2008). The influence of match location, quality of opposition, and match status on technical performance in professional association football. *Journal of Sports Sciences*, *26*(9), 885–895. http://doi.org/10.1080/02640410701836887

Tenga, A., & Sigmundstad, E. (2011). Characteristics of goal-scoring possessions in open play: comparing the top, in-between and bottom teams from professional soccer league. *International Journal of Performance Analysis in Sport*, *11*(3), 545–552. http://doi.org/10.1080/24748668.2011.11868572

Tenga, A., Holme, I., Ronglan, L. T., & Bahr, R. (2010a). Effect of playing tactics on achieving score-box possessions in a random series of team possessions from Norwegian professional soccer matches. *Journal of Sports Sciences, 28*(3), 245–255. http://doi.org/10.1080/02640410903502766

Tenga, A., Holme, I., Ronglan, L. T., & Bahr, R. (2010b). Effect of playing tactics on goal scoring in Norwegian professional soccer. *Journal of Sports Sciences, 28*(3), 237–244. http://doi.org/10.1080/02640410903502774

Tenga, A., Ronglan, L. T., & Bahr, R. (2010). Measuring the effectiveness of offensive match-play in professional soccer. *European Journal of Sport Science, 10*(4), 269–277. http://doi.org/10.1080/17461390903515170

Valter, D. S., Adam, C., Barry, M., & Marco, C. (2006). Validation of prozone®: a new video-based performance analysis system. *International Journal of Performance Analysis in Sport, 6*(1), 108–119.

Vogelbein, M., Nopp, S., & Hökelmann, A. (2014). Defensive transition in soccer – are prompt possession regains a measure of success? A quantitative analysis of German Fußball-Bundesliga 2010/2011. *Journal of Sports Sciences, 32*(11), 1076–1083. http://doi.org/10.1080/02640414.2013.879671

Wade, A. (1996). Principles *of Team Play*. Pennsylvania: Reedswain Inc.

Wright, C., Atkins, S., & Jones, B. (2011). An analysis of elite coaches' engagement with performance analysis services (match, notational analysis and technique analysis). *International Journal of Performance Analysis in Sport, 12*(2), 436–451. http://doi.org/10.1080/24748668.2012.11868609

Wright, C., Atkins, S., Jones, B., & Todd, J. (2013). The role of performance analysts within the coaching process: performance analysts survey. *International Journal of Performance Analysis in Sport, 13*(1), 240–261. http://doi.org/10.1080/24748668.2013.11868645

Wright, C., Atkins, S., Polman, R., Jones, B., & Sargeson, L. (2011). Factors associated with goals and goal scoring opportunities in professional soccer. *International Journal of Performance Analysis in Sport, 11*(3), 438–449. https://doi.org/10.1080/24748668.2011.11868563

Yi, Q., Jia, H., Liu, H., & Gomez, M.-Á. (2018). Technical demands of different playing positions in the UEFA champions league. *International Journal of Performance Analysis in Sport, 18*(6), 926–937. http://doi.org/10.1080/24748668.2018.1528524

Yiannakos, A., & Armatas, V. (2006). Evaluation of the goal scoring patterns in European Championship in Portugal 2004. *International Journal of Performance Analysis in Sport, 6*(1), 178–188.

Yue, Z., Broich, H., & Mester, J. (2014). Statistical analysis for the soccer matches of the first Bundesliga. *International Journal of Sports Science & Coaching, 9*(3), 553–560. http://doi.org/10.1260/1747-9541.9.3.553

# 18 Monitoring training

*Barry Drust and Laura Bowen*

## Introduction

Monitoring training is a key aspect of soccer science. It is commonly researched by academics as well as ubiquitously implemented in most sport science support programmes in elite-level clubs. The shared interest provides opportunity for conceptual and pragmatic discussions amongst those interested in providing effective solutions to the challenge of understanding the demands associated with preparation strategies (and performance). In this chapter, we attempt to present content that is indicative of current scientific thinking and contemporary practice. By presenting these diverse viewpoints, we provide a broad perspective on current opinions and the future challenges that may exist in the field.

## The importance of monitoring training

Superior systems and organisational approaches to training have the potential to provide important competitive advantages. As training is a process-effective training requires regulation (Sands et al., 2017). The monitoring of training represents an important feedback tool by which "data" can be collected to determine if individuals are, in general terms, both completing and adapting to the training that is planned by the coach/practitioner (Impellizzeri et al., 2020). Over the last decade, the interest in training monitoring in elite soccer has risen exponentially with monitoring used to support the planning of training at both team and individual levels (Buchheit & Simpson, 2017). This information is, therefore, a key component of both short- and long-term decision-making in relation to both the exercise that players need to be prepared for competition and an understanding of their subsequent response to that exercise (West et al., 2021). As such, the effective monitoring of training load is an important part of the sports science support strategy of most elite teams to both improve performance and reduce injury risk.

## Scientific and conceptual considerations for the monitoring of training

Training monitoring should involve describing both the exercise (what the player does) and response (how the player changes behaviour or perceives the exercise (Impellizzeri et al., 2020; see Figure 18.1). These outcomes are often operationalised as the external and internal load (Brink et al., 2010). The external load is the physical activity prescribed in the training programme (the quality, quantity, and organisation of the

DOI: 10.4324/9781003148418-22

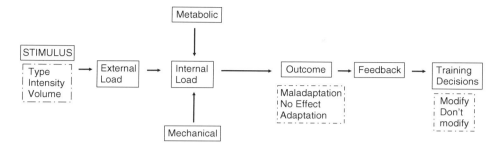

*Figure 18.1* A schematic representation of the role on monitoring training in supporting the training process.

exercises selected) that ultimately induces a specific psychophysiological response (i.e., internal load). Assessing these components allows the practitioner to understand whether the external load has induced the planned acute psychophysiological response (internal load) and whether that load has induced the expected adaptations (indirectly assessed by measuring the training outcome). Impellizzeri et al. (2020) and Gray et al. (2018) have suggested that less is frequently understood about the internal than the external load. This state of play may be a consequence of the increased difficulty in capturing these internal responses compared to the relative ease with which the external load can be captured (West et al., 2021). Traditional approaches to assessing the internal response have focussed on variables that are broadly classified as "metabolic" (e.g., cardiovascular variables, indications of the energy systems used to support the activity). Soccer activities also lead to "mechanical" stresses on tissues in the musculoskeletal system (e.g., cartilage, bone, muscle, and tendon tissue; Vanrenterghem et al., 2017). This mechanical stress is considered important for structural and functional adaptations of the musculoskeletal system (Kjaer, 2004). This mechanical load-adaptation pathway has previously been largely overlooked in approaches to monitoring (Vanrenterghem et al., 2017), but its importance is now recognised. Failure to meet the target internal responses in either system represents a training error that can be used as feedback to modify the training plan (feedback loop) (see Figure 18.1). By applying these processes, the effectiveness of training can be enhanced. These improvements are, however, a direct consequence of the ability of the information to be operationalised by the coach and athlete (Viru & Viru, 2000).

## Important principles for monitoring training

The application of these general concepts and principles to the specific demands of soccer is important. Boullosa et al. (2020) identified several important considerations that are key to monitoring training load in sports such as soccer compared to more individual sports that have traditionally been the focus of research related to training load. Team sports don't require players to maximise their fitness levels as is common in some individual sports that are determined largely by time to completion. The multifactorial nature of performance and the requirements to constantly peak and taper due to the competitive schedule require an approach that is more associated with optimising performance across prolonged timescales than supporting periodic one-off maximal efforts. Training is also a collective activity and is not frequently planned in detail around individual needs. The large number of contextual factors (e.g., playing position) further complicate the relationship between the internal and external load for any individual (Boullosa et al., 2020) compared to more individual athlete-centred approaches. Although the rationale for monitoring training may be similar in soccer to those used with individual athletes, the nuances do combine to necessitate an approach that is specific to the sport.

Attempts to individualise training load monitoring are an important consideration in soccer. Individualising training load monitoring might include tailoring the approach used to collect, analyse, and interpret data based on the type of training completed. For example, different approaches may be important for more gym-based sessions or those associated with the rehabilitation process than those used for field-based training. Individualisation from the perspective of training monitoring approaches for distinct players is also key. Researchers suggest that the response to both an exercise stimulus and to the period immediately following that exercise is highly individual (Becker et al., 2020). This conclusion suggests that relying on group approaches, especially with respect to data analysis and interpretation may be limited due to the loss of specific detail around the data associated with players (Helms et al., 2020; Sands et al., 2017). Such attempts represent a more systematic approach to defining the selection and use of markers of specific stress and adaptation processes of the player in question than adopting more general guidelines (Sands et al., 2017). West et al. (2021) argued that both the internal and external responses may be important to consider at the individual level. The extent to which an individualised approach to training load monitoring can be adopted is probably a function of pragmatics such as cost and time. While it is obvious that it will not be practically possible to employ a strategy that is 100% bespoke, some aspects of individuality are important for an effective protocol.

Individualising training load monitoring may provide the basis for the diversification of monitoring approaches to include methodologies that do not evaluate the players' response to training per se but rather a broader range of factors that relate to issues that have the potential to impact the adaptive process (by influencing either the response to exercise or the that in the acute phase following the completion of exercise; Boullosa et al., 2020). The competitive schedule exposes players to high levels of background stress (e.g., public and media attention) as well as frequent travel to play games (often across international borders and time zones). Such things are in themselves a source of "stress" as they can create an environment for the elite player where important lifestyle factors such as dietary routines and sleep habits are non-conventional. It may, therefore, be important to consider the implementation of approaches that can provide objective information on more general lifestyle factors as experienced by players. Such multi-dimensional approaches could include sleep, nutrition, and general life stress (Pelka et al., 2017). The specific nature of the strategy for these modifiable factors may not be uniform across the season and could change as a function of the specific challenge that may be relevant to the team and/or individual player at a specific point in the preparation/competition cycle.

From a conceptual perspective, an effective strategy to monitor training load need to be flexibly applied and involve multiple methods and outcome variables. Approaches should not be "one size fits all" but rather should be tailored in relation to the context (Impellizzeri et al., 2020) as no single measure captures training load effectively (Maughan et al., 2020; Wiig et al., 2020). Any measurement variable or method may provide useful information if the approach makes logical sense and is well understood

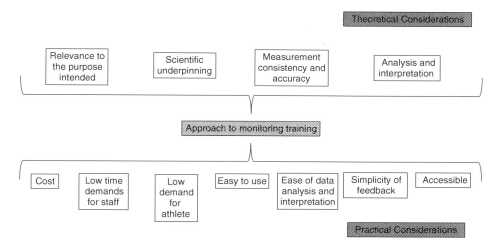

*Figure 18.2* Some theoretical and practical considerations in monitoring training.

by the practitioner (Maughan et al., 2020). This understanding should include a critical appraisal of the reliability, validity, and utility of the data being collected. Depending on resources and context, this may be done through several routes, such as: (i) existing independent validation; (ii) partnering with universities or industry to perform new validation work; or (iii) internal validation work (West et al., 2021).

## Potential approaches for monitoring training

The previous section outlined some of the important conceptual considerations that are important to any training monitoring strategy. This section outlines broad approaches that are commonly used within soccer. While there is typically always a focus on the latest theoretical information in the choice of method used, pragmatics play just as important a part in the strategy (see Figure 18.2).

The specifics of training load monitoring strategies and techniques used in elite soccer are often not publicly available as such information is thought to provide a competitive advantage. This fact makes it difficult to accurately report the exact procedures used by clubs. The widespread availability of practice-based information (professional articles and podcasts) and scientific articles (Akenhead & Nassis, 2016; Weston, 2018) provide some insight into both current industry practices and the usefulness of a given technique for tracking training load (Benson et al., 2020). While a consensus seems to exist on the potential approaches used to collect data, thoughts on their relative effectiveness are a little less coherent. This section briefly describes the methods commonly used as opposed to providing an in-depth critical evaluation of each of these approaches.

### Wearable devices

Wearable devices, particularly those that measure the movement characteristics of players are seen as fundamental for training monitoring. Wearable devices

## 296  *Barry Drust and Laura Bowen*

essentially include sensor(s) and associated firmware to collect the data and software to analyse and store information (Sperlich et al., 2020). Devices may include a single sensor or more commonly multiple sensors such as global positioning or local positioning system and an IMU (which frequently consists of an accelerometer (senses segmental acceleration), a gyroscope (senses angular displacement), and a magnetometer (senses orientation); Willy, 2018). It is important to adhere to recommended guidelines for data collection, processing, and reporting when using wearables (Malone et al., 2017). These include the use of suitable garments in which to wear the device, consistent use of the same unit and quality control procedures for data collection (e.g., number of satellites connected and appropriate horizontal dilution of precision) and analysis (e.g., consistent use of the same manufacturer firmware and threshold bands used for calculation of metrics) (Malone et al., 2020). The use of data from these devices is a major area of research and discussion for scientists and practitioners, respectively (Buchheit & Simpson, 2017) with uncertainty around the most appropriate metrics to use and how information can be most effectively reported back to key stakeholders (i.e., coaches and athletes) (Malone et al., 2020). Current research (Kalkhoven et al., 2020) also continues to critically evaluate the usefulness of data from these systems in reflecting the actual loads experienced by the body's tissues during exercise.

### Evaluating physiological responses

Another popular approach for training monitoring is based on evaluating physiological responses. These internal responses may be assessed within an exercise session (to evaluate the demand associated with the activity) or may be completed post-exercise (to attempt to evaluate the impact that the exercise has had on the individual). Post-exercise responses are typically measured at a variety of time points that could range from immediately post-exercise up to 72 h after the session has finished. Heart rate-related assessments remain a very popular example of this type of approach as the equipment is easily accessible, cheap, and easy to administer.

Measuring concentrations of biomarkers in body fluids (e.g., blood and saliva) represent another popular approach. Pedlar et al. (2019) have suggested that such approaches can be used to assess both the efficacy of training interventions and the capacity to tolerate training load. A wide range of parameters (e.g., creatine kinase, glutamine, and C-reactive proteins) can be typically measured. Such approaches are thought to be effective when they involve frequent measurements and interpretation that is individualised (Becker et al., 2020). Considerations related to sample collection, such as the control of pre-testing conditions (such as the time of day, posture, and fasting/hydration status) and the analysis and storage of samples are important (Pedlar et al., 2019). The development of robust procedures for these types of testing programmes can, therefore, result in significant operational considerations and costs.

Another approach that can broadly be fitted under this category is performance assessments. These approaches are useful as a tool for monitoring training as the performance on a given task broadly reflects the status of the physiological system(s) of an individual following exercise. In some cases, these data may reflect aspects of the psychological state of the individual (e.g., motivation). This may mean that such approaches may give a more holistic indication of the player's status. Common assessments include neuromuscular assessments such as the counter-movement jump or assessment of specific relevant muscle groups (hamstrings, groins, etc.) (Halson, 2014). They may also include sub-maximal running tests (Rago et al., 2020) that incorporate other physiological data, such as heart rate collected during and post-exercise.

## Questionnaires and subjective evaluations

These approaches use scales or short questionnaires to enable the player to provide subjective feedback to coaches/practitioners on either the demands associated with exercise or their specific feelings about the impact of exercise on their physiological status post-exercise. Rating of perceived exertion is probably the most popular approach to subjectively evaluating the physical demands of a training session or a match using a simple scale. This subjective rating is then frequently multiplied by the session duration to provide an indication of the overall training load (Thorpe et al., 2016). Other approaches that are developed to provide more specific information about the demands placed on specific aspects of the body (e.g., muscular, breathlessness, and cognitive) are becoming popular as these have the potential to provide more detailed information on the exact nature of the training demand (Macpherson et al., 2019). Questionnaires are the other subjective tool frequently used to monitor the response to training (e.g., the Hooper scale; Hooper & Mackinnon, 1995). These questionnaires often comprise brief, single-question measurement of an aspect of wellbeing, such as rating of general fatigue on a Likert scale (Duignan et al., 2020). There is evidence for the appropriateness of such approaches in the process of training monitoring (Moalla et al., 2016) (Table 18.1).

## Monitoring training in practice

While there is a plethora of research regarding the approaches and outcomes of training processes, less is known about the implementation of training monitoring within the practice.

Consequently, monitoring is rapidly becoming a minefield. As a sport scientist in the elite game, it is no longer enough to be able to create a few graphs. Top clubs are now recruiting data engineers and programmers to handle the mass of information available. However, translating those pages of numbers and code to something that positively effects on-pitch performance is still the job of practitioners. Therefore, effective implementation of training load monitoring strategies would appear to be important for future research, to inform player support and development, as well as injury prevention.

In soccer, it is very unlikely that the person who decides what information to monitor is also the player being monitored. Quite often, the person making those decisions is also not designing and coaching the practice. Therefore, coach and player buy-in are as important as what information to use. When trusting relationships with staff and players are built, and the value of the information is collectively understood, an effective monitoring environment can be created. The aim of this environment is to inform performance optimisation and injury risk reduction. The only purpose of monitoring is to affect practice. Processes and data sources must be constantly reviewed to ensure that this is the case. In the next section, we cover the application of player monitoring in practice, including streamlining the useful information, creating an effective environment, and most importantly impacting performance.

## 298 Barry Drust and Laura Bowen

*Table 18.1* Potential approaches for training load monitoring including outcome measures

| Approach | Category | Example outcome measure(s) |
|---|---|---|
| Micro-electrical mechanical system (MEMS) devices (e.g., GPS) | Wearable device | • Total distance covered<br>• High-speed running distance/sprint distance<br>• Accelerations/decelerations<br>• Accelerometry-derived load (e.g., playerload) |
| Heart rate | Physiological | • Heart rate during exercise (average, peak, time above a given %)<br>• Heart rate recovery |
| Blood | Physiological | • Blood lactate during/after exercise<br>• Creatine kinase |
| Saliva | Physiological | • IgA<br>• Cortisol |
| Neuromuscular assessments (e.g., counter-movement jump, isometric strength assessment) | Physiological | • Rate of force development<br>• Peak force<br>• Fatigue index<br>• Peak velocity<br>• Impulse |
| Sub-maximal assessments (e.g., sub-maximal running tests) | Physiological | • Peak heart rate<br>• Heart rate at a given time period following exercise |
| Subjective rating scales | Subjective | • RPE<br>• Differential RPE<br>• Muscle soreness<br>• Sleep quality<br>• Fatigue<br>• Recovery |
| Questionnaires | Subjective | • Muscle soreness<br>• Sleep quality<br>• Fatigue<br>• Recovery |

## Streamlining data sources

With the wealth of data now available, practitioners may slip into the trap of thinking "what can we measure?" rather than "what do we need to know?". The first step should be to establish performance questions, specific to the athletes, the club, and the competition. Knowing the answer to the questions should have the potential to affect performance.

The next step should be to identify the tools or measures available to answer the question. These tools should be evidence-based, rather than purely commercially driven. While it may be a cliché, if it seems too good to be true, that usually is the case. A gold standard strategy should include the most accurate equipment, rather than the best packaged. Technological advances are providing evermore detailed information that is of practical value. However, limitations in terms of validity and on-field usefulness are still present and often overlooked (Buchheit & Simpson, 2017). The key measurement principles of validity and reliability, as well as their practical efficacy, should be core foundations upon which choices are based. This fact can be illustrated by the challenges faced when measuring the mechanical loads that exist within applied settings. Most commonly, GPS units with in-built accelerometers are used to quantify these mechanical loads. Yet, existing research has found a lack of precision with which these units measure certain spatio-temporal variables, such as changes in velocity (Roe et al., 2017) or high-speed running (Coutts & Duffield, 2010), as well as other potentially relevant activities such as collisions (Naughton et al., 2020).

Conversely, GPS has been found to be a valid and reliable measure of movement patterns over lower speeds and greater distances (Jennings et al., 2010; Portas et al., 2010). The development of custom algorithms which use the data from integrated 100-Hz accelerometers to improve accuracy (Coutts & Duffield, 2010) alongside technological advancements and greater sampling frequencies have helped to reduce measurement errors at higher velocities. For example, the recent release of 18-Hz units has resulted in a further increase in the validity and reliability of distance measurements and sprint mechanical properties than earlier units with lower sampling rates (Hoppe et al., 2018). Thus, understanding the limitations is vital when determining the best tool for answering a performance question. In the case of GPS, descriptions of basic measurements such as distance and speed during training and match play can be answered with a sufficient level of certainty (Aughey, 2011). However, the quantification of high-velocity movements and changes of direction must be interpreted with varying levels of caution, depending on the device used. Accordingly, GPS does not provide a feasible proxy measure of the mechanical loads experienced by specific tissues. These shortcomings likely contribute to the many inconsistent results associating GPS data with injury (Kalkhoven et al., 2021).

Regardless of the tool, if the validity or reliability is not known, it should not be used. Monitoring can be expensive, and some accuracy may have to be traded off for affordability. Regardless, accuracy still must be tested, to ascertain the error of measurement. Ultimately, if you do not know if it measures what it says it does, you may as well just guess the answer to your performance question. Validity and reliability are not the only factors to consider; soccer is a fast-paced environment; and the information must be analysed and fed back within an effective time frame to impact performance. It is also ever-changing so can the information be collected repeatedly without a detrimental time cost? For example, a counter-movement jump on a force platform can provide a valid and reliable measure of jump performance (Heishman et al., 2020). This testing can be done semi-regularly (e.g., weekly or fortnightly) within a squad gym session, resulting in minimal disturbance to the training schedule. Improvements in jump performance over a season can be determined using a number of evidence-based metrics (e.g., concentric impulse (Ns), jump height (cm), and eccentric peak force (N); Merrigan et al., 2021), and the information can be feedback in real time. However, to use the output measures of a counter-movement jump to indicate neuromuscular fatigue, players would have to be tested multiple times, including a baseline measure and various post-exercises time points (e.g., 0 h, 24 h, 48 h, and 72 h) (Gathercole et al., 2015). How many times a week would a coach allow for a squad to be jump tested, at the sacrifice of time on the pitch? The cost-reward decision of what and how often should always be made in relation to impact on performance. Streamlining information to ensure the optimal impact is a process that requires constant review, reflection, and amendment. The process itself should include three questions. First, and most importantly, will it make a difference to performance? Second, does it accurately measure what it says it does? Third, can the information be used effectively within environmental constraints?

## Building trust and coach buy-in

Sub-optimal integration with coaches has been highlighted as one of the main factors affecting the impact of monitoring in elite soccer (Akenhead & Nassis, 2016). Effective communication, supported by applied research and knowledge, may facilitate the relationship between coach and practitioner, increasing the chances of monitoring being impactful (Ward et al., 2019).

Player buy-in is also vital in ensuring consistency and accuracy of measurement. To enhance compliance, players should have a basic understanding of why they are being monitored and how the information is beneficial. Feedback should be consistent, objective, and individualised where possible. To increase the chance of individual buy-in, a basic understanding of how the player likes to receive information (e.g., verbally and visually) is recommended. Simple psychometric tests, such as the DISC assessment (Marston, 1928) may be used in practical settings to identify personality traits in athletes or coaches which can aid with relationship building. These tests may give an indication of how feedback is best received by the individual, what motivates them, and how they might respond to stress or pressure. This type of information, along with the personal insights of the practitioner about players, may provide a basis for personal communications that can add important additional information about the players' status. These conversations, often dependent on relationships, can provide opportunities for a player to communicate when they feel they can push harder, and when they need thereby providing a useful insight for programming.

Irrespective of the approach used, the purpose of training load monitoring is to influence the training processes completed by the players to impact both the short-term response and the long-term training outcome. To impact this process, the data collected must inform the decisions made by key stakeholders in the management of players. It is important to consider the process by which information use is made effective. One of the major challenges for scientists and coaches who collect training data is to be able to make meaningful inferences on the efficacy of the training processes for players and coaches (Bourdon et al., 2017). Coach and player education, focused mainly on how monitoring will improve performance, provides a platform for effective communication and implementation. Their input on how the information is fed back and used is vital to ensure support. Building relationships should increase the impact of monitoring, only if this relationship consists of mutual trust and understanding. Practitioners should provide clarity on what the information means and how it will be used, highlighting the potential performance benefits, to maximise adherence.

Monitoring should be used to inform decisions, not dictate them. There may be times when information is ignored, as there is an alternative that is considered more beneficial for performance. As elite sporting environments are performance-focused, in those instances, it is the role of the sports science and medical staff to ensure the players are prepared as best as possible for the required demands. Ideally, monitoring tools should not be used to withdraw athletes from sessions part way through. Clarity and trust between coach and practitioner should mean that monitoring can guide the plan prior to execution and provide future recommendations if initial guidelines are not adhered to. Consequently, monitoring solutions must be adaptable and considered a part of the wider picture.

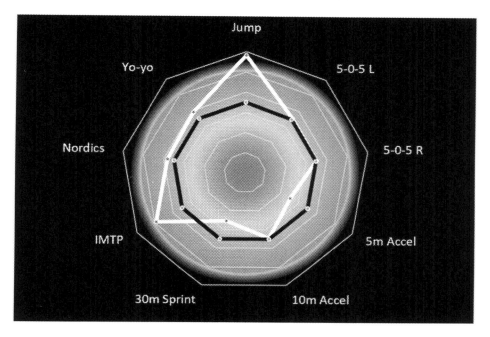

*Figure 18.3* A female player's physical "profile" compared to the squad average. The white line is the player. The black line is the squad average. All testing scores have been converted to z-scores to allow comparison on the same axis.

## Monitoring for performance vs. injury prevention

As well as building relationships with coaches and players, the support staff should have a level of trust between them to provide the best service to the players. Sports scientists will typically prescribe high training loads which are aimed at enhancing performance through physiological adaptation to stress. Conversely, the medical staff advocate lower loads with the aim of reducing the risk of injury (Ekstrand et al., 2019). Both approaches have equal importance in maximising team success, however, the demands must be planned in synergy to be effective (Gabbett & Whiteley, 2017).

Quantification of training allows you to push the boundaries of what the players can achieve, without it being beyond what they can tolerate. The ability to progress training safely is hugely advantageous; players with developed physical qualities can tolerate higher training demands, and exposure to larger amounts of training develops physical qualities (Gabbett et al., 2019). Therefore, not only is it important to monitor training but also to test and monitor the physical qualities of the players. Strength, aerobic capacity, speed, power, and agility are key attributes needed to excel as a player. Baselines should be established and revisited to ensure that the training programmes are effectively developing the players. As mentioned earlier, the tests used to ascertain this must be relevant, accurate, and practical. Some of the field- and gym-based tests regularly used to measure the key physical attributes include whole body or specific muscle strength assessments such as the isometric mid-thigh pull or hamstring strength tests (e.g., Nordbord), tests of aerobic capacity (maximal oxygen consumption or Yo–Yo intermittent recovery test level), sprint and agility tests (e.g., 505 test), and evaluations of horizontal and vertical power such as the counter-movement jump.

These tests can be completed in a day, or individually throughout the pre-season and competitive calendar with very little disruption to the training schedule. Once all the tests are complete, this information can be collated to "profile" the players, identifying their strengths and areas for improvement to help inform training processes. Figure 18.3 shows an example of a female player's results from one testing day. Her results are compared against the squad average to display which attributes she excels at, and which may be improved through a specific training programme.

Testing these attributes also highlights anything that might pre-dispose a player to injury. Injury prevention should not be considered separate from performance, but rather a contributing factor. Researchers have shown that team success is directly related to player availability (Hagglund et al., 2013). Monitoring processes should, therefore, reflect this fact. Choosing tests that can be repeated regularly increases sensitivity to significant changes in results, which may indicate an injury risk. For example, regularly testing limb strength and symmetry during a Nordic hamstring fall allows you to establish individual normative values. From this, you can identify significant changes that may imply hamstring fatigue, or conversely improvements in strength.

## Monitoring in daily practice

The readiness of a player to perform on the pitch is multi-factorial, making it almost impossible to predict. However, collecting relevant and accurate information that span the many factors associated with performance, allows an informed estimate of player readiness. Wellness or self-report questionnaires have proven to be one of the most effective and sensitive monitoring tools (McCall et al., 2016). They provide an internal measure of player readiness and fatigue, with very little cost, and very high applicability across populations. Most often players will be required to answer these questionnaires daily, within an actionable time frame prior to training. Depending on the questionnaire used, the players rate certain variables such as sleep quality, stress, and soreness on a given scale. The literature recommends that these scores are used to detect meaningful change for an individual, rather than allocating an arbitrary "red flag" at a given value (Saw et al., 2016).

Figure 18.4 is an example of a well-being report used daily in a team sport setting to inform player readiness. The colour coding highlights the arbitrary score, whilst icon to the right indicates a significant change from the player's average score for that variable based on the smallest worthwhile change (e.g., if a player scores 5 for soreness, but always scores 5 for soreness, the icon will not appear).

When monitoring female players, it is also important to track the menstrual cycle. Tracking it in a similar way to wellness, to establish individual norms is recommended. While still a relatively new area of research, it is accepted that there is large variation in symptoms at different times in the cycle between people. While is very unlikely that an athlete would have to withdraw from training or competition, some modification or consideration may be required.

The daily training load is most often monitored using GPS. These data are mainly used to provide feedback live and post-session to coaches and players regarding the physical demands of training/match. Most commonly metrics such as total distance, distance at different intensities, accelerations, decelerations, and speed are used to describe physical outputs. More recently, daily GPS data are used to guide training

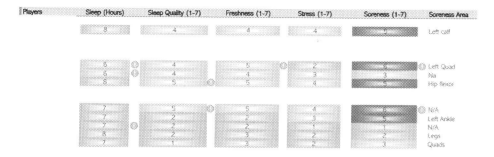

*Figure 18.4* An example well-being report illustrating shading coding and marks to help inform player readiness.

programming and identify potential increases in injury risk through poor programming. GPS is often combined with heart rate monitoring to determine both the external and internal stress on the body. Post-session-rated perceived exertion (RPE) scores are commonly recorded. This requires the players to rate how hard the session felt, usually out of ten. These scores can then be multiplied by the session duration to give an idea of subjective load on the body. The advantage of this monitoring tool is that it is no cost and can be used for any activity. However, scores can be influenced by mood and peers, amongst other factors. Ultimately, there are a multitude of monitoring tools that can be used to understand the factors affecting player readiness to perform. These tools have a much more important role than to provide an objective result on a test. Those results should indicate changes that can be made in practice to promote optimal performance.

## Long-term athlete monitoring

It is rare that a one-off data point can give enough information to properly understand player status. Monitoring of any measure is usually done on a long-term basis to provide a greater understanding of player norms. Long-term monitoring allows you to track progression or improvement, training tolerance, and growth and maturation, as well as enhancing talent identification and benchmarking against other players. Fitness testing is a good example of long-term athlete monitoring. Physical qualities are often tested at the start of pre-season to identify player strengths and weaknesses and to benchmark them against teammates. These tests are then repeated throughout the season, usually every 6–8 weeks, to ascertain progression and, therefore, the effectiveness of training programmes. Repeating these tests can also give an indication of the effects of growth and maturation on physical qualities in youth players.

Long-term training monitoring using GPS is now also widely used. One of the more recent methods of monitoring is known as the acute chronic training load ratio (ACWR). This typically involves the assessment of the absolute 1-week training load (acute training load) relative to 4-week chronic training (4-week average acute training load) (Hulin, Gabbett, Lawson et al., 2016). A training load can then be calculated indicating whether the individual's acute workload is greater, less than or equal to the preceding chronic workload they have been prepared for. If the chronic workload is

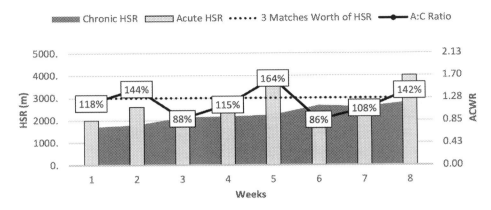

*Figure 18.5* A graphical representation of the progressive increase of a player's chronic high-speed running (training load metric) over the course of 8 weeks. The player begins with a chronic training load of 1,700 m representing a two-match training load and is trained with the goal of progressively increasing his chronic training load to the equivalent of three matches per week. The periodisation model used a three-weekly cycle including a maintenance week with an acute:chronic workload ratio (ACWR) of ~1.0–1.2, an overload week (~1.4–1.7), followed by a de-load (~0.85). Adapted from "Recommendations for hamstring injury prevention in elite football: translating research into practice" (Buckthorpe et al., 2018).

high and the acute workload is low, the player is well-prepared. However, if the acute workload "spikes" beyond the chronic workload, the player is in a state of fatigue which could be both detrimental to performance and increase the risk of injury (Hulin, Gabbett, Caputi et al., 2016). The idea is to fluctuate training to allow both stimulus and recovery, without the current (acute) training being too high, or too low, versus their normal (chronic) training. Over time, the aim is to progressively increase the chronic workload to improve tolerance. However, training at consistently high chronic training demands may result in stress-related injuries (Drew & Finch, 2016) and, therefore, a workload "ceiling" must be set. Below is an example of how the ACWR can be used to plan and monitor training. The players may have two games within a week maximum, interspersed with light training. Thus, the equivalent of three games worth of activity a week was used as the workload ceiling (considered worst-case scenario). In addition to the progressive increases in training, training content was periodised in 3-week blocks (based on (Bowen et al., 2017), involving a de-load week, a maintenance week, and an overload week (Figure 18.5). The ACWR thresholds for each of these weeks were set at ~0.85 for a de-load, ~1.0–1.2 for a moderate week, and ~1.4–1.7 for a high week (Bowen et al., 2020) regardless of the external load metric used. Players who did not regularly play in matches or were returning from injury, were provided with top-up conditioning across the required metrics to maintain sufficient acute and chronic workloads.

## Conclusions and future directions

It is clear from the information presented in this chapter that training load monitoring is now a very important component of any sport strategy used within football.

This is largely the case irrespective of the population of interest (e.g., children, females, and adult males) or level of play (international player, elite players in the highest league or those playing in lower divisions). While there are a range of monitoring strategies available to practitioners they are all primarily focused on evaluating the activities that players complete and the responses of individuals to these external demands. These insights have the potential, when part of an effective decision-making system, to help support the performance of players as well as reduce the potential for injury. While such outcomes have some support within the scientific literature the relative newness of both the available technology and the process of training load monitoring still requires research studies to fully evidence base effective implementation.

As the rewards for successful performances continue to increase there will continue to advance in training monitoring. These developments will likely take many forms and be associated with data collection, data analysis/interpretation, and reporting. It is inevitable that new technologies and approaches will become available, which may facilitate the "invisible monitoring" suggested by West et al. (2021). Advances in data analysis may include better connections across different data streams and provide opportunities to both describe and predict performance outcomes across a variety of key performance metrics. Faster and more detailed data visualisation techniques enable this information to be more efficiently and effectively communicated to players and coaches across multiple platforms. The rapid pace that technology develops makes the exact nature of these developments difficult to predict. It is also unclear if these changes will be a function of the need to better support performance and protect the health of players or be primarily driven by the commercial considerations of the sport and/or a need to continue to impact the spectator experience. It will be important in the future, as it is now, to ensure that any information on training that is provided is useful to support decision-making.

## References

Akenhead, R., & Nassis, G. P. (2016). Training load and player monitoring in high-level football: current practice and perceptions. *Int J Sports Physiol Perform, 11*(5), 587–593. https://doi.org/10.1123/ijspp.2015-0331

Aughey, R. J. (2011). Applications of GPS to field sports. *Int J Sports Physiol Perform, 6*, 295–310.

Becker, M., Sperlich, B., Zinner, C., & Achtzehn, S. (2020). Intra-individual and seasonal variation of selected biomarkers for internal load monitoring in U-19 soccer players. *Front Physiol, 11*, 838. https://doi.org/10.3389/fphys.2020.00838

Benson, L. C., Raisanen, A. M., Volkova, V. G., Pasanen, K., & Emery, C. A. (2020). Workload a-wear-ness: monitoring workload in team sports with wearable technology: a scoping review. *J Orthop Sports Phys Ther, 50*(10), 549–563. https://doi.org/10.2519/jospt.2020.9753

Boullosa, D., Casado, A., Claudino, J. G., Jimenez-Reyes, P., Rave, G., Castano-Zambudio, A., Lima-Alves, A., de Oliveira, S. A., Jr., Dupont, G., Granacher, U., & Zouhal, H. (2020). Do you play or do you train? insights from individual sports for training load and injury risk management in team sports based on individualization. *Front Physiol, 11*, 995. https://doi.org/10.3389/fphys.2020.00995

Bourdon, P. C., Cardinale, M., Murray, A., Gastin, P., Kellmann, M., Varley, M. C., Gabbett, T. J., Coutts, A. J., Burgess, D. J., Gregson, W., & Cable, N. T. (2017). Monitoring athlete training loads: consensus statement. *Int J Sports Physiol Perform, 12*(Suppl 2), S2161–S2170. https://doi.org/10.1123/IJSPP.2017-0208

Bowen, L., Gross, A. S., Gimpel, M., Bruce-Low, S., & Li, F. X. (2020). Spikes in acute:chronic workload ratio (ACWR) associated with a 5–7 times greater injury rate in English premier

## 306 *Barry Drust and Laura Bowen*

league football players: a comprehensive 3-year study. *Br J Sports Med*, *54*(12), 731–738. https://doi.org/10.1136/bjsports-2018-099422

Bowen, L., Gross, A. S., Gimpel, M., & Li, F. X. (2017). Accumulated workloads and the acute:chronic workload ratio relate to injury risk in elite youth football players. *Br J Sports Med*, *51*(5), 452–459. https://doi.org/10.1136/bjsports-2015-095820

Brink, M. S., Nederhof, E., Visscher, C., Schmikli, S. L., & Lemmink, K. A. (2010). Monitoring load, recovery, and performance in young elite soccer players. *J Strength Cond Res*, *24*(3), 597–603. https://doi.org/10.1519/JSC.0b013e3181c4d38b

Buchheit, M., & Simpson, B. M. (2017). Player-tracking technology: half-full or half-empty glass? *Int J Sports Physiol Perform*, *12*(Suppl 2), S235–S241.

Buckthorpe, M., Gimpel, M., Wright, S., Sturdy, T., & Stride, M. (2018). Hamstring muscle injuries in elite football: translating research into practice. *Br J Sports Med*, *52*(10), 628–629. https://doi.org/10.1136/bjsports-2017-097573

Coutts, A. J., & Duffield, R. (2010). Validity and reliability of GPS devices for measuring movement demands of team sports. *J Sci Med Sport*, *13*(1), 133–135. https://doi.org/10.1016/j.jsams.2008.09.015

Drew, M. K., & Finch, C. F. (2016). The relationship between training load and injury, illness and soreness: a systematic and literature review. *Sports Med*, *46*(6), 861–883. https://doi.org/10.1007/s40279-015-0459-8

Duignan, C., Doherty, C., Caulfield, B., & Blake, C. (2020). Single-item self-report measures of team-sport athlete wellbeing and their relationship with training load: a systematic review. *J Athl Train*, *55*(9), 944–953. https://doi.org/10.4085/1062-6050-0528.19

Ekstrand, J., Lundqvist, D., Davison, M., D'Hooghe, M., & Pensgaard, A. M. (2019). Communication quality between the medical team and the head coach/manager is associated with injury burden and player availability in elite football clubs. *Br J Sports Med*, *53*(5), 304–308. https://doi.org/10.1136/bjsports-2018-099411

Gabbett, T. J., Nielsen, R. O., Bertelsen, M. L., Bittencourt, N. F. N., Fonseca, S. T., Malone, S., Moller, M., Oetter, E., Verhagen, E., & Windt, J. (2019). In pursuit of the 'unbreakable' athlete: what is the role of moderating factors and circular causation? *Br J Sports Med*, *53*(7), 394–395. https://doi.org/10.1136/bjsports-2018-099995

Gabbett, T. J., & Whiteley, R. (2017). Two Training-load paradoxes: can we work harder and smarter, can physical preparation and medical be teammates? *Int J Sports Physiol Perform*, *12*(Suppl 2), S250–S254. https://doi.org/10.1123/ijspp.2016-0321

Gathercole, R. J., Sporer, B. C., Stellingwerff, T., & Sleivert, G. G. (2015). Comparison of the capacity of different jump and sprint field tests to detect neuromuscular fatigue. *J Strength Cond Res*, *29*(9), 2522–2531. https://doi.org/10.1519/JSC.0000000000000912

Gray, A. J., Shorter, K., Cummins, C., Murphy, A., & Waldron, M. (2018). Modelling movement energetics using global positioning system devices in contact team sports: limitations and solutions. *Sports Med*, *48*(6), 1357–1368. https://doi.org/10.1007/s40279-018-0899-z

Hagglund, M., Walden, M., Magnusson, H., Kristenson, K., Bengtsson, H., & Ekstrand, J. (2013). Injuries affect team performance negatively in professional football: an 11-year follow-up of the UEFA champions league injury study. *Br J Sports Med*, *47*(12), 738–742. https://doi.org/10.1136/bjsports-2013-092215

Halson, S. L. (2014). Monitoring training load to understand fatigue in athletes. *Sports Med*, *44*(Suppl 2), S139–S147. https://doi.org/10.1007/s40279-014-0253-z

Heishman, A. D., Daub, B. D., Miller, R. M., Freitas, E. D. S., Frantz, B. A., & Bemben, M. G. (2020). Countermovement jump reliability performed with and without an arm swing in NCAA division 1 intercollegiate basketball players. *J Strength Cond Res*, *34*(2), 546–558. https://doi.org/10.1519/JSC.0000000000002812

Helms, E. R., Kwan, K., Sousa, C. A., Cronin, J. B., Storey, A. G., & Zourdos, M. C. (2020). Methods for regulating and monitoring resistance training. *J Hum Kinet*, *74*, 23–42. https://doi.org/10.2478/hukin-2020-0011

Hooper, S. L., & Mackinnon, L. T. (1995). Monitoring overtraining in athletes. Recommendations. *Sports Med*, *20*(5), 321–327. https://doi.org/10.2165/00007256-199520050-00003

Hoppe, M. W., Baumgart, C., Polglaze, T., & Freiwald, J. (2018). Validity and reliability of GPS and LPS for measuring distances covered and sprint mechanical properties in team sports. *PLoS One*, *13*(2), e0192708. https://doi.org/10.1371/journal.pone.0192708

Hulin, B. T., Gabbett, T. J., Caputi, P., Lawson, D. W., & Sampson, J. A. (2016). Low chronic workload and the acute:chronic workload ratio are more predictive of injury than between-match recovery time: a two-season prospective cohort study in elite rugby league players. *Br J Sports Med*, *50*(16), 1008–1012. https://doi.org/10.1136/bjsports-2015-095364

Hulin, B. T., Gabbett, T. J., Lawson, D. W., Caputi, P., & Sampson, J. A. (2016). The acute:chronic workload ratio predicts injury: high chronic workload may decrease injury risk in elite rugby league players. *Br J Sports Med*, *50*(4), 231–236. https://doi.org/10.1136/bjsports-2015-094817

Impellizzeri, F. M., Menaspa, P., Coutts, A. J., Kalkhoven, J., & Menaspa, M. J. (2020). Training load and its role in injury prevention, part i: back to the future. *J Athl Train*, *55*(9), 885–892. https://doi.org/10.4085/1062-6050-500-19

Jennings, D., Cormack, S., Coutts, A. J., Boyd, L., & Aughey, R. J. (2010). The validity and reliability of GPS units for measuring distance in team sport specific running patterns. *Int J Sports Physiol Perform*, *5*(3), 328–341. https://doi.org/10.1123/ijspp.5.3.328

Kalkhoven, J. T., Watsford, M. L., Coutts, A. J., Edwards, W. B., & Impellizzeri, F. M. (2021). Training load and injury: causal pathways and future directions. *Sports Med*, *51*(6),1137–1150. https://doi.org/10.1007/s40279-020-01413-6

Kalkhoven, J. T., Watsford, M. L., & Impellizzeri, F. M. (2020). A conceptual model and detailed framework for stress-related, strain-related, and overuse athletic injury. *J Sci Med Sport*, *23*(8), 726–734. https://doi.org/10.1016/j.jsams.2020.02.002

Kjaer, M. (2004). Role of extracellular matrix in adaptation of tendon and skeletal muscle to mechanical loading. *Physiol Rev*, *84*(2), 649–698. https://doi.org/10.1152/physrev.00031.2003

Macpherson, T. W., McLaren, S. J., Gregson, W., Lolli, L., Drust, B., & Weston, M. (2019). Using differential ratings of perceived exertion to assess agreement between coach and player perceptions of soccer training intensity: an exploratory investigation. *J Sports Sci*, *37*(24), 2783–2788. https://doi.org/10.1080/02640414.2019.1653423

Malone, J. J., Barrett, S., Barnes, C., Twist, C., & Drust, B. (2020). To infinity and beyond: the use of GPS devices within the football codes. *J Sci Med Footb*, *4*(1), 82–84.

Malone, S., Hughes, B., Roe, M., Collins, K., & Buchheit, M. (2017). Monitoring player fitness, fatigue status and running performance during an in-season training camp in elite Gaelic football. *J Sci Med Footb*, *1*(3), 229–236. https://doi.org/10.1080/24733938.2017.1361040

Marston, W. M. (1928). *Emotions of Normal People*. London: Routledge.

Maughan, P., Swinton, P., & MacFarlane, N. (2020). Relationships between training load variables in professional youth football players. *Int J Sports Med*, *42*(7), 624–629. https://doi.org/10.1055/a-1300-2959

McCall, A., Dupont, G., & Ekstrand, J. (2016). Injury prevention strategies, coach compliance and player adherence of 33 of the UEFA elite club injury study teams: a survey of teams' head medical officers. *Br J Sports Med*, *50*(12), 725–730. https://doi.org/10.1136/bjsports-2015-095259

Merrigan, J. J., Tufano, J. J., & Jones, M. T. (2021). Potentiating effects of accentuated eccentric loading are dependent upon relative strength. *J Strength Cond Res*, *35*(5), 1208–1216. https://doi.org/10.1519/JSC.0000000000004010

Moalla, W., Fessi, M. S., Farhat, F., Nouira, S., Wong, D. P., & Dupont, G. (2016). Relationship between daily training load and psychometric status of professional soccer players. *Res Sports Med*, *24*(4), 387–394. https://doi.org/10.1080/15438627.2016.1239579

Naughton, M., Jones, B., Hendricks, S., King, D., Murphy, A., & Cummins, C. (2020). Quantifying the collision dose in rugby league: a systematic review, meta-analysis, and critical analysis. *Sports Med Open*, *6*(1), 6. https://doi.org/10.1186/s40798-019-0233-9

Pedlar, C. R., Newell, J., & Lewis, N. A. (2019). Blood biomarker profiling and monitoring for high-performance physiology and nutrition: current perspectives, limitations and recommendations. *Sports Med*, *49*(Suppl 2), 185–198. https://doi.org/10.1007/s40279-019-01158-x

Pelka, M., Schneider, P., & Kellmann, M. (2017). Development of pre- and post-match morning recovery-stress states during in-season weeks in elite youth football. *Sci Med Footb*, *2*(2), 127–132. https://doi.org/10.1080/24733938.2017.1384560

Portas, M. D., Harley, J. A., Barnes, C. A., & Rush, C. J. (2010). The validity and reliability of 1-Hz and 5-Hz global positioning systems for linear, multidirectional, and soccer-specific activities. *Int J Sports Physiol Perform*, *5*(4), 448–458. https://doi.org/10.1123/ijspp.5.4.448

Rago, V., Krustrup, P., Martin-Acero, R., Rebelo, A., & Mohr, M. (2020). Training load and submaximal heart rate testing throughout a competitive period in a top-level male football team. *J Sports Sci*, *38*(11–12), 1408–1415. https://doi.org/10.1080/02640414.2019.1618534

Roe, G., Darrall-Jones, J., Black, C., Shaw, W., Till, K., & Jones, B. (2017). Validity of 10-HZ GPS and timing gates for assessing maximum velocity in professional rugby union players. *Int J Sports Physiol Perform*, *12*(6), 836–839. https://doi.org/10.1123/ijspp.2016-0256

Sands, W. A., Kavanaugh, A. A., Murray, S. R., McNeal, J. R., & Jemni, M. (2017). Modern techniques and technologies applied to training and performance monitoring. *Int J Sports Physiol Perform*, *12*(Suppl 2), S263–S272. https://doi.org/10.1123/ijspp.2016-0405

Saw, A. E., Main, L. C., & Gastin, P. B. (2016). Monitoring the athlete training response: subjective self-reported measures trump commonly used objective measures: a systematic review. *Br J Sports Med*, *50*(5), 281–291. https://doi.org/10.1136/bjsports-2015-094758

Sperlich, B., Holmberg, H. C., & Aminian, K. (2020). *Wearable Sensor Technology for Monitoring Training Load and Health in the Athletic Population* Swiss: Frontiers. https://doi.org/10.3389/978-2-88963-462-0

Thorpe, R. T., Strudwick, A. J., Buchheit, M., Atkinson, G., Drust, B., & Gregson, W. (2016). Tracking morning fatigue status across in-season training weeks in elite soccer players. *Int J Sports Physiol Perform*, *11*(7), 947–952. https://doi.org/10.1123/ijspp.2015-0490

Vanrenterghem, J., Robinson, M. A., Nedergaard, N. J., & Drust, B. (2017). Training load monitoring in team sports: a novel framework separating physiological and biomechanical load-adaptation pathways. *Sports Med*, *47*(11), 2135–2142.

Viru, A., & Viru, M. (2000). Nature of training effects. In W. E. Garrett & D. T. Kirkendall (Eds.), *Exercise and Sport Science*, Philadelphia: Lippincott Williams & Wilkins (pp. 67–95).

Ward, P., Windt, J., & Kempton, T. (2019). Business intelligence: how sport scientists can support organization decision making in professional sport. *Int J Sports Physiol Perform*, *14*(4), 544–546. https://doi.org/10.1123/ijspp.2018-0903

West, S. W., Clubb, J., Torres-Ronda, L., Howells, D., Leng, E., Vescovi, J. D., Carmody, S., Posthumus, M., Dalen-Lorentsen, T., & Windt, J. (2021). More than a metric: how training load is used in elite sport for athlete management. *Int J Sports Med*, *42*(4), 300–306. https://doi.org/10.1055/a-1268-8791

Weston, M. (2018). Training load monitoring in elite English soccer: a comparison of practices and perceptions between coaches and practitioners. *Sci Med Footb*, *2*(3), 216–224. https://doi.org/10.1080/24733938.2018.1427883

Wiig, H., Andersen, T. E., Luteberget, L. S., & Spencer, M. (2020). Individual response to external training load in elite football players. *Int J Sports Physiol Perform*, *15*(5), 696–704. https://doi.org/10.1123/ijspp.2019-0453

Willy, R. W. (2018). Innovations and pitfalls in the use of wearable devices in the prevention and rehabilitation of running related injuries. *Phys Ther Sport*, *29*, 26–33. https://doi.org/10.1016/j.ptsp.2017.10.003

# 19 Utilising training and match load data

*Patrick Ward and Barry Drust*

## Introduction

To enhance player performance and mitigate injury, sports scientists have tried to understand player-generated data and explore underlying phenomena and hypotheses within the applied setting. These types of investigations have commonly been directed at evaluating the physical profiles of players, monitoring training, understanding periodization, planning, and attempting to quantify the risk of injury. However, despite a large amount of data being collected, there appears to be a disconnect between science and practice. Prior research has indicated that sports scientists often lack "buy-in" from relevant decision-makers when it comes to the application of their findings (Akenhead & Nassis, 2016).

The void between science and practice is likely multi-factorial, however, one potential challenge is the lack of a framework to guide sports scientists within the applied environment (Bartlett & Drust, 2021). Scientists are trained in academia where the approach to data analysis and reporting of findings is a well-documented process. However, in the applied setting, the process of successful knowledge transfer appears less clear. The consumers of information – coaches – are often comprised of, from a scientific perspective, a non-technical audience (Bartlett & Drust, 2021). This issue can be problematic as coaches are the primary decision-makers within sport and any scientific reporting that gets "lost in translation" will lead to a lack of application.

Another potential issue to the successful integration of science into practice is that research within the sport is frequently driven by questions which are interesting to the scientists as opposed to solving a problem that is relevant to the coach (Bishop, 2008). In the applied setting, the coach is the domain expert and primary decision-maker. Therefore, rather than attempting to impart their own scientific agenda or interests on the team, the sports scientist should embrace a role more akin to that found in the business intelligence setting (Ward et al., 2019). The sports scientist should begin by understanding the problems and questions that are *relevant* to the coach. From there, an infrastructure is created for data collection, cleaning, analysis, and reporting of findings that helps to engage the coach in the scientific process. This type of engagement can encourage an appreciation for the research process and hopefully lead to greater application of the findings (Hendricks, 2021).

Technological advances have made player-generated data common place in professional sports. In a survey of 41 elite professional soccer clubs, Akenhead and Nassis (2016) found that all teams are collecting data such as Global Positioning System (GPS), Rating of Perceived Exertion (RPE), and Heart Rate (HR) daily (Akenhead &

DOI: 10.4324/9781003148418-23

## 310  Patrick Ward and Barry Drust

Nassis, 2016). The collection of such data is often directed at specific goals including profiling players (e.g., strength, speed, and fitness) or monitoring training loads to help plan training sessions or identify injury risks. While the analysis of such data is warranted, it is important to consider what the findings might mean to a coach and the players, opening dialogue with them and trying to understand how such information would help in daily practice. Key questions are: (i) How will this information be used in decision-making? and (ii) How should the information be reported to be impactful and meaningful to cause action?

Once the answer to these questions has been articulated, a clear plan for the project lifecycle can be constructed. This plan can direct how the sports scientist will identify the appropriate data, conduct analysis, and communicate their findings in a concise and interpretable manner. Unfortunately, collecting large amounts of data alone does not equate to success in sports. Success comes from the integration of science into practice and the operationalization of findings in a way that allows the coach to access relevant insights that help them make better decisions (Alamar, 2013). To this point, the focus of this chapter is to help applied sports scientists develop a data reporting framework for enhancing "buy-in" with coaches and decision-makers and ultimately improving their contribution to the sports organisation. Although this chapter provides a framework for assessing training and matching physical load, it is also applicable to other areas of sports science, such as performance analysis or psychology.

## Problem, plan, data, analysis, and conclusion cycle (PPDAC)

Applied Sport Science Frameworks have previously been proposed providing suggestions on exploring scientific questions in sport (Bishop, 2008), working in the fast and slow environment of pro-sport to generate insights (Coutts, 2016), creating an underpinning business intelligence role for sports scientists (Ward et al., 2019), and methods of transferring knowledge to decision-makers (Bartlett & Drust, 2021). While each of these frameworks offers a different view as to how sports scientists can operate within a team sport, they only deal with single components within the applied setting. In the team sport environment, the sports scientist is required to perform all these tasks in a succinct manner while allowing the primary decision-makers to participate in the process. In this way, the sports scientists can offer substantial value by overseeing the project lifecycle from generating the problem statement through a method of sharing results.

A formalized, end-to-end approach for answering research questions has been conceptualized within the curriculum called the Problem, Plan, Data, Analysis, and Conclusion (PPDAC) cycle (Wild & Pfannkuch, 1999; MacKay & Oldford 2000). As seen in Figure 19.1, each step of the PPDAC cycle builds on the information gained from the subsequent step, ensuring that the project progresses in a logical order. This type of framework adds value by clearly defining the process, allowing for real-time communication with the decision-maker and, if necessary, iterating the process as additional information or objectives becomes available. The framework helps to set expectations about the project timeline as non-technical audiences may underestimate or be unaware of the length of time it takes for data acquisition, data cleaning, analysis, and model validation before arriving at a conclusion worthy of dissemination.

*Utilising training and match load data* 311

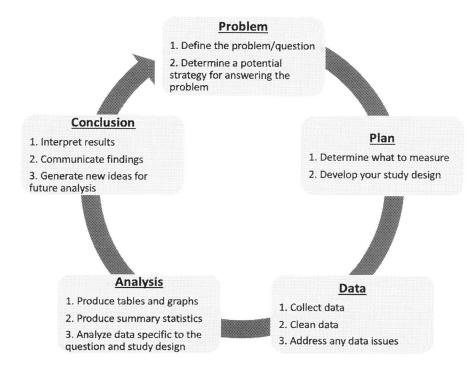

*Figure 19.1* The Problem, Plan, Data, Analysis, and Conclusion (PPDAC) cycle.

## *Problem and plan phases*

Identifying problems to solve and establishing relevant questions should be done in conjunction with the primary decision-makers (e.g., sports coaches, fitness coaches, and medical professionals) to ensure that the analysis and presentation of findings are directed towards issues that are meaningful. Allowing domain experts to participate in shaping the research question can also make communicating results easier, as they feel as if they have been part of the process and had a contributory role in planning the project. This type of back and forth, between the sports scientist and decision-maker, is essential in the Problem and Planning phases of the project lifecycle as decision-makers may not always be adept at asking questions in a clear and formal manner. Obtaining clarity about the question being investigated ensures that time is not wasted collecting meaningless data, which can be burdensome for the players and coaches, or spending time performing analysis that is not specific to the question (i.e., failing to answer the correct question). The sports scientist should feel they can comfortably *question the questions* of the decision-maker. This dialogue helps to refine the question to a point where the results of the ensuing analysis are incorporated into the decision-making process as the decision-maker has been forced to think deeply about that which they are asking and how they might use such information going forward.

Along with defining the question or problem statement, the way in which the question is being asked is an important consideration. Understanding the type of question being posed is necessary to help direct the analysis required to meet the intended goal. For example, there is a distinction between descriptive, explanatory, and predictive questions and the corresponding analyses designed to explore them (Shumeli, 2010). Shumeli (2010) differentiates between the three by defining descriptive analysis as that which summarizes data without having an explicit causal theory underpinning their interpretation. In comparison, the explanatory analysis seeks to test causal hypotheses and explain reasons for outcomes, whereas predictive analysis is directed towards developing statistical models to predict future outcomes. Discussing these differences with the decision-maker during the planning phase of the project lifecycle helps to direct the project towards an analysis that is specific to how they will be using the results in practice. For example, the question: "How have the physical abilities of centre backs changed over the past 10 years?" requires a different type of analysis compared to the question: "Has the pace of the game changed over the past 10 years, requiring centre backs to perform more high-speed distance?". These in turn differ to: "Given the athletic qualities and previous performance of this centre back, what would we forecast his next 4 years to look like if we were to acquire him?". The first question is purely descriptive and lacks any explicit causal mechanism, simply summarizing changes within a positional group over time. The second is more explanatory, where there is a potential causal hypothesis to be tested (What game changes have led to different ergonomic demands in the position?). The final question is more predictive in nature, attempting to forecast the future ability of a player, ultimately aiding the decision-makers with determining if the valuation of the player is worth the current market price of acquiring him.

To illustrate these concepts, a soccer coach may initially want to know the fitness level of their players when starting training camp. Rather than simply conducting a Yo–Yo fitness test and reporting the amount of distance covered and HR response for each player, the sports scientist might ask the coach if they have considered how they would like to apply the findings generated from the test. After some thought, the coach might state they would like to use the information to not only identify those players who require extra conditioning, but to decide upon the style of play the coach would like to employ this season with these players, such as high pressing when out of possession requiring frequent high-intensity running and sprinting. Following this discussion, the sports scientist might perform a separate analysis on data of teams in the league who played a similar style in prior seasons, attempting to understand the physical requirements of those players within that type of system. Such information allows for deeper conversations with the coach regarding the findings from the fitness tests and additional analysis, which can then help to shape discussions around training and match planning.

### Data phase

Once the Problem and Planning phases of the project lifecycle have been agreed upon, identifying data sources that are suitable to answer the question is the next step. When acquiring such data, the sports scientist needs to ensure that it is clean and free from error. This step is important as data in the applied environment can often be "noisy", leading to false signals and wrong conclusions, and causing decision-makers to lose trust in the system. The increased interest in player-generated data in professional sports has given rise to a substantial number of technology providers. Unfortunately, just because something can be measured, does not mean that it is valuable and not all available technology offers the same level of fidelity when it comes to the data provided. Returning to our example of the soccer coach attempting to set their team's style of play, the sports scientist should not only ensure that the pre-season tests are valid and reliable but also that the data are being collected in a standardized manner by the staff. Additionally, analysis performed on previous seasons of league-wide tracking data should be appropriately cleaned and pre-processed so that any insights gleaned from the analysis are accurate.

## Validity

Valid tests or valid data are those that represent the construct that they purport to measure (Thomas et al., 2015). There are a few forms of validity that sports scientist should be aware of, some of which are reviewed in Table 19.1. In the applied sport setting, measures of criterion validity (concurrent or predictive validity), are highly applicable as they evaluate the relationship between the test and some form of criterion measure.

## Reliability

A measurement with good reliability is one that exhibits a high level of repeatability when the activity is performed multiple times. Reliability is essential in applied sports given that a measure cannot be valid if it is not reliable (Thomas et al., 2015). For the sports science practitioner, establishing the reliability of physical tests that will be performed throughout the season is essential. A test that is not repeatable and consists of high variability or "noise" will have little utility when making decisions in practice, as the *signal* for what is being measured will be difficult to identify.

For example, determining the reliability of the Yo–Yo intermittent fitness test and calculating its typical error of measurement (TEM) is the first step in evaluating how useful the test will be in practice. The TEM can be quantified as the standard deviation of the

*Table 19.1* Some examples of different forms of validity that a sport scientist might encounter in the applied environment (Thomas, Nelson, Silverman, 2015)

| Validity type | Definition | Example |
| --- | --- | --- |
| Logical/face validity | Face validity is validity that visually appears to measure the performance it reports. | A 30-m sprint test has face validity for measuring player speed as the coaches and players can clearly see that players are running as fast as possible. |
| Construct validity | Construct validity describes the way in which a test measures an underlying construct. | Construct validity for session-RPE is defined by how well it measures the psycho-biological state of players following exercise. |
| Concurrent validity | Concurrent validity defines the correlation between the test and a criterion measure, often a gold standard measurement. | Player-worn GPS units have been shown to have concurrent validity when compared to laser timing (the criterion measure). |
| Predictive validity | Predictive validity refers to the ability of certain variables to be able to predict some form of criterion measure. | Predictive validity of the Yo–Yo intermittent fitness test could be established by evaluating whether the player's results from the test, in some way, predict match physical output (the criterion of interest). |

## 314  *Patrick Ward and Barry Drust*

*Table 19.2* Example of calculating typical error measurement and minimal difference for a test-retest trial

| Player | Test score 1 | Test score 2 | Difference |
|--------|--------------|--------------|------------|
| A | 1,045 | 1,073 | 28 |
| B | 991 | 973 | −18 |
| C | 1,062 | 1,084 | 22 |
| D | 1,075 | 1,109 | −66 |
| E | 1,064 | 1,145 | 81 |
| F | 1,083 | 1,101 | 18 |
| G | 1,107 | 1,069 | −38 |
| | | Standard deviation of difference (SD) | 48.6 |
| | | TEM = SD$^2$ | 34.3 |
| | | Minimal Difference (MD) = TEM × 1.96$^2$ | 95.2 |

difference scores divided by the square root of two (Table 19.2) (Hopkins, 2000; Weir, 2005). Using the Yo–Yo IR2 test as an example, the off-season period would be a good time to evaluate its test-retest reliability. To perform this analysis, the players would run the Yo–Yo IR2 test once and then wait 1–2 weeks and run it again. It is important to ensure that the players are in similar physical states when performing the test (e.g., performing both tests on Monday morning following a weekend off from training). Assessing reliability under these more stable environments is important as the goal is to attempt to remove as much noise from the test as possible. If the Yo–Yo IR2 test displays a large error in this controlled testing environment it might be difficult to extract meaningful information from the test in the setting in which it is being applied, such as when using the test multiple times during the season to evaluate whether player fitness is improving.

Quantifying validity and reliability not only verifies the quality of the data being collected but also offers the ability to identify meaningful signals in measured outcomes, called the minimum difference (MD). Briefly, the MD is the smallest difference that would need to be observed to be deemed important or relevant from a practical standpoint (Weir, 2005). Using the TEM from the reliability analysis, the minimum difference can be calculated as: MD = TEM× 1.96$^2$. The multiplier, 1.96, is a critical $z$-score specific to the 95% confidence level; however, the practitioner could adjust this value if a different level of confidence were desired. For example, a multiplier of 1.65 is used to represent a 90% confidence level, whereas a multiplier of 2.58 would correspond to a 99% confidence level.

An example of calculating the TEM and MD in a test-retest trial can be seen in Table 19.2. The test has a typical error of 34.3 m and an MD of 95.3 m. The MD indicates that an improvement of at least 95.3 m would need to be observed for the practitioner to be confident at the 95% level as this shows a real change has occurred in the test score because a change of this magnitude incorporates the test measurement error.

Once the data sources have been assessed for validity and reliability, and the quality of the data has been assured, data analysis and communication of findings are the final two steps of the project lifecycle.

### *Data analysis*

Data analysis can range from basic to advanced statistical modelling, depending on the complexity of the question being asked and the structure of data available. Statistics and data science are fields unto themselves, and sports teams often employ analytics staff to handle projects requiring more advanced data skill sets. However, applied sports scientists working in the fast, day-to-day environment of professional sports should be familiar with basic statistical analysis. A *fast* approach to sports science is dependent on quickly producing simple, often descriptive, analysis that the coaches can query, learn from, and integrate immediately into the weekly training structure (Coutts, 2016). For example, once the soccer team begins playing matches with their new style, a post-game report can be generated that quickly provides the coach with details about the high-speed running volume performed by each player during the game. Such information can be used to shape the upcoming weekly training plan.

Summarizing data is often a first step in exploring the underlying characteristics of the data; however, such summary analysis can often answer questions that are relevant to the decision-makers and provide information to foster new questions or hypotheses. This is particularly so when the question being asked is deceptive in nature. The two most common descriptions of data are measures of *central tendency* and measures of *spread*.

### Central tendency

Measures of central tendency are statistics that serve to describe an entire dataset using a single parameter, the middle or centre, value of the data. Two of the more commonly used measures of central tendency are the *mean* and *median*. These measures are valuable for identifying the most likely value within the data and for comparing changes in an individual or group. The mean is simply the arithmetic average and is the most frequently used measure of central tendency when describing a dataset. The mean is calculated by summing all the observations and dividing by the total number of observations in the sample. In Example 19.1, the distance completed for five players during training is summed together and then divided by the number of observations ($N = 5$ players) to obtain a group average of 11,297 m. Because the mean uses the entire dataset, one of its main limitations is that it can be sensitive to outliers because it can be pulled towards those values which are substantially higher or lower than the main concentration of the data.

| Athlete | Score |
|:---:|:---:|
| A | 11618 |
| B | 9763 |
| C | 12042 |
| D | 11291 |
| E | 11771 |
| N = | 5 |
| Sum of Scores = | 56485 |
| Average = | 11297 |

*Example 19.1* The mean is calculated as the sum of all scores divided by the number of samples.

316   *Patrick Ward and Barry Drust*

| Athlete | Score |
|:---:|:---:|
| C | 12042 |
| E | 11771 |
| **A** | **11618** |
| D | 11291 |
| B | 9763 |

*Example 19.2* The median represents the centre value of the data, whereby 50% of the data is above it and 50% of the data is below it.

Conversely, the median value is the middle of the observations and represents the 50th percentile, where 50% of the data reside below and 50% of the data reside above this value. Calculating the median is done by ranking the observations from highest to lowest and identifying the middle value. In Example 19.2, once the data from Example 19.1 are organized in ascending order, the median is identified as 11,618 m (Player A), as this score is directly in the middle of the five observations. Because the median only identifies the middle and does not consider other values within the data it is less sensitive to outlier observations than the mean. When the data are normally distributed the mean and the median will be nearly identical.

*Spread*

Measures of spread are used to represent the amount of variability within the dataset. Measures of variance are frequently used to complement the single parameter measures of central tendency to provide a more complete representation of the data. The four most common measures of spread are the variance, standard deviation, range, and interquartile range. The first two are usually associated with the mean of the data, whereas the latter two are often reported alongside the median.

Variance is used to describe the distance or deviation of each point relative to the mean. The variance is calculated as the average of squared difference of each observation to the mean, as seen in Example 19.3. Because the differences are squared, the variance is not on the same scale as the original data and is thus not directly interpretable. As such, taking the square root of the variance produces the standard deviation, which is now on the scale of the raw data and easier to understand. The data in Example 19.3 can be reported with a mean ± standard deviation of 11,297 ± 899.4 m. Another way to report the standard deviation is to reflect it as a percentage, termed the coefficient of variation, which is 8.0% for this dataset. To calculate the coefficient of variation, divide the standard deviation by the mean and multiply that result by 100, allowing the variability in data to be reported on a percentage scale (Example 19.3).

Unlike the variance, which looks at the relationship of each value to the mean, the range simply reports the smallest and largest values observed within the data. In this way, the range is a very crude measure of variability. Alternatively, the interquartile range (IQR) is used to provide a range of the largest concentration of the data. The lower bound of IQR represents the 25th quartile, whereas the 75th quartile represents the upper bound of the IQR. The middle of the IQR is the median value (50th

| Athlete | Score | Diff = Score - Avg | Diff² |
|---|---|---|---|
| A | 11618 | 321 | 103041.0 |
| B | 9763 | -1534 | 2353156.0 |
| C | 12042 | 745 | 555025.0 |
| D | 11291 | -6 | 36.0 |
| E | 11771 | 474 | 224676.0 |
| N = | 5 | Variance = | 808983.5 |
| Sum of Scores = | 56485 | Standard Deviation = | 899.4 |
| Average = | 11297 | Coefficient of Variation% = | 8.0% |

*Example 19.3* Calculation of variance, standard deviation, and coefficient of variation.

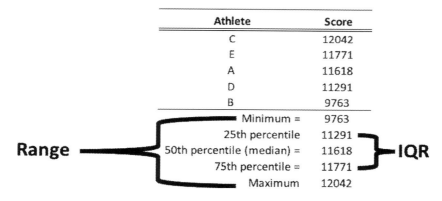

*Example 19.4* The range and interquartile range (IQR) for describing the spread of data.

percentile). Collectively, the IQR represents the inner 50% of the data and is, therefore, less sensitive to outliers. Both the range and IQR of the above data can be seen in Example 19.4.

*Normal distribution*

The shape of the data distribution can explain much about its underlying features and help to put the above summary statistics into a better context. One of the more frequently observed data distributions is that of the normal or bell-shaped distribution. Understanding the properties of the normal distribution provides an appreciation for the role the standard deviation plays in explaining how individual data points relate to the population. Additionally, these properties can be used to calculate further descriptive statistics that can be of value when visualizing and reporting data. The normal distribution is represented by a single, central peak and data evenly distributed around that peak with little or no bias in one direction or the other. Figure 19.1 shows a normal distribution of the data from the total running distance in training for a soccer team. Most of the scores are concentrated in the middle of the distribution, around the mean

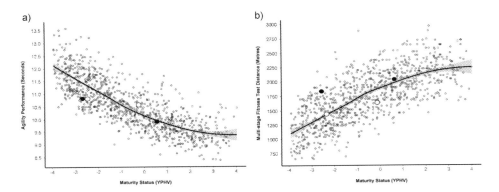

*Figure 19.2* The normal distribution represented as a density plot and a box plot.

(1,016.2 m), represented by the red dashed line. Notice that there is less density of data as the distribution moves further away from the centre (mean). Because the standard deviation considers the relationship of each data point to the mean, 68% of the data reside ±1 standard deviation around the mean, 95% around ±2 standard deviations from the mean, and 99.7% around ±3 standard deviations from the mean. Given these properties of the normal distribution, it is easy to see why values larger than two or three standard deviations are less frequent.

The bottom plot of Figure 19.2 visualizes the same data using a box plot, a common visual used to accompany the median and IQR. The data in this example were simulated to be normally distributed, and therefore, the median value is nearly identical to the mean of the distribution, as both values are right around a score of 1,016 m. Visually this is seen by the black line in the middle of the box, the median value (50th percentile) being directly in line with the red dashed line (mean) in the density plot above it. The IQR, representing the data between the 25th and 75th percentiles, make up the entire area of the box with points outside of the IQR being represented as the "whiskers" of the boxplot.

In addition to describing the properties of data, measures of central tendency and spread can be utilized to convert the raw data into standardized scores. In this way, data that are measured on different scales can now be compared equally. For example, match total distance is substantially larger than match high-speed running distances, making it challenging to interpret these measurements, together, in their raw form and determine how different the player is in both metrics relative to the group. However, on a standardized scale, each data point is reflected relative to the central tendency and variability of the sample data, allowing for a more direct comparison and easier interpretation. Three common standardized scores use to report data in sport science are percentile rank, $z$-scores, and $t$-scores.

*Percentile rank*

Percentile rank reports the data on a percentage scale (0–100%) where 50% represents the measure of central tendency. The percentile rank represents the amount of data in the population that is below the given score for the individual player. For example,

*Utilising training and match load data* 319

*Table 19.3* An example of transforming raw scores into percentile rank, *z*-score, and *t*-scores

| Athlete | Score | Percentile rank | Z-score | T-score |
|---------|-------|-----------------|---------|---------|
| A | 11,618 | 0.64 | 0.4 | 53.6 |
| B | 9,763 | 0.04 | –1.7 | 32.9 |
| C | 12,042 | 0.80 | 0.8 | 58.3 |
| D | 11,291 | 0.50 | 0.0 | 49.9 |
| E | 11,771 | 0.70 | 0.5 | 55.3 |

a soccer player who is reported to be in the 80th percentile for match-day high-speed running has performed more high-speed running than 80% of the population of soccer players they are being compared to. To calculate the percentile rank for Player B in the data above (Table 19.2), first sort the scores from highest to lowest. Count the number of scores below the score of interest. In this case, only one player (Player D) scored below Player B. Divide the number of scores below the score of interest by the total number of observations in the dataset to determine the percentile rank for that individual (1/5 = 20%). The percentile rank for each player's score is shown in Table 19.3.

## Z-scores and t-scores

Z-scores are standardized scores where zero represents the mean and values above or below zero represent the distance from the mean in standard deviation units. To convert raw scores to *z*-scores, subtract the observed value from the average of the group and then divide it by the standard deviation of test scores. An example of how *z*-scores reflect the raw data can be seen in Table 19.3. Because the data is in standard deviation units, observation for Player B (*z*-score = –1.7), is interpreted to be 1.7 standard deviations below the group mean.

While *z*-scores are common in science, they might not always resonate well with coaches who have limited statistical knowledge. A way to make the z-score more palatable is to convert them into a *t*-score. Like a *z*-score, a *t*-score represents the raw data in standard deviation units but does so on a 0–100-point scale where 50 represents average with each 10-point increment representing a one standard deviation change. For example, 40 and 60 represent one standard deviation below and above the mean, respectively. The relationship between *t*-scores and *z*-scores can be seen in column 3 of Table 19.3. Here, we notice that Player B's –1.7 *z*-score is converted into a *t*-score of 32.9.

Although data analysis and statistical modelling can be complicated, often requiring sophisticated approaches to handle various interactions and relationships, understanding the properties of the normal distribution, and calculating descriptive statistics can be useful for the applied sport scientist. Moreover, converting the raw data into standardized scores can aid decision-makers in comparing metrics that are on different scales. Collectively, these basic approaches offer tremendous value when reported in a clear way that is specific to the question posed.

## *Reporting findings*

Unlike the academic environment, where the study findings are often communicated in the form of a peer-reviewed publication, reporting conclusions in the applied setting

320 *Patrick Ward and Barry Drust*

needs to occur within appropriate time frames, depending on the nature of the information and when it is required for decision-making. The soccer environment moves at a fast pace, as coaches who are preparing players for weekly competitions require information to be delivered in a timely manner so that decisions can be made for planning the training process. Three of the most important time frames that the applied sport scientist should be aware of are: (1) baseline; (2) weekly; and (3) monthly reporting.

1  **Baseline testing:** At the start of a training camp or the pre-season, data are collected to establish a baseline for players in various physical measurements, compare players to each other or to some established norm, and to help with planning the first phase of training and designing programs that are directed at improving any identified limitations.
2  **Weekly testing:** Weekly testing is conducted to assess the ways in which players might vary from one week to the next to mitigate any unwanted trends that could predispose them to illness, injury, or poor performance. Examples of such testing include counter-movement jumps to evaluate neuromuscular output, isometric muscle testing to expose any declines in strength or reporting of pain during maximal contraction, and salivary measures, to identify any negative endocrine changes.
3  **Daily (serial) testing:** Daily testing is the most frequent representation of player training demands. Data collected daily provides practitioners with an immediate glimpse into how the player performs each session. The type of training load-specific measurements that occur in daily testing have often been dichotomized into external and internal loads. External load reflects the actual demands of the session, quantified with variables such as distance, speed, high-speed running, or accelerations, whereas internal load represents the psychological or physiological response of players to the session, as quantified by measures such as HR, training impulse (TRIMP) scores, and session-rating of perceived exertion (Halson, 2014).

Presenting data across these time frames requires an understanding of how to convey that which is meaningful. As such, reporting study findings should aid the reader in deciphering the message and be void of superfluous information. The goal should be to make it easy for those reading the report to orient themselves to the key takeaway messages, ensuring that the data can complement future decisions.

One way to direct reader attention to the results of an analysis without using confusing technical words or scientific jargon is through data visualisation. Common types of data visualisation can be seen in Figure 19.3. Each of these approaches conveys data in a different way, specific to the message that needs to be communicated. The selection of one approach over another depends on the type of data and the underlying question. Often, the type of question being answered in an analysis is specific to the data collection time frames discussed above. For example, weekly testing data would be visualized in some form of comparison from 1 week to the next or from the current week to baseline, whereas serial measurement data would be visualized as a time series in which shifts and trends of data can be seen across the season.

Plots A and B in Figure 19.3 are two methods of displaying the distribution of data, as discussed in a previous section. Plot A represents the density of match-day running volumes for a professional soccer club. The distribution here can be described as

*Utilising training and match load data*  321

bimodal (having two modes, or peaks), with most players performing around 11,000 m per match and a handful of players having less locomotor activity (just under 5,000 m), most likely due to less playing time or injury during the match. Boxplots are an alternative way to show the distribution of data and are particularly useful when trying to compare distributions across different groups. The actual observations can be overlayed, in the form of dots, to convey the sample size and more directly show the density of data within the IQR. In Plot B, we can see that across the training weeks, the median running distance is similar on Game Day –3 and Game Day –2, however, Game Day –2 has more variance around the mean. Game Day –1 is clearly lower than the other two training days, as it is closest to match day. Additionally, the reader can observe that Game Day –2 and Game Day –1 have much larger sample sizes compared to Game Day –3.

When attempting to convey the relationship between two continuous variables data can be visualized using a xy-plot, as in Plot C. A linear relationship between training duration and total distance run can easily be observed. The regression line allows the reader to decipher this relationship more clearly. The upward slope indicates a positive correlation between the two variables, whereby as training time increases so does total running distance. A regression model can underpin this type of plot, allowing the decision-maker to input expected values for the training duration of upcoming sessions and obtain a forecasted amount of total running distance, which can aid with planning future training sessions. Such an approach represents a simple example of predictive modelling that an applied sport scientist may be asked to develop. For example, a regression model could be developed to create a training load calculator to assist the coach in planning training. Using various features from historically collected data, such as the training drills being prescribed for the upcoming session and the expected duration for each drill, the sports scientist can build a model that estimates the expected training load for the upcoming training session. A discussion with the coach about whether that expected load is appropriate for the players may transpire, leading to adjustments to the training session.

Baseline testing data that aims to compare a player to the rest of the team or to some physical standard is often visualized in a manner where player test scores are standardized for the purpose of displaying all measurable data points on the same scale, as discussed in the prior section. Plots D, E, and F show three ways of reporting the same standardized data. Plots D and E as *z*-score plots radar and bar chart formats, respectively, and Plot F as a *t*-score. The straight line in the two bar charts and the inner circle of the radar plot represent the population average while the bar charts provide additional context by using a grey-shaded region to show one standard deviation above and below the average. This type of data visualization allows staff to quickly identify the areas where each player is outside of normal. Because the data are scaled, all variables can be represented on the same chart, enhancing communication between staff members about player performance in a variety of physical qualities.

Reporting serial measurements and corresponding changes in players over the course of a season is common in sport science. To provide context around time series data of this nature, for example, comparing a player to their baseline or comparing a player in a week-to-week test, the changes should be reflected relative to the change in the measurement along with its corresponding typical error measurement and the MD for a real change. For example, the weekly percentage change in high-speed running distance during training is visualized in Figure 19.3. Plot A provides a single overview

322 *Patrick Ward and Barry Drust*

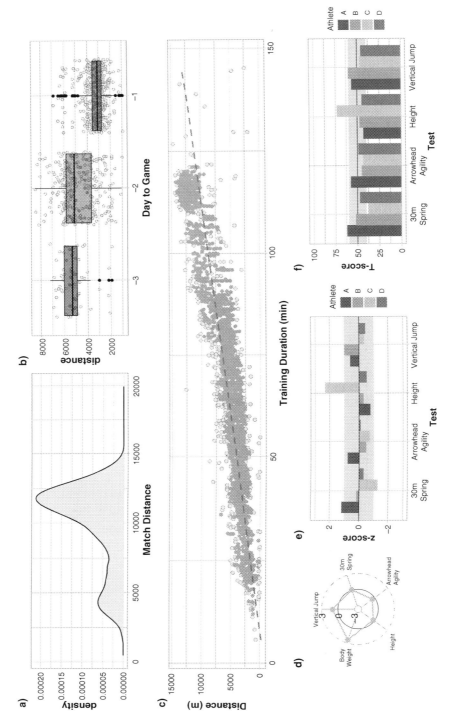

*Figure 19.3* Some examples of common data visualization approaches.

*Utilising training and match load data* 323

of each player relative to the TEM and MD. The point represents the observed percentage change for the player from one week to the next and the error bars indicate the typical error measurement of weekly high-speed running. The shaded region represents the minimal difference, above and below no change (zero difference) compared to the individual player baseline scores. The players exhibiting a change outside of the shaded MD region are of interest in the report. The certainty that the change is real can be further investigated by evaluating the error bars (TEM) around the observed change and how far they are outside of the MD region. This plot allows the staff to quickly identify those players that display weekly changes that are outside of normal, aiding discussions about planning training for those individuals in the upcoming training week.

Aside from looking at a single value of weekly change for the team, Plot B of Figure 19.4 provides a method of visualizing data for an individual player over time. The visual representation of the data is like that of the team view above it (Plot A) so that the coach does not need to re-orient themselves to new information. The only change in Plot B is the *x*-axis now represents each week's score for a single individual across the season. Such information provides a way to investigate any unwanted or

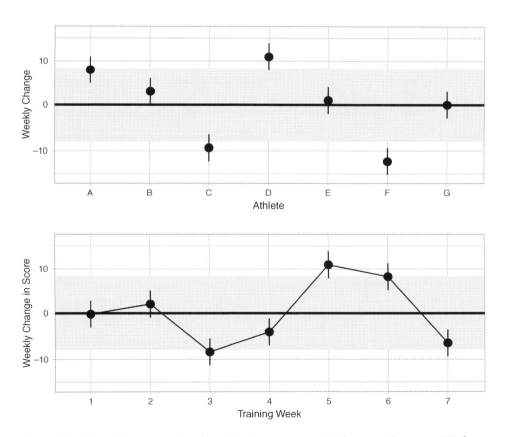

*Figure 19.4* Visualizing analysis of weekly change scores (A) for an entire team, (B) for a single individual from week to week, or (C) for an individual player for each week relative to baseline.

324 Patrick Ward and Barry Drust

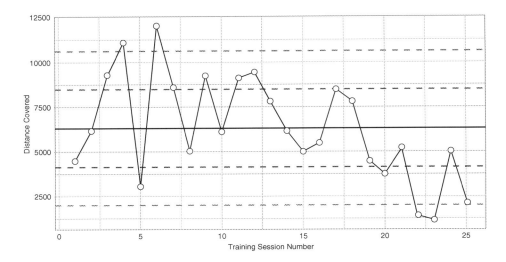

*Figure 19.5* An example of a run chart for a professional soccer player. Total match distance is represented along with 1 and 2 standard deviation bands to alert the viewer to sessions that are outside of normal ranges.

unplanned trends that might require special attention regarding managing the training process of individuals.

The visualization of trends in serial measurements, explained above, can be further shown using a run chart, as seen in Figure 19.5 (Perla et al., 2011; Anhøj & Olesen, 2014). Run charts provide further context in the form of threshold lines above and below the average training distance for this individual; one standard deviation in blue and two standard deviations in red.

Run rules are used to supplement run charts, as seen in Figure 19.6, as a means of drawing attention to important points or patterns (Callahan & Barisa, 2005; Mohammed et al., 2008; Orme & Cox, 2001). Some of the commonly used run rules to include are: (1) an astronomical point, which is a data point falling outside of a specified magnitude, for example, three SD (either above or below the mean); (2) two out of three points beyond the two SD threshold; (3) a run of six or more points on the same side of the centre line; and, (4) a run of five or more points all trending in the same direction. A visual of these rules can be seen in Figure 19.6(a)–(d) where the respective rules are *flagged* for high-speed running in training by changing the colour of the data point.

Evaluating charts as those seen in Figures 19.5 and 19.6 provide the sports scientist and coach with a complete view of the training process and a method of assessing for any divergent trends that may warrant further investigation or intervention from the performance staff. Additionally, such approaches can be structured for daily reporting whereby the run rules that the sports scientist would like to be alerted about can be automatically highlighted without spending too much time reviewing the charts for each player. This automated form of reporting allows the final reporting of the analysis to be operationalized within the daily workflow of the soccer club.

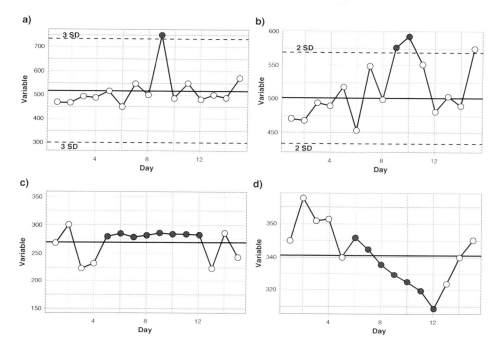

*Figure 19.6* (A) Astronomical point above or below the three SD control limits. (B) Two out of three points above or below the two SD control limits. (C) Six or more points on the same side of the centre line. (D) Six or more points all going in the same direction.

## Future directions and conclusions

The PPDAC cycle provides sports scientists with an easy-to-implement framework for establishing a workflow within the soccer environment, taking them from developing a question to reporting the results of the analysis in a meaningful way that can enhance decision-making within the club. To improve "buy-in" with coaches, sports scientists need to engage them in the scientific process by allowing them to be active from the question development and planning stages of the project lifecycle. Such an approach not only gives the coach some level of ownership in the process but allows the sports scientist to obtain clarity on the specific question they are trying to answer. Once the question has been developed, the sports scientist needs to ensure that the data used for analysis is clean and free from errors and meets some basic requirements with respect to validity and reliability. The type of analysis that is used will depend largely on the available data, the type of data, and the specific nature and goals of the question. Once the final analysis is complete, the sports scientist needs to share the results in a meaningful way. Reporting findings should be specific to the time frames of the weekly cadence for which the information is required to aid decision-making. Importantly, the sports scientist should develop a reporting strategy that provides the coach with easy-to-interpret visuals that are free from "clutter" and scientific jargon, concisely summarizing the most relevant pieces of information from the analysis.

## References

Akenhead, R., & Nassis, G. P. (2016). Training load and player monitoring in high-level football: current practice and perceptions. *Int J Sports Physiol Perf*, *11*(5), 587–593.

Alamar, B. C. (2013). *Sports Analytics: A Guide for Coaches, Managers, and Other Decision Makers*. New York, NY: Columbia University Press.

Anhøj, J., & Olesen, A. V. (2014). Run charts revisted: a simulation study of run chart rules for detection of non-random variation in health care processes. *PLoS One*, *9*, 1–13.

Bartlett, J. D., & Drust, B. (2021). A framework for effective knowledge translation and performance delivery of sport scientists in professional sport. *Eur J Sport Sci*, *21*(11), 1579–1587.

Bishop, D. (2008). An applied research model for the sport sciences. *Sports Med*, *38*(3), 253–263.

Callahan, C. D., & Barisa, M. T. (2005). Statistical process control and rehabilitation outcome: the single-subject design reconsidered. *Rehabil Psychol*, *50*, 24–33.

Coutts, A. J. (2016). Working fast and working slow: the benefits of embedding research in high performance sport. *Int J Sports Physiol Perf*, *11*(1), 1–2.

Halson, S. (2014). Monitoring training load to understand fatigue in athletes. *Sports Med*, *44 Suppl 2*(Suppl 2):S139-47, S139–S147.

Hendricks, S. (2021). Rethinking innovation and the role of stakeholder engagement in sport and exercise medicine. *BMJ Open Sport & Exer Med*, *7*, 1–4.

Hopkins, W. G. (2000). Measures of reliability in sports medicine and science. *Sports Med*, *30*, 375–381.

MacKay, R. J., & Oldford, R. W. (2000). Scientific method, statistical method, and the speed of light. *Stat Sci*, *15*(3), 254–278.

Mohammed, M. A., Worthington, M. A. P., & Woodall, W. H. (2008). Plotting basic control charts: tutorial notes for healthcare practitioners. *Qual Saf Health Care*, *17*, 137–145.

Orme, J. G., & Cox, M. E. (2001). Analyzing single-subject design data using statistical process control charts. *Soc Work Res*, *25*, 115–127.

Perla, R. J., Provost, L. P., & Murray, S. K., (2011). The run chart: a simple analytical tool for learning from variation in health care processes. *BMJ Qual Saf*, *20*, 46–51.

Shumeli, G. (2010). To explain or to predict? *Stat Sci*, *25*(3), 289–310.

Thomas, J. R., Nelson, J. K., & Silverman, S. J. (2015). *Research Methods in Physical Activity*, 7th Ed. Champaign, IL: Human Kinetics.

Ward, P., Windt, J., & Kempton, T. (2019). Business intelligence: how sport scientists can support organization decision making in professional sport. *Int J Sports Physiol Perf*, *14*(4), 544–546.

Weir, J. P. (2005). Quantifying test-retest reliability using the intraclass correlation coefficient and the SEM. *J Strength Cond Res*, *19*(1), 231–240.

Wild, C. J., & Pfannkuch, M. (1999). Statistical thinking in empirical enquiry. *Int J Stat Review*, *67*(3), 223–248.

# Section E

# Talent Identification, Growth, and Development

# 20 Growth and maturation

*Sean P. Cumming, Megan Hill, David Johnson, James Parr, Jan Willem Teunnisen and Robert M. Malina*

## Introduction

Soccer players are traditionally grouped by age for training and competition. Age groups are easy to administer, generally aligned with the school year, and allow children to play with their immediate peers. They are also ideal for matching players on developmental attributes, such as experience, training age, and cognitive, motor-neural, and social development (Malina et al., 2019). Yet, age groups are not without their limitations. Chronological age and physical development do not necessarily proceed in parallel (Malina et al., 2004). Youth of the same age can demonstrate marked variation in physical development, with some individuals growing and maturing well in advance or behind their peers (Johnson et al., 2017).

Individual differences in growth and maturation impact physical and psycho-behavioural development (Cumming et al., 2012). These consequences are especially salient in sports such as soccer where greater size, strength, speed, and power are considered desirable attributes (Malina et al., 2015). Maturity has been shown to impact physical fitness, match performance, and competitive equity in soccer; ultimately impacting talent identification and development (Cumming, 2018; Meylan et al., 2010). Maturity is important to consider in the design, implementation, and evaluation of training/conditioning programmes, and in the prevention of injury (Lloyd & Oliver, 2012; McKay et al., 2019).

## Growth

Growth refers to specific changes in body size, physique, and/or composition, and can be considered in terms of the whole body or specific parts. Increases in body size result from three processes: (i) increases in cell numbers (hyperplasia); (ii) increases in cell size (hypertrophy); and (iii) increases in cellular substances (accretion) (Malina et al., 2004). As children grow, they become taller and heavier, gaining lean and fat tissue, and their organs increase in size. Parts of the body grow at different rates and times, resulting in changes in physique and body proportions. The legs, for example, grow faster than the trunk during childhood; hence, the child becomes relatively long-legged for their height. Heart volume and mass follow a growth pattern like weight, whereas the lungs and lung functions grow proportionally to height.

The most assessed features of growth in soccer are stature (height) and weight (mass), which are often expressed as mass-for-stature (BMI). Measures of height, weight, and BMI provide valuable insight into the growth, maturity, and health status

DOI: 10.4324/9781003148418-25

330  *Sean P. Cumming et al.*

of players (Malina et al., 2015). Routine monitoring of growth status (i.e., longitudinal data) can be used to estimate growth rates (i.e., height and weight velocity) (Johnson, 2015); helping practitioners identify and confirm when players enter important stages of development (e.g., adolescent growth spurt). Rapid increases in growth rates may also be indicative of a high maturation tempo and have been linked to increased injury risk (Kemper et al., 2015).

Mean heights and weights of male soccer players aged 10–18 years in studies spanning 1978–1999 were, on average, consistently shorter and lighter compared to those of players in studies spanning 2000–2015. Mean height of youth players in the recent samples approximate the reference median (50th percentile) of U.S. growth charts at about 10 years of age but was consistently above the reference median through to age 18 years. In contrast, the mean weights of soccer players were consistently between the reference median and 75th percentile. Youth soccer players thus present, on average, greater weights for height, likely reflecting a generally muscular physique.

In contrast to males, secular change in the heights and weights of female players spanning 1992–2020 was negligible. Heights and weights of adolescent players classified as skilled or local did not differ. The composite mean heights of female players were above the U.S. reference median at 9 and 10 years of age, approximated the median at 11–14 years, and were then above the median and approximated the 75th percentile of the reference at 17–18 years of age. In contrast, body weights of female players were consistently above the reference median and were approximately midway between the median and 75th percentiles of the reference from 12 to 18 years of age.

Measures of height and weight, combined with assessments of skeletal age or mid-height of the biological parents, can be used to predict the adult height of a player. Predicted adult height is of potential relevance to those involved in the identification of future adult players. Above average height is an increasingly desired attribute for centre backs and goalkeepers (Carling et al., 2012). The limitations and errors of the prediction equations should be noted, and 90% confidence intervals should be generated for predicted values. Any decisions pertaining to predicted adult height should consider repeated measures over a sustained period of time and 'best case' scenarios (i.e., upper limits of 90% confidence interval) (Johnson, 2015).

### *Maturation*

Biological maturation is the process of progress towards the adult state (Malina et al., 2004). It occurs, and can be assessed, within a range of biological systems, including somatic, skeletal, sexual, endocrinal, and dental. Maturation can be defined in terms of status, tempo, and timing. Status refers to the state of maturity attained at the time of observation (e.g., pubertal stage, skeletal age, or pre-pubertal versus pubertal). Timing refers to the age at which maturational events occur (e.g., age at menarche, age at peak height velocity (PHV), and age at attaining a specific pubertal stage). Tempo refers to the rate at which maturation proceeds.

Methods for assessing maturity status, timing, and tempo vary; each with its advantages and limitations (Malina et al., 2004). Skeletal age is the most objective index of maturity and can be estimated from birth to adulthood (Gilli, 1996). Skeletal age is normally evaluated from a standard hand-wrist radiograph, although DEXA/MRI scans can be used (Romann & Fuchslocher, 2016). Several methods for estimating skeletal age exist, specifically the Greulich-Pyle, Fels, and Tanner-Whitehouse methods.

*Growth and maturation* 331

Skeletal age provides an estimate of maturity status, but not timing. However, the discrepancy between skeletal and chronological age indicates whether a child is advanced, average, or delayed in maturity status. Limitations of this method include expense, the need for specialised equipment, and a low dose of radiation exposure. With modern technology, exposure to radiation is, however, minimal.

Sexual maturation refers to the development of secondary sex characteristics such as pubic hair, breast development, changes in penis/testes, and testicular volume. When performed by a trained assessor, stages of each characteristic provide a valid and reliable indicator of maturity status at the time of observation. Concerns regarding player welfare and safety have, however, led most soccer academies to exclude these methods.

Non-invasive estimates of maturity status and timing based on anthropometry, labelled somatic maturation, are increasingly popular. Common methods include predicted maturity offset (Mirwald et al., 2002) and percentage of predicted adult height (Malina et al., 2005). These methods can be implemented with routine measures of growth status. Predicted maturity offset and percentage of predicted adult height operate on the logic that the closer a player is to, respectively, PHV or predicted mature stature, the more advanced they are in maturity status.

Maturity offset (i.e., predicted time before or after PHV) is predicted with sex-specific equations that require chronological age, height, weight, sitting height, and estimated leg length. Researchers examining the accuracy of the offset equations have raised concerns about the suitability of this method in the general population (Kozieł & Malina, 2018; Malina et al., 2016, 2020; Malina & Kozieł, 2014a, 2014b) and in soccer players (Parr, Winwood, Hodson-Tole, Deconinck, Parry et al., 2020; Teunissen et al., 2020). These studies compared predicted age at PHV with observed age at PHV derived from several longitudinal data series. The prediction equations under- and over-estimated actual age at PHV in younger and older children, respectively, with the error in prediction of age at PHV accentuated in early and late maturing youth.

Percentage of predicted adult height (PPAH) at the time of observation assumes that individuals who are closer to their adult height are more advanced in maturity status. The use of PPAH as a maturity indicator was proposed by Roche and colleagues (Roche et al., 1983), while Malina and colleagues (Malina et al., 2005, 2007, 2012) first applied the protocol with young athletes. The method utilises height prediction equations based on the Fels Longitudinal Study (Khamis & Roche, 1994, 1995). The equations require age, height, and weight of the child and heights of their biological parents. As parental heights are generally reported, they are adjusted for overestimation (Epstein et al., 1995). After predicting adult height, the current height of the player is expressed as a percentage of their predicted adult height. Using this approach, maturity status can be expressed in absolute (percentage of predicted adult height or biological age) or relative (z-score relative to age- and sex-specific standards) terms. More recently, this protocol was modified to include age- and gender-specific reference data from the UK 1990 set to produce a proxy of 'biological age' (Gillison et al., 2017). With a similar intention, protocols to convert PPAH, based on the Tanner Whitehouse 2 and Khamis-Roche height prediction equations have been used to estimate 'skeletal age' in youth (Olivares et al., 2020). PPAH can be used to approximate when a player enters the adolescent growth spurt, for example, age at take-off ($\approx$85%), if they are currently in the interval of PHV ($\approx$91%), or the beginning of the deceleration phase of the adolescent growth spurt ($\approx$96%) (Sanders et al., 2017). This percentage band ($\approx$85–96% of PPAH) was shown to correctly identify 91% of players as being within or outside the

332   *Sean P. Cumming et al.*

pubertal growth spurt in a longitudinal study of academy soccer players (Parr, Winwood, Hodson-Tole, Deconinck, Parry et al., 2020).

### *Growth and maturation screening programmes*

Youth soccer programmes should establish systematic policies and procedures for monitoring the growth and maturation in youth players. Player heights and weights should be measured every 3–4 months and the heights of their biological parents should be assessed or self-reported and adjusted to the tendency for overestimation (Epstein et al., 1995). Measurement frequency is often increased during periods of rapid growth; however, inter- and/or intra-observer measurement variability can influence the accuracy of the estimated increments. To optimise the consistency and accuracy of the measurements, players should be measured with standardised procedures in the morning and prior to training sessions (Johnson, 2015).

The English Premier League launched a 'Growth and Maturation Screening Programme' in 2015 to monitor the growth and maturity status of all registered academy players (U9–U16) (Cumming, 2018). Player data are entered into the Premier League's Player Management Application (PMA) which produces immediate estimates of predicted adult height (with 50% and 90% confidence intervals), PPAH, estimated age at PHV, and maturity offset timing and status. This information is used to: (i) create individual player reports and team audits; (ii) identify players entering periods of rapid growth; (iii) inform training design and delivery; (iv) adjust fitness assessments for maturity status; and (v) group players by maturity status for training and competition (i.e., bio-bands). It should be noted that most PMA outputs utilise PPAH rather than maturity offset as the preferred index of maturation.

## Talent identification, evaluation, and development

As noted, the talent identification process is greatly impacted by individual variance in maturation (Carling et al., 2012; Hill, Scott, Malina et al., 2020; Johnson, 2015). As children, boys who mature early are taller and heavier than their peers, however, it is not until puberty that they possess marked advantages in both size and athleticism. Benefitting from an earlier and more intense growth spurt, early maturing boys are heavier, taller, and possess greater absolute and relative lean mass. As a result of these changes, early maturing boys perform better on tests of strength, power, upper and lower body speed, agility, and aerobic/anaerobic capacity. The physical and functional advantages associated with early maturity in boys are maintained through adolescence (Malina et al., 2004) and it is only in adulthood that these effects are attenuated, and in some cases reversed (Lefevre et al., 2000).

As with boys, girls who mature early are taller and heavier in childhood, yet do not present any noticeable advantages in functional capacities (Malina et al., 2004, 2021). They also experience a more intense adolescent growth spurt, but pubertal gains in lean mass are accompanied by relatively large gains in fat mass. Adolescent gains in physical fitness in girls are, on average, not as marked as those observed in boys. Although longitudinal data are limited, the impact of pubertal timing on physical fitness in girls is mixed and less consistent. Early maturation does afford an advantage in activities that require greater size or absolute strength (Myburgh et al., 2016), yet appears less conducive to tasks that demand relative strength, endurance, and/or movement of the body through space (Malina et al., 2004).

*Growth and maturation* 333

The physical and functional advantages associated with advanced maturation are well-documented in male soccer (Meylan et al., 2010; Murtagh et al., 2018; Parr, Winwood, Hodson-Tole, Deconinck, Hill et al., 2020; Vandendriessche et al., 2012). Youth players advanced in maturity status outperform their peers on tests of strength, speed, power, agility, and endurance. The magnitude of these effects varies from small to moderate, yet is substantial at the extremes of the maturity continuum (Figueiredo et al., 2010). As with the general population, the physical and athletic advantages associated with advanced maturity status in soccer that emerge with puberty are maintained through adolescence before attenuating in late adolescence (Towlson et al., 2018). The earlier attenuation likely reflects the systematic exclusion of late maturing players who lack the necessary physical qualities to succeed (de Silva et al., 2010; Konarski et al., 2020). The physical and functional advantages of advanced maturity status are most likely to impact selection in mid-adolescence when variance in maturity is greatest; yet appear less relevant in late adolescence. For example, among academy soccer players aged 16–18 years, three factors correctly classified about 70% of the players as selected or de-selected, in order: technical skill (ball handling); tactical skill (positioning and deciding); and functional skill (peak shuttle sprinting – a measure of speed and agility). The selected and de-selected players did not differ in size, task, and ego orientation and motivation (Huijgen et al., 2014).

The English Premier League PMA provides age and maturity standards for all physical fitness tests; enabling academy staff to accommodate maturity status when evaluating player fitness, better identify player strengths and weaknesses, and adjust training programmes accordingly. For example, an early maturing player who is 12 years of age may record a 30-m dash time that places them at the 75th centile for their age group, yet only the 30th centile for their maturational status (Cumming et al., 2017).

Research investigating maturity-associated variance in the fitness of female players is limited and most studies have employed the offset method. As such, caution is warranted in interpreting the results of these studies. That said, absolute and relative peak force appears to increase successively in female players across the pre-, circa, and post-PHV stages (Emmonds et al., 2017). Performances on tests of strength (isometric mid-thigh pull), speed (10- to 30-m sprint), agility (505 test), lower body power (counter-movement jump), and aerobic capacity (Yo–Yo test) also improve with advancing maturity in females (Emmonds et al., 2020). There was, however, a decline in relative peak force that occurred between –0.5 and + 0.5 years of PHV, which may have reflected pubertal gains in fat mass. Reduction in relative strength during the growth spurt may increase injury risk in female players, especially those associated with acceleration, deceleration, and/or change of direction.

Emerging evidence suggests that the physical and functional advantages associated with advanced maturity status in males generalise to the soccer field. This research is largely limited to males competing in more select and/or academy programmes. Using GPS to examine maturity-associated variation in match running performance among U14 players, the early maturing players (defined by predicted maturity offset) covered the greater distance at high speed (>16 Km h$^{-1}$), achieved higher peak speeds, and engaged in more high- and repeated high-intensity actions per minute (>1) than late maturing peers (Buchheit & Mendez-Villanueva, 2014). Similarly, advanced maturity status based on percentage of predicted adult stature among U14 male players was associated with greater distance covered, total distance at high speed, total distance at very high speed; maximum speed, and the number of accelerations from zone 4 to zone 6 (Parr et al., 2021). The associations were, however, attenuated when nesting of repeated performances across matches was statistically controlled. In terms of the match performance, academy players advanced in maturity status based on PPAH, played more match minutes and, controlling for minutes played, engaged in more attacking actions, produced more shots and goals, and had higher percentages of successful passes and long passes (Johnson, 2021).

Maturity status in boys has been shown to impact coach evaluations of performance (Hill, Scott, McGee et al., 2020b). Specifically, coaches rated more mature U14–U16 players as performing better than their later maturing peers in matches. This bias coincided with the emergence of a selection gradient for players advanced in maturity status that increased with age. In contrast, later maturing U12 players were awarded higher match grades by coaches. Further analysis suggested that earlier maturing U12 players experienced a temporary decrement in performance associated with the onset of the growth spurt. More specifically, a general decline in match performance was observed across all players categorised as 'circa PHV' (86–95% PPAH), regardless of age, before returning to previous standards when exiting this phase of development (>96% PPAH) (Hill, Scott, McGee et al., 2020a). The preceding observations highlight the need to consider both maturity status and timing when evaluating players. In this context, it is important to compare the match performances and grades of adolescent players when they compete as the most and least mature players within a competitive age-group and note when players are in the middle of a growth spurt.

A selection gradient exists in youth soccer towards boys advanced in maturation. It emerges at the onset of the adolescent growth spurt and increases with age and level of competition. A study of academy players in England and Qatar found 60–80% of U16–U17 players to be advanced in maturation, with only 2–3% being late (Johnson et al., 2017) (Figure 20.1). The bias is most evident amongst goalkeepers, defenders,

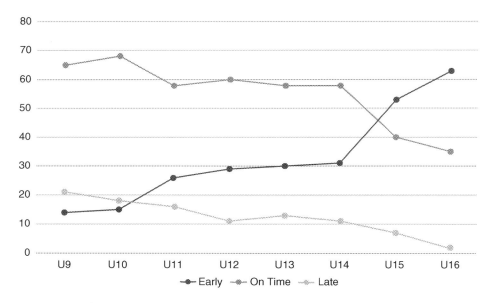

*Figure 20.1* The percentages of male academy players by maturation status across competitive age groups. Adapted from Johnson et al., 2017.

*Growth and maturation* 335

forwards, and those playing central positions. The presence of a bias does vary relative to the method used to estimate maturity. Studies employing PPAH (Hill, Scott, Malina et al., 2020), sexual maturity status (Malina et al., 2013), or Greulich-Pyle, Fels, and TW2 RUS skeletal ages (Malina et al., 2011) have consistently observed a selection bias towards more mature players (Malina, 2011). In contrast, TW3 RUS skeletal ages were systematically lower than TW2 RUS skeletal ages by about 1 year beginning at 11 years; as a result, the number of players classified as late maturing increased while the number classified as early maturing decreased (Malina et al., 2018; see also Malina, 2017).

The impact of maturity status on the selection and retention of female soccer players is unclear (Malina et al., 2021). Most studies suggest that adolescent female soccer players tended to be 'on time' or slightly delayed. Mean ages at menarche based on the retrospective method in seven studies of soccer players ranged from 12.7 to 13.0 years of age, whereas the median age at menarche based on the status quo method was 12.9 years; standard deviations of between 0.7 and 1.3 years (Malina et al., 2021). The mean ages of menarche in the soccer players were within the expected ranges for European and North American populations. Studies of skeletal age in female soccer players are limited. An early study suggested average or 'on-time' maturity status (Novotny, 1981), while a recent study showed variation between the Greulich-Pyle and Fels methods of assessment (Martinho et al., 2021). Among U13–U17 players, skeletal age was, on average, advanced relative to chronological age with the Fels method, whereas skeletal age was advanced among U13 and U14 players, equal to chronological age among U15 players, but delayed relative to chronological age among U16 and U17 players with the Greulich-Pyle method.

### *Maturity status and training*

To optimise training effects and reduce injury risk, practitioners should recognise and accommodate for individual differences in growth and maturity status. Training gains are most efficacious when they complement the physiological adaptations that occur with normal growth and maturation, a concept labelled as *synergistic adaptation* (Lloyd & Oliver, 2012). Prior to puberty, gains in speed, power, and strength are best achieved through activities that promote enhanced neuromuscular adaptation and co-ordination. By inference, training activities for pre-pubertal players should focus on the development of technique and functional competence. Maximum gains in speed, strength, and power post-puberty are, however, best achieved through a combination of neuromuscular and structural (i.e., hypertrophy) adaptation, with the latter resulting from the hormonal and metabolic changes that accompany puberty.

The Youth Physical Developmental Model provides a logical and evidence-based framework for designing and implementing training and conditioning programmes for young athletes (Llyod & Oliver, 2012). Separate models exist for male and female athletes with each identifying the specific ages and stages of maturity when various fitness components and training modalities should be emphasised. Allowing for technical competence and psychological readiness, young athletes should be grouped relative to maturity status. Prior to puberty (e.g., <85% PPAH), boys and girls should engage in low-structured activities that facilitate neural adaptations in speed, strength, power, agility, and sport-specific skills through neuromuscular adaptation in low-structured activities, with a reduced emphasis upon hypertrophy, endurance and/or metabolic

336  *Sean P. Cumming et al.*

conditioning. However, with the onset of the adolescent growth spurt (89–95% PPAH), and especially during its latter stages (>95% PPAH), a greater emphasis can be placed on activities that promote hypertrophy and adaptation of the anaerobic system.

### Maturity status and injury

The interval of the adolescent growth spurt is a period of development when athletes are more susceptible to overuse and growth-related injuries (Johnson et al., 2020; van der Sluis et al., 2014; Wik et al., 2020). With an accelerated rate of linear growth, the physes, apophyses, and articular surfaces are less resistant to compressive, shear, and tensile forces than immature or mature bone due to a lack of collagen or calcified tissue (McKay et al., 2019). Age-adjusted decreases in bone mineral content during the growth spurt may also contribute to a greater risk of injury in adolescent players (Jackowski et al., 2009). Furthermore, rapid and differential timing growth of different segments of the body during adolescence differentially influences limb lengths, muscle mass, and moments of inertia (Adirim & Cheng, 2003), leading some youth to experience delays or regressions in motor control that may adversely impact injury risk; a phenomenon commonly referred to as 'adolescent awkwardness'.

Non-contact injuries are prevalent in youth sports and comprise 53–72% of injuries in high-level male youth soccer players of age 9–21 years (Jones et al., 2019). Moreover, growth and overuse injuries accounted for 6.6% of all injuries among a combined sample of players from six youth academies (Read et al., 2018). Common examples of overuse injuries related to growth among youth soccer players include chondromalacia, Sinding-Larsen-Johansson syndrome, Osgood-Schlatter disease, Sever's disease, osteochondritis dissecans, and lower body stress fractures. A retrospective study of maturity status based on percentage of attained adult height at the time of observation and injury in academy players in Spain suggested a specific pattern related to the incidence of overuse injuries and stages of the growth spurt. Following a gradient of distal to proximal growth, cases of Sever's disease clustered around the start of the growth spurt (85% PPAH), whereas the majority of Osgood-Schlatter's cases approximated the peak of the growth spurt (89% PPAH) (Monasterio et al., 2021). Growth-related injuries related to the spine, lower back (spondylolysis), and hip (e.g., ischial tuberosity) occurred following the peak of the growth spurt and during the deceleration phase.

Puberty is a developmental stage that sees increases in other injuries, such as anterior cruciate ligament (ACL) injuries. ACL injuries are three and a half times more likely in female athletes compared to males with these gender differences occurring at the onset of puberty (Voskanian, 2013). The exact stage of puberty at which this gender discrepancy arises is unclear and further research is warranted to better understand this process. Gender differences in hormonal profiles in addition to functional and structural differences, such as the Q angle and knee ligament laxity, are likely contributors to this increased likelihood of knee injury in females. The mechanism of ACL injuries is often cutting or landing, therefore, consideration of neuromuscular recruitment patterns and landing techniques is paramount (Voskanian, 2013). Monitoring the tempo and timing of the growth spurt could have a meaningful impact on understanding the risk between early and late maturing girls and the age at which specific injury prevention programmes are introduced. Such programmes should include activities emphasising the lower body and core strength,

*Growth and maturation*  337

balance, coordination, fundamental movement skills, and sport-specific techniques of jumping and landing to mitigate the risk of knee-related injuries during this stage of development.

Research investigating the impact of growth and maturation upon injury in youth soccer is limited, yet suggests a heightened risk during periods of rapid growth (Price et al., 2004). Available data suggest that injuries among male adolescent players were associated with an estimated higher rate of growth at the time of injury compared to non-injured players (Rommers et al., 2020). Other data suggest an association between estimated rates of growth in height and leg length with a greater risk of bone and growth plate injuries in adolescent track and field athletes (Wik et al., 2020). The interval of the adolescent growth spurt is also associated with an increased likelihood of injury (Bult et al., 2018; van der Sluis et al., 2014); although most of the studies have used the offset method and should, and thus should be interpreted with caution. Using PPAH as the indicator of maturity status, players with percentages of predicted adult height between 88% and 95% (interpreted as circa PHV) presented a significantly higher incidence and burden of injury compared to players estimated as pre-PHV (Johnson et al., 2020).

A reduction in injury incidence and burden through the growth spurt should be possible through regular assessment of growth and maturity status, consideration of training load and content, and careful monitoring of injury symptomology (McKay et al., 2019). The onset of the growth spurt (i.e., age at take-off) typically occurs at 85% of PPAH, before peaking at 91% of PPAH, and decelerating at 95% of PPAH. Rates of growth in both stature and mass accelerate during the growth spurt from 5–6 cm and 2–3 kg per year, to 9–10 or 8–9 cm and 9–10 kg per year in boys and girls, respectively. An example of how to identify 'at-risk' players is presented in Figure 20.1. The maturity status/growth velocity heat map developed by Johnson and colleagues at AFC Bournemouth illustrates the interaction between growth rate and percentage of predicted adult height on injury incidence (Figure 20.2a) and injury burden (Figure 20.2b) in academy players across a competitive season. Risk for injury incidence peaks at approximately 92–93% of PPAH and among players growing at a rate of 10–15 cm per year, whereas injury burden is greatest post-PHV and among players in the declaration phase of the growth spurt.

Jan Willem Teunnisen, a movement scientist and performance coach at AFC Ajax, proposed a strategy to reduce injury risk and better manage player development as youth enter and transition through puberty (Wormhoudt et al., 2017). The strategy involves the modification of training load and content (exercise diversification per phase: pre-, during, and post-PHV) and is implemented as players enter the growth spurt. Modifications include a reduction in training load and activities that involve significant amounts of acceleration and deceleration; coupled with increased emphasis upon activities that develop and/or maintain coordination, balance, core control and strength, mobility, and the re-training of fundamental and sport-specific skills. These strategies are described in a model presented by Towlson and colleagues (2021) (Figure 20.3). Applying these strategies across a competitive season, sports scientists at AFC Bournemouth reported marked reductions in injury incidence and burden among players identified as being within the growth spurt. Although these results are encouraging, further research is required to validate these findings and better understand the mechanisms underlying the benefits and most appropriate training loads and content to reduce injury risk in adolescent players.

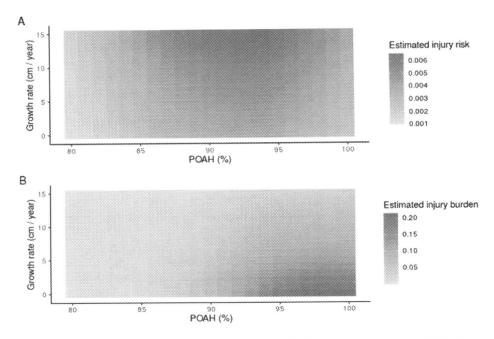

*Figure 20.2a and b* Heat maps showing the combined effects of growth rate and POAH on estimated (A) injury likelihood and (B) injury burden.

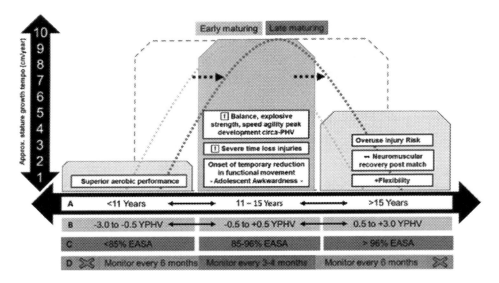

*Figure 20.3* Use of percentage of predicted adult stature to determine location in adolescent growth curve in young athletes.

Source: Reproduced with permission. Towlson, C., Salter, J., Ade, J. D., et al. (2020). Maturity-associated considerations for training load, injury risk, and physical performance in youth soccer: one size does not fit all. *J Sport Health Sci*. Published online September 19, 2020. Copyright© [2020]. doi: 10.1016/j.jshs.2020.09.003.

*Growth and maturation*   339

### *Maturity status and fitness testing*

Fitness testing is employed for the purposes of talent identification, monitoring player development, and evaluating the effectiveness of training programmes. Variance in maturation status can enhance or confound performance on fitness tests, with more mature players outperforming their later maturing peers. As part of their Elite Player Performance Plan, the English Premier League developed academy-wide age- and maturity-specific standards for all physical fitness tests, including 30-m sprint, counter-movement jump, 505 agility tests and Yo–Yo test of aerobic endurance. Academy staff have the capacity to judge players relative to age and maturity standards and, therefore, are better able to identify player strengths and weaknesses. A boy who has matured early may perform at the 90th centile for his age groups in the 30-m sprint, yet place at the 30th centile when compared against players of similar maturity status. Thus, an apparent strength is a weakness when considered from a developmental perspective and coaches should consider adjusting the training for this player to place a greater emphasis on speed work.

### *Maturity status and competition: bio-banding*

As discussed previously, variance in maturation status can create competitive inequity within age groups. Inequity in competition disadvantages both early and late maturing boys. The pressure to win encourages early maturing boys to play to their physical and functional strengths, neglecting the use and development of the technical, tactical, and psychological skills that are necessary to succeed at the professional level. Conversely, the equally, if not more talented late maturing players are less able to succeed and/or demonstrate their ability/potential and, thus, more likely to be overlooked or excluded.

To accommodate individual differences in growth and maturity, it has historically been suggested that youth should be grouped based on their physical development, often labelled as maturity-matching. Bio-banding is a current manifestation of the maturity-matching strategy (Malina et al., 2019). Bio-banding in soccer was first implemented in England in the early 1990s where a bio-banding metric based on size and weight was employed to group players relative to their physical development. Although this strategy was successfully implemented within the Football Association (FA) School of Excellence at Lilleshall, any application outside of the centre was limited.

The English Premier League recently revisited the concept of bio-banding in 2015 as part of its Elite Player Performance Plan (Cumming, 2018). It was hoped that bio-banded games would promote competitive equity and provide new learning opportunities and challenges for early and late maturing youth, whilst providing coaches with the opportunity to better evaluate players in different contexts. Working with the Premier League, the academies used the percentage of predicted adult height to group players relative to maturity status. Bio-bands of 5% of predicted adult stature were used to group players (i.e., 85–90% PPAH; 90–95% PPAH) across a series of bio-banded festival tournaments delivered as part of the academy games programme (Cumming et al., 2018).

The bio-banded format was received positively by the players, with 47 of 48 players interviewed post-tournament recommending the inclusion of bio-banding within the existing games programme. Early and late maturing players did, however, support the

340  *Sean P. Cumming et al.*

initiative for different reasons (Cumming et al., 2018). Players advanced in maturity described the bio-banded games as physically more challenging, better learning experiences and an opportunity to compete with and learn from older, more experienced players. They found they were unable to rely on their physical advantages, placing greater emphasis on technical, tactical, and psychological skills. They described the game as faster, noting less time to make decisions and receive and release the ball. In contrast, late maturing players described their bio-banded games as less physically challenging yet appreciated having greater opportunity to use and demonstrate their physical, technical, and tactical abilities. The older late maturing boys took positions of leadership, organising, motivating, and mentoring their younger peers. Of note, both early and late maturing players described the games as being less physical and more technically and tactically oriented, and as an opportunity to meet and make new friends.

Since the English Premier League's inaugural tournaments, a number of studies have investigated the benefits and challenges of bio-banding, often using GPS and video analysis technology (Abbott et al., 2019; Bradley et al., 2019; Reeves et al., 2018; Romann et al., 2020; Thomas et al., 2017; Towlson et al., 2020). Collectively, these studies supported the tenets of bio-banding, highlighting benefits for early and late maturing players, and changes in game demands. Bio-banded formats encourage a more technical/tactical style of play that involves more short passes and touches (particularly within the defensive half), greater frequencies of tackles, duels, and set pieces. The bio-banding format also led to less long passing, heading, dribbling, distance covered in jogging, running and high-speed running, yet greater physical exertion among early maturing players. In small-sided games, bio-banding resulted in greater equity in terms of physical and psychological challenges (Towlson et al., 2020). In an investigation of the perceived benefits and disadvantages of bio-banding among stakeholders within a professional English Academy, several psychological, social, and technical/tactical advantages associated with the bio-banded format were noted (Reeves et al., 2018). Late maturing players benefitted in terms of confidence and technical and tactical development, whereas early maturing players benefitted from the novel and more physical challenges. Potential negatives of bio-banding were noted, notably, the social stigma associated with asking players to train and compete with youth that were chronologically younger. The latter observation highlights the need to educate players, parents, and coaches on the purpose and potential benefits of bio-banding and to remove stigma associated with the process of 'playing up or down' age groups. Overall, results of studies of bio-banding are interesting and promising, but the need for further research is essential.

### *Future programmes*

To provide greater equity and opportunity for late maturing and/or relatively young players, the Belgian FA developed a 'Futures' programme. This strategy groups players based on developmental status, limiting age, and maturity-associated variance in size and athleticism. To identify talented late developers, coaches and scouts observing fixtures are encouraged to identify players that demonstrate a winning mindset, future physical potential, insight into the game, body, and ball control, learning ability, and self-development. These players are selected for a national future team that trains in parallel with national junior age group teams and compete against smaller nations. Since

Its inception, several other European nations have adopted and implemented equivalent Futures programmes, including Ireland, the Czech Republic, Denmark, and Sweden.

### Future directions and conclusions

Variance in maturity status and timing has important implications for the identification and development of youth players. Although maturity status and timing are genotypic characteristics of individual players, coaches, and practitioners can assess, monitor, and accommodate these individual differences by altering training, content, competition, behaviours, and expectations. In doing so, we can overcome the challenges presented by individual differences in growth and maturation, optimising the opportunities and challenges for early, on-time and late maturing youth. Bio-banding, though still in its infancy, represents one strategy that may help coaches, scouts, and practitioners deal with these challenges. It should not be considered as a replacement for age group competition but should be viewed as an adjunct to and perhaps as part of a diverse and dynamic approach to games programmes. Further research is required to determine the effectiveness of various bio-banding strategies in youth soccer and the ages at which these strategies should be introduced. That said, bio-banding represents an important first step in addressing some of the challenges presented by the individuality of physical growth and biological maturation, and the journey towards an efficient and effective model of talent identification and development.

## References

Abbott, W., Williams, S., Brickley, G., & Smeeton, N. J. (2019). Effects of bio-banding upon physical and technical performance during soccer competition: a preliminary analysis. *Sports*, *7*(8), 193.

Adirim, T. A., & Cheng, T. L. (2003). Overview of injuries in the young athlete. *Sports Medicine*, *33*(1), 75–81.

Bradley, B., Johnson, D., Hill, M., McGee, D., Kana-Ah, A., Sharpin, C., Sharp, P., Kelly, A., Cumming, S. P., & Malina, R. M. (2019). Bio-banding in academy football: player's perceptions of a maturity matched tournament. *Annals of Human Biology*, *46*(5), 400–408.

Buchheit, M., & Mendez-Villanueva, A. (2014). Effects of age, maturity and body dimensions on match running performance in highly trained under-15 soccer players. *Journal of Sports Sciences*, *32*(13), 1271–1278.

Bult, H. J., Barendrecht, M., & Tak, I. J. R. (2018). Injury risk and injury burden are related to age group and peak height velocity among talented male youth soccer players. *Orthopaedic Journal of Sports Medicine*, *6*(12), 2325967118811042.

Carling, C., Le Gall, F., & Malina, R. M. (2012). Body size, skeletal maturity, and functional characteristics of elite academy soccer players on entry between 1992 and 2003. *Journal of Sports Sci*, *30*(15), 1683–1693.

Cumming, S. P. (2018). A game plan for growth: how football is leading the way in the consideration of biological maturation in young male athletes. *Annals of Human Biology*, *45*(5), 373–375.

Cumming, S. P., Brown, D. J., Mitchell, S., Bunce, J., Hunt, D., Hedges, C., Crane, G., Gross, A., Scott, S., & Franklin, E. (2018). Premier League academy soccer players' experiences of competing in a tournament bio-banded for biological maturation. *Journal of Sports Sciences*, *36*(7), 757–765.

Cumming, S. P., Lloyd, R. S., Oliver, J. L., Eisenmann, J. C., & Malina, R. M. (2017). Bio-banding in sport: applications to competition, talent identification, and strength and conditioning of youth athletes. *Strength & Conditioning Journal*, *39*(2), 34–47.

Cumming, S. P., Sherar, L. B., Pindus, D. M., Coelho-e-Silva, M. J., Malina, R. M., & Jardine, P. R. (2012). A biocultural model of maturity-associated variance in adolescent physical activity. *International Review of Sport and Exercise Psychology*, *5*(1), 23–43.

de Silva, M. C., Figueiredo, A. J., Simoes, F., Seabra, A., Natal, A., Vaeyens, R., Philippaerts, R., Cumming, S. P., & Malina, R. (2010). Discrimination of u-14 soccer players by level and position. *International Journal of Sports Medicine*, *31*(11), 790–796.

Emmonds, S., Morris, R., Murray, E., Robinson, C., Turner, L., & Jones, B. (2017). The influence of age and maturity status on the maximum and explosive strength characteristics of elite youth female soccer players. *Science and Medicine in Football*, *1*(3), 209–215.

Emmonds, S., Scantlebury, S., Murray, E., Turner, L., Robinon, C., & Jones, B. (2020). Physical characteristics of elite youth female soccer players characterized by maturity status. *The Journal of Strength & Conditioning Research*, *34*(8), 2321–2328.

Epstein, L. H., Valoski, A. M., Kalarchian, M. A., & McCurley, J. (1995). Do children lose and maintain weight easier than adults: a comparison of child and parent weight changes from six months to ten years. *Obesity Research*, *3*(5), 411–417.

Figueiredo, A. J., e Silva, M. J. C., Cumming, S. P., & Malina, R. M. (2010). Size and maturity mismatch in youth soccer players 11-to 14-years-old. *Pediatric Exercise Science*, *22*(4), 596–612.

Gilli, G. (1996). The assessment of skeletal maturation. *Hormone Research in Paediatrics*, *45*(Suppl. 2), 49–52.

Gillison, F., Cumming, S., Standage, M., Barnaby, C., & Katzmarzyk, P. (2017). Assessing the impact of adjusting for maturity in weight status classification in a cross-sectional sample of UK children. *BMJ Open*, *7*(6), e015769.

Hill, M., Scott, S., Malina, R. M., McGee, D., & Cumming, S. P. (2020). Relative age and maturation selection biases in academy football. *Journal of Sports Sciences*, *38*(11–12), 1359–1367.

Hill, M., Scott, S., McGee, D., & Cumming, S. (2020a). Coaches' evaluations of match performance in academy soccer players in relation to the adolescent growth spurt. *Journal of Science in Sport and Exercise*, 1–8.

Hill, M., Scott, S., McGee, D., & Cumming, S. P. (2020b). Are relative age and biological ages associated with coaches' evaluations of match performance in male academy soccer players? *International Journal of Sports Science & Coaching*, *16*(2), 227–235 1747954120966886.

Huijgen, B. C., Elferink-Gemser, M. T., Lemmink, K. A., & Visscher, C. (2014). Multidimensional performance characteristics in selected and deselected talented soccer players. *European Journal of Sport Science*, *14*(1), 2–10.

Jackowski, S. A., Faulkner, R. A., Farthing, J. P., Kontulainen, S. A., Beck, T. J., & Baxter-Jones, A. D. (2009). Peak lean tissue mass accrual precedes changes in bone strength indices at the proximal femur during the pubertal growth spurt. *Bone*, *44*(6), 1186–1190.

Johnson, A. (2015). Monitoring the immature athlete. *Aspetar Sports Medicine Journal*, *4*(4), 114–118.

Johnson, A., Farooq, A., & Whiteley, R. (2017). Skeletal maturation status is more strongly associated with academy selection than birth quarter. *Science and Medicine in Football*, *1*(2), 157–163.

Johnson, D. (2021). *Growth, Maturation and Bio-banding in Youth Football*.

Johnson, D., Williams, S., Bradley, B., Sayer, S., Murray Fisher, J., & Cumming, S. (2020). Growing pains: maturity associated variation in injury risk in academy football. *European Journal of Sport Science*, *20*(4), 544–552.

Jones, S., Almousa, S., Gibb, A., Allamby, N., Mullen, R., Andersen, T. E., & Williams, M. (2019). Injury incidence, prevalence and severity in high-level male youth football: a systematic review. *Sports Medicine*, *49*(12), 1879–1899.

Kemper, G., Van Der Sluis, A., Brink, M., Visscher, C., Frencken, W., & Elferink-Gemser, M. (2015). Anthropometric injury risk factors in elite-standard youth soccer. *International Journal of Sports Medicine*, *36*(13), 1112–1117.

Khamis, H. J., & Roche, A. F. (1994). Predicting adult stature without using skeletal age: the Khamis-Roche method. *Pediatrics*, *94*(4), 504–507.

Khamis, H., & Roche, A. (1995). Predicting adult stature without using skeletal age-the Khamis-Roche method. *Pediatrics*, *95*(3), 457–457.

Konarski, J., Krzykała, M., Skrzypczak, M., Nowakowska, M., Coelho-e-Silva, M., Cumming, S., & Malina, R. (2020). Characteristics of select and non-select U15 male soccer players. *Biology of Sport*, *38*(4), 535–544.

Kozieł, S. M., & Malina, R. M. (2018). Modified maturity offset prediction equations: validation in independent longitudinal samples of boys and girls. *Sports Medicine*, *48*(1), 221–236.

Lefevre, J., Philippaerts, R. M., Delvaux, K., Thomis, M., Vanreusel, B., Eynde, B. V., Claessens, A. L., Lysens, R., Renson, R., & Beunen, G. (2000). Daily physical activity and physical fitness from adolescence to adulthood: a longitudinal study. *American Journal of Human Biology*, *12*(4), 487–497.

Lloyd, R. S., & Oliver, J. L. (2012). The youth physical development model: a new approach to long-term athletic development. *Strength & Conditioning Journal*, *34*(3), 61–72.

Malina, R. M., Bouchard, C., & Bar-Or, O. (2004). *Growth, Maturation, and Physical Activity*. Champaign Human Kinetics.

Malina, R. M. (2011). Skeletal age and age verification in youth sport. Sports medicine, 41, 925–947.

Malina, R. M., e Silva, M. C., & Figueiredo, A. J. (2013). Growth and maturity status of youth players. In Science and soccer (pp. 319–344). Routledge.

Malina, R. M., Figueiredo, A. J., & Coelho-e-Silva, M. J. (2017). Body size of male youth soccer players: 1978–2015. Sports Medicine, 47, 1983–1992.

Malina, R. M., Coelho-e-Silva, M. J., Figueiredo, A. J., Philippaerts, R. M., Hirose, N., Peña Reyes, M. E., ... & Buranarugsa, R. (2018). Tanner–Whitehouse skeletal ages in male youth soccer players: TW2 or TW3?. Sports Medicine, 48, 991-1008.

Malina, R. M., Choh, A. C., Czerwinski, S. A., & Chumlea, W. C. (2016). Validation of maturity offset in the Fels longitudinal study. *Pediatric Exercise Science*, *28*(3), 439–455.

Malina, R. M., Coelho E Silva, M. J., Figueiredo, A. J., Carling, C., & Beunen, G. P. (2012). Interrelationships among invasive and non-invasive indicators of biological maturation in adolescent male soccer players. *Journal of Sports Sciences*, *30*(15), 1705–1717.

Malina, R. M., Cumming, S. P., Morano, P. J., Barron, M., & Miller, S. J. (2005). Maturity status of youth football players: a noninvasive estimate. *Medicine and Science in Sports and Exercise*, *37*(6), 1044–1052.

Malina, R. M., Cumming, S. P., Rogol, A. D., Coelho-e-Silva, M. J., Figueiredo, A. J., Konarski, J. M., & Kozieł, S. M. (2019). Bio-banding in youth sports: background, concept, and application. *Sports Medicine*, *49*(11):1671–1685

Malina, R. M., Dompier, T. P., Powell, J. W., Barron, M. J., & Moore, M. T. (2007). Validation of a noninvasive maturity estimate relative to skeletal age in youth football players. *Clinical Journal of Sport Medicine*, *17*(5), 362–368.

Malina, R. M., & Kozieł, S. M. (2014a). Validation of maturity offset in a longitudinal sample of Polish boys. *Journal of Sports Sciences*, *32*(5), 424–437.

Malina, R. M., & Kozieł, S. M. (2014b). Validation of maturity offset in a longitudinal sample of Polish girls. *Journal of Sports Sciences*, *32*(14), 1374–1382.

Malina, R. M., Kozieł, S. M., Králik, M., Chrzanowska, M., & Suder, A. (2020). Prediction of maturity offset and age at peak height velocity in a longitudinal series of boys and girls. *American Journal of Human Biology*, *33*(6), e23551.

Malina, R. M., Martinho, D. V., Valente-dos-Santos, J., Coelho-e-Silva, M. J., & Kozieł, S. M. (2021). Growth and maturity status of female soccer players: a narrative review. *International Journal of Environmental Research and Public Health*, *18*(4), 1448.

Malina, R. M., Rogol, A. D., Cumming, S. P., e Silva, M. J. C., & Figueiredo, A. J. (2015). Biological maturation of youth athletes: assessment and implications. *British Journal of Sports Medicine*, *49*(13), 852–859.

Martinho, D. V., Coelho-e-Silva, M. J., Valente-dos-Santos, J., Minderico, C., Oliveira, T. G., Rodrigues, I., Conde, J., Sherar, L. B., & Malina, R. M. (2021). Assessment of skeletal age in youth female soccer players: agreement between Greulich-Pyle and Fels protocols. *American Journal of Human Biology*, *34*(1), e23591.

McKay, C. D., Cumming, S. P., & Blake, T. (2019). Youth sport: friend or Foe? *Best Practice & Research Clinical Rheumatology*, *33*(1), 141–157.

Meylan, C., Cronin, J., Oliver, J., & Hughes, M. (2010). Talent identification in soccer: the role of maturity status on physical, physiological and technical characteristics. *International Journal of Sports Science & Coaching*, *5*(4), 571–592.

Mirwald, R. L., Baxter-Jones, A. D., Bailey, D. A., & Beunen, G. P. (2002). An assessment of maturity from anthropometric measurements. *Medicine and Science in Sports and Exercise*, *34*(4), 689–694.

Monasterio, X., Gil, S., Bidaurrazaga-Letona, I., Lekue, J., Santisteban, J., Diaz-Beitia, G., Martin-Garetxana, I., Bikandi, E., & Larruskain, J. (2021). Injuries according to the percentage of adult height in an elite soccer academy. *Journal of Science and Medicine in Sport*, *24*(3), 218–223.

Murtagh, C. F., Brownlee, T. E., O'Boyle, A., Morgans, R., Drust, B., & Erskine, R. M. (2018). Importance of speed and power in elite youth soccer depends on maturation status. *The Journal of Strength & Conditioning Research*, *32*(2), 297–303.

Myburgh, G. K., Cumming, S. P., Silva, M. C. E., Cooke, K., & Malina, R. M. (2016). Maturity-associated variation in functional characteristics of elite youth tennis players. *Pediatric Exercise Science*, *28*(4), 542–552.

Novotny, V. (1981). Veranderungen des Knochenalters im Verlauf einer mehrjahrigen sportlichen Belastung. *Medezin Und Sport*, *21*, 44–47.

Olivares, L. A. F., De León, L. G., & Fragoso, M. I. (2020). Skeletal age prediction model from percentage of adult height in children and adolescents. *Scientific Reports*, *10*(1), 1–10.

Parr, J., Winwood, K., Hodson-Tole, E., Deconinck, F. J., & Cumming, S. P. (in review). *Maturity Associated Differences in Match Running Performance in Elite Male Youth Soccer Players*, Champaign: Human Kinetics.

Parr, J., Winwood, K., Hodson-Tole, E., Deconinck, F. J., Hill, J. P., Teunissen, J. W., & Cumming, S. P. (2020). The main and interactive effects of biological maturity and relative age on physical performance in elite youth soccer players. *Journal of Sports Medicine*, *2020*, 1–11.

Parr, J., Winwood, K., Hodson-Tole, E., Deconinck, F. J., Parry, L., Hill, J. P., Malina, R. M., & Cumming, S. P. (2020). Predicting the timing of the peak of the pubertal growth spurt in elite male youth soccer players: evaluation of methods. *Annals of Human Biology*, *47*(4), 400–408.

Price, R., Hawkins, R., Hulse, M., & Hodson, A. (2004). The football association medical research programme: an audit of injuries in academy youth football. *British Journal of Sports Medicine*, *38*(4), 466–471.

Read, P. J., Oliver, J. L., De Ste Croix, M. B., Myer, G. D., & Lloyd, R. S. (2018). An audit of injuries in six English professional soccer academies. *Journal of Sports Sciences*, *36*(13), 1542–1548.

Reeves, M. J., Enright, K. J., Dowling, J., & Roberts, S. J. (2018). Stakeholders' understanding and perceptions of bio-banding in junior-elite football training. *Soccer & Society*, *19*(8), 1166–1182.

Roche, A. F., Tyleshevski, F., & Rogers, E. (1983). Non-invasive measurements of physical maturity in children. *Research Quarterly for Exercise and Sport*, *54*(4), 364–371.

Romann, M., & Fuchslocher, J. (2016). Assessment of skeletal age on the basis of DXA-derived hand scans in elite youth soccer. *Research in Sports Medicine*, *24*(3), 185–196.

Romann, M., Lüdin, D., & Born, D.-P. (2020). Bio-banding in junior soccer players: a pilot study. *BMC Research Notes*, *13*(1), 1–5.

Rommers, N., Rössler, R., Goossens, L., Vaeyens, R., Lenoir, M., Witvrouw, E., & D'Hondt, E. (2020). Risk of acute and overuse injuries in youth elite soccer players: body size and growth matter. *Journal of Science and Medicine in Sport*, *23*(3), 246–251.

Sanders, J. O., Qiu, X., Lu, X., Duren, D. L., Liu, R. W., Dang, D., Menendez, M. E., Hans, S. D., Weber, D. R., & Cooperman, D. R. (2017). The uniform pattern of growth and skeletal maturation during the human adolescent growth spurt. *Scientific Reports*, *7*(1), 1–9.

Teunissen, J. W., Rommers, N., Pion, J., Cumming, S. P., Rössler, R., D'Hondt, E., Lenoir, M., Savelsbergh, G. J., & Malina, R. M. (2020). Accuracy of maturity prediction equations in individual elite male football players. *Annals of Human Biology*, *47*(4), 409–416.

Thomas, C. H., Oliver, J., Kelly, A., & Knapman, H. (2017). A pilot study of the demands of chronological age group and bio-banded match play in elite youth soccer. *Graduate Journal of Sport Exercise and Physical Education Research*, *1*, s10.

Towlson, C., Cobley, S., Parkin, G., & Lovell, R. (2018). When does the influence of maturation on anthropometric and physical fitness characteristics increase and subside? *Scandinavian Journal of Medicine & Science in Sports*, *28*(8), 1946–1955.

Towlson, C., MacMaster, C., Gonçalves, B., Sampaio, J., Toner, J., MacFarlane, N., Barrett, S., Hamilton, A., Jack, R., & Hunter, F. (2020). The effect of bio-banding on physical and psychological indicators of talent identification in academy soccer players. *Science and Medicine in Football*, *5*(4), 280–292

Towlson, C., Salter, J., Ade, J. D., Enright, K., Harper, L. D., Page, R. M., & Malone, J. J. (2021). Maturity-associated considerations for training load, injury risk, and physical performance in youth soccer: One size does not fit all. *Journal of Sport and Health Science*, *10*(4), 403–412.

van der Sluis, A., Elferink-Gemser, M., Coelho-e-Silva, M., Nijboer, J., Brink, M., & Visscher, C. (2014). Sport injuries aligned to peak height velocity in talented pubertal soccer players. *International Journal of Sports Medicine*, *35*(04), 351–355.

Vandendriessche, J. B., Vaeyens, R., Vandorpe, B., Lenoir, M., Lefevre, J., & Philippaerts, R. M. (2012). Biological maturation, morphology, fitness, and motor coordination as part of a selection strategy in the search for international youth soccer players (age 15–16 years). *Journal of Sports Sciences*, *30*(15), 1695–1703.

Voskanian, N. (2013). ACL Injury prevention in female athletes: review of the literature and practical considerations in implementing an ACL prevention program. *Current Reviews in Musculoskeletal Medicine*, *6*(2), 158–163.

Wik, E. H., Martínez-Silván, D., Farooq, A., Cardinale, M., Johnson, A., & Bahr, R. (2020). Skeletal maturation and growth rates are related to bone and growth plate injuries in adolescent athletics. *Scandinavian Journal of Medicine & Science in Sports*, *30*(5), 894–903.

Wormhoudt, R., Savelsbergh, G. J., Teunissen, J. W., & Davids, K. (2017). *The Athletic Skills Model: Optimizing Talent Development Through Movement Education*. London: Routledge.

# 21 Talented or developmentally advanced? How player evaluation can be improved

*Stephen Cobley, Chris Towlson, Shaun Abbott, Michael Romann and Ric Lovell*

## Introduction

For professional soccer clubs, being able to accurately identify and optimally develop youth potential – commonly known as talent identification and development (TID; Cobley, Schorer, & Baker, 2012; Williams & Reilly, 2000) – is valuable both in performance and financial terms. For instance, if soccer clubs can develop promising youth players and facilitate their transition to higher-level (senior) performance, there are potential performance benefits. Similarly, if developed high-performing players attract interest from other clubs, potential financial benefits may occur from transfer fees. Yet, while TID systems have become progressively systematised and professionalised in practice (Winand, 2010) via club academies (or local 'feeder' programmes), the capability to achieve the professional-level is fraught with complexity and challenges (Cobley, Schorer, Baker, 2020). To illustrate, data across sports contexts highlight only relatively low percentages (~30%) of youth remain within TID systems for ≥3 years (Güllich, 2014; Güllich & Emrich, 2012). In soccer specifically, <1% of boys recruited to player development centres in youth soccer in England go on to forge a professional career (Read, Oliver, De Ste Croix, Myer, & Lloyd, 2016). Such evidence questions the validity and rationality for TID-related early selection, player differentiation, and specialisation (Baker, Cobley & Fraser-Thomas, 2009; Güllich & Cobley, 2017).

There are potentially multiple theoretical and practical explanations as to *why* soccer TID systems presently may not be (acceptably) effective, either in terms of inaccurate identification or sub-optimal (or even inhibitory) training and development practices. More gravitated explanations highlight limitations in considering (and developing) the multi-factorial, holistic, facets of performance (Reilly, Williams, Nevill, & Franks, 2000; Vaeyens, Lenoir, Williams, & Philippaerts, 2008). The complex interactions that occur over time between individual player characteristics and qualities of the development environment have also been highlighted (Cobley, 2016). Here individual characteristics refer to – for example – genetic (e.g., neurological and biological stage of development; gene allele adaptability), physical (e.g., aerobic and anaerobic capacities), and cognitive (e.g., executive functioning: early-age stimulation) characteristics as well as technical (e.g., motor coordination and skill development), social (e.g., quality of family relationships and support), and emotional (e.g., empathetic and responsive to others) skills or constraints. Whereas qualities of the immediate developmental environment refer to factors such as coaching knowledge and expertise; coaching social and interaction skills; and the types of training activities deployed (including volumes and intensities) according to developmental stages of game involvement. On this basis, it can be proposed that variability in developmental environment qualities can lead to group-level differences in development. Likewise, when considering interactions with pre-existing individual characteristics (and constraints), similar environmental qualities and exposure, may lead to varied individualised player response qualities over time [*Note:* wider influential club-organisational and environmental factors could also be listed and considered as impacting player development].

## Inter-player developmental differences: relative age and maturation status

While acknowledging the potential range of multi-factorial interactions related to youth player development, in this chapter, we focus on inter-player biological developmental differences as a foundational concern. Two sources of developmental difference are examined, namely: *relative age* and *maturational status.* We examine these factors, as both independently (and potentially interactively) influence facets of performance, particularly in youth development stages. They both confound the process of youth player selection and evaluation (Pearson, Naughton, & Torode, 2006), when using either subjective (e.g., scout or coach judgement) or objective assessment methods (e.g., standardised measurement testing procedures), leading to relative age (RA) and maturity biases (Cobley & Till, in press). The influence of these factors on performance is not stable, but rather transient over time; with individual players – for instance – illustrating differing maturational development trajectories. In a general sense, their influence increases from childhood to adolescence (9–16 years in boys), with progressive reductions toward adulthood (16+ years), but their effects on future player evaluation, TID de(selection), and game involvement can be long-lasting. In the following sections, we explain the relationships between relative age, biological maturation, and facets of athletic performance with reference to youth and academy-level soccer; and illustrate RA and maturity biases. Importantly, we then outline a strategy to address these relationships and inequalities (i.e., RA or maturation-based corrective adjustment procedures). We explain how these can be deployed to account for player developmental differences; helping improve the accuracy of player evaluation and selection practices.

Relative age refers to the interaction between a player's 'birth date' and dates used for chronological age-grouping. As such, a coincidental individual-environment interaction can generate age-based developmental differences (i.e., up to potentially 364 days for each annual age-group across 8–18 years), assuming players follow a similar, normative growth and maturational trajectory (Cobley, Romann, Javet, Abbott, & Lovell, 2020). Typically, 'relatively older' players are considered as those whose birth-date reside within the 1st quartile (Q1) of a cut-off date (e.g., UK youth soccer = Sept–Nov). By contrast, 'relatively younger' players' birthdates reside in the last quartile (i.e., Q4; UK soccer = June–August). Independently, RA influences soccer-related performance indices in youth ages. However, potential inter-player anthropometric and physiological performance-related differences can be exacerbated (or reduced) when considered alongside maturational status (see Cobley et al., 2020).

Maturation is regarded as a process of growth towards the mature adult state (Malina, 1994), with component features of *timing, tempo,* and *magnitudes of change* in body size and associated capabilities (Malina, Bouchard, & Bar-Or, 2004). Genetically and hormonally driven, the timing of re-accelerated (maturational) adolescent

348  *Stephen Cobley et al.*

growth in Caucasian populations can typically vary between 13 and 15 years in males (i.e., 'normative maturing'), assuming a normatively distributed sample (i.e., where approximately 68% of the sample is represented). Nonetheless, peak maturation-related growth can occur – although observed with less-expected frequency (estimated at 15.85% of a sample) – at 11–12 (i.e., 'earlier maturing') and 15–16 years of age (i.e., 'later maturing'); Philippaerts et al., 2006; Simpkin, Sayers, Gilthorpe, Heron & Tilling, 2017). Body size and feature characteristics (e.g., height, body mass, muscle, and fat tissue composition change) are all affected by re-accelerated growth. For instance, rudimentary height gain for the 'normative maturer' occurs around 14.0 years, with approximately 10–12 cm/year of gain (i.e., peak height velocity – PHV) commonly apparent, before progressive reductions in post-PHV years. For Caucasian females, the 'normative' age range for peak maturation-related growth occurs between 11 and 13 years of age, with potentially 'earlier' and 'later-maturity' timing initiating at 9.5–11 and 13–14 years, respectively. For the 'normative maturing' female, typical height gains have been estimated at 9–10 cm/year peaking at 12 years, before the progressive reduction in post-PHV years (Kelly et al., 2014; Granados, Gebremariam, & Lee, 2015). Similar maturity-timing variations lead to distinct developmental curves across chronological years (e.g., 10–18 years of age) for other anthropometric (weight – see, e.g., Carrascosa et al., 2018) and physiological indices (e.g., strength – see, e.g., Morris et al., 2018; Emmonds et al., 2017). As such, soccer players who reside within similar age-groups (i.e., 11–16 in males; 10–15 in females) *may* differ markedly according to maturation status and correspondingly connected anthropometric and physiological characteristics.

### Relative age and maturation influences on performance facets

Multi-centre studies have identified small, although practically meaningful anthropometric and physiological advantages that are conferred to Q1 vs Q4 players at the earliest stages of the TID cycle (e.g., under 10–13 age-groups) in soccer. These advantages include (although not exhaustive) stature, body mass, sprinting, agility, and jumping (Deprez et al., 2015b; Lovell et al., 2015). The influence of RA upon several physiological qualities is also demonstrated in cross-sectional (Towlson, Cobley, Parkin, & Lovell, 2018) and longitudinal youth soccer studies (Fransen et al., 2017) where performance trajectories were modelled. In Figure 21.1, the chronological and RA relationships with the (a) agility (T-test – Semenick, 1990) and (b) multi-stage fitness test ([20-m MSFT]; i.e., an aerobic capacity test – Leger & Lambert, 1982) are shown. Within the plots, the isolated black solid circles (●) denote two example players in the under 13s age-group ($N$ = 123), with the highest and lowest relative age; note their performance differences. A summary of modelled differences in males in the under 10s age-group – considered a pre-maturation stage – is provided in Table 21.1. The hypothetical, maximal estimated advantages, afforded to the 'relatively oldest' (Q1) player based on two studies reviewed in Table 21.1 correspond (and often exceed) the difference magnitudes observed in studies. That said, superior anthropometric and physiological qualities based on RA have been consistently observed in selected (or more successful) academy players (Deprez, Fransen, Lenoir, Philippaerts, & Vaeyens, 2015a; Patel, Nevill, Smith, Cloak, & Wyon, 2020).

The performance advantages afforded to the relatively older player, due to predicted advances in normative growth, influence positional role allocation (Towlson et al.,

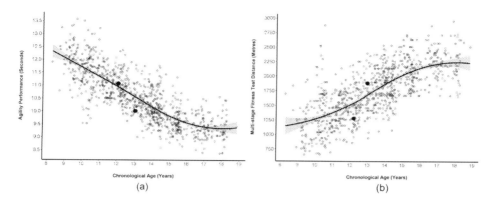

*Figure 21.1a, b* The relationship between chronological and relative age with (a) the agility (T-test), and (b) with the multi-stage fitness test (20-m MFST) in UK soccer academy players (N = 969; Towlson et al., 2018).

Notes: Black solid change the shape here to solid circles (●) denote example individuals (n = 2) with the highest and lowest relative age in the under 13s age-group (N = 123).

*Table 21.1* Modelled differences in physiological performance indices according to relative age between two hypothetical youth male soccer players at the entry point to the talent development process (i.e., under 10 age-group)

| Physiological test | Study | Player A (Q1) (Age = 9.00 years) | Player B (Q4) (Age = 9.99 years) | Difference |
|---|---|---|---|---|
| Agility (T-test) | Fransen et al. | 9.70 s | 9.50 s | 0.20 s |
|  | Towlson et al. | 12.15 s | 11.76 s | 0.39 s |
| Yo–Yo IR1 | Fransen et al. | 621 m | 821 m | 200 m |
| Multi-stage fitness test | Towlson et al. | 1023 m | 1190 m | 167 m |
| 10-m Sprint | Fransen et al. | 2.25 s | 2.19 s | 0.06 s |
|  | Towlson et al. | 1.99 s | 1.95 s | 0.04 s |
| 20-m Sprint | Fransen et al. | 3.94 s | 3.83 s | 0.11 s |
|  | Towlson et al. | 3.64 s | 3.57 s | 0.07 s |
| Vertical jump | Towlson et al. | 21.1 cm | 23.0 cm | 1.9 cm |
| Standing broad jump | Fransen et al. | 151.4 cm | 160.6 cm | 9.2 cm |

Notes: Data estimated via digitisation of published segmented regression plots (physiological test ~ chronological age). IR1 = Intermittent recovery test – level 1.

2017), playing opportunities (Vaeyens, Philippaerts, & Malina, 2005), and performance outcomes (Augste & Lames, 2011) within TID systems. As a stable advantage across youth ages (if dates for age-grouping do not change), RA can thus relate to diverging Q1 vs Q4 player development paths at least until growth differences diminish. There is no data available on the relationships between RA and soccer performance indices in female players. Although it is suspected that such relationships are limited to earlier age-groups, with lower inter-player differences and with more complex relationships (Smith, Weir, Till, Romann, & Cobley, 2018).

In older age-groups, several researchers have either shown RA differences of smaller effect magnitude (Deprez et al., 2013; Lovell et al., 2015) or no distinct disadvantages were apparent for relatively younger players within youth academies (Carling, Le Gall, Reilly, & Williams, 2008; Skorski, Skorski, Faude, Hammes, & Meyer, 2016). While initially seeming to contrast with prior findings, either advanced normative growth (e.g., Patel, Nevill, Cloak, Smith, & Wyon, 2019) or advanced, earlier, biological maturation (Müller, Gonaus, Perner, Müller, & Raschner, 2017) may provide the explanations. In other words, anthropometric and physiological profile homogeneity may have occurred via selection in later age-groups. Lovell et al. (2015), for example, identified that under 10 Q4 players were between the 75th and 91st centile in population stature, whereas Q1 players resided around the 50th centile for their chronological age. While in older age-groups, relatively younger academy players were advanced in biological maturation terms for their respective chronological age.

The potential for substantial inter-player variation in both maturation timing and tempo influences many performance facets. These include aerobic capacity, sprinting speed, agility, and strength (Deprez et al., 2013; Lovell et al., 2015), which collectively can also influence physical match performance outcomes (Lovell et al., 2019). Whilst the influence of maturation has asynchronous relationships across adolescence (Philippaerts et al., 2006; Towlson et al., 2018), maturation is generally associated with accelerated physiological development. Towlson et al. (2018) captured these changing, dynamic, relationships when modelling cross-sectional data across 900+ players who were participating in 23 UK soccer academies (Tiers 2–4). Figure 21.2 shows, for instance, relationships between maturity status and performance in the (a) agility (T-test) and (b) 20-m MSFT. Within the plots, the isolated black solid circles (●) denote two example players in the under 13s age-group ($N = 123$), with the highest and lowest relative age. However, the white markers (○) identify two players with the highest and lowest maturity status at under 13s, but who had the exact same relative age: demonstrating the independent influence of maturation status on performance indices.

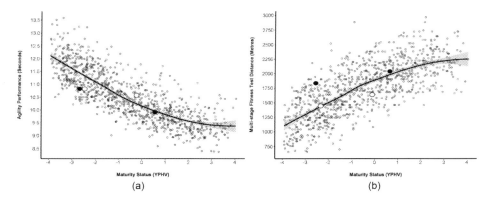

*Figure 21.2a, b* The relationship between maturity status (YPHV) with (a) the agility (T-test) and (b) with the multi-stage fitness test (20-m MFST) in UK soccer academy players ($N = 969$; Towlson et al., 2018).

Notes: Black solid squares (■) denote example individuals ($n = 2$) with the highest and lowest relative age in the under 13s age-group ($N = 123$). White squares (□) denote example individuals ($n = 2$) with the highest and lowest maturity status when chronological age was the same in the under 13s sample ($N = 123$).

*How player evaluation can be improved* 351

*Table 21.2* Modelled differences in physical qualities according to biological maturity between two elite-youth male soccer players within the same chronological age (14.3-years old; i.e., under 15 age-group)

| Anthropometric or physiological test | Player A (YPHV = −0.65) | Player B (YPHV = 1.02) | Difference |
|---|---|---|---|
| Stature | 154.5 cm | 171.3 cm | 16.8 cm |
| Body mass | 46.2 kg | 63.9 kg | 17.7 kg |
| Agility (T-test) | 10.43 s | 9.79 s | 0.64 s |
| Multi-stage fitness test | 1733 m | 2051 m | 318 m |
| 10-m Sprint | 1.77 s | 1.63 s | 0.14 s |
| 20-m Sprint | 3.22 s | 2.95 s | 0.27 s |
| Vertical jump | 29.3 cm | 33.2 cm | 3.9 cm |

Notes: Stature, body mass, and somatic maturity data taken from two national-level youth players. Physiological test data estimated via digitisation of Towlson et al. (2018) segmented regression plots (physiological test ~ YPHV). YPHV = Years from peak height velocity.

Using the derived regression parameters, estimated performance differences can be forecasted between players of similar chronological age (14.3 years), but who were at different stages of biological maturation. In this case, the inter-player differences in maturity timing are relatively modest (1.67 years), considering maturation status within a similar age-group can be as much as six years (Johnson, Doherty, & Freemont, 2009). The anthropometric and physiological differences predicted for the two individual players are summarised in Table 21.2. Comparison of difference magnitudes in Tables 21.1 and 21.2 demonstrates the potential greater impact of maturity status if maturation timing (and thus status) is highly varied between players. Nevertheless, caution is required as these differences are transient, with some athletic capacities in 'late maturing' males often exceeding those of their 'earlier-maturing' peers in late (adult) years (Lefevre, Beunen, Steens, Claessens, & Renson, 2009; Pearson et al., 2006).

## Relative age and maturational biases in youth soccer

Given the relationships between RA and maturation with performance facets and identified (changing) inter-player differences within and across age-groups, it is perhaps not surprising for participation and selection biases to exist in youth soccer. In RA terms, biases are associated with the over-valuing and selection of players born within the first and second quartiles of a given age-group (Cobley et al., 2009; Lovell et al., 2015). For example, in Lovell et al.'s sample (N = 1212) of UK academy soccer players, which spanned adolescence (i.e., under 9–18 age-groups), 48.6% were relatively older (Q1) players. By comparison, only 9.2% of selected academy players were relatively younger (Q4). Of these players, odds ratio (OR) statistics revealed Q1 players were 5.3 (95% CI 4.08–6.83) times more likely to be selected than Q4s, with the bias strongest at under 13–16 age-groups (i.e., OR = 5.45–6.13); time-points coinciding with periods of accelerated growth (Towlson et al., 2018).

Such biases or inequalities are not new or unknown in soccer (Cobley et al., 2009). In fact, the original soccer-related studies were published almost three decades ago (Barnsley et al., 1992), with Helsen et al. (1998) showing clear over-representations of relatively older Q1 (31–46%) compared to Q4 (6.8–18%) within a sample of selected Belgium youth soccer players (6–16 years old). Despite such prevalence, at the turn of the

352 *Stephen Cobley et al.*

millennia (i.e., data from 2000/01) and when again examining a similar context, Helsen et al. (2012) noted that little had changed a decade later (i.e., 2010/11; Q1 = 31.9%, Q4 = 18.4%). Relative age and maturation bias continue to influence soccer player evaluation and selection processes across the globe (see data from Spain – Mujika et al., 2009; France – Delorme, Boiché, & Raspaud, 2010; Brazil – Costa, Albuquerque, & Garganta, 2012; Germany – Skorski et al., 2016; and China – Li et al., 2020).

The robustness of developmental biases likely occurs due to the consistent application of chronological age groupings, which don't account for the often transient large between-player maturity-related differences in anthropometry and physical fitness characteristics (Philippaerts et al., 2006; Towlson et al., 2018). Relatively older players are often – although not always – the beneficiaries of early exposure to normative growth curves (Malina et al., 2004, 2000), possessing superior anthropometrical dimensions (e.g., stature) and performance characteristics (e.g., power, speed, strength, and endurance; Carling et al., 2012, 2009; Vaeyens et al., 2006). This explanation for RA and maturational biases in participation and selection is commonly known as the maturation-selection hypothesis (Cobley et al., 2009; Helsen et al., 2005). Jackson and Comber (2020) also illustrated the cumulative probability of academy retention was higher for relatively older players and correspondingly lower for relatively younger players (i.e., Q4). Thus, relatively younger players are systematically disadvantaged, and implicitly discriminated against in terms of de-selection, particularly in player positions favouring enhanced maturity-related anthropometric and physiological characteristics (Towlson et al., 2017). Such trends stand glaringly opposed to wider knowledge and understanding of inter-player developmental differences being temporary; short-lived within the adolescence timespan; and with reducing/subsiding differences post-maturation (Till, Cobley, O'Hara, Chapman, & Cooke, 2013; Lovell et al., 2015), suggesting biases also reflect TID inaccuracy.

## Removing inter-player developmental differences and biases to improve player evaluation

While RA and maturity-selection biases persist, practical attempts have been suggested or implemented to remove or reduce their impact. These include the creation of shorter (e.g., 9-month) and/or rotating age group cut-off dates in other sports contexts (i.e., ice-hockey – Boucher & Halliwell, 1991; Hurley, Lior, & Tracze, 2001), along with proposals to group players based on stature and body mass classifications (Baxter-Jones, 1995; Musch & Grondin, 2001). In outlining a range of strategies, with reference to team sports, Cobley (2016, 2017) promoted organisational policies targeting: (i) the delay of age time-points for structured competition; and relatedly, (ii) the delay of age time-points when tiers of selective representation occur (i.e., post-maturation). Targeted more specifically to youth soccer, Mann and van Ginneken (2017) illustrated how the use of 'RA ordered' shirt-numbering could help prevent RA bias in coach assessment and player evaluation. Furthermore, maturity status 'bio-banding' (see Cumming et al., 2018) – as opposed to age-grouping – has also been implemented and evaluated in terms of impact upon player game involvement and coach evaluation (see Bradley et al., 2019; Romann, Lüdin, & Born., 2020; Towlson et al., 2021). Meanwhile, developed in the sports contexts of track and field and swimming, 'corrective performance adjustments procedures' (Romann & Cobley, 2015) also show potential for soccer application.

## Relative age and maturation-based corrective adjustment procedures

Corrective Adjustment Procedures (CAPs) refer to the process of purposefully removing the underlying influence of either RA or maturation status differences from age-group performance and player evaluation (Cobley, Abbott, Moulds, Hogan, & Romann, 2020). Whether considering specific sport events (e.g., 100 m in athletics) or as part of performance testing within a sport (e.g., soccer), objective measurements (i.e., centimetres, seconds, etc.; Moesch, Elbe, Hauge, & Wikman, 2011) are used to determine performance relative to others. Therefore, the relationships between RA or maturation status and the performance measure can be directly plotted, and quantified, with reference to multiple or single age-group cohorts. Subsequently, trendline properties in these relationships are utilised to adjust individual performance to a standardised RA (e.g., relatively oldest individual in an age-group) or maturation status (e.g., individual with highest maturity status in an age-group) within the larger cohort. Such adjusting generates a 'correctively adjusted performance' measure (e.g., sprint time in seconds); one which estimates performance based on a RA or maturation-matched status across all individuals within a particular age-group.

CAPs were first utilised by Romann and Cobley (2015) in their examination of 7,000+ Swiss male junior athletic 60-m sprinters aged 8–15 years old. The relatively older were expectedly over-represented as Q1 v Q4 ORs ranged between 2.11 and 1.55 at 9- to 15-year-olds, respectively. But, when examining the 'Top 50–10%' of sprint times (i.e., not the whole sample), Relative age effect (RAE) size increased in each age group (i.e., OR range = 2.61–5.03). To address these biases, the negative linear trendline between decimal age and sprint performance was used (see Figure 21.1 in Romann & Cobley, 2015). The expected difference in performance times from being 1 day to 1 year younger for each age group was calculated. Given sprinter decimal age on the day of participation, each sprinter's performance time was then adjusted relative to the oldest sprinter within an age-group, generating a 'corrected performance time'. Importantly, when re-examining the 'Top 50–10%' of 'corrected sprint times', RAE inequalities were removed in almost all age-groups. Only in isolated younger age-groups at specific performance levels (i.e., under 9 and 10 in 'Top 50%' of sprint times) did typical RAEs remain, likely due to the higher frequency of relatively older individuals volunteering to participate. Since, RA-based CAPs have been successfully tested in youth males (Cobley et al., 2019) and females (Abbott et al., 2020) swimming using substantive longitudinal sampling and more advanced analytical approaches.

More recently, Abbott et al. (2021) trialled the application of Maturation-based (Mat-) CAPs on 700+ Australian male regional/state-level 100 m front-crawl swimmers aged 12–17 years. Abbott and colleagues first identified an overwhelming and consistent over-representation of 'early-maturing' swimmers across all age-groups and section levels ('Top 50%' & 'Top 25%' of swim times). Notably, there was a complete absence of 'late-maturing' swimmers. Using the curvilinear relationship between maturation status and swim performance, Abbott et al., adjusted individual swim performance times relative to the most mature swimmer in each age-group. Then, when maturity distributions of 'corrected performance times' were examined across the 'Top 50%' and '25%', maturity biases within the sample were removed. Thus, RA- and Mat-CAPs provide a strategy to remove respective RA or maturational influences from performance, prevent short-term (de-)selection biases, and increase the accuracy of youth athlete evaluation.

354 *Stephen Cobley et al.*

RA- and Mat-CAPs can be applied to youth soccer. However, determining individual performance in soccer is different to sprinting and swimming. Quantifying individual performance within a team-game context is not easily isolated, with inter-dependence with other 'in-game' team factors relative to the opposition necessary. Instead, individual performance can be indirectly assessed via assessments deemed as facet components of 'in-game' performance (e.g., physiological aerobic and anaerobic capacities, sprint speed etc.). Therefore, to illustrate, we return to Towlson et al.'s (2018) data on 969 youth academy soccer players (aged 8–18 years). In Figure 21.1, the relationships between chronological and RA with (a) agility and (b) 20 m MSFT performance are plotted. The curvilinear trendlines along with 95% confidence intervals (shaded area about the trendline) are shown.

Table 21.3 provides a summary of raw and correctively adjusted Agility performance data for the 'Top-five' raw ranked players; five of the 'relatively youngest' players; and five players with the lowest maturation status in the Under 13 academy sample. For each of these player categories, raw rank; agility time; RA quartile; maturation status; and maturation category (relative to normative population distributions) are shown. In the 'Top-five' performers, the favourable benefit from earlier RA and/or advanced maturation status is descriptively apparent. The next three columns provide the Relative Age-based (RA-CAPS) correctively adjusted agility time; percentage change from the raw time; and adjusted rank, with the relatively oldest individual in the Under 13s age-group used as the reference. The final three columns show the maturation-based (Mat-CAPS) correctively adjusted agility time; percentage change from the raw time; and adjusted rank with the player of the highest maturation status in the Under 13s acting as the reference.

For the 'Top-five' performers, results identify minimal changes in time, percentage change in time, or rank from RA-CAPs, though with slightly greater changes from Mat-CAPs. These changes are somewhat expected, given the increased likelihood of being relatively older and/or of maturation status to attain 'Top-five' performance (i.e., closer proximity to the reference player). Here, recognise the changes in rank order, with some players descending out of the 'Top-five' (e.g., raw rank 5 - rank 15 following Mat-CAPs). In other words, such cases could be potentially 'over-valued' in terms of physical agility, due to advanced developmental differences.

When reviewing the five relatively youngest players, their comparatively slower agility performance time and rank status relative to the 'Top-five' performers can be immediately identified, along with the likelihood of lower maturation status. Following RA-based corrective adjustments, a 3.1–3.3% reduction in performance time was apparent, with increases in rank occurring (rank change range = 5–14). Similarly, when reviewing five players of the lowest maturation status within the academy sample, firstly note the absence of 'later maturing' players in the academy. Second – and expectedly – slower raw agility times and ranks are apparent. But, following Mat-CAPS, individual performance times were reduced by 7.4–9.1%, with rank increases ranging between 9–33. Interestingly, one player jumped from outside the 'Top 20' to being ranked second, suggesting that some case players might be 'under-valued' or less well recognised due to developmental differences. It is in relation to these case players, where RA and Mat-CAPs could have positive, informative, value.

With reference to 20 m MSFT data, Table 21.4 similarly provides a summary of raw and correctively adjusted results for Towlson et al.'s (2018) Under 13 sample. In the 20 m MSFT, the 'Top-five' performing players were not necessarily all relatively older or

Table 21.3 Agility test performance according to 'top-five ranked', 'relatively youngest', and 'lowest maturation status' youth academy football players (under 13 years). Relative age and maturity status *corrective adjustment procedures* determined adjusted performance scores and ranks based on the relatively oldest (*) and most mature male player (†), respectively

| + | Age group | Rank | Agility | Decimal age | Maturity status | Category | RA adj. time* | % Change* | Adj. rank* | Mat. adj. time† | % Change† | Adj. rank† |
|---|---|---|---|---|---|---|---|---|---|---|---|---|
| **Raw top-5 performers** | Under 13 | 1 | 9.63 | 12.59 | −0.31 | Early | 9.49 | −1.47 | 1 | 9.48 | −1.59 | 5 |
| | Under 13 | 2 | 9.83 | 12.82 | −1.09 | Normative | 9.77 | −0.62 | 5 | 9.33 | −5.09 | 1 |
| | Under 13 | 3 | 9.85 | 12.90 | −0.85 | Normative | 9.82 | −0.30 | 7 | 9.45 | −3.96 | 3 |
| | Under 13 | 4 | 9.89 | 12.61 | −0.76 | E.Norm | 9.75 | −1.39 | 3 | 9.54 | −3.50 | 7 |
| | Under 13 | 5 | 9.91 | 12.36 | −0.42 | Early | 9.68 | −2.28 | 2 | 9.71 | −2.01 | 15 |
| **Relatively youngest** | Under 13 | 114 | 11.68 | 12.01 | −1.69 | Normative | 11.32 | −3.08 | 109 | | | |
| | Under 13 | 86 | 11.02 | 12.01 | −1.40 | E.Norm | 10.66 | −3.26 | 74 | | | |
| | Under 13 | 102 | 11.3 | 12.01 | −1.59 | Normative | 10.94 | −3.17 | 93 | | | |
| | Under 13 | 70 | 10.86 | 12.01 | −1.13 | E.Norm | 10.50 | −3.30 | 56 | | | |
| | Under 13 | 71 | 10.88 | 12.03 | −1.61 | Normative | 10.53 | −3.23 | 58 | | | |
| **Lowest maturation status** | Under 13 | 22 | 10.30 | 12.11 | −1.96 | Normative | | | | 9.36 | −9.12 | 2 |
| | Under 13 | 108 | 11.56 | 12.23 | −1.86 | Normative | | | | 10.67 | −7.64 | 99 |
| | Under 13 | 67 | 10.85 | 12.22 | −1.84 | Normative | | | | 9.97 | −8.06 | 34 |
| | Under 13 | 95 | 11.15 | 12.34 | −1.76 | Normative | | | | 10.32 | −7.44 | 66 |
| | Under 13 | 76 | 10.92 | 12.16 | −1.73 | Normative | | | | 10.10 | −7.47 | 44 |
| *Reference 1* – relatively oldest* | *Under 13* | *14* | *10.16* | *12.99* | *−0.68* | *Normative* | | | | | | |
| *Reference 2† – most mature* | *Under 13* | *10* | *10.05* | *12.99* | *0.08* | *Early* | | | | | | |

Notes: E. Norm = Early normative maturity timing based on sample-specific APHV M ± SD.

*Table 21.4* Multi-stage fitness test performance according to 'top-five' ranked', 'relatively youngest', and 'lowest maturation status' youth academy football players (under 13 years). Relative age and maturity status *corrective adjustment procedures* determined adjusted performance scores and ranks based on the relatively oldest (*) and most mature male player (†), respectively

| | Age group | Rank | Distance | Decimal age | Maturity status | Category | RA Adj. distance* | % Change* | Adj. rank* | Mat. Adj. distance† | % Change† | Adj. rank† |
|---|---|---|---|---|---|---|---|---|---|---|---|---|
| **Raw Top-5 Performers** | Under 13 | 1 | 2,400 | 12.96 | −0.77 | Normative | 2,404 | 0.16 | 1 | 2,547 | 6.11 | 1 |
| | Under 13 | 2 | 2,280 | 12.91 | −0.85 | Normative | 2,291 | 0.47 | 5 | 2,441 | 7.06 | 4 |
| | Under 13 | 3 | 2,260 | 12.55 | −1.17 | Normative | 2,341 | 3.57 | 2 | 2,482 | 9.83 | 3 |
| | Under 13 | 4 | 2,260 | 12.44 | −1.29 | Normative | 2,324 | 2.85 | 4 | 2,504 | 10.81 | 2 |
| | Under 13 | 5 | 2,200 | 12.12 | −0.83 | Early | 2,327 | 5.78 | 3 | 2,357 | 7.13 | 6 |
| **Relatively Youngest** | Under 13 | 24 | 1,860 | 12.01 | −1.69 | Normative | 2,004 | 7.75 | 15 | | | |
| | Under 13 | 72 | 1,480 | 12.01 | −1.40 | E.Norm | 1,624 | 9.74 | 61 | | | |
| | Under 13 | 101 | 1,260 | 12.01 | −1.59 | Normative | 1,404 | 11.41 | 99 | | | |
| | Under 13 | 40 | 1,720 | 12.01 | −1.13 | E.Norm | 1,864 | 8.36 | 30 | | | |
| | Under 13 | 46 | 1,640 | 12.03 | −1.61 | Normative | 1,781 | 8.59 | 41 | | | |
| **Lowest Maturation Status** | Under 13 | 70 | 1,500 | 12.11 | −1.96 | Normative | | | | 1,883 | 25.51 | 45 |
| | Under 13 | 56 | 1,540 | 12.23 | −1.86 | Normative | | | | 1,900 | 23.38 | 43 |
| | Under 13 | 56 | 1,540 | 12.22 | −1.84 | Normative | | | | 1,897 | 23.18 | 44 |
| | Under 13 | 90 | 1,380 | 12.34 | −1.76 | Normative | | | | 1,719 | 24.57 | 68 |
| | Under 13 | 37 | 1,740 | 12.16 | −1.73 | Normative | | | | 2,074 | 19.18 | 26 |
| *Reference 1\* - Relatively Oldest* | *Under 13* | *79* | *1,460* | *12.99* | *−0.68* | *Normative* | | | | | | |
| *Reference 2† - Most Mature* | *Under 13* | *22* | *1,880* | *12.99* | *0.08* | *Early* | | | | | | |

Notes: E. Norm = Early normative maturity timing based on sample-specific APHV M ± SD.

How player evaluation can be improved  357

earlier maturing, though advantages were still expectedly gained (see Figures 19.1a, b and 19.2a, b). When RA-CAPs and Mat-CAPs were applied to the 'Top-five', there were again lesser percentage changes in performance via RA-CAPs (0.2–5.8%) versus Mat-CAPs (6.1–10.8%), and there was minimal change in rank order. Nonetheless, when reviewing results on the five relatively youngest players, their distance ran, and rank was expectedly lower. Following RA-CAPs, their performances increased by an estimated 7.7–11.4%, with corresponding rank improvements ranging between 2 and 11 (note: one case rank changed from 24 to 15). When Mat-CAPs were applied to the five players of the lowest maturation status, their correctively adjusted estimated distance ran increased by 19.2–25.5%, with rank order changes ranging between 11 and 25.

## Future directions and conclusions

If advanced inter-individual developmental differences are contra-indicators of youth soccer talent and player evaluation procedures, and CAPs can be considered as a viable strategy to implement, then several future directions can be recommended. Principally, soccer organisations and their practitioners (e.g., youth academy managers, coaches, scouts) should measure (and track) RA and maturity status. These indices should also be integrated within player evaluation and (de-)selection processes. To facilitate a more objective approach, with inter-player developmental differences considered, this chapter recommends assessing relationships between RA and/or maturation status with physical performance indices, and then apply RA- or Mat-CAPs. Nevertheless, whilst pitched as beneficial, existing RA- or Mat-CAP studies also highlight caution.

Within soccer, CAPs appear best placed to be applied as part of fitness testing or physiological assessments. As CAPs estimate an adjusted performance value, measurement accuracy is paramount. Therefore, the accuracy and limitations of somatic-based maturation estimates along with the precision (or error) for each performance measurement must be considered (see e.g., Mills, Baker, Pacey, Wollin, & Drew (2017). The application of the most accurate methods - where feasible – is recommended. Furthermore, a substantially large reference sample must be acquired, with consistent data across (relative) age and/or maturation status necessary to generate accurate reference trendlines and regression parameters (Cobley et al., 2020). To address measurement concerns; non-linearity in maturation-associated growth trajectories (i.e., higher or lower growth tempo in short-time periods); and, the need for validity in correctively adjusted performance estimates, regular testing and CAPs application is recommended (e.g., two to three times per year; Towlson et al., in press). Finally, the respective demands of soccer physiological tests should also be considered. As tests have different underpinning (and inter-acting) anthropometric, physiological, movement coordination (technical) skill and biomechanical demands, the degree to which developmental differences (also at a given age) influences performance should be considered. Such variation will partially explain why RA- and Mat-CAPs may lead to greater or lesser changes in performance adjustment (e.g., see agility vs 20-m MSFT). Change estimates are also expected to vary according to the age and sex of the samples examined.

If precautionary messages are addressed, we predict corrected performance indices will help enable practitioners to: (i) better evaluate physical performance attainment relative to others; (ii) determine which other physiological, biomechanical, technical,

358  *Stephen Cobley et al.*

and psychological factors may be accounting for better or worse performance relative to others; (iii) identify differing developmental trajectories between players; and (iv) identify necessary training interventions (e.g., strength and conditioning) to optimise player development. If achieved, the accuracy of player evaluation in the short term will be improved, which may subsequently contribute toward achieving greater effectiveness in long-term player development programmes.

## References

Abbott, S., Hogan, C., Castiglioni, M. T., Yamauchi, G., Mitchell, L. J., Salter, J., ... & Cobley, S. (2021). Maturity-related developmental inequalities in age-group swimming: The testing of 'Mat-CAPs' for their removal. *Journal of Science and Medicine in Sport*, 24(4), 397–404.

Abbott, S., Moulds, K., Salter, J., Romann, M., Edwards, L., & Cobley, S. (2020). Testing the application of corrective adjustment procedures for removal of relative age effects in female youth swimming. *Journal of Sports Sciences, 38*(10), 1077–1084. https://doi.org/10.1080/0264 0414.2020.1741956

Augste, C., & Lames, M. (2011). The relative age effect and success in German elite U-17 soccer teams. *Journal of Sports Sciences, 29*(9), 983–987. http://doi.org/10.1080/02640414.2011.574719

Baker, J., Cobley, S., & Fraser-Thomas, J. (2009). What do we know about early sport specialisation? Not much! *High Ability Studies, 20*(1), 77–89. https://doi.org/10.1080/13598130902860507

Barnsley, R. H., Thompson, A. H., & Legault, P. (1992). Family planning: football style. The relative age effect in football. *International Review for the Sociology of Sport, 27*(1), 77–87.

Baxter-Jones, A. D. (1995). Growth and development of young athletes. *Sports Medicine, 20*(2), 59–64.

Boucher, J., & Halliwell, W. (1991). The Novem system: a practical solution to age grouping. *Canadian Association for Health, Physical Education, and Recreation, 57*(1), 16–20.

Bradley, B., Johnson, D., Hill, M., McGee, D., Kana-Ah, A., Sharpin, C., Sharp, P., Kelly, A., Cumming, S. P., & Malina, R. M. (2019, Aug). Bio-banding in academy football: player's perceptions of a maturity matched tournament. *Annals of Human Biology, 46*(5), 400–408. https://doi.org/10.1080/03014460.2019.1640284

Carrascosa, A., Yeste, D., Moreno-Galdó, A., Gussinyé, M., Ferrández, Á., Clemente, M., & Fernández-Cancio, M. (2018). Pubertal growth of 1,453 healthy children according to age at pubertal growth spurt onset: the Barcelona longitudinal growth study. *Anales de Pediatria, 89*(3), 144–152. https://doi.org/10.1016/j.anpedi.2017.11.018

Carling, C., Le Gall, F., Reilly, T., & Williams, A. M. (2008). Do anthropometric and fitness characteristics vary according to birth date distribution in elite youth academy soccer players? *Scandinavian Journal of Medicine and Science in Sports, 19*(1), 3–9. http://doi.org/10.1111/j.1600-0838.2008.00867.x

Carling, C., Le Gall, F., Reilly, T., & Williams, A. (2009). Do anthropometric and fitness characteristics vary according to birth date distribution in elite youth academy soccer players? *Scandinavian Journal of Medicine and Science in Sports, 19*(1), 3–9. https://doi.org/10.1111/j.1600-0838.2008.00867.x

Carling, C., Le Gall, F., & Malina, R. M. (2012). Body size, skeletal maturity, and functional characteristics of elite academy soccer players on entry between 1992 and 2003. *Journal of Sports Sciences, 30*(15), 1683–1693. https://doi.org/10.1080/02640414.2011.637950

Cobley, S. (2017). *Growth and Maturation in Athlete Development: An Educational Resource for Sporting Organisations* (pp. 1–29). Canberra, Australia: Australian Institute of Sport.

Cobley, S. (2016). Talent identification and development in youth sport. In K. Green & A. Smith (Eds.), *Routledge Handbook of Youth Sport* (pp. 476–491). Abingdon: Routledge.

Cobley, S., & Till, K. (in press). Talent identification, development, and the young rugby player. In C. Twist & Paul Worsfold (Eds.), *The Science of Rugby* (2nd Ed.). Abingdon: Routledge.

Cobley, S., Baker, J., & Chorer, J. (2012). Identification and development of sport talent: a brief introduction to a growing field of research and practice. In J. Baker, S. Cobley, & J. Schorer (Eds.), *Talent Identification and Development in Sport: International Perspectives* (pp. 1–10). London: Routledge (Taylor & Francis).

Cobley, S. P., Baker, J., Wattie, N., & McKenna, J. (2009). Annual age-grouping and athlete development. *Sports Med, 39*(3), 235–256. https://doi.org/10.2165/00007256-200939030-00005

Cobley, S., Abbott, S., Eisenhuth, J., Salter, J., McGregor, D., Romann, M. (2019). Removing relative age effects from youth swimming: the development and testing of corrective adjustment procedures. *Journal of Science and Medicine in Sport, 22*(6), 735–740. https://doi.org/10.1016/j.jsams.2018.12.013

Cobley, S., Abbott, S., Moulds, K., Hogan, C., Romann, M. (2020). Re-balancing the relative age effect scales: meta-analytical trends, causes, and corrective adjustment procedures as a solution. In J. C. Dixon, S. Horton, L. Chittle, & J. Baker (Eds.), *Relative Age Effects in Sport International Perspectives* (pp. 136–153). New York: Routledge.

Cobley, S., Romann, M., Javet, M., Abbott, S., & Lovell, R. (2020). The shifting sands of time: maturation and athlete development. In J. Baker, S. Cobley, & J. Schorer (Eds.), *Talent Identification and Development in Sport International Perspectives* (2nd Ed.), (pp. 81–98). Abingdon: Routledge (Taylor & Francis) Abingdon, Oxon, United Kingdom: Routledge (Taylor & Francis).

Costa, I. T. D., Albuquerque, R. M., & Garganta, J. (2012). Relative age effect in Brazilian soccer players: a historical analysis. *International Journal of Performance Analysis in Sport, 12*(3), 563–570. https://doi.org/10.1080/24748668.2012.11868619

Cumming, S. P., Brown, D. J., Mitchell, S., Bunce, J., Hunt, D., Hedges, C., Crane, G., Gross, A., Scott, S., Franklin, E., Breakspear, D., Dennison, L., White, P., Cain, A., Eisenmann, J. C., & Malina, R. M. (2018). Premier league academy soccer players' experiences of competing in a tournament bio-banded for biological maturation. *Journal Sports Science, 36*(7), 757–765. https://doi.org/10.1080/02640414.2017.1340656

Deprez, D. N., Fransen, J., Lenoir, M., Philippaerts, R. M., & Vaeyens, R. (2015a). A retrospective study on anthropometrical, physical fitness, and motor coordination characteristics that influence dropout, contract status, and first-team playing time in high-level soccer players aged eight to eighteen years. *Journal of Strength and Conditioning Research, 29*(6), 1692–1704. http://doi.org/10.1519/JSC.0000000000000806

Deprez, D., Buchheit, M., Fransen, J., Pion, J., Lenoir, M., Philippaerts, R. M., & Vaeyens, R. (2015b). A longitudinal study investigating the stability of anthropometry and soccer-specific endurance in pubertal high-level youth soccer players. *Journal of Sports Science and Medicine, 14*(2), 418–426.

Deprez, D., Coutts, A., Fransen, J., Deconinck, F., Lenoir, M., Vaeyens, R., & Philippaerts, R. (2013). Relative age, biological maturation and anaerobic characteristics in elite youth soccer players. *International Journal of Sports Medicine, 34*(10), 897–903. http://doi.org/10.1055/s-0032-1333262

Delorme, N., Boiché, J., & Raspaud, M. (2010). Relative age and dropout in French male soccer. *Journal of Sports Sciences, 28*(7), 717–722. https://doi.org/10.1080/02640411003663276

Emmonds, S., Morris, R., Murray, E., Robinson, C., Turner, L., & Jones, B. (2017). The influence of age and maturity status on the maximum and explosive strength characteristics of elite youth female soccer players. *Science and Medicine in Football, 1*(3), 209–215. https://doi.org/10.1080/24733938.2017.1363908

Fransen, J., Bennett, K. J. M., Woods, C. T., French-Collier, N., Deprez, D., Vaeyens, R., & Lenoir, M. (2017). Modelling age-related changes in motor competence and physical fitness in high-level youth soccer players: implications for talent identification and development. *Science and Medicine in Football, 1*(3), 203–208. http://doi.org/10.1080/24733938.2017.1366039

360 *Stephen Cobley et al.*

Granados, A., Gebremariam, A., & Lee, J. M. (2015). Relationship between timing of peak height velocity and pubertal staging in boys and girls. *Journal of Clinical Research inPediatric Endocrinology, 7*(3), 235–237. https://doi.org/10.4274/jcrpe.2007

Güllich, A. (2014). Selection, de-selection and progression in German football talent promotion. *Eur Journal of Sport Sci, 14*(6), 530–537. https://doi.org/10.1080/17461391.2013.858371

Güllich, A. & Cobley, S. (2017). On the efficacy of talent identification and talent development programmes. In J. Baker, S. Cobley, J. Schorer, & N. Wattie (Eds.), *Routledge Handbook of Talent Identification and Development in Sport* (pp. 80–98). Abingdon: Routledge. (Taylor & Francis).

Güllich, A. & Emrich, E. (2012). Individualistic and collectivistic approach in athlete support programmes in the German high-performance sport system. *European Journal of Sport and Society, 9*, 243–268. https://doi.org/10.1080/16138171.2012.11687900

Helsen, W. F., Baker, J., Michiels, S., Schorer, J., Van Winckel, J., & Williams, A. M. (2012). The relative age effect in European professional soccer: did ten years of research make any difference? *Journal of Sports Sciences, 30*(15), 1665–1671. https://doi.org/10.1080/02640414.2012.721929

Helsen, W. F., Van Winckel, J., & Williams, A. M. (2005). The relative age effect in youth soccer across Europe. *Journal of Sports Sciences, 23*(6), 629–636. https://doi.org/10.1080/02640410400021310

Helsen, W. F., Starkes, J. L., & Van Winckel, J. (1998). The influence of relative age on success and dropout in male soccer players. *American Journal of Human Biology, 10*(6), 791–798. https://doi.org/10.1002/(SICI)1520-6300(1998)10:6%3C791::AID-AJHB10%3E3.0.CO;2-1

Hurley, W., Lior, D., & Tracze, S. (2001). A proposal to reduce the age discrimination in Canadian minor hockey. *Can Public Policy – Analyse de Politiques, 27*(1), 65–75.

Jackson, R. C., & Comber, G. (2020). Hill on a mountaintop: a longitudinal and cross-sectional analysis of the relative age effect in competitive youth football. *Journal of Sports Sciences, 38*(11–12), 1352–1358. https://doi.org/10.1080/02640414.2019.1706830

Johnson, A., Doherty, P. J., & Freemont, A. (2009). Investigation of growth, development, and factors associated with injury in elite schoolboy footballers: prospective study. *BMJ (Clinical Research Ed), 338*, b490. https://doi.org/10.1136/bmj.b490

Kelly, A., Winer, K. K., Kalkwarf, H., Oberfield, S. E., Lappe, J., Gilsanz, V., & Zemel, B. S. (2014). Age-based reference ranges for annual height velocity in US children. *The Journal of Clinical Endocrinology & Metabolism, 99*(6), 2104–2112. https://doi.org/10.1210/jc.20134455

Lefevre, J., Beunen, G., Steens, G., Claessens, A., & Renson, R. (2009). Motor performance during adolescence and age thirty as related to age at peak height velocity. *Annals of Human Biology, 17*(5), 423–435. http://doi.org/10.1080/03014469000001202

Léger, L. A., & Lambert, J. (1982). A maximal multistage 20-m shuttle run test to predict VO2 max. *European Journal of Applied Physiology and Occupational Physiology, 49*(1), 1–12.

Li, Z., Mao, L., Steingröver, C., Wattie, N., Baker, J., Schorer, J., & Helsen, W. F. (2020). Relative age effects in elite Chinese soccer players: implications of the 'one-child' policy. *PloS ONE, 15*(2), e0228611. https://doi.org/10.1371/journal.pone.0228611

Lovell, R., Towlson, C., Parkin, G., Portas, M., Vaeyens, R., & Cobley, S. (2015). Soccer player characteristics in English lower-league development programmes: the relationships between relative age, maturation, anthropometry and physical fitness. *PLoS ONE, 10*(9), e0137238. http://doi.org/10.1371/journal.pone.0137238

Lovell, R., Fransen, J., Ryan, R., Massard, T., Cross, R., Eggers, T., & Duffield, R. (2019). Biological maturation and match running performance: a national football (soccer) federation perspective. *Journal of Science and Medicine in Sport, 22*(10), 1139–1145. http://doi.org/10.1016/j.jsams.2019.04.007

Malina, R.M. (1994). Physical growth and biological maturation of young athletes. *Exercise and Sport Sciences Reviews, 22*, 280–284.

Malina, R. M., Reyes, M. P., Eisenmann, J., Horta, L., Rodrigues, J., & Miller, R. (2000). Height, mass and skeletal maturity of elite Portuguese soccer players aged 11–16 years. *Journal of Sports Sciences, 18*(9), 685–693. https://doi.org/10.1080/02640410050120069

Malina, R. M., Bouchard, C., & Bar-Or, O. (2004). *Growth, Maturation, and Physical Activity.* Champaign: Human Kinetics Publishers.

Mann, D. L., & van Ginneken, P. J. (2017). Age-ordered shirt numbering reduces the selection bias associated with the relative age effect. *Journal of Sports Sciences, 35*(8), 784–790. https://doi.org/10.1080/02640414.2016.1189588

Mills, K., Baker, D., Pacey, V., Wollin, M., & Drew, M. K. (2017). What is the most accurate and reliable methodological approach for predicting peak height velocity in adolescents? A systematic review. *Journal of Science and Medicine in Sport, 20*(6), 572–577. https://doi.org/10.1016/j.jsams.2016.10.012

Moesch, K., Elbe, A. M., Hauge, M. L., & Wikman, J. M. (2011). Late specialisation: The key to success in centimeters, grams, or seconds (cgs) sports. *Scandinavian Journal of Medicine & Science in Sports, 21*(6), 282–290. https://doi.org/10.1111/j.1600-0838.2010.01280.x

Morris, R., Emmonds, S., Jones, B., Myers, T. D., Clarke, N. D., Lake, J., Ellis, M., Singleton, D., Roe, G., & Till, K. (2018). Seasonal changes in physical qualities of elite youth soccer players according to maturity status: comparisons with aged matched controls. *Science and Medicine in Football, 2*(4), 272–280. https://doi.org/10.1080/24733938.2018.1454599

Mujika, I., Vaeyens, R., Matthys, S. P., Santisteban, J., Goiriena, J., & Philippaerts, R. (2009). The relative age effect in a professional football club setting. *Journal of Sports Sciences, 27*(11), 1153–1158. https://doi.org/10.1080/02640410903220328

Müller, L., Gonaus, C., Perner, C., Müller, E., & Raschner, C. (2017). Maturity status influences the relative age effect in national top level youth alpine ski racing and soccer. *PLoS ONE, 12*(7), e0181810. http://doi.org/10.1371/journal.pone.0181810

Musch, J., & Grondin, S. (2001). Unequal competition as an impediment to personal development: a review of the relative age effect in sport. *Developmental Review, 21*(2), 147–167. https://doi.org/10.1006/drev.2000.0516

Patel, R., Nevill, A., Cloak, R., Smith, T., & Wyon, M. (2019). Relative age, maturation, anthropometry and physical performance characteristics of players within an elite youth football academy. *International Journal of Sports Science & Coaching, 14*(6), 714–725. http://doi.org/10.1177/1747954119879348

Patel, R., Nevill, A., Smith, T., Cloak, R., & Wyon, M. (2020). The influence of birth quartile, maturation, anthropometry and physical performances on player retention: observations from an elite football academy. *International Journal of Sports Science & Coaching, 15*(2), 121–134. http://doi.org/10.1177/1747954120906507

Pearson, D. T., Naughton, G. A., & Torode, M. (2006). Predictability of physiological testing and the role of maturation in talent identification for adolescent team sports. *Journal of Science and Medicine in Sport, 9*(4), 277–287. http://doi.org/10.1016/j.jsams.2006.05.020

Philippaerts, R. M., Vaeyens, R., Janssens, M., Van Renterghem, B., Matthys, D., Craen, R., Bourgois, J., Vrijens, J., Buenen, G., & Malina, R.M. (2006). The relationship between peak height velocity and physical performance in youth soccer players. *Journal of Sports Sciences, 24*(3), 221–230. http://doi.org/10.1080/02640410500189371

Read, P. J., Oliver, J. L., De Ste Croix, M. B., Myer, G. D., & Lloyd, R. S. (2016). The scientific foundations and associated injury risks of early soccer specialisation. *Journal of Sports Sciences, 34*(24), 2295–2302. https://doi.org/10.1080/02640414.2016.1173221

Reilly, T., Williams, A. M., Nevill, A., & Franks, A. (2000). A multidisciplinary approach to talent identification in soccer. *Journal of Sports Sciences, 18*(9), 695–702. https://doi.org/10.1080/02640410050120078

Romann, M., Lüdin, D., & Born, D. P. (2020). Bio-banding in junior soccer players: a pilot study. *BMC Research Notes, 13*(1), 240. https://doi.org/10.1186/s13104-020-05083-5

Romann, M., & Cobley, S. (2015). Relative age effects in athletic sprinting and corrective adjustments as a solution for their removal. *PLoS ONE, 10*(4), e0122988. https://doi.org/10.1371/journal.pone.0122988

Semenick, D. (1990). Tests and measurements: the T-test. *Strength & Conditioning Journal, 12*(1), 36–37.

Simpkin, A. J., Sayers, A., Gilthorpe, M. S., Heron, J., & Tilling, K. (2017). Modelling height in adolescence: A comparison of methods for estimating the age at peak height velocity. *Annals of Human Biology, 44*(8), 715–722. https://doi.org/10.1080/03014460.2017.1391877

Skorski, S, Skorski, S., Faude, O., Hammes, D., & Meyer, T. (2016). The relative age effect in German elite youth soccer: implications for a successful career. *International Journal of Sports Physiology and Performance, 11*(3), 370–376. http://doi.org/10.1123/ijspp.2015-0071.

Smith, K., Weir, P., Till, K., Romann, M., Cobley, S. (2018). Relative age effects across and within female sport contexts: a systematic review and meta-analysis. *Sports Medicine, 48*(6), 1451–1478. https://doi.org/10.1007/s40279-018-0890-8

Till, K., Cobley, S., O'Hara, J., Chapman, C., Cooke, C. (2013). A longitudinal evaluation of anthropometric and fitness characteristics in junior rugby league players considering playing position and selection level. *Journal of Science and Medicine in Sport, 16*(5), 438–443. https://doi.org/10.1016/j.jsams.2012.09.002

Towlson, C., Cobley, S., Midgley, A. W., Garrett, A., Parkin, G., & Lovell, R. (2017). Relative age, maturation and physical biases on position allocation in elite youth soccer. *International Journal of Sports Medicine, 38*(3), 201–209. http://doi.org/10.1055/s-0042-119029

Towlson, C., Cobley, S., Parkin, G., & Lovell, R. (2018). When does the influence of maturation on anthropometric and physical fitness characteristics increase and subside? *Scandinavian Journal of Medicine and Science in Sports, 28*(8), 1946–1955. http://doi.org/10.1111/sms.13198

Towlson, C., Salter, J., Ade, J. D., Enright, K., Harper, L. D., Page, R. M., & Malone, J. J. (2020). Maturity-associated considerations for training load, injury risk, and physical performance within youth soccer: One size does not fit all. *Journal of Sport and Health Science.* https://doi.org/10.1016/j.jshs.2020.09.003

Towlson, C., MacMaster, C., Gonçalves, B., Sampaio, J., Toner, J., MacFarlane, N., ... & Abt, G. (2021). The effect of bio-banding on physical and psychological indicators of talent identification in academy soccer players. Science and Medicine in Football, 5(4), 280–292.

Towlson, C., Salter, J., Ade, J. D., Enright, K., Harper, L. D., Page, R. M., & Malone, J. J. (2021). Maturity-associated considerations for training load, injury risk, and physical performance in youth soccer: One size does not fit all. Journal of Sport and Health Science, 10(4), 403–412.

Vaeyens, R., Philippaerts, R. M., & Malina, R. M. (2005). The relative age effect in soccer: a match-related perspective. *Journal of Sports Sciences, 23*(7), 747–756. http://doi.org/10.1080/02640410400022052

Vaeyens, R., Lenoir, M., Williams, A. M., & Philippaerts, R. M. (2008). Talent identification and development programmes in sport. *Sports Medicine, 38*(9), 703–714. https://doi.org/10.2165/00007256-200838090-00001

Vaeyens, R., Malina, R. M., Janssens, M., Van Renterghem, B., Bourgois, J., Vrijens, J., & Philippaerts, R. M. (2006). A multidisciplinary selection model for youth soccer: the Ghent youth soccer project. *British Journal of Sports Medicine, 40*(11), 928–934. http://dx.doi.org/10.1136/bjsm.2006.029652

Williams, A. M., & Reilly, T. (2000). Talent identification and development in soccer. *Journal of Sports Sciences, 18*(9), 657–667. https://doi.org/10.1080/02640410050120041

Winand, M., (2010). The global sporting arms race. An international comparative study on sports policy factors leading to international sporting success (SPLISS). *European Sport Management Quarterly, 10*(5), 613–615, https://doi.org/10.1080/16184742.2010.524242

# 22 Talent identification and talent promotion

*Arne Güllich and Paul Larkin*

## Introduction

Many soccer federations and professional clubs worldwide have established talent identification (TID) and talent promotion programmes (TPPs) at local, regional, and national levels. The most common TPPs are national and regional under-age selection squads (typically ages 12–19 years) and the youth soccer academies of professional clubs (starting at 8–14, operating up to 19 years). Youth academies operate almost year around and provide day-to-day training and competition for players, whereas under-age national and regional selection teams typically gather for training camps and tournaments for several weeks annually. In Germany, there is an additional programme, "talent bases," where regional federations offer practice sessions on the weekend to players who are considered promising but are not among the ~10,000 players selected for an academy. The talent identification and talent promotion processes of these programmes are the focus of this chapter.

The aim of TPPs is to identify and select the most promising talents and promote their long-term performance development into adulthood. TPPs provide extensive resources and interventions to youth players (Ford et al., 2020; Larkin & Reeves, 2018; Larsen et al., 2013, 2020). These include training and competing with equals who have a similar performance level; participation in national and international leagues and tournaments; expanded training volumes; educated, professional full-time and part-time coaches; high-profile facilities and equipment; support staff providing physiotherapy, sports medicine, performance diagnostics, nutritional counselling, psychological support, and academic assistance; school timetables adjusted to the soccer schedule; residency; and transportation. The common belief is that providing a high-profile training environment with a multitude of resources will facilitate the progression of promising talents into the highest professional competitions.

### Key terms

A *soccer talent* is a young player during the early periods of their athletic career who possesses the potential to develop into an elite performer in adulthood (Güllich & Cobley, 2017; Johansson & Fahlén, 2017). Following recent conceptions of talent development (see Fransen & Güllich, 2018; Sarmento et al., 2018), one's potential is cultivated and realised through a multi-year task-related training process. This training process and its effectiveness are moderated by physiological (e.g., responsiveness to stimuli and load tolerance), psychological (e.g., learning, motivation, self-regulation,

DOI: 10.4324/9781003148418-27

and coping), and environmental factors (e.g., opportunities, facilities, teammates, TPPs, family, and school). Accordingly, "talent" is considered as a task-person-environment concept, rather than just a person concept. Talent indicators can thus be in the person and their interaction with the task and the environment.

*Talent search* comprises the scouting activities to discover previously unknown talents. *TID* is the identification of talents and distinction from non-talents; that is, the distinction of young players who possess a greater or lower potential for future, adult high performance. *Talent selection* is the selection of players for admittance to a TPP.

A *TPP* is designed to promote the long-term performance development of selected talents. Scholars and practitioners have used different terms for these programmes. Some labelled them "talent development programmes." We refrain from using this term because talents may develop within and outside these programmes. Furthermore, some used "TID" as an umbrella term referring to all the processes of searching, identifying, selecting, and promoting talents. We suggest that the central purpose of these programmes is to promote talent development, where TID is instrumental to talent selection and selection is instrumental to talent promotion.

In the following sections, we first review the available evidence on TID processes, including coaches' perspectives and the prognostic validity of potential talent indicators, and then review TPPs, including the effects of early TPP involvement and the functioning of TPPs.

## Talent identification and selection

Coaches in TPPs make annual selection decisions among two populations: (i) the selection among new applicants for admittance to the TPP, which may include players preselected and suggested by scouts; and (ii) the selection among TPP participants who are dismissed or retained for the next season. As reflected in Williams and Reilly's (2000) model of soccer talent (updated by Williams et al., 2020), coaches may consider the overall playing performance of players and/or certain potential talent indicators, including physique (e.g., height and weight), physical abilities (e.g., speed, agility, power, endurance, and flexibility), perceptual-technical ball-control skills (e.g., first touch, dribbling, passing, and shooting), perceptual-tactical skills (e.g., orientation, anticipation, and situational decision-making), and psychological and psychosocial characteristics (e.g., motivation, self-regulation, and social skills). These may be assessed by coaches viewing players in matches, training sessions, or invited trials (e.g., invited training sessions or games; "open-door talent days") either with or without standardised tests of potential talent indicators.

### *Coach perspectives on TID*

Researchers have recently started to investigate the factors coaches consider when making talent identification and selection decisions (Larkin et al., 2020). To understand the nuanced thought processes of coaches during this process, researchers used qualitative, descriptive designs, such as interviewing or concurrent verbal reporting of experienced soccer coaches (Christensen, 2009; Larkin & O'Connor, 2017; Lund & Söderström, 2017; Reeves et al., 2019). Coaches value a range of player characteristics including perceptual-technical skills (e.g., first touch; dribbling; passing accuracy; one-versus-one skill; and ball control under pressure); perceptual-tactical skills (e.g., decision-making; game awareness; game intelligence; ability to read the play; and anticipate game-play); and psychological attributes (e.g., character; positive attitude; drive to succeed; winning mindset; willingness to learn; and coachability) as the most important traits when assessing talent (Bergkamp et al., 2022; Christensen, 2009; Larkin & O'Connor, 2017; Lund & Söderström, 2017; Reeves et al., 2019; Saether, 2014; Williams et al., 2020). Lund and Söderström (2017) added that knowledge of current elite player qualities and the values and belief system of a club are also important factors.

It should be acknowledged, however, that these findings can only report the constructs coaches verbalise. Their selection decisions partly rest on some intuitive "gut instinct" (Christensen, 2009; Roberts et al., 2019), and there is perhaps further tacit knowledge that is inaccessible. Furthermore, for several constructs, the relevant studies did not describe what exactly they are, how they manifest, and what exactly the coach evaluates, for example, "character," "positive attitude," "drive to succeed," "winning mindset," "willingness to learn," "game awareness," "game intelligence," and "coachability." In addition, the objectivity and inter-individual consistency of player assessment by coaches were mostly not reported. However, Jokuschies et al. (2017) found that different coaches consider different aspects of a player, which questions the objectivity of these evaluations.

Quantitative, cross-sectional studies compared players selected (i.e., talent-identified) or dismissed by TPPs, thereby describing player characteristics that predict the likelihood to be selected. It has generally been found that selected players were biologically more mature, taller, faster, and stronger, and showed better perceptual-technical ball-control skills, and perceptual-tactical skills, than non-selected counterparts; they also differed in several psychological characteristics (see Murr et al., 2018; Sarmento et al., 2018; Williams et al., 2020). However, being selected does not necessarily imply being talented, and as cross-sectional studies do not consider future performance development, they cannot evaluate TID and the validity of selection decisions. Investigating the *prognostic validity* requires multi-year longitudinal prospective studies.

### *Prognostic validity of potential talent indicators*

The critical quality criterion of TID procedures is their *prognostic validity* for which the central research question is: To what extent do individual differences in talent indicators at the time of TID procedures predict individual differences in later, adult performance? That is, did higher-performing adult players show greater values of childhood/adolescent talent indicators than lower-performing adult players did? These questions are investigated by long-term longitudinal studies that determine potential talent indicators of players during childhood/adolescence and their playing level as adults.

Youth players' current overall playing performance may be relevant in two regards. First, coaches seek to have strong youth players in their team. Second, coaches and scouts search for talents in higher leagues, cups, and tournaments rather than lower ones. Therefore, playing in high youth competitions facilitates the chance to be seen by TPP coaches and scouts.

The extent to which higher youth playing performance correlates with higher adult playing performance, to our knowledge, has not been reported in the literature. Nevertheless, the following data allow for relevant inferences. The annual player turnover within

TPPs suggests that 43% of under-age national-team players are replaced with new, external players every year. Furthermore, of all national-level youth players, 37.7% continued to play at a national level 2 years later, 9.2% after 5 years, and only 4.3% after 8 years (see references in Table 22.1). Out of 636 U16–U21 national team players, 37 (5.8%) went on to play in the senior national team (Schroepf & Lames, 2017); of 283 U15 national team players, one (0.4%) achieved a nomination for the senior national team (Güllich, 2014). Likewise, only 5.9% of all senior national team players had played in the U15 national team and 26.5% in the U19 national team. Furthermore, of all German first Bundesliga players, only 10.1% had played in the highest U15 division, and 37.9% in the highest U19 division (Güllich, 2014).

Twenty-seven studies published between 2009 and 2021 have investigated the prognostic validity of potential talent indicators longitudinally (see Table 22.1). They considered player evaluations by coaches, physique (i.e., height, weight, and % body fat), physical abilities (i.e., speed, agility, power, endurance, and flexibility), perceptual-technical skills (i.e., dribbling, passing, shooting, and juggling), perceptual-tactical skills (i.e., recognition and anticipation of game situations, orientation, and situational decision-making), psychological and psychosocial characteristics (i.e., self-concept, motivation, self-regulation, and parental support), and multidimensional approaches combining various predictors, using linear and non-linear analyses.

All studies were from West-European countries (Austria, Belgium, Finland, France, Germany, the Netherlands, Norway, Portugal, Switzerland, and the UK). Twenty-five studies involved male players and two studies female players. Ten investigations involved baseline samples of under-age national team or youth academy players while the other 17 involved lower-level or more heterogeneous samples involving general primary pupils or youth players from regional teams, bases, or clubs. Five studies recorded potential talent indicators at baseline ages up to 10 years, 21 studies at 11–14 years, and 16 studies at 15 years and older (the sum exceeds the number of studies because several studies considered various ages). Twenty studies involved relatively short prediction periods of up to 4 years, whereas 18 studies included predictions over 5 or more years. Fourteen investigations considered playing performance within youth age groups, with eight studies using the junior-to-senior transition (e.g., U18–U21), and five investigations considered adult peak playing performance. Of the latter, four studies used rather relaxed success criteria, such as obtaining a professional contract or being on the roster of 1st–3rd or 1st–5th league clubs.

A central finding is that the existing evidence on the prognostic validity of potential soccer talent indicators is characterised by great heterogeneity and inconsistency. For each of the potential talent indicators, some studies reported positive predictive effects on later playing performance, whereas these findings were countered by other studies (or the same study).

Table 22.2 summarises quantitative findings on the prognostic validity of the potential talent indicators in terms of the range of reported effects and sample-weighted mean determination coefficients ($r_w^2$) across all studies. The prognostic validity of each potential talent indicator was inconsistent between studies and, synthesising all studies, was generally poor: mean determination coefficients $r_w^2$ ranged from 0.1% to 3.5%. That is, on average, player evaluations by coaches and variables of player physique, physical abilities, ball-control skills, perceptual-tactical skills, and psychological characteristics, each only explained 3.5% or less of the variance of later playing performance.

Player assessment by coaches did not generally have superior or inferior predictive validity compared to standardised tests of the potential talent indicators, but the

## Talent identification and talent promotion 367

*Table 22.1* The effect sizes for studies investigating predictive effects of potential talent indicators of youth soccer players on their later playing performance. Upper half: short prediction periods of 1–4 years. Lower half: longer prediction periods of >4 years. Black figures: baseline samples from youth academies; grey figures: lower-level or more heterogeneous baseline samples (general primary pupils, participants from regional soccer teams, bases, or clubs). Effects reported in original studies as Cohen's $d$, $\eta_p^2$, odds ratio, or AUC were converted to $r$.

| | Positive effect (r ≥ 0.10) | No/negligible/negative effect (r < 0.10) |
|---|---|---|
| **Short period (≤4 years)** | | |
| Coach rating | 14 | |
| Physique | | |
| Body height | 2, 6, 18 | 18, 19, 21, 24 |
| Body mass | 6, 18 | 2, 18, 21, 24 |
| % lean mass | 2, 18 | 18 |
| Physical abilities | | |
| Linear sprint speed | 2, 4, 6, 7, 13, 20, 14, 18, 21, 24 | 4, 13, 20, 18, 19, 21 |
| Agility | 6, 13, 20, 14, 21, 24 | 7, 20, 14, 19, 21 |
| (Jumping) Power | 2, 6, 18, 21 | 7, 18, 21, 24 |
| Aerobic endurance | 1, 4, 6, 14, 18, 24 | 4, 7, 18 |
| Flexibility | | 7 |
| Ball control skills | | |
| Dribbling | 2, 13, 20, 14, 19, 24 | 13, 20, 19 |
| Passing | 13, 20, 14, 24 | 13, 20, 14, 19 |
| Shooting | 20, 14 | 13, 20, 19, 24 |
| Juggling | 14, 24 | |
| Perceptual-tactical skills | 6, 14, 17 | 7, 17 |
| Psychological characteristics | 6, 14, 27 | 6, 10, 14, 27 |
| Multidimensional | 6, 7, 14, 26, 27 | 2, 26, 27 |
| **Longer period (>4 years)** | | |
| Coach rating | 5, 23, 25 | |
| Physique | | |
| Body height | 1, 8, 12, 18, 19 | 3, 5, 12, 18, 21, 22, 23, 24 |
| Body mass | 1, 12, 18, 22 | 3, 5, 8, 12, 18, 21, 22, 23, 24 |
| % Lean mass | 5, 18 | 1, 18 |
| Physical abilities | | |
| Linear sprint speed | 5, 7, 8, 9, 11, 12, 14, 21, 22 | 1, 3, 4, 7, 11, 12, 18, 22, 23, 24 |
| Agility | 5, 7, 11, 12, 15, 21, 22 | 11, 12, 22, 23, 24 |
| (Jumping) Power | 7, 8, 9, 22 | 1, 3, 5, 7, 18, 21, 22, 23, 24 |
| Aerobic endurance | 3, 5, 8, 9, 18, 22 | 3, 7, 8, 18, 22, 23, 24 |
| Flexibility | 8 | 7, 8, 9 |
| Ball control skills | | |
| Dribbling | 5, 11, 12, 15, 23, 24 | 11, 12 |
| Passing | 5, 11, 12, 23, 24 | 11, 12 |
| Shooting | 12, 24 | 5, 11, 12 |
| Juggling | 23, 24 | |
| Perceptual-tactical skills | 7 | 7 |
| Psychological characteristics | 5, 23, 25 | 5, 23 |
| Multidimensional | 7, 8, 9, 12, 23, 25 | |

[1]Carling et al. (2012), [2]Deprez et al. (2015), [3]Dugdale et al. (2021), [4]Emmonds et al. (2016), [5]Figueiredo et al. (2019), [6]Forsman et al. (2016), [7]Gonaus & Müller (2012), [8]Hohmann & Siener (2021), [9]Hohmann et al. (2018), [10]Höner & Feichtinger (2016), [11]Höner & Votteler (2016), [12]Höner et al. (2017), [13]Höner et al. (2019), [14]Höner et al. (2021), [15]Huijgen et al. (2009), [16]Jokuschies et al. (2017), [17]Kannekens et al. (2011), [18]Le Gall et al. (2010), [19]Leyhr et al. (2018), [20]Leyhr et al. (2020), [21]Noon et al. (2020), [22]Saward et al. (2020), [23]Sieghartsleitner et al. (2019a), [24]Sieghartsleitner et al. (2019b), [25]Van Yperen (2009), [26]Zuber et al. (2014), [27]Zuber et al. (2016).

## 368  Arne Güllich and Paul Larkin

*Table 22.2* An overview of predictive effects of potential talent indicators of youth soccer players on their later playing performance (references reported in Table 22.1). Range (minimum, maximum), sample-weighted mean effect ( $r_w^2$ ), and numbers of reported effects (k; greater numbers of effects than studies because several studies reported various effects, e.g., across age categories). Effects reported in original studies as Cohen's d, $\eta_p^2$, odds ratio, or $AUC$ were converted to r.

| Predictor variable | Min r | Max r | Sample-weighted mean $r_w^2$ (%) | k |
|---|---|---|---|---|
| Coach rating | 0.14 | 0.48 | 2.7% | 7 |
| Physique | | | | |
|    Height[1] | −0.18 | 0.35 | 0.7% | 40 |
|    Weight[1] | −0.20 | 0.38 | 0.8% | 40 |
|    % Lean mass | −0.05 | 0.27 | 0.6% | 12 |
| Physical abilities | | | | |
|    Linear sprint speed | −0.09 | 0.55 | 1.0% | 72 |
|    Agility | −0.07 | 0.48 | 0.5% | 49 |
|    Power | −0.22 | 0.23 | 0.4% | 42 |
|    Aerobic endurance[1,2] | −0.61 | 0.59 | 0.3% | 45 |
|    Flexibility | 0.00 | 0.17 | 0.1% | 7 |
| Ball control skills | | | | |
|    Dribbling | 0.00 | 0.58 | 1.3% | 34 |
|    Passing | 0.04 | 0.36 | 0.9% | 31 |
|    Shooting[2] | −0.29 | 0.23 | 0.5% | 30 |
|    Juggling[2] | 0.10 | 0.33 | 1.7% | 9 |
| Perceptual-tactical skills | −0.15 | 0.32 | 3.5% | 14 |
| Psychological characteristics | −0.15 | 0.23 | 1.4% | 9 |
| Multidimensional evaluation[1] | 0.18 | 0.72 | 18.0% | 21 |

[1]Among relatively homogeneous samples (academy players), lower or no predictive effects: body height $r_w^2$ = 0.0%; body weight $r_w^2$ = 0.0%; aerobic endurance $r_w^2$ = 0.0%; and multidimensional evaluation $r_w^2$ = 7.4%.

[2]Across prediction periods >4 years, no predictive effects: $r_w^2$ = 0.0%, respectively.

combination of coach evaluation with standardised motor and/or psychological tests showed better prognostic validity than either alone. Furthermore, multidimensional approaches generally had higher, although mostly still low, predictive effects, with $3.2\% < r_w^2 < 51.9\%$.

The average sensitivity of these multidimensional approaches was 65.4% and the specificity was 65.0% (sample-weighted means). Assuming a *base rate* of 1/1,000 (i.e., 1 of 1,000 youth players becomes a successful adult professional, for example, a national-level player) – quite a realistic estimate based on the figures of the performance development discussed above – the application of these TID approaches yields a *hit rate* for a TPP of 0.2%. That is, two out of 1,000 positively talent-identified players become successful adult players. At the same time, 34.6% of the true talents are dismissed. Even when applying the strongest predictor model reported in the literature (Sieghartsleitner et al., 2019a, "holistic model": sensitivity 90%, specificity 87%), this only increases the *hit rate* of a TPP to 0.7%. These calculations indicate that the low prognostic validity of TID procedures is not due to deficient research or practice, but to the nature of the unsolvable problem (i.e., the impossibility of reliable TID at a young age in association with the low base rate). Table 22.3 summarises major impediments to the prognostic validity of TID in soccer.

Given the inconsistent evidence and generally poor prognostic validity, a recommendation to use any of the considered potential talent indicators in TID procedures

*Talent identification and talent promotion* 369

*Table 22.3* Some impediments to reliable talent identification in youth soccer (following Güllich & Cobley, 2017)

| Constraints | Issues |
|---|---|
| Characteristics of the task | One's success rests on one's own performance relative to other players' performance. Who the competitors will be in the future and what their performance will be is uncertain and cannot be influenced. |
| | Rules, playing tactics, and playing systems may have changed in the future, leading to a demand for different types of players. |
| | High playing performance can be achieved through many different compositions of performance components, including physique, physical abilities, perceptual-technical, and perceptual-tactical skills. The complex components of the match-play performance are mutually compensable. |
| | The effect and weight of different predictors of playing performance change across age and performance levels. (For example, physique and physical abilities predict differences in childhood/adolescent performance, but less so or not at all among the highest levels of adult performance.) |
| Characteristics of the player | The rate of progress of the various performance components differs and also varies intra-individually over time. Inter-individual differences in future long-term individual development of the performance components are difficult to predict. |
| | Initial performance advantages of biologically accelerated and of relatively early-born players (relative age effect, RAE) diminish in adulthood. |
| | The intra-individual development over time of psychological characteristics varies inter-individually; their long-term future development can hardly be predicted. |
| | The participation history of players is typically not considered in TID procedures. Furthermore, individual differences in long-term future training of players, its quality, the player-coach match, and the effectiveness of that training can hardly be predicted. |
| Characteristics of the environment | The intra-individual development over time of parental support, coach-athlete relationship, peer relationships, and athlete services (e.g., performance diagnostics, sports medicine, physiotherapy, nutritional and psychological counselling) and their effects on performance development vary inter-individually. Respective long-term future inter-individual differences can hardly be predicted. |
| Quality of tests | Tests possess imperfect objectivity, reliability, and validity. The objectivity of player evaluation by coaches is widely unstudied (or unpublished) to date. The retest reliability and differential developmental stability of many psychological and psychosocial characteristics are uncertain. Furthermore, several tests of perceptual-technical ball-control skills and perceptual-tactical skills do not measure representative skills. They typically record repeated standardised tasks under standardised conditions (e.g., series of passes against walls and dribbling through a course of cones), tasks that do not occur in games. Critically, these tests do not consider varying skill demands in game situations through varying weather conditions, opponent and organisational pressure (i.e., complexity of game situations), which are crucial to performance in game situations. |

370    *Arne Güllich and Paul Larkin*

would hardly be reconcilable with the ethos of science. Furthermore, some studies reported the reliability of their tests incompletely and some failed to report it at all. Where reported, the reliability was sometimes acceptable and in other cases unacceptable (e.g., Höner et al., 2019; Hohmann et al., 2018; Jokuschies et al., 2017; Leyhr et al., 2018; Sieghartsleitner et al., 2019a, b; Zuber et al., 2016). For psychological and psychosocial constructs, studies typically reported Cronbach's α, but not the retest reliability and differential developmental stability, although these are critical to assessments, especially during childhood/adolescent development. Also, multidimensional approaches were generally more predictive than each predictor alone. However, each of the multidimensional approaches used different combinations of predictor variables and research has not identified an optimal set of predictors to date.

### Talent promotion programmes

The central 'idea' of TPPs is to select the most promising youth players, provide resources and supportive interventions to facilitate their long-term training and competition process, and thereby increase their likelihood to become a nationally or internationally successful adult player (not just a successful junior player). TPPs start selecting players from a young age, mostly from 8–14 years, to secure young talents for that TPP, before other TPPs, and to enable a long period of nurturing until the anticipated age of peak performance.

The general approach of TPPs implies two underlying premises: (i) reliable TID at a young age is possible; and (ii) TPP resources and intervention measures applied to the participants at a young age positively influence their long-term adult performance. The falsification of the first premise (TID) has been reported in the previous section. We discuss the following questions:

1   What are participant perceptions of a TPP?
2   What effects do the TPP resources and intervention measures provided to participants have on their long-term performance development?
3   Does early TPP involvement correlate with long-term adult performance?
    Another question concerns part of the general approach of TPPs. Unlike the central 'idea' of TPPs mentioned above, annual selection and de-selection procedures imply revisions of previous selection decisions and the selection of new 'side-entry players' across age categories. Thus, a critical question is:
4   Does the population of high-performing adult players develop from early selection and long-term continuous TPP nurture, or does this population rather emerge via repeated procedures of selection, de-selection, and replacement of previous participants across age categories?

### Perceptions of TPP participants

Participants of one academy reported positive scores on stress-recovery balance, need satisfaction, psychological and social well-being, and school-related quality of life, and they did not differ from recreational players (Rongen et al., 2020). Furthermore, in several studies, players rated the academy environment as positive (Gangso et al., 2021; Gesbert et al., 2021; Mitchell et al., 2021), typically reporting values of around 4–5 on 6-point scales of the "Talent Development Environment Questionnaire" (TDEQ, Martindale et al., 2010). However, the development of the TDEQ failed to consider whether the

*Talent identification and talent promotion* 371

addressed environmental factors influence player performance development (or other long-term outcomes, such as academic, health, or psychological wellbeing).

Academy players are aware that their clubs see them as an "investment," "commodity," and a "marketable asset" (Christensen & Soerensen, 2009; Larsen et al., 2020; Manley et al., 2012). They are aware that their chances to be promoted to the first team or another professional team are minimal, often implying a permanent feeling of frustration. The players perceive some inconsistency between management talk and action, in that clubs externally display a focus on long-term player development, not immediate success, whereas players perceive the expectation is to "win every day" (e.g., Larsen et al., 2020). Likewise, players report that clubs say they want home-grown players in their first team, but increasingly recruit foreign players (e.g., Larsen et al., 2020; Webb et al., 2020).

Academy players know they need a "back-up plan" implying future employment outside of soccer and are aware of the necessity of academic education (Christensen & Soerensen, 2009; Aalberg & Saether, 2016; Webb et al., 2020). All academies described in the literature had some cooperation with schools providing modified educational programmes for the players (e.g., flexible lesson times; exemption from lessons; individual extra tuition; replacement of school subjects by sports subjects; and transportation service; Christensen & Soerensen, 2009; Aalberg & Saether, 2016; Webb et al., 2020). Nevertheless, players report permanent high levels of stress from the conflicting time demands of soccer and school. They often must make decisions between doing homework and attending a soccer training session or game. Furthermore, a significant decline in exam results and school-related quality of life and premature dropping out of school have been reported (Aalberg & Saether, 2016; Christensen & Soerensen, 2009; Rongen et al., 2020). Players reported that clubs displayed priority of education to them and the public; however, in reality, soccer was clearly prioritised over academic outcomes (Webb et al., 2020).

De-selection – which the vast majority of academy players experience at some time – implies severe immediate and lasting psychological disturbances, including feelings of loss of identity, confidence, and self-esteem; being a failure; depression; uncertainty, disorientation, and anxiety regarding their future life; and of being left alone (O'Halloran, 2019; Wilkinson, 2021). Blakelock et al. (2016) found 55% of deselected players exhibited clinical levels of psychological distress. These effects were exacerbated by the strong, and often exclusive, athletic identity of players (Mitchell et al., 2014; Rongen et al., 2020).

Finally, reports on the player-coach and player-staff relationships are heterogeneous. Players from two Scandinavian academies (Aalberg & Saether, 2016; Larsen et al., 2013) reported a culture of community, mutual respect, and open two-way communication. Coaches and staff created an environment centred around player-staff relationships, where everybody seeks to help players wherever possible regarding their holistic development, self-awareness, and managing soccer and school. They also facilitate the empowerment of players by delegating as much responsibility as possible to the player concerning physical and mental load-recovery balance, nutrition, leisure activities, school, and time management, and by encouraging players to ask questions and make suggestions on the practice design and game tactics.

On the other hand, players from an English academy (Manley, 2012; Manley et al., 2012) reported a culture of "authoritarian environment," "discipline," "control," and "surveillance." This included continuous physical and techno-motor testing and evaluation of each training session and game, with weekly reports to the manager, and data documented in individual player files. Perhaps more significantly, the coaches, assistants, conditioning staff, sports scientists, physiotherapists, teachers, tutors, teammates, and even parents, reported observations of and conversations with players, both within and

## 372   *Arne Güllich and Paul Larkin*

away from the academy, as well as social media entries, to the manager without the player being aware. Therefore, these individuals become the "eyes and ears of the manager," with staff acknowledging they are "monitoring them all the time" (Manley, 2012; Manley et al., 2012). Players thus experienced a "silent mode of surveillance" leading to a culture of "suspicion" and "distrust."

### *Effects of TPP resources and intervention measures*

The effects of TPP resources and intervention measures on long-term player performance development have not been empirically investigated in soccer TPPs. This is interesting given the questions of how to design and organise a TPP and what resources and intervention measures to provide to players are central to these programmes. This has two significant implications. First, managers cannot make evidence-based decisions in the designing and organisation of TPPs. Second, extensive research into TID is opposed by lacking research into the purpose TID is undertaken for: the effects of TPPs. Nevertheless, the following sections allow for respective inferences from empirical evidence, although not individual TPP measures, considering the long-term effects of early TPP involvement and annual player turnover.

### *Effects of early TPP involvement*

Given that TPPs aim to involve participants from very young ages, often 8–14 years, a critical question is whether earlier TPP involvement facilitates higher short-term junior performance and long-term adult performance. Table 22.4 reviews the available evidence. Each study reported comparisons between higher and lower-performing youth or adult players regarding their age of selection for a youth academy or selection team.

For junior performance, the findings are inconsistent and generally inconclusive. Overall, there is no consistent evidence indicating an association of higher junior performance with earlier or later selection age. Results for adult performance are much more consistent because a higher adult performance was associated with a *later* selection for TPPs and lower adult performance was associated with younger selection for TPPs. This finding consistently applied among adult players at regional to national playing levels and adult international-level compared to lower-performing players. Most of the highest-performing adult players were not involved in a TPP at a particularly young age, but developed outside of TPPs until later ages, and late "side-entry players" were over-represented among the highest-performing adult players.

### *Player turnover within TPPs*

TPP coaches and staff review their previous selection decisions at least annually. For each season, they decide which players are retained through the next season and which are dismissed and replaced with new "side-entry players." The question of the extent to which current players are dismissed (i.e., a revision of previous selection decisions) and replaced with new players is critical to understanding the functioning of TPPs. This is commonly calculated for each season-to-season transition by the *annual player turnover* within a TPP using the equation:

$$Annual\ player\ turnover = \frac{(number\ of\ entering\ players + number\ of\ dismissed\ players)/2}{total\ number\ of\ players}$$

Table 22.5 shows the mean annual player turnover within youth soccer academies was 29%. This turnover rate was similar, and did not significantly differ, across age

*Talent identification and talent promotion* 373

*Table 22.4* The effects (Cohen's *d*) of the age of selection for a talent promotion programme on later junior and adult playing performance. Academy = youth soccer academy; L. = league; U-NT = under-age national team; A-NT = senior national A-team. Note the sign of effects (Cohen's *d*): A *positive* effect indicates that higher eventual performance was associated with *higher* (later) entry age.

| Study | Country, sex, sample | n | Entry age | Comparison groups | Cohen's d |
|---|---|---|---|---|---|
| **Junior performance** | | | | | |
| Dugdale et al., 2021 | GBR, m Academy | 537 | Academy | retained vs. dismissed | +0.54 |
| Ford & Williams, 2012 | GBR, m Academy | 32 | Academy | retained vs. dismissed | −0.18 |
| Ford et al., 2009 | GBR, m Academy | 22 | Academy | retained vs. dismissed | +0.27 |
| Hendry & Hodges, 2018 | GBR, m Academy | 102 | Academy | retained vs. dismissed | −0.87 |
| Huijgen et al., 2014 | NED, m Academy | 113 | Academy | retained vs. dismissed | −0.45 |
| Noon et al., 2020 | GBR, m Academy | 76 | Academy | retained vs. dismissed | −0.50 |
| | | | | Sample-weighted mean | +0.10 |
| **Adult performance** | | | | | |
| Güllich, 2014 | GER, m 1st–2nd League | 348 | Academy | 1st vs. 2nd League | +0.18 |
| Hendry & Hodges, 2018 | GBR, m Academy | 28 | Academy | U21 1st L. vs. below | −0.07 |
| Hendry et al., 2019 | CAN, f A-NT, varsity | 45 | Academy | A-NT vs. varsity | +0.89 |
| Roca et al., 2012 | GBR, m Semi-prof. | 32 | Academy | Higher vs. lower skill | +0.36 |
| Hendry et al., 2019 | CAN, f A-NT, varsity | 45 | U-NT | A-NT vs. varsity | +0.59 |
| Hornig et al., 2016 | GER, m 1st BL, 4–6th L. | 102 | U-NT | 1st L. vs. 4th–6th L. | +0.10 |
| Hornig et al., 2016 | GER, m 1st League | 52 | U-NT | A-NT vs. 1st League | +0.33 |
| Güllich, 2014 | GER, m U-NT | 847 | U-NT | 1st vs. 3rd League | +0.61 |
| Güllich, 2014 | GER, m U-NT | 599 | U-NT | 1st vs. 2nd League | +0.71 |
| Güllich, 2014 | GER, m 1st–2nd League | 348 | U-NT | 1st vs. 2nd League | +0.54 |
| Güllich, 2014 | GER, m 1st League | 321 | U-NT | A-NT vs. 1st League | +0.25 |
| Güllich, 2019 | GER, f, 1st League | 29 | U-NT | A-NT vs. 1st League | +0.78 |
| Schroepf & Lames, 2017 | GER, m U-NT | 599 | U-NT | 1st–3rd L. vs. lower | +0.99 |
| Schroepf & Lames, 2017 | GER, m U-NT | 317 | U-NT | A-NT vs. below 3rd L. | +0.81 |
| Schroepf & Lames, 2017 | GER, m U-NT | 389 | U-NT | A-NT vs. 1st–3rd L. | +0.28 |
| | | | | Sample-weighted mean | +0.58 |

374  *Arne Güllich and Paul Larkin*

*Table 22.5* The annual player turnover in TPPs and the proportion of identical players in a squad after 3 and 5 years. Annual player turnover = [(*n* new players + *n* dismissed players)/2]/*n* squad size

| Study | Country, sex, sample | Period of ... | | Mean annual | Persistence after | |
|---|---|---|---|---|---|---|
| | | Observation | Age | player turnover | 3 years | 5 years |
| **Youth soccer academies** | | | | | | |
| Ford et al., 2020 | 15 countries, m; 29 academies, *n* ≈ 7,000 | 1 year | U8–U21 | 29% | 36% | 18% |
| Güllich, 2014 | GER, m; 13 academies, *n* = 1,420 | 10 years | U10–U19 | 25% | 42% | 24% |
| Noon et al., 2020 | GBR, m; 1 academy, *n* = 76 | 5 years | U10–U18 | 47% | 12% | 3% |
| | | Sample-weighted mean | | 29% | 37% | 19% |
| **Under-age national teams** | | | | | | |
| Güllich, 2014 | GER, m; *n* = 1,059 | 13 years | U15–U19 | 41% | 21% | 7% |
| Schroepf & Lames, 2017 | GER, m; *n* = 636 | 13 years | U16–U21 | 46% | 16% | 4% |
| | | Sample-weighted mean | | 43% | 19% | 6% |

categories from U10 to U19. The finding implies that at any age, the odds that a current participant will still be involved in an academy 3 years later is 37% and after 5 years 19%. Within the national under-age selection teams, the mean annual turnover was even higher, 43%. Therefore, the probability an under-age national team player is still in a national team 3 years later is 19% and after 5 years 6%.

Figure 22.1 illustrates the proportions of under-11 participants of youth soccer academies and of under-15 national team players who remained in the programme through subsequent age categories (grey lines). As can be seen, the proportions drop continuously to about 1% in adulthood. The figure also shows the proportion of successful adult players in the first Bundesliga, Premier League, and senior national-team players (black lines) who were involved in a youth soccer academy or a national under-age selection team during junior age categories. A minority of the successful adult players were selected for a youth academy before age 15 years, with only 6% of senior national-team players selected for a U15 selection team, and about half of them playing for an under-age selection team until age 19.

In sum, the observations suggest four inferences:

1    TPP coaches revise most of their previous selection decisions within 3 or fewer years.
2    Most of the young TPP players are "overtaken" by other players who have a better development outside TPPs regarding performance and/or indicators of future potential.
3    Most of the early selected players do not become successful adult players while most of the successful adult players were not selected at a particularly young age. The populations of early selected players and successful adult players are not identical but are widely disparate populations.

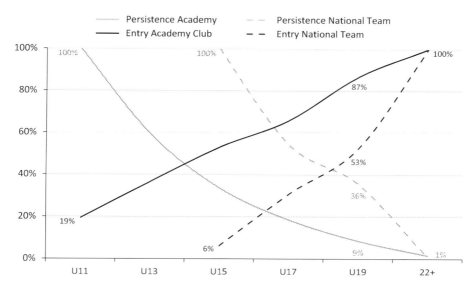

*Figure 22.1* Proportions of members of youth soccer academies and under-age national teams persisting in the programme through subsequent age categories (grey lines) and proportions of senior first Bundesliga/Premier League players involved in youth academies and of senior national team players involved in under-age national teams through previous age categories (black lines). Aggregated data from Anderson & Miller, 2011; Güllich, 2014, 2019; Grossmann & Lames, 2015; Hornig et al., 2016; Schroepf & Lames, 2017.

4   Rather than early identification and long-term continuous nurture of talents, the functioning of the TPPs primarily rests on recurrent selection and de-selection procedures across all age categories.

## Conclusion and future directions

The idea of early identification of talents and their long-term continuous TPP nurture reflects an institutionalised ideology rather than empirical reality. The functioning of soccer TPPs rests on recurrent selection and de-selection procedures rather than long-term player development through continuous nurture. TPPs recruit large numbers of young players and extend this number through high rates of player turnover. Players are "tried out"; some continue through several years to be assigned to the highest-performing and/or most promising players while most are dismissed in the short term and replaced with external players now considered to have higher performance and/or greater future promise. This also implies that TID mostly occurs *a posteriori* rather than *a priori*.

Recent meta-analyses (Güllich et al., 2022; Barth et al., 2022; including 23 studies from soccer) show that some predictor effects differentiating higher *vs.* lower early *junior* performance are different and partly opposite to predictor effects differentiating higher *vs.* lower long-term *adult* performance. Higher-performing juniors had greater amounts of coach-led main-sport practice, less other-sports practice, and earlier achievement of developmental performance milestones (first national or international championships and first nomination for a selection team) than lower-performing juniors. In contrast, adult international-level athletes had less main-sport practice, more childhood/adolescent other-sports practice, and later achievement of performance milestones than adult national-level athletes. Amounts of peer-led play in the main sport or other sports generally had negligible effects on both junior and adult performance. The findings were confirmed by studies comparing higher *vs.* lower-performing youth soccer players and adult international *vs.* national-level players (Güllich et al., 2022; Barth et al., 2022, and Table 22.4).

TPPs preferably select the most advanced young players. Besides being biologically accelerated, most of them have heavily invested in specialised soccer practice prior to selection, with little or no other-sports practice. Once selected, the TPPs seek to further accelerate their development through expanded soccer practice. Increasing childhood/adolescent specialised practice may rapidly improve junior performance but does not facilitate the long-term player development into the highest adult performance levels. At the same time, it magnifies the opportunity costs of players (education, other hobbies, family, and friends) and risks of future motivational decline, burnout, and overuse injuries (Güllich et al., 2022; Barth et al., 2022, for reviews). In contrast, most of the highest-performing adult players had moderate amounts of childhood/adolescent soccer training, practised various sports, and remained unaffected by the potential negative effects of early TPP involvement, thereby buffering long-term costs and risks while growing their long-term potential.

The impossibility of reliable early TID and uncertainty of the effects of TPP measures are associated with pronounced forms of functional decoupling of talk, decisions, and actions of TPP management (Brunson, 2002). Talk: early identification of talents; long-term player development; importance of education over soccer; home-grown players in adult teams. Action: high annual player turnover; emphasis on current team success; priority of soccer over academic outcomes; and increasing recruitment of foreign players.

From an applied perspective, the evidence suggests postponing selection for TPPs to later ages and reduce opportunity costs of players, their well-being-related costs, and long-term risks. Furthermore, one could expect that consistency of management talk and action is a matter of course.

The available evidence has several limitations.

1   The major limitation is that the effects of TPP measures are widely unstudied. The massive body of TID research is opposed by lacking investigation into the purpose TID is done for.
2   Most studies involved West-European male players. It is widely unknown whether reported findings apply to female players and to other soccer cultures.
3   Many TID studies were restricted to relatively short prediction periods within youth ages and those considering adult performance used relatively relaxed success criteria.
4   Many of the highest-performing adult players may not have been involved in studies because they were not considered for TPPs at a young age.
5   The objectivity (i.e., inter-individual consistency) of coaches' player evaluation and the retest reliability and differential stability of childhood/adolescent psychological and psychosocial characteristics were mostly not reported.

The goal for future research is to investigate the effects of TPP resources and interventions provided to players. Such research should consider short- and long-term TPP effects at different ages on future performance development of players but also their academic, health, psychological, and psychosocial development. In this context, researchers may investigate whether prioritising education over soccer or being entirely upfront with players, parents, and the public would hamper the achievement of the goals of TPPs.

The fact that an improvement of TID accuracy from ~65% to ~90% only increases the TPP *hit rate* from 0.2% to 0.7% suggests the practical use of continued research efforts into TID is questionable. If any, it may be interesting to attempt to access the nuanced tacit knowledge of coaches in TID (the content of their "*gut instinct*"), definitions of several undefined constructs they use, and to investigate the objectivity of their player assessment (see also the review of Williams et al., 2020).

Finally, anecdotally, several outstanding players (e.g., Lionel Messi, Andrés Iniesta, Luís Figo, Johan Cruyff, and Franz Beckenbauer) had moderate physical abilities, but outstanding ball control and understanding of game situations. Traditional TID research fails to take account of such patterns. A question for future research may be whether a combination of moderate levels in most characteristics with just one or two outstanding characteristics is a more promising approach to TID.

## References

Aalberg, R. R., & Sæther, S. A. (2016). The talent development environment in a Norwegian top-level football club. *Sport Science Review, 25*(3–4), 159–182.

Anderson, G., & Miller, R. M. (2011). *The Academy System in English Professional Football: Business Value or 'Following the Herd'?* University of Liverpool Management School: Research Paper Series No. 2011/43.

Barth, M., Güllich, A., Macnamara, B. N., & Hambrick, D. Z. (2022). Predictors of junior versus senior elite performance are opposite: a systematic review and meta-analysis of participation patterns. *Sports Medicine, 52*, 1399–1416.

Bergkamp, T. L., Frencken, W. G., Niessen, A. S. M., Meijer, R. R., & den Hartigh, R. J. (2022). How soccer scouts identify talented players. *European Journal of Sport Science, 22*(7), 994–1004.

Blakelock, D. J., Chen, M. A., & Prescott, T. (2016). Psychological distress in elite adolescent soccer players following deselection. *Journal of Clinical Sport Psychology, 10*(1), 59–77.

Brunson, N. (2002). *The Organization of Hypocrisy: Talk, Decision, and Actions in Organizations* (2nd ed.). Oslo: Copenhagen Business School Press.

Carling, C., Le Gall, F., & Malina, R. M. (2012). Body size, skeletal maturity, and functional characteristics of elite academy soccer players on entry between 1992 and 2003. *Journal of Sports Sciences, 30*(15), 1683–1693.

Christensen, M. K. (2009). 'An eye for talent': talent identification and the 'practical sense' of top-level soccer coaches. *Sociology of Sport, 26*(3), 365–382.

Christensen, M. K., & Søerensen, J. K. (2009). Sport or school? Dreams and dilemmas for talented young Danish football players. *European Physical Education Review, 15*(1), 115–133.

Deprez, D., Fransen, J., Boone, J., Lenoir, M., Philippaerts, R., & Vaeyens, R. (2015). Characteristics of high-level youth soccer players: variation by playing position. *Journal of Sports Sciences, 33*(3), 243–254.

Dugdale, J. H., Sanders, D., Myers, T., Williams, A. M., & Hunter, A. M. (2021). Progression from youth to professional soccer: a longitudinal study of successful and unsuccessful academy graduates. *Scandinavian Journal of Medicine & Science in Sports, 31*(Suppl. 1), 73–84.

Emmonds, S., Till, K. A., Jones, B., Mellis, M., & Pears, M. (2016). Anthropometric, speed and endurance characteristics of English academy soccer players: do they influence obtaining a professional contract at 18 years of age? *International Journal of Sports Science & Coaching, 11*(2), 2212–2218.

Figueiredo, A. J., Coelho-e-Silva, M. J., Sarmento, H., Moya, J., & Malina, R. M. (2019). Adolescent characteristics of youth soccer players: do they vary with playing status in young adulthood? *Research in Sports Medicine, 28*(1), 72–83.

Ford, P. R., Bordonau, J. L. D., Bonanno, D., Tavares, J., Groenendijk, C., Fink, C., ... & Di Salvo, V. (2020). A survey of talent identification and development processes in the youth academies of professional soccer clubs from around the world. *Journal of Sports Sciences, 38*(11–12), 1269–1278.

Ford, P., Ward, P., Hodges, N. J., & Williams, A. M. (2009). The role of deliberate practice and play in career progression in sport: the early engagement hypothesis. *High Ability Studies, 20*(1), 65–75.

Ford, P., & Williams, A. M. (2012). The developmental activities engaged in by elite youth soccer players who progressed to professional status compared to those who did not. *Psychology of Sport & Exercise, 13*(3), 349–352.

Forsman, H., Blomqvist, M., Davids, K., Liukkonen, J., & Konttinen, N. (2016). Identifying technical, physiological, tactical and psychological characteristics that contribute to career progression in soccer. *International Journal of Sports Science & Coaching, 11*(4), 505–513.

Fransen, J., & Güllich, A. (2018). Talent identification and development in game sports. In R. F. Subotnik, P. Olszewski-Kubilius, & F. C. Worrell (Eds.), *The Psychology of High Performance* (pp. 59–92). Washington, DC: American Psychological Association.

Gangsø, K., Aspvik, N. P., Mehus, I., Høigaard, R., & Sæther, S. A. (2021). Talent development environments in football: comparing the top-five and bottom-five-ranked football academies in Norway. *International Journal of Environmental Research & Public Health, 18*(3), 1321.

Gesbert, V., Crettaz von Roten, F., & Hauw, D. (2021). Reviewing the role of the environment in the talent development of a professional soccer club. *PloS One, 16*(2), e0246823.

Gonaus, C., & Müller, E. (2012). Using physiological data to predict future career progression in 14-to 17-year-old Austrian soccer academy players. *Journal of Sports Sciences, 30*(15), 1673–1682.

Grossmann, B., & Lames, M. (2015). From talent to professional football – youthism in German football. *International Journal of Sports Science & Coaching, 10*(6), 1103–1113.

Güllich, A. (2014). Selection, de-selection and progression in German football talent promotion. *European Journal of Sport Science, 14*(6), 530–537.

Güllich, A. (2019). "Macro-structure" of developmental participation histories and "microstructure" of practice of German female world-class and national-class football players. *Journal of Sports Sciences, 37*(12), 1347–1355.

Güllich, A., & Cobley, S. (2017). On the efficacy of talent identification and talent development programmes. In J. Baker, S. Cobley, J. Schorer, & N. Wattie (eds.), *Routledge Handbook of Talent Identification and Talent Development in Sport* (pp. 80–98). London: Routledge.

Güllich, A., Macnamara, B. N., & Hambrick, D. Z. (2022). What makes a champion? Early multidisciplinary practice, not early specialization, predicts world-class performance. *Perspectives on Psychological Sciences, 17*(1), 6–29.

Hendry, D. T., & Hodges, N. J. (2018). Early majority engagement pathway best defines transitions from youth to adult elite men's soccer in the UK: a three time-point retrospective and prospective study. *Psychology of Sport & Exercise, 36*, 81–89.

Hendry, D. T., Williams, A. M., Ford, P. R., & Hodges, N. J. (2019). Developmental activities and perceptions of challenge for national and varsity women soccer players in Canada. *Psychology of Sport & Exercise, 43*, 210–218.

Hohmann, A., & Siener, M. (2021). Talent identification in youth soccer: prognosis of U17 soccer performance on the basis of general athleticism and talent promotion interventions in second-grade children. *Frontiers in Sports and Active Living, 3*:625645.

Hohmann, A, Siener, M., & He, Renye (2018). Prognostic validity of talent orientation in soccer. *German Journal of Exercise and Sport Research, 48*, 478–488.

Höner, O., & Feichtinger, P. (2016). Psychological talent predictors in early adolescence and their empirical relationship with current and future performance in soccer. *Psychology of Sport & Exercise, 25*, 17–26.

Höner, O., Leyhr, D., & Kelava, A. (2017). The influence of speed abilities and technical skills in early adolescence on adult success in soccer: a long-term prospective analysis using ANOVA and SEM approaches. *PloS One, 12*(8), e0182211.

Höner, O., Murr, D., Larkin, P., Schreiner, R., & Leyhr, D. (2021). Nationwide subjective and objective assessments of potential talent predictors in elite youth soccer: an investigation of prognostic validity in a prospective study. *Frontiers in Sports & Active Living, 3*, 115.

Höner, O., Raabe, J., Murr, D., & Leyhr, D. (2019). Prognostic relevance of motor tests in elite girls' soccer: a five-year prospective cohort study within the German talent promotion program. *Science & Medicine in Football, 3*(4), 287–296.

Höner, O., & Votteler, A. (2016). Prognostic relevance of motor talent predictors in early adolescence: a group- and individual-based evaluation considering different levels of achievement in youth football. *Journal of Sports Sciences, 34*(24), 2269–2278.

Hornig, M., Aust, F., & Güllich, A. (2016). Practice and play in the development of German top-level professional football players. *European Journal of Sport Science, 16*(1), 96–105.

Huijgen, B. C., Elferink-Gemser, M. T., Lemmink, K. A., & Visscher, C. (2014). Multidimensional performance characteristics in selected and deselected talented soccer players. *European Journal of Sport Science, 14*(1), 2–10.

Huijgen, B. C., Elferink-Gemser, M. T., Post, W. J., & Visscher, C. (2009). Soccer skill development in professionals. *International Journal of Sports Medicine, 30*(08), 585–591.

Johansson, A., & Fahlén, J. (2017). "Simply the best, better than all the rest?" Validity issues in selections in elite sport. *International Journal of Sports Science & Coaching, 12*(4), 470–480.

Jokuschies, N., Gut, V., & Conzelmann, A. (2017). Systematizing coaches' 'eye for talent': player assessments based on expert coaches' subjective talent criteria in top-level youth soccer. *International Journal of Sports Science & Coaching, 12*(5), 565–576.

Kannekens, R., Elferink-Gemser, M. T., Visscher, C. (2011). Positioning and deciding: key factors for talent development in soccer. *Scandinavian Journal of Medicine & Science in Sports, 21*(6), 846–852.

Larkin, P., Marchant, D., Syder, A., & Farrow, D. (2020). An eye for talent: the recruiters' role in the Australian football talent pathway. *PloS One, 15*(11), e0241307.

Larkin, P., & O'Connor, D. (2017). Talent identification and recruitment in youth soccer: recruiter's perceptions of the key attributes for player recruitment. *PloS One, 12*(4), e0175716.

Larkin, P., & Reeves, M. J. (2018). Junior-elite football: time to re-position talent identification? *Soccer & Society, 19*(8), 1183–1192.

Larsen, C. H., Alfermann, D., Henriksen, K., & Christensen, M. K. (2013). Successful talent development in soccer: the characteristics of the environment. *Sport, Exercise, & Performance Psychology, 2*(3), 190.

Larsen, C. H., Storm, L. K., Saether, S. A., Pyrdol, N., & Henriksen, K. (2020). A world class academy in professional football: the case of Ajax Amsterdam. *Scandinavian Journal of Sport and Exercise Psychology, 6(2),* 33–43.

Le Gall, F., Carling, C., Williams, M., & Reilly, T. (2010). Anthropometric and fitness characteristics of international, professional and amateur male graduate soccer players from an elite youth academy. *Journal of Science & Medicine in Sport, 13*(1), 90–95.

Leyhr, D., Kelava, A., Raabe, J., & Höner, O. (2018). Longitudinal motor performance development in early adolescence and its relationship to adult success: an 8-year prospective study of highly talented soccer players. *PloS One, 13*(5), e0196324.

Leyhr, D., Raabe, J., Schultz, F., Kelava, A., & Höner, O. (2020). The adolescent motor performance development of elite female soccer players: a study of prognostic relevance for future success in adulthood using multilevel modelling. *Journal of Sports Sciences, 38*(11–12), 1342–1351.

Lund, S., & Söderström, T. (2017). To see or not to see: talent identification in the Swedish football association. *Sociology of Sport Journal, 34*(3), 248–258.

Manley, A. (2012). *Surveillance, Disciplinary Power and Athletic Identity: A Sociological Investigation into the Culture of Elite Sports Academies*. Doctoral dissertation, Durham University.

Manley, A., Palmer, C., & Roderick, M. (2012). Disciplinary power, the oligopticon and rhizomatic surveillance in elite sports academies. *Surveillance & Society, 10*(3/4), 303–319.

Martindale, R. J., Collins, D., Wang, J. C., McNeill, M., Lee, K. S., Sproule, J., & Westbury, T. (2010). Development of the talent development environment questionnaire for sport. *Journal of Sports Sciences, 28*(11), 1209–1221.

Mitchell, T. O., Gledhill, A., Shand, R., Littlewood, M. A., Charnock, L., & Till, K. (2021). Players' perceptions of the talent development environment within the English premier league and football league. *International Sport Coaching Journal, 8(3),* 362–370.

Mitchell, T. O., Nesti, M., Richardson, D., Midgley, A. W., Eubank, M., & Littlewood, M. (2014). Exploring athletic identity in elite-level English youth football: a cross-sectional approach. *Journal of Sports Sciences, 32*(13), 1294–1299.

Murr, D., Feichtinger, P., Larkin, P., O'Connor, D., & Höner, O. (2018). Psychological talent predictors in youth soccer: a systematic review of the prognostic relevance of psychomotor, perceptual-cognitive and personality-related factors. *PloS One, 13*(10), e0205337.

Noon, M. R., Eyre, E. L., Ellis, M., Myers, T. D., Morris, R. O., Mundy, P. D., ... & Clarke, N. D. (2020). The influence of recruitment age and anthropometric and physical characteristics on the development pathway of English academy football players. *International Journal of Sports Physiology & Performance, 16*(2), 199–207.

O'Halloran, L. M. (2019). *The Lived Experience of 'Critical Moments' in Premier League Academy Football: A Descriptive Psychological Phenomenological Exploration*. Liverpool: John Moores University (United Kingdom).

Reeves, M. J., McRobert, A. P., Lewis, C. J., & Roberts, S. J. (2019). A case study of the use of verbal reports for talent identification purposes in soccer: a Messi affair! *PloS One, 14*(11), e0225033.

Roberts, A. H., Greenwood, D. A., Stanley, M., Humberstone, C., Iredale, F., & Raynor, A. (2019). Coach knowledge in talent identification: a systematic review and meta-synthesis. *Journal of Science & Medicine in Sport, 22*(10), 1163–1172.

Roca, A., Williams, A. M., & Ford, P. R. (2012). Developmental activities and the acquisition of superior anticipation and decision making in soccer players. *Journal of Sports Sciences, 30*(15), 1643–1652.

Rongen, F., McKenna, J., Cobley, S., Tee, J. C., & Till, K. (2020). Psychosocial outcomes associated with soccer academy involvement: longitudinal comparisons against aged matched school pupils. *Journal of Sports Sciences, 38*(11–12), 1387–1398.

Saether, A. S. (2014). Identification of talent in soccer – what do coaches look for? https://idrottsforum.org/sather140319/ (retrieved Aug. 14, 2021).

Sarmento, H., Anguera, M. T., Pereira, A., & Araújo, D. (2018). Talent identification and development in male football: a systematic review. *Sports Medicine, 48*, 907–931.

Saward, C., Hulse, M., Morris, J. G., Goto, H., Sunderland, C., & Nevill, M. E. (2020). Longitudinal physical development of future professional male soccer players: implications for talent identification and development? *Frontiers in Sports & Active Living, 2*, 578203.

Schroepf, B., & Lames, M. (2017). Career patterns in German football youth national teams–a longitudinal study. *International Journal of Sports Science & Coaching, 13*(3), 405–414.

Sieghartsleitner, R., Zuber, C., Zibung, M., & Conzelmann, A. (2019a). Science or coaches' eye? – Both! Beneficial collaboration of multidimensional measurements and coach assessments for efficient talent selection in elite youth football. *Journal of Sports Science & Medicine, 18*(1), 32.

Sieghartsleitner, R., Zuber, C., Zibung, M., Charbonnet, B., & Conzelmann, A. (2019b). Talent selection in youth football: specific rather than general motor performance predicts future player status of football talents. *Current Issues in Sport Science, 4*, 011.

Van Yperen, N. W. (2009). Why some make it and others do not: identifying psychological factors that predict career success in professional adult soccer. *The Sport Psychologist, 23*(3), 317–329.

Webb, T., Dicks, M., Brown, D. J., & O'Gorman, J. (2020). An exploration of young professional football players' perceptions of the talent development process in England. *Sport Management Review, 23*(3), 536–547.

Wilkinson, R. J. (2021). A literature review exploring the mental health issues in academy football players following career termination due to deselection or injury and how counselling could support future players. *Counselling & Psychotherapy Research, 21*, 859–868.

Williams, A. M., Ford, P. R., & Drust, B. (2020). Talent identification and development in soccer since the millennium. *Journal of Sports Sciences, 38*(11–12), 1199–1210.

Williams, A. M., & Reilly, T. (2000). Talent identification and development in soccer. *Journal of Sports Sciences, 18*, 657–667.

Zuber, C., Zibung, M., & Conzelmann, A. (2014). Motivational patterns as an instrument for predicting success in promising young football players. *Journal of Sports Sciences, 33*(2), 160–168.

Zuber, C., Zibung, M., & Conzelmann, A. (2016). Holistic pattern as an instrument for predicting the performance of promising young soccer players – a 3-years longitudinal study. *Frontiers in Psychology, 7*, 1089.

# 23 Modern approaches to scouting and recruitment

*David Piggott and Bob Muir*

## Introduction

Talent scouts are an essential part of talent identification and development systems in all sports though their effectiveness has often been questioned by academics (Baker et al., 2019). In soccer, relatively little is known about the activities of scouts or the processes by which they reach judgements about talent (Bergkamp et al., 2021). Nevertheless, one emerging recommendation in the literature is that more structured systems with more explicit reasoning may support more accurate predictions (Bergkamp et al., 2021; Johnston & Baker, 2020; Larkin & O'Connor, 2017). In this chapter, we describe and explain the process of developing and delivering such a system for identifying young soccer players for international selection. Specifically, we describe a process that took place within the 'Team Strategy and Performance' department at the English FA (The FA) between 2018 and 2020, initiated by the then 'Player Insights' team, who was responsible for collecting information about players to inform selection and development decisions. Some of the most important information used in this process came from a team of dedicated scouts, or 'talent reporters'[1], whose main role was to attend live games and submit reports on a small number of players who were under consideration for international selection. Talent reporters typically covered games in either the 'youth development phase' (YDP, U15s–U17s) or the 'professional development phase' (PDP, U18s and U23s) and made reports for the men's pathway squads (U15–U21). During the lifetime of the project, the first author (David Piggott) was a full-time employee in the Player Insights department and the second author (Bob Muir) was a consultant commissioned to design and deliver a Continuing Professional Development (CPD) programme for talent reporters.

## Understanding scouts and scouting

Despite their centrality and obvious importance in the talent identification process, the activities of scouts have been almost entirely overlooked by academics. To our

---

1 In international soccer, we use the term 'talent reporter' as opposed to 'scout' in recognition of the different roles they perform. In club soccer, a 'scout' is searching for talent: they are seeking to *detect* or *identify* talent. In international soccer, players of interest have already had some level of talent *confirmed* by the academy system, so a 'talent reporter's' role is to *describe*, in more detail, the specific nature of the talent they see and consider if this will transfer into senior international soccer.

DOI: 10.4324/9781003148418-28

Reeves et al. (2018) interviewed 37 professionals working across recruitment roles in category-one academies in the United Kingdom with the broad aim of understanding the nature and function of their work. They revealed a reflective group of professionals who had deep and extensive knowledge of the grassroots context; an awareness of biases towards early maturing players; and a holistic approach to talent prediction, based on an attempt to consider (albeit tacitly) multiple characteristics and environmental factors (e.g., a player's family background). Similar conclusions were reached by Bergkamp et al. (2021) in their survey of 125 recruiters working in professional soccer in the Netherlands. They found that scouts working across the age groups tended towards a structured approach to making predictions, combining assessment of different attributes (principally technical skills), but ultimately making holistic appraisals in the final analysis. These scouts, too, seemed to be aware of the dangers of making early assessments based on physical attributes, ranking them well below technical, tactical, and psycho-social attributes when evaluating adolescent players. Finally, in their Delphi poll of 20 selectors working in the regional system in Australia, Larkin and O'Connor (2017) found that selectors made holistic appraisals based on an assessment of a wider range of technical, tactical, and psychological attributes. Perhaps due to the age of the players involved (i.e., U13), they ranked technical skills as relatively more important and tended to place less value on physical attributes.

This portrait is highly consistent with the popular work of British journalist, Michael Calvin, whose seminal book, *The Nowhere Men* (Calvin, 2014), is another important source of information about scouts working in English soccer. Calvin outlines an industry in transition, as 'big data' and video analysts steadily invade the territory that scouts have occupied for years. The scouts with whom Calvin spent time were underpaid (relative to other professionals in clubs), increasingly anxious about the future of their industry and increasingly insecure and marginal, despite their experience, passion, and undoubted skill. Calvin also detailed the careful record keeping of many scouts, a practice that enabled them to engage in thoughtful reflection about their successes and 'the ones that got away'. These reflective capacities are the same as those documented by Reeves et al. (2018) though they also cast some doubt as to the degree to which these reflections are systematic and, therefore, of limited impact in a wider talent ID system.

An important conclusion common to these studies is that the deeper processes and 'decision rules' applied by scouts to make predictions are largely implicit and, therefore, difficult to scrutinise. Whilst many scouts use structures such as checklists and forms to help increase the reliability of assessments, the process by which the more general holistic appraisal is made – how they weight and combine the assessment of a variety of attributes, in context – seems to be tacit and, therefore, potentially inconsistent (Bergkamp et al., 2021). A strong recommendation from this small body of research, therefore, is that talent ID systems in soccer should seek to adopt a more structured and consistent approach to scouting, with more explicit rules and reasoning applied to decision-making to enable more effective critical appraisal (also see Johnston & Baker, 2020).

## 384 *David Piggott and Bob Muir*

The accounts offered by these researchers and authors certainly resonate with our own experiences in interacting directly with international talent reporters in our own programme, and indirectly with scouts and recruiters from a range of professional clubs (through delivery on numerous FA talent ID courses). In our experience, scouts are often aware of the biases they bring to the job (e.g., Christiensen, 2009); are increasingly (if tacitly) knowledgeable about the multidimensional indicators of talent or potential (e.g., Jokuschies et al., 2017); and are often active in seeking support and professional development to refine their craft. It was with an attitude of openness and optimism, then, that we started this project: one in which we considered the scouts to be the subject 'experts' with a very deliberate aim of drawing on (and drawing out) their tacit knowledge to inform a new system of reporting on talent. The project also aimed to address the recommendations from the research, in supporting scouts (or talent reporters) to develop and more explicit and consistent approach to the complex process of identifying future international players.

### The problem situation

At the time we began the project in the summer of 2018, a new 'Player Insights' team had recently been created at The FA. This team was tasked with creating systems for collecting and making sense of a wider set of data about players. This included data generated from a range of internal activities, such as physical testing data and psycho-behavioural notes, but also included externally generated performance analysis data and scouting reports from live games. The Player Insights team was, therefore, positioned at the 'hub' of a wheel, with multiple forms of player data being fed into coaches (who still made executive decisions over squad selection) with the support of 'phase leads' who oversaw selection meetings for each age group and constantly updated the data available to coaches. In this sense, the team had been created in line with recent recommendations improving talent forecasting (cf., Johnston & Baker, 2020).

As the flow of player data into and through the department began to increase, the live game reporting was still deemed to be of central importance to the decision-making process. Coaches were keen to know how players were performing week to week, and keen to pick up on 'soft intelligence' that a talent reporter may have gleaned from being present at the game (e.g., specific instructions a coach may have given, or a chat with a parent that might reveal a player was about to move clubs). The systems for recording and reporting this information, however, had changed almost annually over the preceding 3 or 4 years, and it was felt that the system was not supporting or enabling talent reporters to best use their considerable professional resources.

Like many scouting systems that operate in clubs, the existing system was a mixture of numerical scales (to rate a player's abilities in different domains), often referenced to an ideal type 'positional profile' (cf., Towlson et al., 2019), followed by summary statements where talent reporters were asked to make a holistic judgement about a player's potential (Christiensen, 2009). This would typically lead to unhelpful abstract generalisations of a player's ability, such as 'he has a good first touch' or 'moves well for a big lad'. This type of system, applied in international soccer, was deemed problematic for two main reasons, which we summarise below as: (1) the future game problem and (2) the surrogate selector problem.

*Modern approaches to scouting and recruitment*  385

### The future game problem

Systems that reference positional profiles, with scales for ranking key abilities (e.g., a full-back needs: to be able to cross the ball, stamina, 1v1 defensive skills), assume that current senior players and the skills they possess, are appropriate 'models' for the players of the future. However, as the FA's own Dick Bate noted over a decade ago: 'The game will evolve dramatically over the next two decades and it is critical that those responsible for the development of our young players prepare for what is ahead. Thinking forward and devising both programmes and practice to equip our players for the future is paramount now' (The FA, 2010, p. 20). The ongoing evolution of the game is clear in the scientific research (Harper et al., 2020), with significant changes to, for example, the physical performance of players in different positions (Bush et al., 2015). Looking for current senior qualities in the players of the future, when the future game will pose different challenges, seems to be based on flawed logic. This is one of the many factors that makes forecasting talent very difficult (Baker et al., 2019; Johnston & Baker, 2020), and, therefore, posed a challenge to us in developing the new system. We explain our response to this challenge in the next section.

### The surrogate selector problem

In asking talent reporters to write summarised holistic judgements about players (irrespective of the quality or veracity of those judgements), they interfere with the selector's ability to come to informed judgements themselves. In club scouting, this is often necessary given the large number of players they will have under consideration. Coaches and heads of recruitment do not have time to scrutinise hundreds of reports and prefer a simple 'referral' from a scout: should we bring them in for a trial or not? In international selection, however, there are far fewer players in the frame, and international coaches have far more time to carefully consider detailed reports (at the FA, coaches were also heavily involved in talent reporting). Moreover, it is arguably a more difficult task to identify international potential from a homogenous group of highly talented players, than to identify a talented player in a grassroots setting (Bergkamp et al., 2019). Hence, more detailed, and carefully compiled reports, are necessary to make this difficult distinction between a potential professional and a potential international player.

In addition to these specific problems, it was also the case that the talent reporters had developed their own style of reporting, leading to a high degree of variability in the length and quality of reports. Some of these 'styles' were preferred by coaches; others were not. So, in summary, this is the situation we found ourselves in as we embarked on the project: (1) we had a varied group of highly experienced and expert talent reporters who were constrained and frustrated by the current systems; (2) we had to find a way to overcome the 'future game' and 'surrogate selector' problems; and (3) we had to develop a system and framework that enabled the talent reporters to express their individual expertise but with a higher degree of consistency across the group.

## The solution: CPD and a framework for talent reporting

As noted above, the brief for the development of a new system was clear: we needed to help create a more consistent method of reporting that generated richer, more detailed, contextualised information to assist coach decision-making in the selection and development of youth international players. It was also clear that, as two people with no prior experience in scouting, we would need to draw heavily on the expertise of the talent reporters to inform this new system. We, therefore, couched the programme of work within a CPD programme for the talent reporters, who were grateful for the investment in them and eager to have a say in the development of the new system.

### Design principles

In designing the CPD programme, we made several informed assumptions about the talent reporters. First, we assumed they had a high level of professional expertise – deep tacit knowledge about talent, but also about the context and mechanisms surrounding that talent in the English professional system (Christiensen, 2009; Lund & Söderström, 2017; Reeves et al., 2018) – that was not being maximised under the current system. Second, we assumed that the talent reporters could and would respond positively to educational activities that would help them become more aware of the 'biases' influencing their judgements (cf., Mann & van Ginneken, 2017). And third, we knew that programmes with similar goals, working to create more consistent and coherent talent selection criteria among scouts in international soccer, had led to successful outcomes (cf., Jokuschies et al., 2017). Working with these assumptions, we drew on Gary Klein's triple path model of insight generation (Klein, 2013) in designing the programme.

Klein (2013) argues that when organisations try to improve performance, they often focus on 'error reduction' strategies (e.g., introducing standards, controls, checklists, and procedures), and neglect 'insight generation' strategies. Insight generation, by contrast, involves raising awareness of and discussing connections and contradictions between views and 'changing the frame' (ways of looking at players), to replace flawed explanatory stories with better ones. In our context, we, therefore, aimed not to introduce new scouting forms and checklists, but to create opportunities for experts to generate new insights about talent, and better explanations for how international potential comes to be fulfilled (or not).

### Programme delivery

The CPD programme was delivered over an 18-month period via semi-regular weekend workshops (i.e., every 2–3 months) and occasional larger events (e.g., visits to international camps and tournaments). The participants were 16 male part-time talent reporters working for the FA, all of whom held a range of full-time and part-time jobs in addition to their reporting roles. Among the group, there were teachers, sales executives, coaches, taxi drivers, and university and college lecturers. All had extensive coaching and scouting qualifications and experience working as scouts in the professional game, often for multiple Premier League clubs. The CPD programme was split into three broad phases, outlined in Figure 23.1.

In the first phase, our goal was to get to know the group, to share stories reflecting beliefs and ideas about international talent, and to *cultivate curiosity* based on exploring the differences in ideas (contradictions). Towards the end of the phase, we created very deliberate opportunities to notice clashes and contradictions by asking multiple reporters to report on the same player, without consulting, before juxtaposing their reports in the room. In this way, these early sessions served to surface and problematise

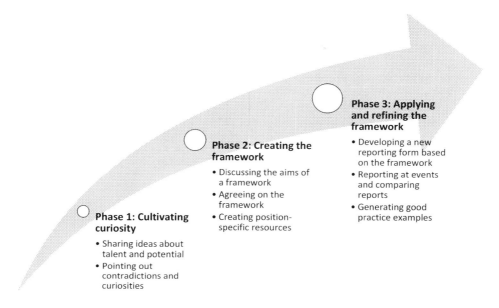

*Figure 23.1* A three-phase approach to talent reporter CPD.

the various biases and heuristics (some helpful, some unhelpful) that the talent reporters held (Miller et al., 2012).

By the second phase of the programme, we had developed some trust and rapport with the group, surfaced some of the main socially constructed theories (and biases and heuristics) used by the reporters (Christensen, 2009), and provoked some curiosity in the differences that existed between their emerging judgements. We, therefore, agreed that it would be helpful to co-create a framework to help the group collectively channel its insights and reduce inconsistences in reporting (again, in line with the recommendations from the literature).

## *Developing the talent reporting framework*

As we approached the challenge of developing a new framework, we had the future game problem and surrogate selector problems in mind. We wanted the talent reporters to be able to communicate their deep knowledge about players and their potential without having to do so in a simplified summarised judgement. We also wanted to encourage the reporters to observe players in a different way to that informed by the 'player profile' model, which runs afoul of the future game problem. The core idea we introduced and discussed in phase 2, then, was very fundamental: it took us back to a discussion of the basic demands of soccer and led us to a new, broader definition of talent as 'the emerging ability to find effective solutions to the problems of the game'.

This thinking was directly influenced by the American philosopher, Bernard Suits, and his famous definition of games as 'the voluntary attempt to overcome unnecessary obstacles'. Suits (1978) defines games as goal-directed activities with rules (the unnecessary obstacles) that prevent you from achieving the goal in the most efficient way. Games

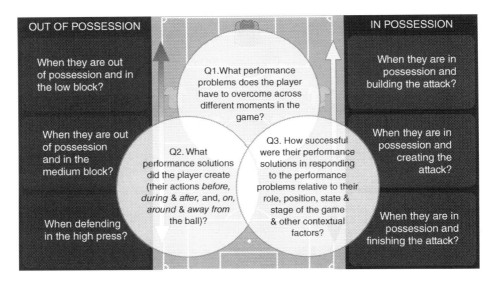

*Figure 23.2* The new talent reporter framework.

therefore present players with *performance problems*, that emerge in the conflict between goals, rules, and opposition. In the early 1980s, Len Almond took this idea and used it to classify sports into families, based on similarity in the goals, rules, and thus problems they pose (Harvey et al., 2017). For example, all invasion games require players, when in possession, to solve the problems of 'keeping the ball', 'moving it up the field/court', and 'penetrating a compact defensive unit to score in a central goal' (Mitchell et al., 2013). We have used this idea elsewhere to support coaches to deepen their understanding of their sports (Piggott & Jones, 2020), and felt it could be usefully transferred to help us solve the future game problem. So, we took Suits' idea of sport as a problem-solving activity and combined it with an existing framework that was used widely at the FA to classify six 'moments of the game' (The FA, 2021) to build the framework (see Figure 23.2).

The framework was developed through a 2-day consultation with the group of talent reporters who developed drafts and experimented with it in a live reporting setting. The framework (Figure 23.2) asks reporters to observe and locate player's actions in different moments (three in possession, three out of possession) in relation to the performance problems they faced (Q1) and describe the solutions they created, both on and off the ball (Q2), before judging their success *in context* (Q3).

The basic idea of the framework, then, was that it invited a different way of thinking about talent or potential that wasn't bound to a fixed profile; it simply asked reporters to consider how well players solved the problems of the game, in context (e.g., relative to their stage of development, the quality of the opposition, and the state of the game). We reasoned that, as the problems of the game change in the future, the best players would be those that could find the best solutions. This was our short-hand definition of potential, and one that is referenced by international coaches elsewhere (cf., Jokuschies et al., 2017).

As we began to experiment with the framework the first thing we noticed is that it invited reporters to observe in much more detail than they had previously. For example, where a scout's attention may naturally drift away from a central defender during the 'finish the attack' moment, the new framework required them to continuously observe the individual's actions throughout a game. Because talent reporters were frequently required to report on two or three players in a game, the new framework posed a serious challenge to the talent reports' attention-switching and note-taking abilities. Despite the challenge it posed, early attempts yielded promising reports and there was a collective belief that we could get faster and more efficient in applying the new framework as it became internalised.

An additional resource we created during phase 2 was a set of position-specific performance problems to ensure we were observing players in broadly the same way (see Q1 in Figure 23.2). These position-specific problems were generated through small 3-hr workshops, conducted with three to four talent reporters, collectively observing video clips of a single position (across all moments), with talent reporters noting down and discussing the main performance problems the players faced. The goal of each workshop was to agree on a small number of draft problems in each moment. An example of the output generated from the workshops is presented in Figure 23.3.

### Reporting with the framework

In the third and final phase of the programme, we ran events where the talent reporters applied the new framework in live reporting situations. Typically, this would involve groups of three reporters attending a game, watching the same player independently (equipped with Figures 23.2 and 23.3, printed in small cards as an *aide memoir*), then working together after the game to construct a joint report, based on a shared understanding of the principles. These discussions would often generate new insights through making connections, noticing contradictions, and encouraging reporters to consider players from different perspectives (Klein, 2013).

Table 23.1 contains an example report that was produced after one of these events. In this case, it is a short report on a YDP player (these reports were typically shorter as it is typical to report on more players per game in the YDP). The report is clearly

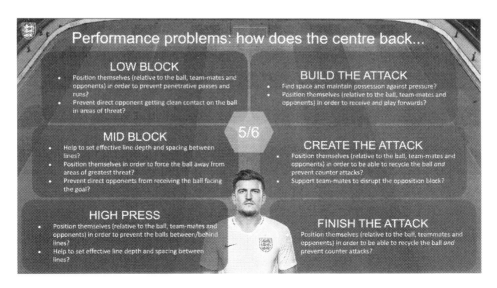

*Figure 23.3* An example of performance problems by position (central defender).

## 390  *David Piggott and Bob Muir*

broken down into sections for: match details and context; in-possession actions; out-of-possession actions; and a summary and recommendation. The additional section labelled '4-corner sensemaking' was a section in which the reporters we asked to interpret player actions through a developmental lens: in short, were some of the players' actions strongly influenced by their state and stage of development (physical, psychological, social, and technical)? This was a difficult section to complete and relied heavily on reporters' knowledge of adolescent development and their ability to observe these characteristics in the field (e.g., that a player might be close to peak growth, based on observation of limb length and torso length and breadth).

In the final section – the summary and recommendation – the summary is intended to capture the main points from the report, and the recommendation is made against four categories: *recommend* (this individual clearly has potential to be an international player); *monitor +* (this individual has potential that needs to be confirmed); *monitor* (this player has potential but there are reasons why it is not appropriate to report on him/her immediately); and *not recommend* (there were no signs that this individual has potential to be an international player). In the case of the player featured in the report above, the recommendation was 'monitor' because they had signs of potential (positioning, concentration, and leadership) but made mistakes that could have been due to rapid growth, a situation that would not change if they were observed again in the following month.

By the end of the programme, the Player Insights team were pleased with the progress made in reforming the talent reporting system. As a direct illustration of the impact of the system on reporting quality, Table 23.2 compares extracts from two reports generated on the same player, under the old and new systems. Hopefully, it is clear how much more useful and specific information is present in the second report. Again, to repeat what we said in the introductory sections, the flaws of the first report reflect the system, not the resources or capability of the individual reporters. When provided with support and a clear and flexible framework – one that encouraged them to make use of their deep personal resources – we found that talent reporters responded very positively.

## Future directions and conclusions

In line with recommendations from the extant literature on scouting in soccer (Bergkamp et al., 2021), our project aimed to support talent reporters to raise their extensive tacit knowledge to be more explicit and to develop and apply a flexible framework to create a more consistent, systematic, and detailed approach to talent assessment. In helping scouts and selectors to better understand their own processes and theories about talent and potential, we aimed to create a 'method for checking the accuracy of our forecasts' (Johnston & Baker, 2020, p. 7). This process of recording forecasts and the reasoning behind them as a basis for later scrutiny and improvement was in its infancy at the FA. Forecasting in this context is a complex business involving the assessment of multiple sources of information (scouting report being just one among many) about multiple interacting variables by a range of professionals over developmental time. There can be, of course, no algorithm for prediction in such circumstances, so the best we can do is to create a framework to support the consistent collection and interpretation of information about players, use it to make predictions, and then revisit those predictions to test and adjust the theories on which they are based.

*Modern approaches to scouting and recruitment* 391

*Table 23.1* An example short report (for a YDP player) [team names redacted]

| Player details | *Billy Tackle\* (born 2005, U15) #5 (left-sided CD)*<br>*\*this is a pseudonym* |
|---|---|
| Match details and context | This report covers performances in $2 \times 50$-min group games in the premier league U15s international tournament. The first a hard-fought 2–1 win against Derby and the second a must-win 3–0 performance against Olympiakos to win a place in the semi-final. The pitch was slick and a little heavy in both games. |
| In possession | **Finish the attack/create the attack**<br>Billy found good support positions, always available to recycle when on the left and playing some dangerous deep crosses into the box on occasion.<br>**Build the attack**<br>Billy showed good composure under pressure, often playing the right pass and showing a good range of passing on his left side. He only misplaced two passes, but one was in a dangerous position. He also showed an ability to step-in and break lines when appropriate. In the Olympiakos game, it was his header, pick-up and calm pass (under pressure) to the right that started the counter-attack for the first goal. |
| Out of possession | **High press**<br>Billy marshals his defence well, maintaining and policing the line depth and communicating constantly. When in the high press, he moves well in relation to the ball and is almost constantly in a good position to respond to direct balls (i.e., side-on body position, tracking the opposition #9).<br>**Mid-block**<br>Billy showed a tendency to step-in aggressively to shut out passed through the middle or into the opposition CF/10. He misjudged this a few times and was left exposed, with teammates having to cover behind.<br>**Low block**<br>Here he showed excellent bravery and determination to win defensive headers, block shots and organised the line well. He was occasionally caught out in 1v1s, especially against Derby's fast and strong CF, who was able to 'pin and spin' on Billy twice. He also struggled when squared up 1v1, failing to stop two shots on goal. |
| 4-Corner sensemaking (what did you notice that helps to explain the solutions reported on above?) | Billy looks like he is around peak growth (upright and awkward in his movements), which may explain his aggression and perception of risk when attacking balls in midfield, and also his lack of mobility when in 1v1s. This needs to be confirmed, but if it is the case it may be worth waiting 3–6<br>months before reporting on him again. |
| Summary and recommendation | Billy showed good bravery and leadership in these games, was calm under pressure with the ball and determined in his low-block defending. His positioning and concentration were always good, but he was too aggressive in going to meet the ball on occasion and got caught out. His 1v1 defending was the main weakness but his mobility may improve with time.<br>Recommendation (on this occasion): Monitor<br>(Recommend – Monitor + – **Monitor** – Not recommend) |

## 392 David Piggott and Bob Muir

*Table 23.2* Extracts of reports of the same player (U21 #9) under the old and new systems

| System | Old | New |
|---|---|---|
| In possession | Movement was very good. Great pace and sharp in his movement but didn't quite come off for him. Pace and reactions both ways are excellent. He was a key outlet over the top and in the channels as soon as they won the ball but the quality into him wasn't great. | *Build the attack* From a high central position, he tended to either drift into space between lines to receive or make sharp inside-out diagonal runs between CDs and FBs. Early in the game the timing of these runs was excellent, and he frequently received in threatening positions in the final third, protected the ball and won two free kicks in dangerous areas. |
| Out of possession | As a striker he was isolated and led the line well; his desire to close down and defend was good. | *High press* His team rarely attempted to press high up the pitch, except when they went behind in the last 15 min. He occupied a central position, loosely screening the ball to stop penetration through the centre. Really this was token pressure and he rarely pressed from behind once the ball had been played into midfield. When the team went behind and (another CF) came on to make a front two, he closed down with much greater intensity, forcing the ball back to the GK who turned the ball over twice as a result. |

The framework we developed (which is still very much in use) offers a basis for such consistent observation across a large team of professionals involved in the talent selection process. We offer this account as potential inspiration and illustration for other national associations and clubs seeking to invest in the development of scouts. It will take many years for such systems to mature and for predictions to be scrutinised (e.g. even in the case of the most precocious players, such as Jude Bellingham, there is a 5-year gap between our initial report and his senior England selection). Future evaluation work must, therefore, be planned and undertaken across long periods of time (i.e., 5–10 years, at least). Moreover, because of the complexity of the decisions and decision-making process, evaluation methodologies need to be sensitive enough to unpick the multi-layered mechanisms at play (how sources of information influence thinking) and the outcome patterns that emerge (decisions about selection) (Pawson, 2013). Whilst the exploratory research focusing on the practices and processes of soccer scouts has been useful, we would also argue that future research needs to locate the activity of scouts in a much broader context. Almost all professional clubs and major national associations generate and have access to extensive multifaceted data on players, with scouting reports representing just one vector among many.

## References

Baker, J., Wattie, N., & Schorer, J. (2019). A proposed conceptualization of talent in sport: the first step in a long and winding road. *Psychology of Sport and Exercise, 43*, 27–33.

Bergkamp, T., Frencken, W., Neissen, S., Mejer, R., & den Hartigh, R. (2021). How soccer scouts identify talented players. *European Journal of Sport Science.* https://doi.org/10.1080/17461391.2021.1916081

Bergkamp, T., Nielssen, A., den Hartigh, R., Frencken, W., & Meijer, R. (2019). Methodological issues in soccer talent identification research. *Sports Medicine, 49*(9), 1317–1335.

Bush, M., Barnes, C., Archer, D., Hogg, B., & Bradley, P. (2015). Evolution of match performance parameters for various playing positions in the English premier league. *Human Movement Science, 39*, 1–11.

Calvin, M. (2014). *The Nowhere Men: The Unknown Story of Football's True Talent Spotters.* London: Penguin Books.

Christiensen, M. (2009). "An eye for talent": talent identification and the "practical sense" of top-level soccer coaches. *Sociology of Sport Journal, 26*, 365–382.

Harper, D., Sandford, G., Clubb, J., Young, M., Taberner, M., Rhodes, D., Carling, C., & Keily, J. (2020). Elite football of 2030 will not be the same as that of 2020: what has evolved and what needs to evolve? *Scandinavian Journal of Medicine & Sport Science, 31*, 493–494.

Harvey, S., Pill, S., & Almond, L. (2017). Old wine in new bottles: a response to claims that teaching games of understanding was not developed as a theoretically based pedagogical framework. *Physical Education & Sport Pedagogy, 23*(2), 166–180.

Johnston, K., & Baker, J. (2020). Waste reduction strategies: factors affecting talent wastage and the efficacy of talent selection in sport. *Frontiers in Psychology, 10*(2925), 2–11.

Jokuschies, N., Gut, V., & Conzelmann, A. (2017). Systematising coaches' 'eye for talent': player assessments based on expert coaches' subjective talent criteria in top-level youth soccer. *International Journal of Sport Science & Coaching, 12*(5), 565–576.

Klein, G. (2013). *Seeing What Others don't: The Remarkable Ways We Gain Insights.* New York: Public Affairs.

Larkin, P., & O'Connor, D. (2017). Talent identification and recruitment in youth soccer: recruiters' perceptions of the key attributes for player recruitment. *PLoS ONE, 12*(4), e0175716.

Lund, S., & Söderström, T. (2017). To see or not to see: talent identification in the Swedish football association. *Sociology of Sport Journal, 34*, 248–258.

Mann, D., & van Ginneken, P. (2017). Age-ordered shirt numbering reduces the selection bias associated with relative age effect. *Journal of Sport Sciences, 35*(8), 784–790.

Miller, P., Rowe, L., Cronin, C., & Bampouras, T. (2012). Heoristic reasoning and the observer's view: the influence of example availability on *ad-hoc* frequency judgements in sport. *Journal of Applied Sport Psychology, 24*, 290–302.

Mitchell, S., Oslin, J., & Griffin, L. (2013). *Teaching Sports Concepts and Skills.* Champaign, IL: Human Kinetics.

Pawson, R. (2013). *The Science of Evaluation: A Realist Manifesto.* London: Sage.

Piggott, D., & Jones, R. (2020). The practical application of immersive games-based narratives, in S. Pill (Ed.), *Perspectives on Games-based Coaching.* London: Routledge.

Reeves, M., Littlewood, M., McRobert, A., & Roberts, S. (2018). The nature and function of talent identification in junior-elite football in English category one academies. *Soccer & Society, 19*(8), 1122–1134.

Suits, B. (1978). *The Grasshopper: Games, Life and Utopia.* Ontario, CA: Broadview Press.

The FA. (2010). *The Future Game: The FA's Guide for Young Player Development.* London: The FA.

The FA. (2021). *The England DNA: How We Play.* Burton: The FA. https://thebootroom.thefa. com/resources/england-dna/how-we-play

Towlson, C., Cope, E., Perry, J., Court, D., & Levett, N. (2019). Practitioners' multi-disciplinary perspectives of soccer talent according to phase of development and playing position. *International Journal of Sport Science & Coaching, 14*(4), 528–540.

# Section F

# Some Key Organizational Roles at Clubs

# 24 Working as a director of sports science or high-performance director

*Tony Strudwick*

## Introduction

Soccer is played by 250 million people in more than 200 countries making it the world's most popular sport. The worldwide influence and daily interest attract ever-increasing attention and intelligent focus into the sport. Many academic institutions around the world now offer programmes of study specifically related to soccer. In an applied setting, a major shift has occurred towards scientific methods of preparing soccer players for competition. Many soccer teams now routinely employ practitioners from the various sub-disciplines of sports science with the aim of improving sporting performance.

Throughout the past few decades, the demand for soccer scientists and performance directors has been growing because of the ever-increasing focus in the soccer world on achieving the best results possible. The establishment of advanced scientific support models is evidence that high performance is being taken seriously. Although the field of sport management has been widely defined, the sub-field of managing high-performance sports is relatively new and has emerged from elite sports (Sotiriadou & De Bosscher, 2018). A multitude of titles have been assigned to those practitioners leading and managing high-performance departments, such as the Head of Medical Services, Director of Performance, Human Performance Manager, and Head of Performance. For the purpose of this chapter, the Director of Sports Science and High-Performance Director will be used to identify those individuals leading and managing departments and performance processes.

Ultimately, the roles and functions of support staff have been examined more closely, to the benefit of the soccer profession. The increase in qualification-led employment has led to an examination of the traditional role of the head coach and support team. To facilitate these changes, a new era of high-performance directors and managers have evolved. These practitioners with a diverse range of skills are trained and educated to think and work in a multidisciplinary environment. Moreover, these practitioners have the relevant skills for appreciating the coaching process and its associated elements.

The key objective of this chapter is to explore the role of Director of Sports Science/High-Performance Director and highlight some of the key issues involved in leading and managing contemporary high-performance when working at a professional club or with a national team. This chapter also focuses on translating into practice the requirements of leading and managing high-performance teams, with special reference to the cultural and organisational structures pertinent to real working practices in soccer.

DOI: 10.4324/9781003148418-30

## The rise of soccer science and sports medicine

On-field Soccer performance has always been the chief concern for all soccer clubs throughout the professional era. The methods employed, however, have changed considerably over the past few decades. Throughout the early professionalisation of the sport, the players were mostly left in the charge of the trainer. Trainers were responsible for maintaining both discipline and physical fitness. Initially, besides having fitness duties, the trainer provided day-to-day medical care and treated and managed player injuries. Initially, ideas on what constituted training for soccer players were limited, and the first generation of trainers was largely made up of professional athletes and athletic trainers. From the 1960s, soccer players were becoming increasingly critical of the medical treatment they received, and players began to seek second opinions outside their clubs without permission. Although the image of the soccer trainer with a bucket and sponge has been both mythologised and derided, the role needs to be seen in context. Moreover, it does provide insight into the history of the relationship between soccer and medicine, as well as the evolution of soccer science in the professionalisation of the game (Carter, 2010).

Throughout the later stages of the 21st Century, soccer clubs appointed doctors, physiotherapists, soft tissue therapists, fitness coaches, and sports scientists to maximise player preparation. Over these years, the trainer began to take on a more physiotherapeutic role and medical support teams increased in numbers and complexity. Demand was growing for greater support services with greater accountability amongst support staff.

In 1992 the establishment of the English Premier League signalled a change in the relationship between soccer and science. Greater intensity emerged as the commercialisation of soccer increased. The value of players increased exponentially, as did financial rewards for staying in the Premier League. As a result, these developments necessitated a greater investment in medical and scientific facilities and resources. In many ways, little had changed from the dawn of professional soccer in the early 1900s. Clubs had always invested in the welfare of their players, but the nature of the process and organisational structure was shaped by the prevailing cultural context – commercial, soccer, and social (Carter, 2016).

Contemporary players have now been exposed to scientific approaches in preparation for competition. Certainly, examples of best practices can be seen in Elite English soccer. Coaching practice that for many years was based largely on tradition, emulation, and intuition is now giving way to an approach based on scientific evidence. This shift has resulted in better-informed practitioners working with teams, stronger links with scientific institutes, and more coaches willing to accept the changing role of sports science in elite soccer. More importantly, it is against this backdrop, that through the evolution of soccer science and increased professionalisation, we witness the emergence of Directors of Sports Science and High-Performance Directors.

## The role of the high-performance director

With the need to maximise individual and team performance, High-Performance Directors are required to manage and identify the key parameters that are required for elite participation. High-performance sport operates in a fast-paced, complex environment and the skills required for successful practitioners are multifaceted and

*Working as a director of sports science* 399

*Table 24.1* Some of the key responsibilities of a High-Performance Director

| *Responsibilities* |
| --- |
| Provide leadership and strategic vision to team functions, including medical services, sports science, psychology, and performance analysis. |
| Manage all stakeholders involved in the delivery of the performance strategy; ensuring all stakeholders clearly understand their roles and responsibilities and that all are delivering to the required standard. |
| Maintain an effective, collaborative, and continuous relationship with the management team, sharing and co-creating on best practice methods and research that can be deployed across the organisation and partners. |
| Oversee the delivery of a multi-disciplinary team approach to the management of long-term athletic development considering injury management, player load and development. |
| Ensure the performance trajectory of the players is positively impacted by contemporary research and innovation initiatives. |
| Understand and manage risk/compliance requirements; be an expert in compliance and protocol, ensure that the department abides by regulations and activities in scope and is always compliant. |
| Champion continuous process improvement; drive operational efficiency and effectiveness by identifying opportunities for improvement in processes and ways of working, establishing measurement and KPIs where relevant. |
| Set, deliver, and report to senior management on the strategic and operational plans and budgets for the performance team. |

multidisciplinary. To make sense of the requirements of the High-Performance Director in a sporting context, it is perhaps useful to define the components of the role that are relevant in shaping the performance environment. While there are many areas of focus when delivering high-performance services, the key responsibilities of the Director role are provided in Table 24.1.

Successful soccer performance is undoubtedly multidisciplinary in nature. High-Performance Directors need to be aware of the physiological, biomechanical, psychological, nutritional, medical, and other types of issues that can affect competition. When all these factors work as an integrated system, excellence in high-performance soccer is possible. Coaching is about problem-solving. Practitioners who are trained to think critically about all aspects of performance will gain an advantage over competitors.

If the role of the coach is to assimilate information and drive the coaching process, then the role of the High-Performance Director is to lead a team to monitor, manage, record, and deliver performance insights. Just as modern coaches need to be familiar with the significant contributions that sports science can offer, High-Performance Directors need to be familiar with the complexities of the demands of soccer and the appropriate methods of communicating with athletes, coaches, and stakeholders involved in elite participation. While many factors need to be considered when working as a Director of Sports Science or a High-Performance Director, there are four key areas that need to be appreciated and understood to shape the performance environment:

- High-Performance;
- Sports Science;
- Talent Development;
- Organisational Culture.

## High performance

High-performance can be considered as producing results above and beyond standard norms over a long-term. High performance is used to describe a product that is faster, more efficient, and superior in functioning than other products. In a sporting context, high performance is competition at the highest level of participation, where the emphasis is on winning and success. A high-performance culture is a set of behaviours and norms that leads an organisation to achieve superior results. In other words, it's a culture that drives a high-performance organisation. In a high-performance sporting environment, organisations offer training in specialised facilities, coaching, and skill development and transition to higher levels of competition (Rees et al., 2016). In addition, athletes operating within a high-performance environment are offered advanced sports science support to maximise individual and team performance to achieve the best results possible.

The intensive training and frequent competition in elite soccer induce a high degree of stress upon the player. An analysis of the stress and injuries that may result is helpful in identifying risk factors associated with soccer-related activities. In addition, players must meet the requirements of the game with a demonstration of appropriate coping strategies. It is, therefore, prudent for the High-Performance Director to focus on the 'High-Performance Status' of individual participants so that appropriate strategies can be implemented to maximise performance. In addition, key metrics for performance can be established and used as evidence to demonstrate the impact of service.

The underlying philosophy behind 'High-Performance Status' is that coping strategy and overall success is reflected in a player's ability to sustain the load associated with training and match-play at the highest level. Clearly, the athlete and the environment per se are critical to achieving sustained success. Coaches and athletes need to understand the 'Performance v Cost/Benefit' profile of elite participation and how to manage/mitigate these risks on a team and individual basis through proactive monitoring and the implementation of preventative strategies.

In introducing this approach to monitoring high performance, it is important to identify the objectives most critical to success. Moreover, it is important to identify the critical few metrics to track high performance and alignment. High-performance status factors along with metrics used to track these parameters are listed in Table 24.2. These parameters can also be used as individual and team selection criteria and form a basis for squad selection and rotation. Additionally, there is a need to look at the performance reliability of players, which is based on the following equation:

$$\text{Performance Reliability} = \left( \frac{\text{Match Availability} \times \text{Percentage time on pitch}}{1000} \right)$$

This metric has been introduced because it represents a player's ability to not only cope with the demands of training but also of high-performance games. That is, it reflects how constitutional factors of the athlete interact with how teams employ the player during matches.

## Sport science

Sports science is a discipline that studies the application of scientific principles and techniques and has the aim of improving sporting performance. The study of sports

*Working as a director of sports science* 401

*Table 24.2* High-performance status of elite players

| High-performance factors | How the factor is measured |
| --- | --- |
| Remain injury free | Days missed through injury |
| Capable of sustaining high-performance work rates | Work-rate profiles during elite match-play based on objective match analysis data |
| Capable of playing 50 games per season | Games played – Percentage used during in-season competition |
| Window of opportunity (22–30 years old) | Player age – number of playing seasons in professional league |
| Capable of playing a game every 4 days over a 5-game period | Number of days per game over 5 game period (90 min played) |
| Ability to demonstrate sound recovery on objective markers | Objective markers as employed by sports science department |
| Demonstrate seasonal match availability of 90% | See equation below* |
| Demonstrate seasonal training availability of 85% | See equation below** |

Where:
* Squad availability match = 100 – ((# of matches absent/Total no of matches) * 100)
** Squad availability training = 100 – ((# of training sessions absent/Total no of training sessions) * 100)

science traditionally incorporates areas of physiology, psychology, and biomechanics but also includes other topics such as performance analysis and nutrition. Sports science also helps practitioners understand the physical and psychological effects of sports, thereby providing the best techniques for a sport and the most appropriate methods of preventing injuries to an athlete involved in the performance of the sport. Key areas of research in soccer include the effect of nutrition and training on performance and recovery from participation, the effect of training volume on the immune system, the biomechanics and motor control of elite sporting performance, talent identification and development, cognition and muscle function, and motivation and mental toughness.

The application of soccer science has a self-evident part to play in improving soccer performance. Important features of the performance model, such as devising training programmes, monitoring performance, and establishing preparation for competition, are informed by such knowledge. The primary role of sports science in elite soccer is to utilise scientific principles to maximise individual performance and player availability. Clearly, the role of the Director of Sports Science is to manage the delivery of the key components of the sports science model.

## Talent development

In sports research, the process of talent development is discussed with the purpose of producing athletes that can attain a consistent world-class level of performance (Li et al., 2014). Although the area of talent identification and development has been a subject of research for over 50 years, definitive definitions of talent have rarely been offered (Tranckle, 2004). In the literature, it is widely believed that the likelihood of becoming an elite performer depends on the presence of innate gifts. Moreover, talent is the expression of innate gifts and is influenced by a series of internal and external developmental processes (Gagné, 1985).

402  *Tony Strudwick*

Much of the contemporary research on talent development has focused on individual athletes and their micro-environment (Henriksen et al., 2010). Researchers have emphasised either innate prerequisites (talent detection and selection) for excellence or the amount and quality of training required to reach the highest level of elite participation (talent development). While talent, innate abilities, and chance are recognised (Gagné, 1998, 2005) as significant elements to excellence, there is limited evidence to support how these areas interact with each other.

More recently, the psychological perspective has been developed in a new trend regarding talent development environment models and a social perspective in understanding athletic talent (Stambulova, 2009). The focus shifts from the individual athlete per se to the environment itself. Martindale et al. (2005) introduced the term Talent Development Environment (TDE). TDE refers to all aspects of the coaching/learning situation and focuses on the coaching context. Using this approach, Martindale et al. (2005) identified five properties of effective TDEs:

- Long-term aims and methods clearly identified;
- Wide-ranging coherent support and messages;
- Emphasis on appropriate development rather than early selection;
- Individualised and ongoing development;
- An integrated, holistic, and systematic development.

The emphasis becomes not on identifying individual talent, but rather on how best to develop talent (Ivarsson et al., 2014). Moreover, the focus is on the interaction between the individual athletes and their environment. Henriksen (2010) has applied a holistic approach to talent development, which also considers the macro-environment (organisational culture and sports systems). By applying a holistic approach to talent development, it is easier to understand the challenges associated with it, such as recruitment, retention, and transitions (Henriksen, 2010).

It is against this backdrop of contemporary research that modern-day High-Performance Directors and Directors of Sports Science need to appreciate the key facets of talent development when shaping the high-performance environment. Given the exponential growth of emerging departments associated with talent development and sports performance, there will be tensions and challenges in managing and coordinating the input of each area. The High-Performance Director must also recognise that managing the co-existence of the 'talented' athletes alongside other experts across the various disciplines and departments is also a critical component of their role (Littlewood et al., 2018).

## Organisational culture

According to Littlewood et al. (2018), it is imperative that the figure leading and shaping high-level performance must have an intimate knowledge and appreciation of the organisational culture in which he/she operates. Moreover, change is best achieved through a process that involves attending to daily working practices and helping the broader culture to evolve. To make sense of the influence of culture in a sporting setting (within a developmental and performance environment) it is useful to understand the culture and organisational structure that exist between groups of people or members of a group.

Sport participation in many countries cannot be appreciated aside from the Nation's culture, traditions, and values. Sport reflects national culture because it permeates all levels of society. These cultural systems influence talent development, methods of preparation, and organisational structures that form a durable template by which ideas are transferred from one generation to the other. In seeking to ascertain how the culture of a society may affect the development of methods of soccer preparation, we need to recognise that culture itself is an extremely complex phenomenon.

Culture is typically referred to as a pattern of behaviours and basic assumptions that are invented, discovered, or developed by a given group as it learns to cope with its problems of external adaptation and internal integration (Schein, 1991). At a more visible level, culture describes ideas and images that are transferred from one generation or group to another. On a soccer level, we can assume that methods of player preparation and daily interactions of stakeholders have become so deeply entrenched in organisational structure that any attempt to challenge traditional practice is often received with caution and resistance. Nonetheless, the increasing concern with financial profit and professionalisation has inevitably led to evolving methods of player preparation and move away from overreliance on traditional methods.

A strong culture is one that is shared by all employees. However, one limitation of a strong culture is the difficulty changing that culture. In an organisation where certain values are widely shared, unlearning the old values and learning the new ones will be challenging because employees (and other key stakeholders) will need to adopt to new ways of thinking. This is a critical role for the High-Performance Director, where there is a requirement to satisfy all the stakeholders within the business, while at the same time navigate change management.

## Building an organisational structure to facilitate high performance

High-performance sport operates in a fast-paced, highly dynamic environment that is influenced by the social, cultural, and economic conditions of the community in which it operates (Chelladurai, 2009). As such, managing the organisational structure of a High-performance team is a complex process shaped by several factors (De Bosscher et al., 2006).

Sports organisations use structures to determine relationships in the workplace. An organisational structure is a system that outlines how certain activities are directed to achieve the goals of an organisation. These activities can include rules, roles, and responsibilities. The structure also determines how information flows between levels within the company. There are a variety of structures to choose from, and it's important to choose one that best fits the company's needs. The structure can be both horizontal and vertical in nature and it is the role of the High-Performance Director to characterise the dimensions of the performance support structure and levels of decision-making. When deciding on the most appropriate organisational structure to deliver high-level performance, the following elements will impact on the structure:

- Levels of decision-making;
- Number of managers;
- Level of employee input;
- Flow of communication;
- Level of efficiency;

## 404 Tony Strudwick

---

**Differences between horizontal and vertical structures**

Vertical structures have clearly defined roles with specific responsibilities for each person, reducing the level of employee autonomy. Horizontal structures have less structure, often providing employees with equal opportunities. However, this may result in a lack of guidance or lead to internal conflict.

---

- Level of creativity;
- Amount of collaboration;
- Willingness to take risks.

The horizontal structure is related with the number of departments, divisions, and sub-divisions within the organisation and to the work broken down into narrow tasks (Slack, 1997). Sports organisations with these structures often have few managers, and they allow employees to make decisions without needing manager approval. Providing employees with autonomy often helps employees feel empowered and motivated, increasing their connection to the organisation and its goals. The relaxed structure of horizontal organisational structures also often naturally encourages collaboration.

The vertical structure is related to the number of levels in a sports organisation. Vertical organisational structure is a pyramid-like top-down management structure. These organisations have clearly defined roles with the highest level of leadership at the top, followed by middle management than regular employees. Decision-making often works from top to bottom, but work approval will work from bottom to top.

Vertical organisational structures define a clear chain of command. The highest levels of managers make decisions about sales, marketing, customer service, and other standards and communicate them to middle managers. Middle managers assign work to employees and communicate processes and goals. Employees complete the work, and the work goes through middle management and upper management for approval.

The first important step in gaining an advantage through sports science support is to ensure the organisational structure and staffing are efficient. Traditionally, a soccer team has a head coach and coaching staff, fitness or strength and conditioning coach, sports scientist, physiotherapist, and medical doctor. All too often, this structure is disjointed and has multiple avenues of coordination. Moreover, the head coach often receives information referring to a player's status from several sources, and this information is often clouded by personal and occupational bias (Duncan & Strudwick, 2016). Over the past few years, there has been major growth in the support services around professional soccer players, and this has led to the development of the 'Human Performance Team'. While the Human Performance Team is constituted as a set of people from different sub-disciplines of soccer science, the impact of the service provision is reliant on the organisational structure. A more contemporary model is shown in Figure 24.1. The High-Performance Director may have a medical, sports science, physiotherapy or strength, and conditioning background and report directly to the Head Coach and/or Director of Soccer.

Given the complexity of modern soccer and the various sub-disciplines operating within the 'Human Performance Team', High-Performance Directors may consider developing a hybrid strategy that incorporates elements of both vertical and horizontal

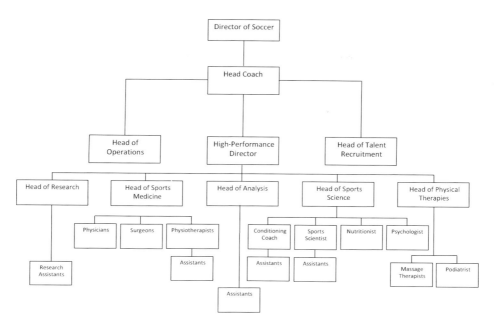

*Figure 24.1* Example organisational model associated with the operation of a modern elite soccer team.

organisational structures. The hybrid organisational structure establishes clear departments related to specific topics with individual vertical structures. In this hybrid structure, the performance team brings members together from each department to collaborate. Here, each employee has vertical accountability to their specific department and horizontal accountability to their teammates. For efficient delivery across the Performance Team, rules, regulations, job descriptions, and procedures need to be well-defined.

## The role of director of sports science

The application of scientific support models has a self-evident part to play in improving elite performance. Important features of the model such as devising training programmes, monitoring performance, and establishing preparation for competition, are informed by such knowledge. The primary role of the Director of Sports Science is to utilise scientific principles to maximise individual performance and player availability. Practitioners must effectively manipulate the training process to achieve these objectives. Moreover, the dimensions of the training programme must be established, and detailed planning carried out to positively influence both the coaching process and the resultant player performance risk management.

An elite soccer player attempting to reach the highest level requires a systematic approach to all areas of performance management. Such an approach can be achieved by identifying critical component parts of the coaching process and the relationships between the sub-processes. There are several critical components that impact on player performance management as detailed in Figure 24.2. While many of the

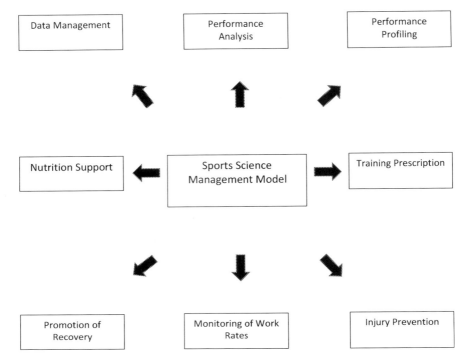

*Figure 24.2* A typical sports science performance management model.

components overlap, successful implementation is dependent on a sound organisational support structure developed between players and staff. Critically, the Head of Sports Science must have an appreciation of all the key components in the delivery of high-performance support.

### *Data management*

Information is the fuel that drives the performance management process. Planning, decision-making, monitoring, and performance analysis all depend on the availability of the necessary information. A critical concept for the Director of Sports Science is distinguishing between which data are important and which are not. Data gathering for the sake of it can be very expensive and futile unless it is used to drive action during the coaching process. While technology on its own cannot guarantee success at an elite level, time and effort focussed on developing robust analytical processes have great potential. Only recently has data begun to transform the management of professional soccer.

### *Performance analysis*

To gain a correct impression of the physiological loads imposed on soccer players during competitive matches, observations must be made during real match-play. Performance analysis entails determining work-rate profiles of players within a team and classifying activities in terms of intensity, duration, and frequency (Reilly, 1994). In this way, an overall picture of the physiological demands of soccer can be gathered. The application of performance analysis to soccer has enabled the objective recording and interpretation of match events, describing the characteristic patterns of activity in soccer. Improvement in performance is the central purpose of the coaching process and a detailed knowledge at the behavioural level of performance is essential for almost all stages of the performance management model.

### Performance profiling

To ensure that elite players are well-prepared, the Director of Sport Science should use performance profiling as a means of providing information on current performance status. A performance profile of a player provides a benchmark of the overall state of his/her level of conditioning. A player's level of conditioning may vary due to the stage of the season, the effectiveness of the training programme, game frequency, or the maturity status of the player. Quite simply, performance profiling should provide information for analysis and subsequent action by both coach and player. To achieve this end, assessment needs to be built into the training plan at regular and appropriate intervals. In this way, performance profiling will assist the design and regulation of a high-performance programme.

### Training prescription

In the preparation of elite players, it is important that the training programme is well-planned. The training programme needs to be specific and objective, taking into consideration the player's potential and rate of development. Any training programme adopted should encompass relevant experiences accumulated over the years together with applied research findings. Such a programme needs to be versatile, enabling it to be utilised as a model of training, being easily applied to individuals with their own specific characteristics and goals. The consistency and knowledge of workloads during each of the training categories means that two of the most important training principles can be applied during field-based conditioning, namely, progression and periodisation. Progression refers to gradually increasing the training load over time as fitness gains are incurred. Periodisation can be defined as a logical, phasic method of manipulating training variables to increase the potential for achieving specific performance goals.

### Injury prevention

In the preparation of elite athletes, the Director of Sports Science has a responsibility to implement a comprehensive and planned training programme that allows for gym-based injury prevention strategies. The athlete must be trained in such a way that the body will be prepared for optimum response to the physical demands of competition. Strength training has been increasingly employed in the holistic management of contemporary soccer players. In simple terms, strength training involves increasing the ability of the athlete to apply force. The ultimate objectives of strength training are to develop the capacity to reproduce forceful bursts of energy and withstand the forces of physical impact, landing, and deceleration. Following specific screening protocols

408   *Tony Strudwick*

for local muscles as well as joints and lower back/pelvis, preventative gym-based programmes in the form of core stability, balance, proprioception, muscular strength, and power should be implemented to address the increasing issues of muscle strains in contemporary elite soccer.

### Monitoring of work-rates

To develop a successful training programme, the physical demands of training and competition need to be fully understood. The physiological requirements of match-play vary from match to match (Gregson et al., 2010) and depend upon playing position, tactical role, and team success amongst other factors (Bradley et al., 2009; Di Salvo et al., 2009; Rampinini et al., 2007). Consequently, the subsequent volume and intensity of training and/or recovery should be individually prescribed according to the players' previous loadings and future requirements to optimise their readiness to perform in the next match. A continual system of monitoring is essential to ensure the correct decisions are made with regard to individual player requirements.

### Promotion of recovery

A chronic problem in high-performance sport remains the continual risk of an imbalance between the training, competition, and recovery components (Budgett, 1990). Successful training must involve overload while avoiding the combination of excessive overload plus inadequate recovery (Meeusen et al., 2006). Because of intense training and competition, players may experience acute feelings of fatigue which temporarily reduces functional capacity and performance. During the subsequent rest period, positive adaptations may follow. This process of overcompensation should be considered as the foundation of all functional increases in athletic efficiency. However, if the optimal balance between training stress and adequate recovery is miscalculated the adaptation process will lessen, leading to overtraining.

### Nutritional support

To maximise adaptations from training and enhance recovery after match play, it is essential that players follow an effective individual nutritional support strategy. Moreover, a systematic approach to providing the appropriate nutritional-based strategies will yield favourable results in terms of training adaptations, recovery, and match performance.

## Key challenges managing high performance at international level

The focus of international soccer is exclusively on elite performance. Therefore, a performance support model needs to be well-informed and deliver high-level results. As a practitioner working at this level, the critical areas of focus include:

- Ensure the team(s) are physically prepared to compete successfully during major tournaments;
- Maximise selection of players for every competitive game;
- Create concepts that reflect the Federation's approach to training and preparation;

*Working as a director of sports science*  409

*Table 24.3* Some key challenges at an international level of competition

| Key challenges | Factors |
|---|---|
| Environment | Events played at environmental extremes |
| Nutrition | Diverse range of individual nutritional requirements |
| Immunity | Travel, exercise, and tournament stress |
| International fixtures | Multiple fixtures during major tournaments |
| Tactics and systems of play | Changing demands of international play |
| Contact time | Reduced preparation time with players |
| Lines of communication | Managing communication with clubs and players |
| Club v country priorities/agendas | Managing requirements of club and country |
| Individual player requirements | Tailored training v generic team training |
| Individual player differences | Managing players with different periodisation plans |
| Head coach communication | Making sure head coach receives information |
| Load management | Create an efficient strategy to manage load |
| Identifying player readiness/freshness | Need to quickly establish the status of players |
| Information sharing | Ensuring close communication with clubs |

- Facilitate high levels of motivation and organisation during training;
- Create a performance model that satisfies the needs of all stakeholders, including players, coaches, and staff;
- Ensure close communication and liaison with clubs.

With countless variables influencing success at elite-level international match-play, high-performance practitioners must appreciate how their athletes will be challenged during competition. International soccer presents a unique set of challenges and opportunities. These challenges must be appreciated, confronted, and quantified for soccer success. An example of some of these challenges is presented in Table 24.3.

In addition to these challenges, practitioners need to have knowledge and understanding of the physical and physiological demands of participation in different environmental conditions, heat and altitude acclimation, optimisation of recovery strategies, the impact of travelling across multiple time zones, and an appreciation of dense fixtures during the international calendar.

The physical requirements at the international level vary from match to match, depending on playing style, tactical organisation, and location of the match. Soccer players at the international level are regularly called on to travel large distances to participate in competitive games. Although international travel is routine for many elite performers, it is not without issues for the travelling player, a circumstance that should be recognised and managed by support staff. When journeys entail a 2- to 3-hour time zone transition and a short stay (2 days), staying at home time may be feasible. Such an approach is useful if the stay in the new time zone is 3 days or less and adjustment of circadian rhythms is not essential. A European team that is to compete in the morning in Japan or in the evening in the United States will require an adjustment of the body clock because these timings would otherwise be too difficult to cope with.

The key is planning and advance preparation. By doing so, player health can be maintained and negative influences on physical performance can be minimised. Players and teams that do not plan will approach international competitions with inadequate preparation and will be less likely to achieve a successful outcome.

The preparation and training programme must be well-organised considering individual differences, physiological capabilities, and diversity of periodisation templates

410 *Tony Strudwick*

athletes are exposed to at their respective clubs. A system of continual monitoring is essential to ensure that all athletes perform the required volume, intensity, and frequency of training. Training load should be prescribed to ensure optimal team preparation for the upcoming fixture, but also based on each individual athlete's previous training history and current physiological status. Careful planning between the coach and sports scientist will allow the training process to be maximised reducing the risk of injury occurrence or overtraining.

For coaches and high-performance practitioners to make effective use of time available, a series of steps must be followed. First, the coach must appreciate the technical and tactical elements of successful performance, including physiological considerations and time on task. Second, the coach needs to translate this information into soccer-specific training drills. Third, the organisation, design and prescription of relevant training methods must consider the major conditioning principles (specificity, overload, and recovery). The application of these principles in a planned manner is the key to effective physiological preparation, enhanced motivation, and improved execution of technical performance.

At an elite level of participation, the coach builds cooperation between sports scientists and soccer players. Moreover, the coach with sports science guidance assimilates information, analyses the effectiveness of the training plan, and constructs the training sessions. Planning, decision-making, monitoring, and performance analysis all depend on the availability of the necessary information. Prior to arrival at an international training camp, High-Performance Directors/Directors of Sports Science collaborate with host clubs to share data on athletes' physiological status. This information provides the platform to drive discussions and make informed decisions to maximise individual and team preparation. Although situational variables such as quality of opposition, game location, and congested fixture periods must be taken into consideration, key performance insights may be identified.

When planning for international fixtures a 'Tactical Preparation' methodology is recommended to control training variables and maximise tactical input from the coaching staff. This methodology will allow for multiple scenarios, diverse individual management strategies and tactical planning. Some facets of a tactical preparation methodology are listed below.

- All soccer training decisions are based on tactical preparation.
- There should be a direct relationship between practices and the tactical emphasis of the upcoming fixture.
- Weekly training pattern with alternating loads and complexity to cope with recovery demands.
- Always combing tactical principles and physical components in training.
- Managing the physical components and tactical complexity to ensure the recovery from previous sessions.
- Practices designed by manipulating constraints such as time, space, number of players and rules.
- Practices designed so that their specific requirements (tactical, physical, and mental) are higher or lower than game.
- Recognising that the concept of periodisation is non-linear and an individual approach will be required.
- Adopting an agile approach to planning and decision-making where complexity is embraced.

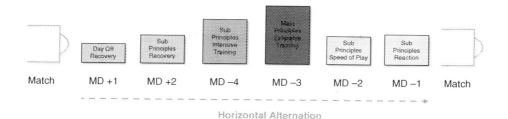

*Figure 24.3* Model showing a potential periodisation strategy for player and team preparation for a international soccer team.

The Tactical Preparation methodology shares many of the concepts defined in The Tactical Periodisation approach (Oliveira, 2014), where a framework is provided to organise training sessions to create 'actions' that players expect during the next competitive match. Here, 'principles' and 'sub-principles' of the different phases of the game are delivered to the players over different types of training sessions (Intensive, Extensive, Speed, and Reaction). This methodology does not separate any component of the game model (physical, technical, tactical, and psychological) and is delivered as an integrated approach to preparation. The consistency and knowledge of workloads during each of the training sessions means that two important principles can be applied, namely, the principle of specificity and the principle of horizontal alternation.

The principle of specificity relates to training sessions designed to replicate situations of the game to improve the decision-making of the players. The principle of horizontal alternation relates to weekly training patterns with alternating loads and complexity to cope with recovery demands. Moreover, it is necessary to develop levels of play with an organisation by varying the complexity of the training throughout the week. To achieve this end, it is necessary to horizontally alternate the type of dominant contraction of the muscle, such as tension, duration, and speed. An example of an international working week incorporating the principle of horizontal alternation is presented in Figure 24.3.

To optimise player freshness and maximise performance in competition, players exposed to a Tactical Preparation approach are exposed to different stimuli daily, thus avoiding monotony and/or overwork. The inclusion of low-intensity and recovery training will help achieve this aim. In practice, the weekly training plan is dictated by several variables including, current physical status, load coming into the training camp, number of games and individual differences. Therefore, a logical approach is to include flexibility in the training plan and tailor weekly templates to the specific requirements of the team and individual. But to follow some generic guidelines.

## Future directions and conclusions

We can assume that genuine endeavours are now being undertaken to improve coach education, knowledge of soccer science and professionalisation. Organisational and cultural factors that have previously conspired against a move towards high-performance environments (i.e., reluctance to embrace change, professionalisation,

412 *Tony Strudwick*

and the development of scientific framework) are now being overcome. Coaches and players operating at an elite level understand the small increments in performance standards that are possible at the highest level require training programmes that are extensive in scale and need to be conducted at a high intensity. For this reason, the Director of Sports Science or High-Performance Director needs to have an enhanced appreciation of the processes that are involved in the holistic management of elite players.

At the elite level of soccer, the next decade will observe continued enhancement in sports science innovation and player management. The exponential growth in tactical development, player development, and the rise in technology to support high performance will be fully explored. Elite soccer teams will move towards high-performance environments where the development of systematic performance models and increased accountability will be commonplace. Innovations in player preparation are more challenging by the year and expectations go on rising. Therefore, player preparation must be sharper and better informed. All in all, these factors call for superior sports science support models and deeper insights, driven by empirical data, into issues relating to the management of elite performance.

An enormous amount of data is now generated about a team's performance on a constant basis. Some coaches now have first-hand experience of how to use 'sports analytics' to improve player and team performance. In the future, high-performing teams (those that substantially outperform their competitors over the long term) will turn to analytics as a competitive strategy. While technology on its own cannot turn a soccer organisation into a high performer, time and effort focused on developing robust analytical processes has great potential.

The key deliverable of the analytics process will be an increasing emphasis on using data to make better decisions. A critical concept in the process of data collection is distinguishing between which information/data is important and which is not. Data gathering for the sake of gathering data can be very expensive and futile unless it is used to drive action during the coaching process. While technology on its own cannot guarantee success at an elite level, time and effort focused on developing robust analytical processes has great potential.

There is no doubt that successful soccer performance is multi-disciplinary in nature. The Director of Sports Science or High-Performance Director will need to be aware of the physiological, biomechanical, psychological, nutritional, medical, and other issues that can impact on competition. When all these factors come together and work as an integrated system, excellence in high-performance soccer is possible. Elite sport is above all about problem-solving. Practitioners who are trained to think critically about all aspects of performance and how they interact and influence each other will be rewarded with success by gaining an advantage over competitors.

## References

Bradley, P. S., Sheldon, W., Wooster, B., Olsen, P., Boanas, P., & Krustrup, P. (2009). High-intensity running in English FA premier league soccer matches. *J Sports Sci, 27,* 159–168.

Budgett R. (1990). Overtraining Syndrome. *Br J Sports Med*, 24 (4), 231–6.

Carter, N. (2010). The rise and fall of the magic sponge: medicine and the transformation of the football trainer: *Social History Med, 23*(2), 261–279.

Carter, N. (2016). Evolution of soccer science. In Tony Strudwick (Ed.), *Soccer Science* (pp. 3–14). Champaign: Human Kinetics.

Working as a director of sports science 413

Chelladurai, P. (2009). *Managing Organisations for Sport and Physical Activity: A Systems Perspective*. Scottsdale, AZ: Holcomb Hathaway Publishers.

De Bosscher, V., De Knop, P., Van Bottenburg, M., & Shibli, S. (2006). A conceptual framework for analysing sports policy factors leading to international sporting success. *European Sport Management Quart*, 6(2), 185–215.

Di Salvo, V., Gregson, W., Atkinson, G., Tordoff, P., & Drust, B. (2009). Analysis of high intensity activity in premier league soccer. *Int J Sports Med, 30*, 205–212.

Duncan, C. & Strudwick, T. (2016). National and cultural differences. In Tony Strudwick (Ed.), *Soccer Science* (pp. 15–36). Champaign: Human Kinetics.

Gagné, F. (1985). Giftedness and talent: a re-examination of the definitions. *Gifted Child Quart, 29*, 103–112.

Gagné, F. (1998). A proposal for subcategories within the gifted or talented populations. *Gifted Child Quart*, 42, 87–95.

Gagné, F. (2005). From gifts to talents: The DMGT as a developmental model. In R. J. Sternberg & J. E. Davidson (Eds.), *Conceptions of Giftedness (2nd ed.)*, (pp. 98–119). New York: Cambridge University Press.

Gregson, W., Drust, B., Atkinson, G., & Di Salvo, V. (2010). Match-to-match variability of high-speed activities in premier league soccer. *Int J Sports Med, 4*, 237–42.

Henriksen, K., Stambulova, N., & Roessler, K. K. (2010). A holistic approach to athletic talent development environments: A successful sailing milieu. *Psychol Sport Exer, 11*, 212–222.

Ivarsson, A., Stenling, A., Fallby, J., Johnson, U., Borg, E. & Johansson, G. (2014). The predictive ability of the talent development environment on youth elite football players' well-being: a person-centered approach. *Psychol Sport Exer, 16*, 15–23.

Li, C., Wang, J. K. C. & Pyun, Y. D. (2014). Talent development environmental factors in sport: a review and taxonomic classification. *Rev Taxon Classification, 66*(4), 433–447.

Littlewood, M., Richardson, D. & Nesti, M. (2018). Shaping the performance culture: the role of the performance director. In Warren Gregson & Martin Littlewood (Eds.), *Science in Soccer Translating Theory into Practice* (pp. 3–15). London: Bloomsbury Sport.

Martindale, J.J.R., Collins, D. & Daubney, J. (2005). Talent development: a guide for practice and research within sport. *Quest, 57*(4), 353–375.

Meeusen, M., Duclos, M., Gleeson, M., Rietjens, G., Steinacker, J., & Urhausen, A. (2006). Prevention, diagnosis and treatment of the overtraining syndrome. *Eur J Sports Sci, 6*(1), 1–14.

Oliveira, R. (2014). *Tactical Periodization: The Secrets of Soccer Most Effective Training Methodology.*

Rampinini, E., Coutts, A. J., Castagna, C., Sassi, R., & Impellizzeri, F. M. (2007). Variation in top level soccer match performance. *Int J Sports Med, 28*, 1018–1024.

Rees, T., Hardy, L., Gullich, A., Abernathy, B., Cote, Core., Woodman, T., Montgomery, H., Laing, S. & Warr, C. (2016). The Great British medalists project: a review of current knowledge on the development of the world's best sporting talent. *Sports Med, 46*(8), 1041–58.

Reilly, T. (1994). Physiological aspects of soccer. *Biol Sport, 11*, 3–20.

Schein, E. (1991). *Organisational Culture and Leadership* (2nd Ed). San Francisco, CA: Jossey-Bass.

Slack, T. (1997). *Understanding Sport Organizations: The Application of Organization Theory*. Champaign: Human Kinetics.

Sotiriadou, P. & De Bosscher, V. (2018) Managing high-performance sport: introduction to past, present and future considerations, *Eur Sport Manag Quart*, 18:1, 1–7.

Stambulova, N. (2003). Symptoms of a crisis-transition: a grounded theory study. In N. Hassmen (Ed.), *SIPF Yearbook 2003* (pp. 97–109). Orebro, Sweden: Orebro University Press.

Tranckle, P. (2004). Understanding giftedness and talent in sport. *The Coach, 21*, 61–73.

# 25 Working as a sporting director

*Daniel Parnell, Rebecca Caplehorn, Kevin Thelwell, Tony Asghar and Mark Batey*

## Introduction

The soccer industry has a problem with stability, helped little by Covid-19 (Parnell et al., 2020a). The approach of regularly dismissing head coaches and their entire backroom staff, may bring rapid short-term results, but is not a paradigm regularly employed in industries outside the sporting sphere. The high turnover of senior staff within the club sporting hierarchy leads to a myriad of policy changes and inconsistency of strategy and in culture (Bridgewater, 2010; Kelly, 2017). This context has created an environment of employment instability and vulnerability, which is, in turn, detrimental to organisational performance and success (Relvas et al., 2010; Gibson & Groom, 2018, 2019; Roderick & Schumacker, 2017). Traditionally, this instability has created problems for club owners who have often focused on delivering success on the pitch, and a 'win on a Saturday', rather than strategically protecting their investment. As owners have clamoured for quick-fix solutions, entrenched in the short-term thinking and solutions, rather than the medium-to-long-term horizon, a vicious circle of decision-making, intensified by the risk and reward of success or failure, has created even greater instability and more Head Coach turnover (Bridgewater, 2010; Gammelsæter, 2013; Kelly, 2017). One strategy considered and adopted by some clubs to address these issues has been the introduction of a Sporting Director (Parnell et al., 2018a).

In this chapter, we seek to examine the role of the Sporting Director in soccer. Historically, we can broadly categorise two main groups of clubs depending on where the majority of power was congregated. Those clubs who were run mainly by the First Team Manager, who generally had the final say on all aspects of the club and team, or those clubs who were run by an Owner, President or Chief Executive who maintained power for many aspects of how the club functioned, leaving the Head Coach to work within the parameters he/she was given. Yet, the ever-growing complexity and commercialisation of the sport, increasing demands on performance for players, backroom staff, consultants, and managers, has challenged this conventional leadership structure. It appears an important time to review the Sporting Director role and how this role can help support the Head Coach and help deliver the goals of the organisation.

## Defining a sporting director

As an emerging role within the soccer management landscape, there exists considerable ambiguity regarding the title or definition of a Sporting Director. We use the term Sporting Director in this chapter, but clubs seemingly use the title 'Director of

DOI: 10.4324/9781003148418-31

Football', 'Technical Director', 'Director of Football Operations', and even 'Chief Soccer Officer' to describe individuals with strategic management responsibilities. The inconsistency in terminology regarding the Sporting Director role has and will continue to impede scholarly research into this area. For the purposes of clarity, and in the absence of an existing definition, using descriptions from Parnell et al., (2018a, b) we propose that a Sporting Director may be defined as the individual with strategic management responsibility for soccer operations.

Figures 25.1–25.3 provide representations of management structures that incorporate a Sporting Director. Typically, Sporting Directors adopt a position in between that of the Head Coach and Chair/Owner in the hierarchy (Figures 25.1 and 25.3), but may in a flatter structure make up a management team alongside the Head Coach (Figure 25.2). In some circumstances, the Sporting Director will report to a CEO (Figure 25.1), at others directly to the board or owner. At highly-developed, elite clubs with many sporting departments, there may be a clearer demarcation of management responsibilities for the Sporting Director and Head Coach or heads of departments (Figure 25.2) each with their own complex reporting structures. In smaller clubs, the

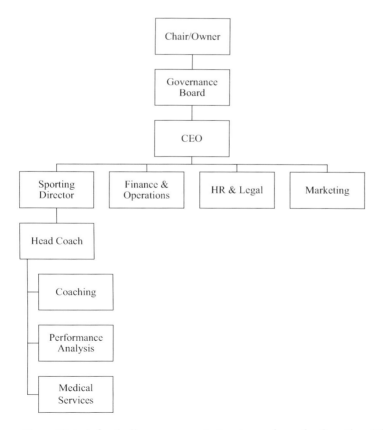

*Figure 25.1* A football management structure where the Sporting Director reports to a CEO.

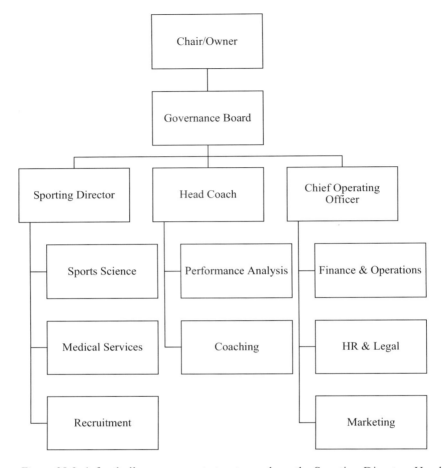

*Figure 25.2* A football management structure where the Sporting Director, Head Coach, and CEO report to the Governance Board/Chair/Owner.

hierarchy may be simplified with the Sporting Director taking a wide range of responsibilities including player recruitment (Figure 25.3). In effect, the position taken by the Sporting Director varies from club to club and will be impacted by such factors as the size of the club, the scope and scale of the club's administrative functions and the existence of other technical roles (e.g. Head of Recruitment) and sometimes the desires of the owner or powerful stakeholders.

Given our proposed definition above, the Sporting Director is characterised as having the direct responsibility of overseeing the core business pertaining to soccer operations, and in some clubs, entails the responsibility for Head Coach recruitment, succession-planning, and dismissal (Nissen, 2014; Parnell et al., 2021). In addition, the Sporting Director as an architect or custodian of culture ensures the creation and maintenance of a sustainable high-performance environment from the academy to the first team (Wagstaff & Burton-Wylie, 2018).

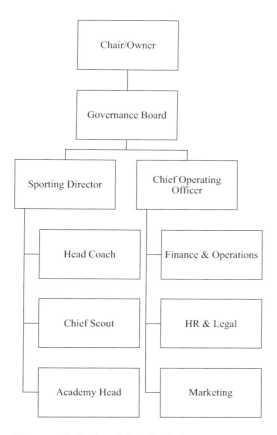

*Figure 25.3* A simplified football management structure where the Sporting Director would take responsibility for player recruitment.

## The rise of the sporting director role

Professional soccer (and sport) has undergone dramatic changes over the past two decades. These changes have arisen primarily due to media rights, with most professional clubs now operating as complex business institutions in dynamic pursuit of an ever greater share of the significant monies that media rights provide (Morrow & Howieson, 2014). The English Premier League (EPL) has been at the forefront of these changes and is embedded within a European and international marketplace of clubs, fans, sponsors, governing bodies, and partner commercial organisations. The European market is thought to be worth ~£25 billion, with combined league revenues for the 'Top-5' leagues across Europe valued at ~£13 billion for the 17/18 season (Deloitte, 2019). Much of this growth is due to the hyper-commercialisation and commodification of soccer across Europe. At present, it is common for global investment funds, multi-national conglomerates, sovereign wealth funds, and even royalties, to be part of ownership structures and linked to club acquisition (Parnell et al., 2020b). A complex stakeholder environment within which a Sporting Director may expect to operate and negotiate.

During the past 30 years of the EPL, many factors in the soccer ecosystem have evolved. Notably, the financial rewards and consequences of success or failure have intensified. At

418   *Daniel Parnell et al.*

the end of each EPL season, the bottom three teams are relegated to the division below – The Championship. This relegation has significant negative financial ramifications on the club's income, including broadcast, matchday, and commercial revenue streams (Maguire, 2021). While the consequence of demotion is partially mitigated by the protection of 'parachute payments' (see Wilson et al., 2021), the chances of a prompt return to the EPL are slim, despite the recent success of Norwich City FC, who were relegated from the EPL to the Championship in 2019/20, only to bounce-back immediately in the 2020/21 season. Notably, given the focus of this chapter, Norwich City FC implemented a Sporting Director model, recruiting Stuart Webber in 2017. The EPL has also seen an influx of foreign ownership and majority of clubs in the EPL (2021/22) are foreign-owned. We have also seen how the role of the contemporary manager (or Head Coach) has considerably expanded during this period (Bridgewater, 2010; Kelly, 2017). Gone are the days of a kitman and a handful of trusted coaches, to be replaced with a multi-layered high-performance team of internal employees working alongside specialists, advisors, and analysts sometimes from external providers, the Sporting Director will expect to manage and influence within and across formal and informal boundaries with diverse, skilled colleagues.

The implementation of a Sporting Director model has been commonplace in Europe and is gaining popularity worldwide. Many senior leaders occupy these positions across Europe, including major clubs such as AFC Ajax, AS Roma, Atletico Madrid, Barcelona, Bayern Munich, Borussia Dortmund, Inter Milan, Juventus, Lille OSC, Paris Saint-Germain FC, PSV Eindhoven, RB Leipzig, and Real Madrid. Sporting Directors can be found extensively in Major League Soccer and across the continent at clubs such as Club Bolivar in Bolivia and Guadalajara in Mexico. The United Kingdom-based Association of Sporting Directors caters for in excess of 500 members from every continent (see: https://associationofsportingdirectors.com). There is undoubtedly a rise in the popularity of Sporting Directors in soccer globally, much of which remains under the radar with regard to research. Given the position and pre-eminence of the English Premier League, and the reticence with which the role was adopted, there has been a focus on the role in this context.

English clubs are often accused of being resistant to change and slow to adopt modern management methods. However, researchers have identified the multiple challenges of making the switch to the Sporting Director model, including hostility, and distrust (Kelly & Harris, 2010). Many head coaches harboured these feelings due to what they perceived to be interference in their role, by owners and directors, all with their own agenda (Kelly, 2017) and none facing the pressure of losing their job if there were to be a 'bad run' of results. Therefore, and despite the challenges, many clubs now seek strategies to best focus the talents of a Head Coach, who could easily be subsumed by a vast array of responsibilities in the new complex, fixture-congested, highly contested, and commercial era of modern soccer. The Sporting Director model seeks to minimise the Head Coach's non-essential duties and find a more sensible and parsimonious 'division of labour' of leadership. While some have criticised clubs in England for being slow in adopting the role, others have argued this is simply a re-brand of an existing structure. Researchers have identified that perhaps Liverpool FC, had an early version of the model, where Bob Paisley (who became manager of Liverpool in 1974) had some of the administrative duties previously undertaken by Bill Shankly (his predecessor) given to Peter Robinson (Liverpool FC club secretary). Paisley was relieved of player contract duties, allowing him to focus on the day-to-day management of the first team (Lawrence, 2018). Lawrie McMenemy, Southampton FC

Working as a sporting director    419

manager between 1973 and 1985 was asked to do a role similar to the Sporting Director (Lawrence, 2018). We could argue that one of the most successful managers in history, Sir Alex Ferguson operated as a quasi-Sporting Director, fulfilling responsibilities associated with the role. As is often the case, the role may have existed long before it became popularised and given a formal title.

A report considered the 'Technical Director' (which as we have discussed is a term akin to the Sporting Director) role in England, compared and contrasted this to the same role in European clubs (Church, 2012). Church implied the role would become more popular in England and outlined several reasons for this expected growth in popularity. These reasons include: (1) new ownership bringing in new working models; (2) a more 'business-like' approach by clubs, meaning the link between the technical staff and the board will become increasingly vital; (3) the Premier League's Elite Performance Plan (EPPP) would cause a change to current staffing structures, and these changes would need to be developed and managed; (4) an increase in mandatory qualifications, professionalism, and accountability within clubs would also be a driver for the uptake of the role; and (5) it seems to be the modern trend for clubs to employ a Sporting Director, and the likelihood is that other clubs will replicate this model for fear of being 'laggards' in adopting innovative practices. Since the report, England has slowly shifted its governance structures towards a Sporting Director model and Church maintains a leadership position within The FA overseeing their flagship Level 5 Technical Directors course. For example, in season 2016/17 only 13 out of 20 EPL clubs had someone in a similar role to a Sporting Director, however, in the 2021/22 season, 17 out of 20 have such appointments. Sporting Directors within clubs are becoming a mainstay, with greater clarity now possible regarding their primary roles and responsibilities.

## The roles and responsibilities of sporting directors

The initial appointment of a Sporting Director, by an owner or board, is often in the pursuit of change, or a new (or better) way of doing things. The Sporting Director often includes an aspiration to give a club a 'way of doing things', through a cohesive and joined-up structure, a greater sense of stability and a 'road-map' to deliver upon a long-term strategy (Parnell et al., 2018b). The Sporting Director is often someone who has overall responsibility for the performance of various sporting departments within a club. We have described this as someone who can deliver a strategic plan and operate as a custodian of the club. They often have responsibilities for the first team, the academy, recruitment and scouting, sport science, and medical departments (Parnell et al., 2018a, 2021). The Sporting Director will often act as the intermediary between the strategic apex of a club (i.e., the board) and sporting departments (Parnell et al., 2018b). As a more 'permanent fixture' within a club's hierarchy, the Sporting Director is instrumental in shaping the long-term vision, strategy, and culture to support sustainable high performance. They can act as a custodian of the 'way we do things around here' against the backdrop of (relatively) regular changes to the Head Coach and backroom staff.

The priorities of the Sporting Director may include supporting numerous assistants across the first team and academy departments (Parnell et al., 2018b). They are also responsible for developing a positive working relationship with the owners and Board, the recruitment of the best talent (on and off the pitch) within budget (Parnell et al., 2021) and, developing and maintaining a club-wide philosophy to support its

420   *Daniel Parnell et al.*

sporting strategy. The Sporting Director is often renowned for recruitment practice taking players in and out of the club (Parnell et al., 2021), which is vital in the globalised race for talent (Bond et al., 2018, 2019). Recruitment of talent is undoubtedly a key task, however, an overreliance on this capability may constrain the effectiveness of introducing someone into the role. At present, little attention is given to the support the Sporting Director may give to medical and sports sciences, or the academy environment – all of which can be critical for achieving short- and long-term sporting objectives and ensuring a cohesive core of how 'we do things round here' from top to bottom.

Our intention is not to provide an exhaustive list or description, merely a nod to important areas of consideration. Sporting Directors should: know the football industry (Renton, 1999); understand the context within which the business operates (Renton, 1999); possess strategic awareness (Renton, 1999); and a breadth of perspective, professional reputation, and expertise (Ingley & Van der Walt, 2003); exercise interpersonal and communicational skills (Ingley & Van der Walt, 2003; Pye & Pettigrew, 2005; Roberts et al., 2005); bring motivation and commitment (Ingley & Van der Walt, 2003); and the ability to question and challenge (Roberts et al., 2005). As a consequence, the recruitment of Sporting Directors raises considerations around their skill set and capabilities.

The emergence of the Sporting Director role has been fraught with challenges. Like any change or disruption is an innovation that changes the world (or in our case, the soccer industry) in such a way, that if successful organisations keep on doing what they always did, they are likely to fail. As such, the Sporting Director often demands a new organisational structure. In this respect, there are mixed views and practices on whether a Sporting Director should sit on the board (apex) of the club or elsewhere (for example, above the first team Head Coach, but below the board). Yet, when asked Sporting Directors have stated:

> "A director needs to sit on the board. A director is a director and clubs need to commit to that so you can do the job. I don't understand why anyone would take a [Sporting] Director role in title and not insist on being on the board."…"In a football club, key decisions related to strategy are decided in the board room. If you don't sit round a table with the CEO and Director for Finance, how can you possibly ensure your strategy is presented correctly, to influence decisions, to ensure you get the support you need? You can't. You can't really lead properly as a Sporting Director without being on the board".
>
> (See Parnell et al., 2018a, p. 162)

Although many Sporting Directors know the importance of sitting on the board of the club, it is often negotiable as candidates seek opportunities in old organisations who refuse to change and continue to face an uphill struggle despite their past success. Architectural innovation refers to structural change to the organisation to embrace the innovation and is worth consideration (Henderson & Clark, 1990). Yet, if a club brings in a new strategy (i.e., a Sporting Director), fitting this new innovation into old structures offers very little scope for change – little influence, power, and resources – the hierarchies remain intact. An existing board may see the introduction of a Sporting Director as someone seeking to make a grab for power and challenge the leadership's decision-making status quo.

New change requires experimentation and the introduction of a Sporting Director is a change that appears to require architectural innovation (i.e., organisational and structural change). This change will create consequences for clubs, people, power dynamics, resource division, and decision-making responsibilities. There has been much experimentation on how this should work or be implemented (or not) in any club at any moment in time. This issue will remain a key item on the agenda for boards examining the Sporting Director model for implementation in what we can consider as the current experimentation period. We have seen and can expect vast amounts of trial and error. Some clubs may view an unsuccessful attempt to implement a Sporting Director model as an indication to completely end their experimentation with the role. This period of experimentation is fraught with challenges as boards are engaged with the management of stakeholder expectations, politics, influence, and power dynamics. However, we hope this experimentation leads to learning, improvements, and success. This period will naturally come to an end as a dominant design emerges.

## Successes associated with sporting directors in the role

Clubs have made progress on the journey of change with the introduction of different Sporting Directors models. While we can accept that errors have been made by all involved in the decision-making processes with respect to initiating this new role, there has also been plenty of success. This is often unique to the club context as this can vary from club to club based on ownership, governance, and organisational structure. The following section provides the reader with two selections of successful people. It does not serve to identify every successful Sporting Director, person or club, nor does non-inclusion allude to unsuccessful practice. These examples serve to provide a road map for the reader for further exploration and analysis.

### *Dan Ashworth – Technical Director at Brighton Hove Albion FC*

Dan Ashworth joined West Bromwich Albion (WBA) originally to help develop the academy structure – later becoming Academy Director, where he formed a relationship with the WBA Chairman Jeremy Peace. Within 3 years of joining WBA, Dan was appointed Technical Director. Dan then moved to the English FA where he oversaw the development of the 'England DNA' strategy. During his time at the English FA, he would see World Cup victories at U17 and U20 age groups, along with senior World Cup semi-finals with both the men's and women's teams. Part of this success was developing an enhanced competitive games programme and teams that could compete within these fixtures. Those who have worked with Dan regularly speak about his management skills as being one of his biggest strengths. Dan is known for being inclusive and democratic in his decision-making. He described his role at Brighton as being the hub in the centre of a wheel – around him are the seven heads of department. He described his job as connecting those seven areas and recruiting the right person to lead the department and overseeing succession planning in the result that someone leaves. Dan is committed to a development culture, getting the best out of people, and helping them grow. This links to his inclusive approach, through allowing people to express themselves and allowing the space to succeed. This role included non-playing and playing talent. For example, there were ongoing discussions between Dan and Graham Potter (the first team Head Coach) to explore ways to improve their game,

## 422    *Daniel Parnell et al.*

the focus would be on internal players in their own system (i.e., peripheral squad, loan, and/or academy players), rather than to look immediately outwards for playing talent. Dan's recruitment of Graham aligns both of their desires to develop people, whether staff or players. Dan was naturally well-placed to support talent pathways within Brighton given his experience at WBA and The FA. However, he also has key staff and quality people around him. For example, David Weir, a former player, assistant manager of Rangers FC and Brentford FC as loan manager. David (alongside the other heads of departments) would work with Dan to deliver on the club's strategy, in this case, it may include achieving 30% of playing minutes attributed to academy players in the English Premier League, alongside finishing in the top 10 places. There is of course much more to say, to discuss and analyse, including Dan's commitment to the health and well-being of his staff and women's game. Most recently, Dan joined Newcastle United Football Club as their new Sporting Director. Dan is a leader and one of the 'go-to' people within the inudstry.

### *Monchi – current Sporting Director at Sevilla FC and former sporting director @ Roma FC*

Monchi was a goalkeeper at Sevilla and spent most of his time as the number two choice. When Sevilla was relegated from La Liga, Monchi was recruited as Sporting Director to develop an elite scouting system and improve talent pathways from the academy to the first team. During his time as Sporting Director of Sevilla, he oversaw an incredible six Europa League trophies, along with a reputation for producing large profits on undervalued talent who come to Sevilla and move on to some of Europe's top clubs. For example, Julio Baptista £1.5m to £15m, Dani Alves £435k to £27m, and Ivan Rakitic £1.8m to £44m. Monchi believes in attention to detail rather than luck. He views clubs that have opted for a Sporting Director model as being advantaged over those that do not. Monchi describes his role as sitting between the Chairman, who gives him the economic information, and the Head Coach, who outlines what he needs with the first team, while also focusing on internal player development. He outlines an ongoing tension between short- and long-term goals and the need to continue to focus on player pathways. Monchi describes three pillars for success as having a united direction, planning, and teamwork. During his 30 years at Sevilla, the two times he experienced relegation was a result of internal division, as such its key to have a united direction of work. Each club also needs a strategic and operational plan, to ensure role clarity, and objections, which requires detailed planning. Finally, he believes in the power of the collective and avoids individualism, as such teamwork is key for successful organisations. Operationally, Monchi stays close to the players (e.g., staff and Head Coach), describing himself as a 'locker-room' Sporting Director, to know the people, challenges, issues, and how he can help. Monchi utilises data analytics (i.e., big data, artificial intelligence, and machine learning) to inform his recruitment, alongside an extensive professional scouting network. There is much more to discuss on recruitment, but to close this short feature, here are the areas Monchi identifies as important for Sporting Directors to consider:

- Do not avoid risk when making decisions – it is impossible to do great things without taking big risks;
- If you want to go fast, go alone, but if you want to go far, go together;

*Working as a sporting director*   423

- Continual investment in personal development and do not be afraid of failure;
- Being able to adapt is the difference between success and failure.

## Challenges that face sporting directors

A number of challenges impact the success of implementing a Sporting Director approach. The flexibility in the role title and lack of clarity with respect to the role can create tensions internally and externally with stakeholders (including fans and media), which can influence the effectiveness of the club. The position of a Sporting Director in a club's hierarchy (i.e., on the board or otherwise) impacts the influence and effectiveness of anyone in the role. This is a relatively new role, and like any new innovation, it takes time to find the best way to implement and change ways of doing things. Therefore, managing existing hierarchies and power dynamics is key. This process must be managed carefully when implementing a new Sporting Director, as this is undoubtedly a complex change. More broadly, there are a wide variety of challenges facing Sporting Directors in practice that should inform continued professional development and education programmes (see Table 25.1). The challenges pertain to the role and responsibilities of a Sporting Director as we have reviewed in this chapter, in addition to the myriad of macro issues that soccer organisations must adapt to. To 'bridge the gap' between the challenges faced and the skills required, we provide a suggestive set of skills and competencies that Sporting Directors should look to develop – and which providers of formal and informal education should cater for.

## Future directions and conclusions

There are a number of key considerations we have drawn from our analysis and experience. The title used for the Sporting Director role is flexible, but with definitional clarity provided in this chapter, we hope to support focused and rigorous research in this area. A Sporting Director may be defined as an individual with strategic management responsibility for soccer operations.

The job role varies across clubs, and therefore the knowledge, expertise, and skill required to perform the role may vary. Sporting Directors currently do not always assume a board-level position. Internal and external stakeholders do not appear to fully understand the Sporting Director role and can lead to ambiguity both internally and externally to the organisation. The role is new and innovation will take time and involve trial and error. We are still learning the best ways for a Sporting Director to maximise his/her working relationship with the Head Coach and the wider network of influential stakeholders. How best to support innovation and change in both operations and cultures will remain an issue. The challenges facing Sporting Directors are plenty, as such we need a shift in how we support Sporting Directors to prepare for internal and external changes (i.e., technology, social, media, data, and political).

If the Sporting Director role is to be successful, we need to think and work for organisational structures that give those in the role the genuine position to influence. While each club context is unique, this will likely result in a Sporting Director assuming a board-level position and influence. Once a dominant effective design is established for the Sporting Director, the initial set of components will need to be refined and elaborated, and progress takes the shape of improvements in the components within the framework of a stable organisation. This process should allow clubs to focus on

424    *Daniel Parnell et al.*

*Table 25.1* Some challenges facing the Sporting Director in practice and the skills and competencies required to address them

| Challenges | Skills and competencies |
| --- | --- |
| The formulation and implementation of successful strategies | Strategic thinking<br>Commercial acumen<br>Change and innovation management<br>Operations management skills |
| Leading high-performing teams comprised of highly-skilled, diverse professionals | Leadership and management skills<br>Change and innovation management |
| Building culture – taking a leading role as a 'custodian of culture' | Leadership and management skills<br>Change and innovation management<br>Strategic thinking |
| Ensuring good governance – ethics, transparency, trust, and compliance | Commercial acumen<br>Governance, legal and financial skills<br>Operations management skills |
| Managing and influencing across formal and informal boundaries – including complex supply chains of specialists – e.g., outsourcing | Leadership and management skills<br>Commercial acumen<br>Contract management<br>Strategic thinking |
| Building trust and influence in complex club hierarchies – navigating 'cultures of ownership' | Leadership and influencing skills<br>Emotional intelligence |
| Talent identification and recruitment (players and staff) including regulations, contracts, and negotiation. | Commercial acumen<br>Leadership and influencing skills<br>Emotional intelligence |
| Data analytics (to inform performance, talent development and recruitment) | Industry-specific data analytics skills |
| Industry regulations (i.e., financial fair play, loan regulation changes) | Commercial acumen<br>Governance, legal and financial skills |
| TV rights and resultant financial implications | Commercial acumen |
| Health and well-being of staff and players | Emotional intelligence<br>Human resource skills |
| Continued professional development, training, qualifications and education for Sporting Directors and all staff | Emotional intelligence<br>Human resource skills |
| Succession planning (backroom staff) | Strategic thinking<br>Leadership and management skills<br>Human resources skills |
| Communication – internal and external, fans, liaison committees, and social media | Emotional intelligence<br>Communication skills<br>Digital and media skills |
| Emergent technology – industry 4.0 or 4th industrial revolution (world economic forum); e.g., how will blockchain and cryptocurrency effect transfers? | Strategic thinking<br>Commercial acumen<br>Change and innovation management |
| Navigating the external environment (i.e., Brexit, COVID-19, climate change) | Strategic thinking<br>Leadership and management skills<br>Commercial acumen<br>Change and innovation management<br>Operations management |
| Navigating a football club through complex societal change (for example: black lives matter, LGBTQ+, national politics, religious observance) | Emotional intelligence<br>Leadership and management skills<br>Strategic thinking<br>Commercial acumen<br>Change and innovation management<br>Governance, legal and financial skills |
| Horizon scanning to ensure prepared and ready for continued improved practice and innovation | Strategic thinking<br>Leadership and management skills<br>Commercial acumen |

continuous improvement, development, and progress – in the systems, people, and processes – in line with the principles of total quality management. Ultimately, this change will take time, there will be stumbles and there will be successes. The components and practices associated with these successes must be acknowledged and shared with key decision-makers and where possible implemented.

To further enhance the implementation of the role of Sporting Director within soccer, additional work is required. This includes ensuring clearly defined role descriptors for the Sporting Director role for employers and employees. Clubs need to position the Sporting Director with an appropriate level of power and influence. This conceptual clarity will avoid role ambiguity. We require enhanced professional education and qualifications to support those seeking to gain a Sporting Director role. In this respect, we need to develop clear pathways for the recruitment and development of future Sporting Directors. We require a distinct body of research to inform decision-making and practice. For example, optimal Head Coach recruitment strategy, how to best onboard a Head Coach, how to identify the best-fit between the club, Sporting Director, and Head Coach, change preparation and management as a result of promotion or relegation, and strategic alliances across clubs and ownership groups. The collective work of formal and informal education bodies will be vital for the ongoing professionalisation of sport and Sporting Directors. The unique Master of Sport Directorship (MSD) qualification at Manchester Metropolitan University provides a formal executive qualification in this regard. Furthermore, the Association of Sporting Directors is key to providing an independent and inclusive professional membership body to provide continued support and guidance. Closing some of these gaps will help ensure the growth and effectiveness of implementing a Sporting Director model in clubs.

## Acknowledgements

We would like to thank our colleagues at the Association of Sporting Directors for their support with this research. Alongside our many colleagues in the industry who have supported our work.

## Disclosure statement

Daniel Parnell is CEO of the Association of Sporting Directors, Rebecca Caplehorn is on the Technical Committee of the Association of Sporting Directors and Kevin Thelwell is a member of the Association of Sporting Directors. Mark Batey is Programme Leader of the Master of Sport Directorship (MSD) at Manchester Metropolitan University, UK.

## References

Bond, A. J., Widdop, P., & Chadwick, S. (2018). Football's emerging market trade network: ego network approach to world systems theory. *Managing Sport and Leisure, 23*(1–2), 70–91. doi: 10.1080/23750472.2018.1481765.

Bond, A. J., Widdop, P., & Parnell, D. (2019). Topological network properties of the European football loan system. *European Sport Management Quarterly, 20*, 1–24. doi:10.1080/16184742.2019.1673460

Bridgewater, S. (2010). *Football Management*. Basingstoke: Palgrave Macmillan.

426  *Daniel Parnell et al.*

Church, P. (2012). Technical director report (pp. 70–98).

Deloitte. (2019). Annual Review of Football Finance 2019. *Deloitte Football Finance.* Retrieved from: https://www2.deloitte.com/uk/en/pages/sports-business-group/articles/annual-review-of-football-finance.html.

Gammelsæter, H. (2013). Leadership succession and effectiveness in team sport. A critical review of the coach succession literature. *Sport, Business and Management: An International Journal, 3*(4), 285–296. doi: 10.1108/SBM-06–2013–0015

Gibson, L., & Groom, R. (2018). Ambiguity, manageability and the orchestration of organisational change: a case study of an English premier league academy manager. *Sports Coaching Review, 7*(1), 23–44. doi: 10.1080/21640629.2017.1317173

Gibson, L., & Groom, R. (2019). The micro-politics of organizational change in professional youth football: towards an understanding of 'actions, strategies and professional interests'. *International Journal of Sports Science & Coaching, 14*(1), 3–14. doi: 10.1177/1747954118766311

Henderson, R., & Clark, K. (1990). Architectural innovation: the reconfiguration of existing product technologies and the failure of established firms. *Administrative Science Quarterly, 34*(1) 35. Doi: 10.2307/2393549

Kelly, S. (2017). *The Role of the Professional Football Manager.* Routledge: London.

Kelly, S., & Harris, J. (2010). Managers, directors and trust in professional football. *Sport in Society, 13*(3), 489–502. doi: 10.1080/17430431003588150

Lawrence, I. (2018). *Football Club Management: Insights From the Field.* Routledge: London.

Maguire, K. (2021). *The Price of Football Second Edition: Understanding Football Club Finance.* Agenda Publishing: London.

Morrow, S., & Howieson, B. (2014). The new business of football: a study of current and aspirant football club managers. *Journal of Sport Management, 28*(5), 515–528. doi: 10.1123/jsm.2013–0134

Nissen, R. (2014). Playing the game: how football directors make sense of dismissing the coach. *International Journal Sport Management and Marketing, 15*(3/4), 214–231. doi: 10.1504/IJSMM. 2014.072009

Parnell, D., Groom, R., Widdop, P., & Ward, S. (2018a). The sporting director: exploring current practice and challenges within elite football. In S. Chadwick, D. Parnell, D. Widdop, & C. Anagnostopoulos (Eds.), *Routledge Handbook of Football Business and Management* (pp. 155–170). London: Routledge.

Parnell, D., Widdop, P., Groom, R., & Bond, A. (2018b). The emergence of the sporting director role in football and the potential of social network theory in future research. *Managing Sport and Leisure, 23*(4–6), 242–254.

Parnell, D., Bond, A.J., Widdop, P., & Cockayne, B. (2020b). Football worlds: business and networks during COVID-19. *Soccer & Society, 22*(1–2), 19–26. Doi: 10.1080/14660970.2020.1782719

Parnell, D., Widdop, P., Bond, A., & Wilson, R. (2020a). COVID-19, networks and sport. *Managing Sport and Leisure, 2020,* 1–7. https://www.tandfonline.com/doi/full/10.1080/23750472. 2020.1750100

Parnell, D., Bond, A.J., Widdop, P., Groom, R., & Cockayne, D. (2021). Recruitment in elite football: a network approach, *European Sport Management Quarterly.* https://doi. org/10.1080/16184742.2021.2011942

Pye, A., & Pettigrew, A. (2005). Studying board context, process and dynamics: Some challenges for the future. *British Journal of Management, 16*(1), 27–38. doi: 10.1111/j.1467–8551.2005.00445.x

Relvas, H., Littlewood, M., Nesti, M., Gilbourne, D., & Richardson, D. (2010). Organizational structures and working practices in elite European professional football clubs: understanding the relationship between youth and professional domains. *European Sport Management Quarterly, 10*(2), 165–187. doi: 10.1080/16184740903559891

Renton, T. (1999). *Standards for the Board: Improving the Effectiveness of your Board.* London: Institute of Directors.

Roberts, J., McNulty, T., & Stiles, P. (2005). Beyond agency conceptions of the work of the non-executive director; creating accountability in the boardroom. *British Journal of Management, 16*(1), 5–26. doi: 10.1111/j.1467–8551.2005.00444.x

Roderick, M., & Schumacker, J. (2017). 'The whole week comes down to the teamsheet': a footballer's view of insecure work. *Work, Employment and Society, 31*(1), 166–174. doi: 10.1177/0950017016672792

Wagstaff, C., & Burton-Wylie, S. (2018). Organizational culture in sport: a conceptual, definitional, and methodological review. *Sport and Exercise Psychology Review, 14*(2), 32–52.

Wilson, R., Plumley, D., Mondal, S., & Parnell, D. (2021). Challenging parachute payments and unmasking English football's finances. *Managing Sport and Leisure, 27*, 93–98. Doi: 10.1080/23750472.2020.1792745

# Index

active recovery 95
adaptive expertise 189
aerobic training 34, 39
anaerobic speed endurance training 42
anaerobic speed training 41
anaerobic training 34, 36, 41
analysis: free kicks 280; open play 278; penalty kicks 280; set play 279
ASPIRE 147–148

bio-banding 339–340
biomechanics toolbar 243

carbohydrates 67–74; in-game 71–72; post-game 72; pre-match 71
career transitions 168
central tendency 315–316
challenge point hypothesis 148–149
coach-athlete relationship 158–160
coach development pathways 185
cognitive function and heat 55
compression garments 99–100
concussion 215–218
confidence 114–115
constraints-led approach 149
contextual priors 130
cooling strategies 60
Covid-19 231–232
creatine phosphate 37
cryotherapy 97–98
cultural background 160–161
cultural diversity 160

data management 406
decision-making 131–132
dehydration 76–78
deliberate practice 147–148
de-selection 371
developmental pathways 141–145
diagnosis of infectious diseases 229–230
Director of Football Operations 415
Director of Sports Science 397

electromyography 241–243
elite player performance plan 155
emotions 115
expertise in coaching 183
EXPERTS 147–148

factor analysis 281–283
family 156–158
fatigue 90–91, 257; transient 258
Female Athlete Triad 78
FIFA (11+) 7, 10, 11
financial fair play 155
fluid requirement 76
formal learning 186–189
future game problem 385
future programmes 340–341

game intelligence 124
game performance evaluation tool 131
games-based approaches 149–150
gastrointestinal tract infection 224
gaze behaviours 125–129
GPS 253, 273, 299, 302
growth 329–332

heat acclimatation 59
heat-related illness 55
high-performance director 398–399
high-speed running 255
home advantage 113–114
home grown players 160
hyperthermia 7

ill-being 170
Index of Game Control 281
Index of Offensive Behaviour 281
infections 223
infectious diseases 223–229
informal learning 185–186
injury 201–203; ankle 208–210; bone 212–214; cruciate ligament 204–208; epidemiology 199; joint 203–210; knee 204; medial

430 *Index*

collateral ligament 208; meniscus 204; mitigation 200; prevention 301–303, 264–265; screening 200, 246; tendon 210–212
international soccer 408–411
isokinetic dynamometer 243–244
isometric exercises 17, 21

jumping performance 238–239; Sargent jump 239; vertical jump 239

key performance indicators 277

load: external 293; internal 293
long-term athlete monitoring 303–304
LPS 253, 273

massage 96
match analysis 273
match day routines 5
match demands 254–257
maturation status 330–332, 347–351; fitness testing 339; injury 336–338; screening programme 332; training 335–336
maximum voluntary contraction 243
menstrual cycle 57
mental health 168–174; literacy 173
micronutrients 80–81
microstructure of practice 145–146
monitoring training 44, 292–305
muscle: biopsies 37; concentric contraction 11, 245; damage 93; eccentric contraction 11, 245; lactate 38
myofascial release 96

needs analysis 22
nutritional considerations 78–80; adolescent players 79–80; female players 78

pattern recognition 129–130
peak height velocity 330–331
percentile rank 318–319
perceptual-cognitive skills 124
performance analysis and coaching 274
performance profiling 407
periodisation strategies 26
physical capabilities of players 36
physical conditioning strategies 261
Player Insights team 382
player monitoring and management 261, 263–264
position specific match demands 257
Possession Effectiveness Index 281
post-activation: performance enhancement 4; potentiation 4
pre-cooling 67–74

protein 74–75
psychological momentum 112

rate limiters 149
reading the game 125
recovery 91; kinetics 24
recovery strategies 90
red zone 40
reflective practice 190
relative age 347–351; maturation biases 351–357
reliability 313–314
repeated bout effects 20, 24, 93
repeated sprint training 256
resistance training 15, 16
retirement 175

scanning 126–127
scouts 382–384
self-care 172
simulation training 133–135
situational probabilities 130
skeletal age 330–331
sleep 100–101
small-sided games 5
social identity 115
social network analysis 283
socioeconomic background 161–162
sporting director 414
streamlining data 298–299
strength: assessment 243; training 9
stretching 96; dynamic 6; exercises 6; static 6
supercompensation 23
surrogate selector problem 387

tacit knowledge 365
tactical preparation approach 411
tactics 276
talent 363; development environment questionnaire 370; identification indicators 351–357; promotion programmes 370–375; recruiting framework 387–389
tanner-whitehouse method 330
tapering 15
teaching games for understanding 149–150
time motion analyses 253
tolerance model 16

upper respiratory tract infection 223–224

vaccination 225–226
validity 313
video feedback 119
virtual reality 133–135

warm up 3; active 4; passive 4
wearable devices 295–296
wellbeing 168–174